DIAGNOSING LEARNING DISORDERS

Also Available

Explaining Abnormal Behavior:
A Cognitive Neuroscience Perspective
Bruce F. Pennington

Pediatric Neuropsychology, Second Edition:
Research, Theory, and Practice
Edited by Keith Owen Yeates, M. Douglas Ris,
H. Gerry Taylor, and Bruce F. Pennington

The Development of Psychopathology:
Nature and Nurture
Bruce F. Pennington

Diagnosing Learning Disorders

From Science to Practice

THIRD EDITION

Bruce F. Pennington
Lauren M. McGrath
Robin L. Peterson

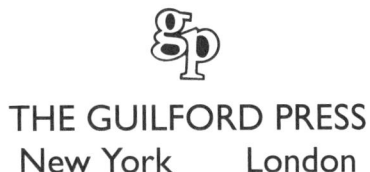

THE GUILFORD PRESS
New York   London

Copyright © 2019 The Guilford Press
A Division of Guilford Publications, Inc.
370 Seventh Avenue, Suite 1200, New York, NY 10001
www.guilford.com

All rights reserved

No part of this book may be reproduced, translated, stored in a retrieval system, or transmitted, in any form or by any means, electronic, mechanical, photocopying, microfilming, recording, or otherwise, without written permission from the publisher.

Printed in the United States of America

This book is printed on acid-free paper.

Last digit is print number: 9 8 7 6 5 4 3 2 1

The authors have checked with sources believed to be reliable in their efforts to provide information that is complete and generally in accord with the standards of practice that are accepted at the time of publication. However, in view of the possibility of human error or changes in behavioral, mental health, or medical sciences, neither the authors, nor the editors and publisher, nor any other party who has been involved in the preparation or publication of this work warrants that the information contained herein is in every respect accurate or complete, and they are not responsible for any errors or omissions or the results obtained from the use of such information. Readers are encouraged to confirm the information contained in this book with other sources.

Library of Congress Cataloging-in-Publication Data

Names: Pennington, Bruce Franklin, 1946– author.
Title: Diagnosing learning disorders : from science to practice / Bruce F.
    Pennington, Lauren M. McGrath, Robin L. Peterson.
Description: Third edition. | New York : The Guilford Press, [2019] |
    Includes bibliographical references and index.
Identifiers: LCCN 2018052173 | ISBN 9781462537914 (hardback)
Subjects: LCSH: Learning disabilities—Diagnosis. | Autism in
    children—Diagnosis. | Attention-deficit hyperactivity
    disorder—Diagnosis. | BISAC: PSYCHOLOGY / Neuropsychology. | MEDICAL /
    Psychiatry / Child & Adolescent. | EDUCATION / Special Education /
    Learning Disabilities. | PSYCHOLOGY / Psychotherapy / Child & Adolescent.
Classification: LCC RJ496.L4 P46 2019 | DDC 618.92/85889—dc23
LC record available at *https://lccn.loc.gov/2018052173*

For Linda, Amy, Luke, Della, and Dorothy
—B. F. P.

*For my parents, Todd and Mary Ann.
Their educational values and strong work ethic
continue to inspire my career.*
—L. M. M.

*In loving memory of my father, Bob Leonhardt.
His commitment to knowledge, education, and the dignity
of all people provided a model that continues to guide me.*
—R. L. P.

About the Authors

Bruce F. Pennington, PhD, is Distinguished University Professor Emeritus in the Department of Psychology at the University of Denver. He has conducted extensive research on learning disorders and their comorbidity, using genetic and neuropsychological methods. Dr. Pennington is a recipient of Research Scientist, MERIT, and Fogarty awards from the National Institutes of Health; the Samuel T. Orton Award from the International Dyslexia Association; and the Emanuel Miller Memorial Lecture from the British Association for Child and Adolescent Mental Health.

Lauren M. McGrath, PhD, is Assistant Professor in the Department of Psychology at the University of Denver. Her expertise is in child clinical psychology, developmental neuropsychology, and psychiatric and behavioral genetics. Dr. McGrath's research focuses on children with learning disabilities along two main themes: comorbidity between learning and behavioral disorders, and genetic risk factors and gene–environment interactions.

Robin L. Peterson, PhD, ABPP, is a pediatric neuropsychologist and Assistant Clinical Professor at Children's Hospital Colorado/University of Colorado School of Medicine. She has clinical and research interests in learning disorders, pediatric traumatic brain injury (including concussion), and spina bifida. Dr. Peterson is board certified in clinical neuropsychology. She lives in Denver with her husband, Eric, and daughters, Cordelia and Beatrix.

Laura M. McGrath and Robin L. Peterson made equal contributions to this book. The order of their authorship was determined alphabetically.

Preface

This book is about the science and practice of learning disorders, which are prevalent and impairing conditions that for too long were neglected by mainstream psychology and medicine. For much of the 20th century, learning disorders were relegated to the margins of science, characterized by various myths, and treated with controversial alternative therapies.

Some of these myths are still prevalent today, such as the myth that dyslexia is a visual disorder that causes a person to see things backward. Or there is the myth that vaccines cause autism (this myth has even reached the White House!). Not too long ago, it was even popular to claim that some learning disorders *themselves* were myths. For instance, it was argued that attention-deficit/hyperactivity disorder (ADHD) did not exist as a disorder, that it was just a medicalization of normal childhood exuberance. Or when one of us (BFP) first entered the field, it was seriously proposed that learning disabilities did not exist, that instead they were a middle-class myth to protect the self-esteem of parents whose children were not meeting high educational expectations. Or if they agreed that learning disabilities did exist, clinical psychologists proposed Freudian explanations of learning disabilities based on unconscious conflicts. For instance, they hypothesized that mathematical problems with addition were caused by oral issues, problems with subtraction were caused by castration anxiety, problems with multiplication were caused by sexual conflicts, and so on. It is our hope that all readers of this book agree that learning disorders *do* exist and can see how ludicrous these Freudian explanations of math problems are, but it may take a little more understanding of science to understand why the other myths are wrong.

The fact that we have been able to refute all these myths about learning disorders demonstrates how science works. Various hypotheses about how and why things happen in the world can be rigorously examined to determine whether they are true, and science progresses by rejecting wrong ideas about how the world works. The dustbin of scientific history is filled with curious ideas such as the earth is flat, the sun revolves around the earth, the stars are mounted on crystalline spheres (hence, "the music of the spheres" that some of us sang about in church), the mind is in the heart, invisible ether is needed to transmit light, and combustion occurs when objects give up their phlogiston. It is our hope that all readers of this book recognize that these ideas are wrong, and can even explain why most of them are wrong.

The ultimate goal of scientific research on learning disorders, like all biomedical research, is to improve public health by improving early detection, intervention, and ultimately prevention. This is a "virtuous cycle" between science and practice: Practice leads to scientific questions, and scientific research improves practice, which in turn leads to new scientific questions. This book illustrates this virtuous cycle in the domain of learning disorders.

To achieve this goal, the book is divided into two major parts. Part I, "Scientific Foundations," is concerned with both scientific methods used to understand learning disorders and key issues for practice. It has chapters dedicated to specific methods (i.e., genetics, neuroimaging, neuropsychology) that will be useful for individuals interested in these methods. Part II, "Reviews of Disorders," is concerned with what these scientific methods have taught us about six learning disorders and how to diagnose, treat, and possibly prevent them: speech and language disorders (Chapter 9), dyslexia (Chapter 10), mathematics disorder (Chapter 11), ADHD (Chapter 12), autism spectrum disorder (Chapter 13), and intellectual disability (Chapter 14). Each chapter reviews the history, definition, and prevalence of each disorder, as well as current knowledge of their underlying developmental neuropsychology, brain mechanisms, and etiology. Each disorder-specific chapter contains a section on diagnosis and treatment that reviews current assessment and treatment recommendations, and their scientific basis. To illustrate the principles reflected in these sections, we provide case presentations that include data tables that describe assessment results and a description of the differential diagnostic process. Last, each disorder-specific chapter contains a summary table of the entire chapter.

The main target audience for this book is psychologists who assess children, including clinical psychologists, clinical neuropsychologists, school psychologists, and counseling psychologists. However, this book is also relevant for educators, pediatricians, neurologists, speech–language pathologists, occupational and physical therapists, and researchers in developmental psychology, educational psychology, and cognitive neuroscience. We also hope that parents of children with learning disorders as well as adolescents and adults with learning disorders will find the content useful.

Lay readers may want to start with the Preface, Chapter 1, and the summary tables for each disorder in Chapters 9–14. Clinicians will find the diagnosis and treatment sections in Chapters 9–14 most relevant for their applied work. Readers who are interested in the science of learning disorders will want to familiarize themselves with scientific methods with which they are less familiar in Part I before proceeding to the scientific sections of each disorder-specific chapter in Part II.

All readers will benefit from the summary tables that accompany each disorder-specific chapter.

In the nearly 30 years since the first edition of this book was written, there has been enormous scientific progress in our understanding of learning disorders. The biggest scientific advances have been in the fields of genetics and brain mechanisms, where much more powerful methods have displaced old findings and have made it clearer how much remains to be understood. More than ever before, there is a new appreciation that both the genome and the developing brain are complex systems whose functioning needs to be understood in network terms. In terms of practice, diagnostic definitions of learning disorders have evolved, their extensive comorbidity is better understood, and we have much better data questioning the validity of some learning disorders (e.g., Asperger syndrome, the hyperactive–impulsive subtype of ADHD, and disorders of written expression).

There have also been major advances in the science and practice of learning disorders in the decade since the second edition of this book was published; thus, this third edition is considerably different from its predecessor. We have extensively revised and updated all of the main chapters of the previous volume. For example, genetic and neuroimaging technologies have advanced considerably in the past decade, and these advancements are reflected in the chapters on etiology (Chapter 2) and brain mechanisms (Chapter 3). For each of the disorder-specific chapters in Part II, the genetics, brain mechanisms, and developmental neuropsychology of each disorder have advanced to such an extent that each chapter was nearly fully rewritten. The case presentations that accompany each chapter in Part II were also revised to be consistent with DSM-5 and current assessment techniques. In addition to these extensive revisions, we have added four entirely new chapters on comorbidity (Chapter 5), on differential diagnosis of specific learning disorders using DSM-5 (Chapter 6), on evidence-based practice in assessment (Chapter 7), and on achievement gaps (Chapter 8). We believe that readers who are familiar with the second edition will find that this third edition is not merely an incremental update, but nearly a completely new book.

Acknowledgments

Several colleagues provided very useful comments on earlier drafts of the chapters in this book, including Anne Arnett, David Baker, Amy Connery, Jamie Edgin, Deborah Fein, Mike Kirkwood, Sarah Lukowski, Allison Meyer, Joel Nigg, Sally Ozonoff, Nancy Raitano-Lee, Sally Rogers, Miriam Rosenberg, and Greg Wallace.

Preparation of this book was supported by a Colorado Learning Disability Research Center (CLDRC) grant (P50HD027802) from the National Institute of Child Health and Human Development (NICHD) and an R15 grant (R15HD086662) from the NICHD. Suzanne Miller and Sarah Pollard provided invaluable help in preparing the manuscript.

Contents

PART I. Scientific Foundations

CHAPTER 1.	How Learning Disorders Develop	3
CHAPTER 2.	Etiology of Learning Disorders	14
CHAPTER 3.	Brain Mechanisms of Learning Disorders	24
CHAPTER 4.	Neuropsychological Constructs	41
CHAPTER 5.	Comorbidity	54
CHAPTER 6.	Specific Learning Disorder: DSM-5 and Beyond	69
CHAPTER 7.	Evidence-Based Practice in Assessment	77
CHAPTER 8.	Understanding Achievement Gaps	93

PART II. Reviews of Disorders

CHAPTER 9.	Speech and Language Disorders	111
CHAPTER 10.	Reading Disability (Dyslexia)	156
CHAPTER 11.	Mathematics Disorder	190

CHAPTER 12. Attention-Deficit/Hyperactivity Disorder — 217

CHAPTER 13. Autism Spectrum Disorder — 258

CHAPTER 14. Intellectual Disability — 312

Conclusions — 343

References — 349

Index — 387

PART I
SCIENTIFIC FOUNDATIONS

CHAPTER 1

How Learning Disorders Develop

This chapter provides an overview of the issues and methods necessary for understanding learning disorders. It is important to realize that the scientific methods explained in Part I are absolutely generic to all of psychiatry and, with a few modifications, to all of medicine. At a more general level, these methods characterize all of science. All of science begins with a *description* of phenomena that humans want to understand, whether they be rainbows or heart attacks. The first step in the scientific method is to carefully describe the phenomenon at hand. What are rainbows, when and where do they occur, are myths about them accurate (pots of gold, Noah's flood insurance), and so forth? This description needs to be objective and replicable, so that all observers can agree that this is indeed a rainbow (and not the Northern Lights or dirty eyeglasses). So too with heart attacks.

Once the careful description of the phenomenon is complete, science moves on to *explaining* how and why the phenomenon occurs. So *description* and *explanation* are separate parts of the scientific method, and it is important that the description not covertly sneak in a preformed explanation. Hence, when we apply the scientific method to human disorders, the first step is to describe the given disorder in an objective and reliable way.

As we will see, this initial step of describing learning disorders is still not complete. As explained in Chapters 5 and 6, our current *nosology* (classification system) of learning disorders in the fifth edition of the *Diagnostic and Statistical Manual of Mental Disorders* (DSM-5; American Psychiatric Association, 2013) includes some diagnostic constructs (e.g., written language disorders) that currently lack discriminant validity because they are not clearly distinct from other learning disorders. The seven learning disorders covered in Chapters 9–14 are the ones that current research best supports as valid and distinct disorders.

One goal of this book is to make the emerging science of learning disorders accessible to practitioners who help children with learning disorders. The other goal is to show concretely how science informs practice by thoroughly presenting actual examples of diagnosis and treatment planning. We begin with an overview of what learning disorders are and how they develop.

DEFINING LEARNING DISORDERS

So what are *learning disorders*? This term is broader than the more familiar term *learning disabilities*. As used here, learning disorders are a subset of *neurodevelopmental disorders*, namely, those that mainly produce atypical cognitive development. Neurodevelopmental disorders are genetically influenced variations in brain development that are distinct from brain disorders acquired later in childhood or in adulthood, like traumatic brain injury (TBI). The category of neurodevelopmental disorders is broad and also includes some neurologically or medically defined conditions (e.g., spina bifida or lissencephaly), as well as psychiatric disorders such as major depression, bipolar disorders, anxiety disorders, and schizophrenia. Psychiatric disorders are not usually thought of as learning disorders, because either their peak age of onset is later in development or their main symptoms are not problems in learning, even though cognition is disrupted in these disorders as well. The neurodevelopmental disorders covered in this book include virtually all the disorders contained in the neurodevelopmental disorders section of DSM-5, with the exception of stuttering, tic disorders, and stereotypic movement disorder, again because they are not primarily learning disorders. Neurological conditions are not the focus of this book, but many individuals with these conditions exhibit at least some features of the more prevalent DSM-5 behaviorally defined learning disorders that we cover in detail.

While one can draw distinctions among these different kinds of disorders (i.e., neurodevelopmental vs. acquired; psychiatric vs. learning disorders; neurological vs. behavioral), the distinctions are not absolutely clear-cut and partly derive from the history of different disciplines rather than from current science. All disorders that affect behavior, regardless of age of onset or etiology, are brain disorders that modern neuroscience is beginning to understand, with similar concepts and methods (see Pennington, 2014). Hence, in our view, traditionally defined learning disabilities such as dyslexia or mathematics disorder are a subset of learning disorders that also includes disorders such as autism spectrum disorder, intellectual disability (formerly called *mental retardation*), speech sound disorder (SSD), language impairment, and attention-deficit/hyperactivity disorder (ADHD). All these disorders are covered in this book. So, learning disorders are a subset of neurodevelopmental disorders, which in turn are a subset of neurological disorders (some would say neuropsychiatric disorders or central nervous system [CNS] disorders). We turn next to key theoretical issues in the science of learning disorders.

EXPLICIT AND IMPLICIT MEMORY

The word *learning* in the term *learning disorders* has two meanings: learning in early development and later learning of academic skills, such as reading, writing, and mathematics. Every learning disorder affects a particular kind of early learning that undermines the acquisition of precursor skills necessary for academic learning. An important part of the new perspective in this third edition is identifying which type of early learning is impaired in each learning disorder.

Recent research aimed at accomplishing this goal is based on an important distinction in the neuropsychology of learning and memory, namely, that between explicit or declarative learning and long-term memory, and implicit or procedural learning and long-term memory. To understand this distinction, it is important to realize the brain has multiple memory systems, each specialized for different learning tasks, and each dependent on somewhat different brain structures. The explicit memory system is dependent on the hippocampus and related cortical structures; it is specialized for both remembering specific episodes and for slowly learning semantic information, both of which can be explicitly recalled. In contrast, the implicit memory system is dependent on subcortical structures, mainly the basal ganglia and cerebellum, and is specialized for learning new skills and statistical patterns in the world, neither of which can be explicitly recalled but can be measured by changes in behavior. As a concrete example, consider taking a tennis lesson. One uses explicit memory to remember when and where the lesson is, but much of what one learns in the lesson depends on implicit memory to learn new motor skills for hitting a serve, a backhand, a dropshot, and so on. If one has hippocampal amnesia, one could still learn these new motor skills, even though one wouldn't remember anything explicit about the lesson. On the other hand, if one had a subcortical dementia, such as Parkinson's or Huntington's, one would learn these new motor skills much more slowly, even while one's memory for the actual episode of taking a tennis lesson was intact.

Turning from adult neuropsychology to developmental neuropsychology, one may ask which parts of early cognitive development depend on which memory system. Infants are prodigious learners, as evidenced by how much their behavior changes in the first few years of life, but little of what they are learning requires the explicit memory system. Instead, they rely on the implicit memory system to learn new motor and social skills, and to perceive and produce speech and language. As we discuss in later chapters, many of the learning disorders in this book begin with early deficits in implicit memory. Hence, learning disorders may be divided into (1) those that mainly affect explicit memory (i.e., various intellectual disabilities, all of which involve a global impairment in learning rate in the acquisition of declarative knowledge) and (2) those that mainly affect various forms of implicit or procedural memory (i.e., all the other learning disorders covered in this book). This new perspective provides a clearer understanding of how early cognitive development goes wrong in various learning disorders, an understanding that points the way to better approaches for early identification and preventive treatment.

HETEROTYPIC CONTINUITY IN DEVELOPMENT

Understanding neurodevelopmental disorders requires a developmental perspective, because each of these disorders has its origin in genetic and environmental risk factors that usually act on prenatal brain development and change early learning in particular ways. As children with a particular learning disorder encounter different developmental tasks, different symptoms emerge. One hallmark of learning disorders is thus *heterotypic continuity,* which means that while the underlying learning impairment remains the same across development, the particular manifestations of that impairment (observable symptoms) vary across ages.

For instance, consider the example of heterotypic continuity provided by dyslexia. Infants who will later be diagnosed with dyslexia likely have a deficit in implicit, statistical learning that manifests early on as a delay in babbling and a problem learning phonological representations necessary for speech perception and production. At the same time, these infants have intact social cognition and declarative memory; thus, their social skills and semantic memory are developing normally. Somewhat later, these children will have some delays in vocabulary development and expressive syntax, likely because of their phonological deficit. Hence, even though vocabulary is part of declarative memory, the mild vocabulary deficit in dyslexia is not caused by a broader problem in forming new declarative memories. By kindergarten, these children will likely be having trouble learning letter names and color names. In first grade, phoneme awareness will nearly always be difficult, as will learning to decode new printed words and reliably recognize familiar ones. In the later elementary grades, problems in reading fluency and comprehension will be more evident, in addition to problems memorizing math facts. Somewhat later, there will likely be problems with math "word" problems, as well as problems with foreign languages. The underlying continuity that explains these diverse symptoms is in the cognitive risk factors that characterize dyslexia (in phonological development and processing speed) and in the altered brain networks necessary for these cognitive skills. So, there is continuity in the cognitive risk factors yet discontinuity in how these risk factors manifest in the face of different developmental tasks.

Another key point concerns the plasticity of brain development, which allows causal influences in neurodevelopmental disorders to be bidirectional. Because brain development is an open process that continues throughout the lifespan, the environment, including the social environment, also affects brain development. So a child without genetic risk factors for dyslexia may end up with a reading problem, because the environment does not provide adequate spoken language and preliteracy input. And a child with genetic risk factors for dyslexia may benefit from compensating environmental protective factors and end up with only a subclinical form of the disorder. This is why the model is probabilistic rather than deterministic, and why the causal influences are bidirectional. This interplay among risk and protective factors in development also means that achieving a complete scientific understanding of why one child has a disorder and another does not is a very ambitious goal, since it requires disentangling complex developmental pathways. Nonetheless, considerable progress toward this ambitious goal has been made in the nearly three decades since the first edition of this book was published in 1991, and that progress is accelerating because of technical advances in both genetics and neuroscience.

Whereas a true science of learning disorders seemed almost unimaginable when one of us (BFP) began his career in 1977, it is now emerging rapidly.

Hence, a key point in this book is that most of what we currently know about these learning disorders at the levels of brain, neuropsychology, and behavior are somewhat static outcomes of a developmental process we do not yet fully understand. We typically diagnose and study many of these disorders at school age, but we know much less about how the neuroimaging or neuropsychological phenotype that we measure at school age actually developed. Hence, another key part of the new perspective in this third edition is to review and evaluate current knowledge about the early development of each of these disorders. We next explain the scientific methods used to understand learning disorders.

A MULTILEVEL MODEL

Multiple levels of analysis are needed to completely explain the different kinds of atypical cognitive development found in learning disorders, and we are very far from a complete neuroscientific explanation of any learning or other psychiatric disorder. Such a complete explanation would begin with a fertilized egg and trace how sequences of gene expression, partly regulated by the environment, change brain development. We are only beginning to identify the genes that affect brain development and how they interact through molecular signaling pathways. There have been a few solid gene discoveries for neurodevelopmental disorders, and they provide fascinating insights into the various ways neurodevelopment may go wrong. We discuss these discoveries in more detail in Chapter 2.

For now, it is important to emphasize a point that may seem strange to psychologists, educators, and parents. That point is that every neurodevelopmental disorder, like every medical disorder, has a physical basis that can be traced to molecular and cellular levels. As is the case in the rest of medicine, discovering the molecular and cellular bases of a disorder can lead to profound insights into how the disorder develops and can be either prevented or treated. Recent advances in molecular biology—specifically, (1) the ability to create pluripotent stem cells by taking cells from a mature human, and (2) very precise gene editing—have now made it possible to study the development *in vitro* of neurons that have the genotype of a particular neurodevelopmental disorder. In other words, we can now observe the earliest stages of brain development in several neurodevelopmental disorders, pinpoint where it first goes wrong, and identify which gene variants associated with the disorder cause which changes in neuronal phenotypes. As we discuss in later chapters, this experiment has already been conducted for some syndromal intellectual disabilities, such as fragile X syndrome (Park et al., 2015) and Williams syndrome (Chailangkarn et al., 2016), but will very likely soon be conducted with others. Strange as it may seem, we potentially have the means to look at the development of "dyslexic" neurons in a petri dish!

The previous paragraph makes it clear why research on the etiology of neurodevelopmental disorders is so important and why this research is included in a book whose main audience consists of clinicians and educators. Hence, in this book, we review what is currently known about the development of each learning disorder covered here, beginning at the most basic level of analysis, etiology.

Other levels of analysis include brain development, neuropsychology, and behavior (Figure 1.1). Other important features of the developmental model used here are that it (1) recognizes bidirectional causal influences across levels, (2) is probabilistic rather than deterministic, and (3) and incorporates multiple factors at each level of analysis. Earlier biological models of the development of disorders have emphasized unidirectional causation and single factors at each level of analysis, as illustrated in the upper half of Figure 1.1, but we have learned that such a model is too simple for most, if not all, neurodevelopmental disorders.

Etiology is concerned with the distal causes of disorders, the particular genetic and environmental risk and protective factors that cause one child to have a disorder and another child *not* to have the disorder. *Distal causes* can also be thought of as the ultimate causes or initial reasons that development gets under way in one direction versus another. These distal causes act on brain development, often *in utero*, changing the wiring and/or the neurotransmitter systems of the brain. These structural and neurochemical changes in the brain are the proximal or immediate causes of learning disorders. They alter brain functions in ways we can detect with neuroimaging studies and neuropsychological tests, and we postulate that these cognitive risk factors result in behavioral symptoms that are often observable by teachers, parents, and peers, and which define various learning disorders in DSM-5 and the 10th revision of the *International Classification of Diseases* (ICD-10; World Health Organization, 1990).

Of course, these four broad levels of analysis can be further subdivided. As indicated earlier, a molecular biologist would subdivide the first two levels into genes, molecules, molecular signaling pathways, cells (neurons and glial cells), and structural and functional brain networks. A cognitive neuroscientist would not only

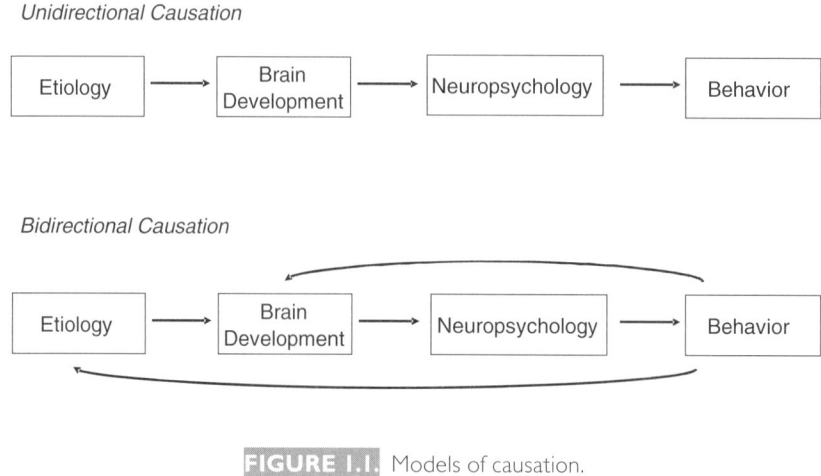

FIGURE 1.1. Models of causation.

use neuroimaging methods to study brain networks, but would also divide the level of neuropsychology into a neurocomputational level and a cognitive level. The neurocomputational level provides the critical link between brain and cognition. A neurocomputational model incorporates key features of atypical brain development in a given disorder (e.g., impaired dopamine signaling in schizophrenia or Parkinson's disease) in a neural network model that learns certain key cognitive tasks and attempts to simulate the resulting cognitive deficits found in that disorder. We may find that there are likely even more levels within these additional levels.

How Our Psychological Constructs Will Change

As scientific progress continues across these various levels of analysis, some of our familiar neuropsychological and diagnostic constructs will be modified or even disappear! As discussed in subsequent chapters, research on the reasons for comorbidities among learning disorders will lead to changes in our neuropsychological and diagnostic constructs, because it will make it clearer which of these constructs need to be lumped with other constructs and which need to be split. As we discuss in Chapter 6, we also already know that some DSM-5 specific learning disorders currently are not valid constructs and will need to be reformulated.

THE MULTIPLE-DEFICIT MODEL

We now turn to an example of an important way in which science has changed our thinking about learning disorders. Unlike the first edition of this book (Pennington, 1991), this third edition and the second edition (Pennington, 2009) that preceded it are based on a multiple-deficit model of the etiology and neuropsychology of learning disorders (Pennington, 2006). The first edition espoused a modular, single-deficit model of the neuropsychological causes of learning disorders (see also Morton, 2004; Morton & Frith, 1995). Since this is the simplest and most parsimonious model, it made sense for the field to test it first. Now, some 25 years later, enough evidence has accumulated to force us to abandon this simple model. The view taken in this book is that *modules* (i.e., brain regions specialized for processing certain kinds of input like language or faces) are not innate but are instead the product of a developmental process that shows considerable plasticity. Moreover, the function of these developed modules is not encapsulated but instead depends on their connections and interactions with other brain structures. Consequently, it is too simplistic to completely localize a complex cognitive operation such as recognizing faces or spoken words in just one part of the brain (see Van Orden, Pennington, & Stone, 2001, for a fuller discussion of these issues).

Another related aspect of the single-deficit paradigm was a focus on "pure" cases, which most clinicians realize are much rarer than mixed cases. This issue of pure versus mixed cases is perhaps even more relevant to neurodevelopmental disorders than it is to acquired ones. If there were evolved cognitive modules, as Fodor (1983) hypothesized, maybe different neurodevelopmental disorders each were due to weaker development in a specific module. Developmental dyslexia was hypothesized by Morton and Frith (1995) to be due to a specific developmental deficit in the phonological module, and autism was hypothesized by them to be due to a specific developmental deficit in the theory-of-mind module. Other scientists (Duchaine, 2000; Kanwisher, 2010) studying *developmental prosopagnosia* (in which children are very poor at recognizing faces of even very familiar people) have hypothesized that it is due to a specific developmental deficit in the face recognition module. The simplicity of this modularity theory was very appealing, but it ultimately proved to be too simple.

Focusing only on the theoretically meaningful or specific cognitive components in a given disorder risks making erroneous claims about what the disorder means. This has happened in the cases of Williams syndrome and the KE family (a British family in which there is a dominantly transmitted speech dyspraxia), and in other disorders, as we discuss later. So the lesson that emerges is that it is important to realize that any particular disorder will present with a mix of both general and specific deficits, *all* of which need to be explained. Overall IQ will be somewhat lower, and some aspects of cognitive development will be slower in virtually any neurodevelopmental disorder compared to population controls selected to not have that disorder. Most neurodevelopmental disorders will also have specific differences in cognitive profile when compared with other neurodevelopmental disorders. Our goal as researchers is to provide an explanation of *both* the general and specific deficits found in the profile of that disorder. In some disorders, such as intellectual disability (ID), the general deficits will predominate, whereas in others, such as dyslexia, the specific deficits will be more striking.

This brings us to another key aspect of the new perspective in this third edition of this book, namely, the importance of both shared and specific risk factors at each level of analysis. At the etiological level, both risk and protective factors vary in how general versus specific their effects are. Alterations in brain development have both general and specific neuropsychological effects.

INSIGHTS FROM COMORBIDITY

It was our own work on the reasons why disorders co-occur (i.e., comorbidity) that forced us to abandon the single-deficit model (Pennington, Willcutt, & Rhee, 2005). We found that there was more generality than specificity in the cognitive profiles of comorbid neurodevelopmental disorders. The single-deficit model posits that a single cognitive deficit is sufficient to explain the symptoms of a given disorder, and that different disorders have different single deficits. We and others have found that the frequent phenomenon of comorbidity is often explained by partially shared etiological and cognitive risk factors. Hence, because neurodevelopmental disorders are frequently comorbid, they are intrinsically mixed rather than pure cases. So, as we review later, dyslexia and ADHD have a partial genetic overlap, as do dyslexia and SSD. This overlap at the etiological level is consistent with the widely accepted multifactorial model of the etiology of behaviorally defined disorders. In the multifactorial model, multiple genetic and environmental risk factors combine to produce a given disorder, and some of these risk factors are shared by multiple disorders, producing the many comorbidities found among learning and other psychiatric disorders.

We came to realize that the multifactorial model of etiology did not fit well theoretically with the single cognitive-deficit model of learning disorders, which was also challenged by the empirical finding of multiple cognitive deficits in *all* the learning disorders considered in this book. If a cognitive deficit is shared by two distinct disorders, it cannot be sufficient to produce either one, but it could act as a cofactor with other cognitive deficits not shared by the two comorbid disorders. So we have proposed and tested a multiple cognitive-deficit model of learning disorders (Figure 1.2).

Similar to the complex disease model in medicine (Sing & Reilly, 1993) and the quantitative genetic model in behavioral genetics (Plomin, DeFries, Knopik, & Neiderhiser, 2013), the current model proposes that (1) the etiology of complex behavioral disorders is multifactorial and involves the interaction of multiple risk and protective factors, which can be either genetic or environmental; (2) these risk and protective factors alter the development of neural systems that mediate cognitive

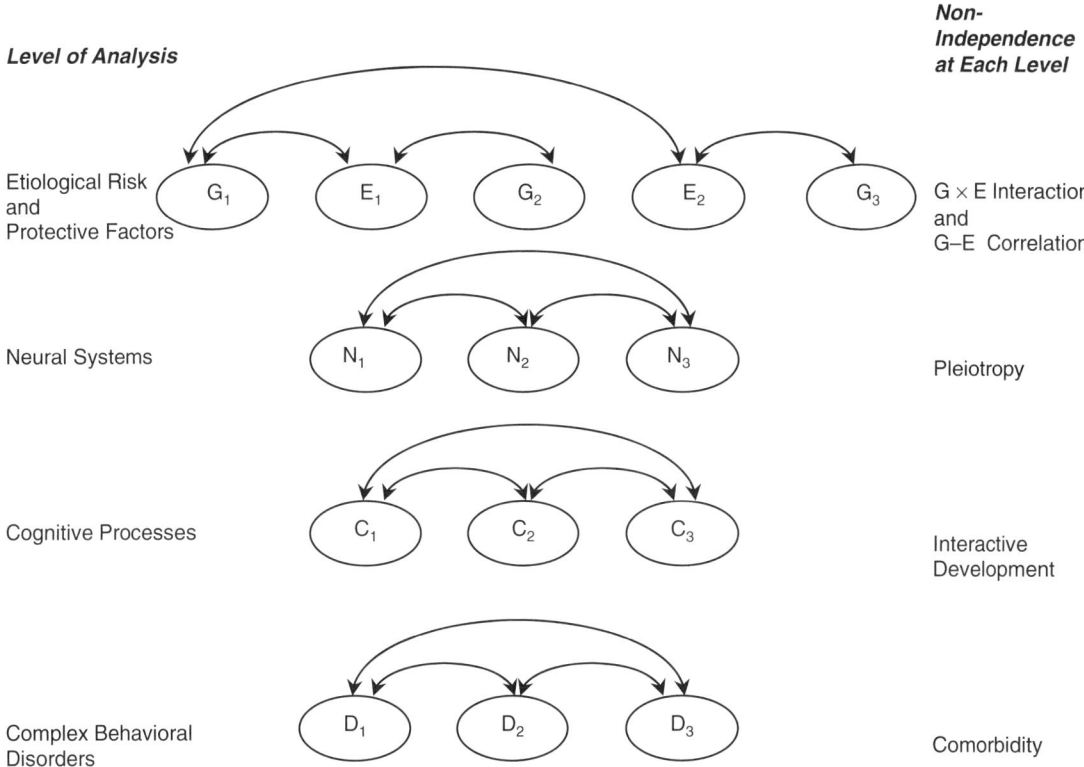

FIGURE 1.2. Multiple-deficit model. G, genetic risk or protective factor; E, environmental risk or protective factor; N, neural system; C, cognitive process; D, disorder.

functions necessary for normal development, thus producing the behavioral symptoms that define these disorders; (3) no single etiological factor is sufficient for a disorder, and few may be necessary; (4) consequently, comorbidity among complex behavioral disorders is to be expected because of shared etiological and cognitive risk factors; and (5) the liability distribution for a given disease is often continuous and quantitative, rather than being discrete and categorical, so that the threshold for having the disorder is somewhat arbitrary. Applying the model to two comorbidities considered in this book (dyslexia + ADHD and dyslexia + SSD), each individual disorder would have its own profile of risk factors (both etiological and cognitive), with some of these risk factors being shared by the other disorder, resulting in comorbidity.

Figure 1.2 illustrates the complex disease model as applied to complex behavioral disorders. Similar to Figure 1.1, there are four levels of analysis in this diagram: etiological, neural, cognitive, and symptom, in which clusters of symptoms define complex behavioral disorders. For any such complex behavioral disorder, it is expected that there will be many more etiological risk and protective factors than the five shown in Figure 1.2. Bidirectional connections at each level indicate that constructs are not independent. For instance, at the etiological level, there are likely to be gene × environment (G × E) interactions and gene–environment (G–E) correlations. At the neural level, a single genetic or environmental risk factor will often affect more than one neural system (*pleiotropy*). Even if the risk factor initially only affects one neural system, this alteration will likely have downstream effects on the development of other neural systems. At the cognitive level, constructs are correlated because their developmental pathways overlap, and because cognition is interactive. Overlap at the cognitive level leads to comorbidity at the symptom level. At the symptom level, there is comorbidity (i.e., greater than chance co-occurrence) of complex behavioral disorders. Omitted from the diagram are the causal connections *between* levels of analyses, some of which would include feedback loops from behavior to brain or even to etiology, as in Figure 1.1. The existence and strength of these various causal connections must be determined empirically. The weights on the connections between levels of analysis will tell us to what extent different etiological and cognitive factors contribute to comorbidity at the symptom level.

This model makes it clear that achieving a complete understanding of the development of disorders such as SSD, dyslexia, or autism will be very difficult because of the multiple pathways involved. But this kind of model is needed, because it is becoming increasingly clear that there are shared processes at the etiological, neural, and cognitive levels across such disorders.

In the chapters on disorders (Chapters 9–14), we consider their comorbidities and discuss how the multiple-deficit model applies to them. For instance, in the case of dyslexia, we used to think a deficit in phoneme awareness (PA) was the single cognitive deficit that caused the disorder in most children. But we have learned that children with SSD can have a similar deficit in PA and not develop dyslexia, questioning whether a single PA deficit is sufficient to produce dyslexia (Peterson, Pennington, Shriberg, & Boada, 2009). Moreover, children with dyslexia compared to children with SSD but not dyslexia (SSD only) have deficits in processing speed, suggesting that intact processing speed is a protective factor for children with SSD, despite having a PA deficit (Pennington & Bishop, 2009). And we have also learned that deficits in processing speed are shared by dyslexia and ADHD (McGrath et al., 2011; Peterson et al., 2017; Willcutt et al., 2010; Willcutt, Pennington, Olson, Chhabildas, & Hulslander, 2005), which helps to explain their comorbidity.

In Chapters 9–14, we apply this multiple-deficit model to specific learning disorders. In each chapter, we provide a research review of what is known about that disorder's etiology, brain mechanisms, neuropsychology, and comorbidities. Then we show how our scientific understanding of each disorder informs its diagnosis and treatment. So the overall goal is to integrate science and practice in the field of learning disorders. In the next three chapters, we explain the levels of analysis in Figure 1.2, beginning with etiology.

SUMMARY

In this chapter, we have explained our multilevel model of how learning disorders develop and why they are often comorbid. We have also explained the new perspective that informs the third edition of this book. There are four aspects of this new perspective:

1. Research on learning disorders is necessarily interdisciplinary.
2. A full understanding of learning disorders will require taking a developmental perspective at each level of analysis and identifying causal links across levels of analysis.
3. We need to identify which aspect of early learning, implicit versus explicit, is impaired in each learning disorder.
4. In our multiple-deficit model, there are both shared and specific risk factors for each learning disorder at the etiological, brain development, and neuropsychological levels of analysis, with the shared risk factors producing comorbidities among these disorders.

CHAPTER 2

Etiology of Learning Disorders

In the preceding chapter, we mentioned that comorbidity among neurodevelopmental disorders derives from partly shared etiological risk factors. In this chapter we delve into what those etiological risk factors are and how to find them. This chapter contains material that was first presented in Pennington (2015) and Pennington and Peterson (2015).

Since the term *etiology* is sometimes used in different ways, it is important to be precise at the outset about what we mean by this term. *Etiology* as used here refers to initial or *distal* causes of individual differences within a species, the early factors that change the trajectory of development in some domain of function so as to produce different outcomes among individuals in a population. So, various health outcomes, both favorable and unfavorable (e.g., not only longevity and physical fitness but also heart disease, cancer, obesity, and cystic fibrosis), all have etiologies, as do various psychological traits (e.g., intelligence, personality, and the various aspects of academic skills discussed in this book) and psychological disorders (e.g., intellectual disability [ID], anxiety, and dyslexia). Some disorders are categorical (one either has the disorder or one does not); these categorical disorders often have a discrete etiology, such as a mutation in a single gene, as is true for cystic fibrosis, phenylketonuria (PKU), and Huntington's disease (HD).

Many other disorders, and especially behaviorally defined disorders, are not categorical, but are just extremes on a continuous distribution that ranges from optimal outcomes to poor outcomes, with the underlying mechanisms being similar across the whole distribution. For instance, many cases of ID (formerly called "mental retardation") are mainly defined by a cutoff on the distribution of intelligence (even though there are forms of intellectual disability that have a known genetic etiology, e.g., untreated PKU, Down syndrome, or fragile X syndrome.) The same is true of reading disability, or dyslexia, which is defined by cutoffs on a distribution of reading scores. For these noncategorical disorders, the etiology is often complex, due to many etiological factors acting together.

Etiology consists of distal genetic and environmental risk and protective factors (and their interplay) that act in development to produce outcome differences among members of a population. If the outcome in question involves behavior, then these etiological factors generally act on brain development in some fashion or another, because our brains produce our behavior. As previously discussed, the resulting changes in the anatomy, physiology, and cognitive processes of the developing brain constitute the proximal or immediate causes of behavior. So the proximal causes of behavior found in brain mechanisms are *not* what we mean by the term *etiology*.

As discussed in Chapter 1, the identification of etiological risk factors, especially genetic ones, can be very informative about the development of individual differences, because different genes act at different times on different processes in brain development. Identifying even one rare gene that influences an outcome can greatly accelerate progress in finding other genes, because there are families of genes that work together in development. As we will see, some of the candidate genes for dyslexia appear to be part of such a gene family.

Etiology is about the distal causes of individual differences within a population or species. There are also universal species-typical behaviors (e.g., language and social behavior in humans) that are caused by evolution, both biological and cultural, but these causes of human universals are also not what we mean by the term *etiology*. Nonetheless, evolved human genes and cultural practices can be very informative about where to look for etiological factors that lead to individual differences in behaviors such as language and social behavior. Hence, the etiology of behaviorally defined disorders is potentially informative about both individual differences in development and human evolution, just as the evolution of human genes and culture may be informative about the etiology of individual differences.

It is these reciprocal relations across levels of analysis that make the study of etiology so exciting and so important for both basic and applied science. For instance, a discovery about the etiology of a rare pathology can lead to the discovery of not only other, related genes but also pathogenetic and evolutionary mechanisms. As a specific example, a mutation in the coding region of the *FOXP2* gene was found in a family (the KE family) with a rare oral–motor coordination disorder (i.e., childhood apraxia of speech [CAS], which is discussed in Chapter 9) that affected their speech and language development (Fisher, Vargha-Khadem, Watkins, Monaco, & Pembrey, 1998; Lai, Fisher, Hurst, Vargha-Khadem, & Monaco, 2001). Subsequently, imaging studies reveal that this gene appeared to act on the basal ganglia in the brain, an important structure in motor control and implicit learning and memory (Lai, Gerrelli, Monaco, Fisher, & Copp, 2003), that this gene evolved recently in human evolution (Enard, 2011), and that an earlier form of this gene is important in audiovocal communication in birds (Konopka & Roberts, 2016; Scharff & Haesler, 2005). As can be seen, etiological research on this rare disorder led to breakthrough discoveries with much wider significance for our understanding of the evolution of human language. Interestingly, the *FOXP2* mutation does not account for most cases of language impairment outside the KE family (Newbury et al., 2002), but there are common noncoding variants of *FOXP2* that affect procedural learning of novel speech sound categories in human adults (Chandrasekaran, Yi, Blanco, McGeary, & Maddox, 2015). Moreover, other genes regulated by *FOXP2*, such as *CNTNAP2*, are turning out to influence other communication disorders besides CAS. In summary, the discovery of the rare mutation of *FOXP2* in the KE family was a breakthrough discovery with widespread implications, many of which remain to be discovered. This is why the study of etiology is so important.

Neither genes nor environments code for behavior directly. As discussed by Oyama (1985), both sides of the nature–nurture debate share the same erroneous assumption that the instructions for behavior are preexistent either in the genome or in the environment and are imposed from without on the developing organisms. Instead, genetic and environmental influences are inputs to a developmental process, and their impact on behavioral outcome depends on their interactions with all the components of that process. Consequently, it is misleading to speak of the genome as a "blueprint" or to think that genes "code" for behaviors. A better metaphor for the genome is that it is a "recipe," a sequence of operations that produces a new form. But even this metaphor is misleading, because there is no "chef" to follow the recipe. Genes simply code for protein structure or regulate other genes, and variations in the structure of a given protein in a particular developmental context may push behavioral outcomes in one direction or another. Thus, genetic and environmental factors are best conceptualized as acting as risk (or protective) factors in the development of individual differences in behavior; their effects are probabilistic rather than deterministic. We next consider various methods scientists use to learn about etiology, beginning with behavioral genetics, then considering molecular genetics.

BEHAVIORAL GENETICS

Behavioral genetic methods rely on twin and adoption samples to identify genetic and environmental influences on behavior. Behavioral geneticists have documented moderate heritability (often around .50) for individual differences in most dimensions of human cognition and personality (Plomin, Haworth, Meaburn, Price, & Davis, 2013), and for behaviorally defined disorders, including the learning disorders discussed in this book. It is important to understand what the technical term *heritability* means and does not mean. Heritability refers to the proportion of variance in a given population that is attributable to genetic influences; the remaining variance is attributable to environmental influences, gene–environment interplay, or just error of measurement. To further illustrate the limits of interpretation, take a heritability estimate of 50% for a disorder such as dyslexia. This estimate is often misinterpreted to mean that 50% of cases with dyslexia are genetic or that there is a 50% chance that a child will inherit the disorder from his or her parents. Both of these interpretations fundamentally misunderstand what the heritability estimate tells us, namely, that it estimates the proportion of variance in a population (in reading or other traits) that can be explained by genetic influences. Because it is dependent on a population estimate, the heritability estimate does not tell us about the cause of an individual's outcome and, because it is population-specific, it can vary across populations. The heritability estimate does indicate that genes contribute to variation in the population, but it does not identify which genes or how many of them. For this, molecular genetic methods are necessary (discussed below). The ACE model for estimating the genetic and environmental variance components is described shortly. Like all behaviorally defined disorders, the cause of learning disorders is thought to be multifactorial and thus due to multiple genes and environmental risk factors. It remains possible, however, that in some individuals or families with a behavioral disorder, the disorder is caused by a single, rare mutation, as was true in the KE family. As will be discussed later, one example of such a rare mutation is a copy number variation (CNV), and it has been discovered that some cases of autism and schizophrenia are caused by rare CNVs, even though the etiology of both disorders at the population level is multifactorial.

Moderate heritability has also been found for other behaviorally defined neurodevelopmental disorders, such as attention-deficit/hyperactivity disorder (ADHD), speech sound disorder (SSD), and language impairment (LI), all of which are comorbid with dyslexia. Because these results come from mainly middle-class twin samples in developed countries, it is important to remember that they may not generalize to other populations (but see Hensler, Schatschneider, Taylor, & Wagner, 2010, who found moderate heritability, > .50, both for dyslexia and typical reading skill in a more ethnically and economically diverse sample).

Heritability estimates are usually derived by applying a very simple variance components model to data from twin or adoption studies. This ACE model estimates main effects of genes acting additively (*A*), common or shared environment (*C*), and nonshared environment (including error) (*E*). Shared environmental influences are shared by siblings in the same family (e.g., the number of books in the home) but differ across families; environmental influences that are shared by all families, such as light and gravity, are crucial to species-universal development but do not contribute to individual differences. Nonshared environmental influences differ among siblings in the same family (e.g., seeking out books from the school library or going to a reading tutor). The *E* component also includes error of measurement *and*, importantly, currently unpredictable variations in development, sometimes called *epigenetic noise* (Molenaar, Boomsma, & Dolan, 1993). So the *E* component is not always necessarily environmental. Because the ACE model only includes these three main effects, it does not tell us about gene–environment interplay, which we discuss next. Although the heritability estimate is usually a point of focus for ACE models, it is important to note that these models also provide support for environmental contributions to complex traits, since heritability estimates are rarely 100%.

BEYOND THE ACE MODEL: GENE–ENVIRONMENT INTERPLAY

Going beyond the main effects of genes and environment captured by the ACE model, we can ask how genetic and environmental risk factors act together in the development of abnormal behavior. As Rutter (2006) discusses, there are many kinds of interplay between genes and environments. Two broad classes of such interplay are gene × environment (G × E) interaction and gene–environment (G–E) correlation. In G × E interaction, the effect of independent genetic and environmental factors is synergistic rather than additive. In other words, the impact of a given genetic risk factor varies in different environments (and vice versa). There are three subtypes of G × E interaction: diathesis–stress, bioecological, and susceptibility. In a diathesis–stress G × E interaction (Caspi et al., 2003), the effects of a risk genotype are increased by an environmental risk factor and vice versa. In a bioecological G × E interaction (Bronfenbrenner & Ceci, 1994), the opposite pattern is observed: The effects of a risk genotype are *stronger* in a protective environment than in a risk environment. Finally, in a susceptibility G × E interaction (Belsky & Pluess, 2009), a susceptibility genotype leads to a worse outcome in a risk environment, but to a *better* outcome in a protective environment, whereas a nonsusceptibility genotype is less affected by either type of environment.

There is also increasing evidence for the importance of transactional processes in atypical development, in which the child and environment mutually alter each other over time. G–E correlation is an example of such a transaction. Such transactions occur because children evoke different kinds of reactions from their environments (Scarr & McCartney, 1983), and select different kinds of environments for themselves. Not surprisingly, the individual characteristics that influence such reactions and selections are genetically influenced. There are three subtypes of G–E correlation: passive, evocative, and active (Scarr & McCartney, 1983). In the case of reading development, an example of a passive G–E correlation is the relation between parents' reading skill and the number of books in the home. Parents' reading skill is partly due to genes, and parents who are better readers on average have more books in their home. Without any action on the part of their biological children, their literacy environment is correlated with their reading genotype on average. In contrast, an evocative G–E correlation occurs when adults in a given child's environment notice the child's interests and talents, and seek to foster them. In the case of reading development, an example of an evocative G–E correlation would be a caregiver taking a child who likes to read to the library. Finally, an active G–E correlation occurs when children on their own initiative seek or avoid environments as a function of their genotype. Dyslexia provides a clear example of an active G–E correlation. Even before formal literacy instruction, young children who will later become dyslexic avoid being read to and spend less independent play time looking at books than their siblings who do not develop dyslexia (Scarborough, Dobrich, & Hager, 1991). As they get older, school-age children with dyslexia read dramatically fewer words per year than do typically developing children (Cunningham & Stanovich, 1998), and this reduced reading experience negatively influences both their reading fluency and their oral vocabularies (Stanovich, 1986; Torgesen, 2005).

MOLECULAR GENETICS

Molecular methods (i.e., ones that rely on measuring DNA variations among individuals) test directly for genetic influences on a phenotype and now allow us to go beyond the indirect methods used in classical behavior genetics, which we just discussed. They also allow a direct test of whether behavior genetics results are valid. Briefly, molecular genetics studies of the etiologies of typical traits and disorders exploit two important facts about the genome. The first fact is that some "rungs" in the DNA "ladder" (where these rungs consist of pairs of the four chemical bases adenine [A], cytosine [C], guanine [G], and thymine [T]) differ across individuals in a species such that one individual may have the pair AG for one rung and another individual may have the pair CT (in humans, about 1 per 300 base pairs show differences across individuals on average; our genome has a total of about 3 billion pairs). Those base pairs that frequently differ across individuals are called *single-nucleotide polymorphisms* (SNPs). The second important fact is that the DNA segments (e.g., SNPs) on chromosomes are "shuffled" by recombination in the process of making individual sperm and egg cells (i.e., *gametes*). As a result of this shuffling, only DNA segments that are close together on the same chromosome will be inherited together or "linked" within families. If the linkage is tight enough, the DNA segments will be associated both within and across families. (We now use genetic association more frequently than genetic linkage to identify candidate genes for disorders.) As a result of recombination, individuals in a species (except for identical twins) differ in their exact DNA sequences, and some of these DNA differences lead to differences in behavior and other traits. By relating trait similarity to DNA similarity, we can eventually discover which DNA variants are important for a given trait.

Several candidate genes for dyslexia have been identified, as we discuss in Chapter 10, and some of these candidate genes contribute to speech and language disorders, consistent with comorbidity between dyslexia and these other disorders. In the case of ID, there are several well-studied genetic syndromes that produce ID, such as Down syndrome and fragile X syndrome, which are discussed in Chapter 14. The greatest genetic progress since the second edition of this book was published in 2009 has been for autism spectrum disorder. That progress is discussed in Chapter 13. In contrast, virtually nothing is known about the genetics of mathematics disorder, partly because there are few molecular studies of this disorder. Finally, despite a considerable amount of molecular research, progress in ADHD has been very slow, though recent large-scale studies might lead to an acceleration of findings in the coming years. We consider in the next section some reasons why genetic progress is easier for some learning disorders than others.

MISSING HERITABILITY?

A potential criticism of twin studies of heritability (Wahlsten, 2012) is that molecular studies have identified only a very few of the many genes needed to account for the moderate to high heritability found by twin studies for common traits such as IQ or reading or height. This problem is called the problem of "missing heritability" (Manolio et al., 2009). Once microarrays (sometimes called gene or SNP "chips") with large numbers of SNPs across the genome became readily available, researchers undertook genomewide association studies (GWAS) of complex phenotypic traits, such as height, IQ, and common diseases. At the outset of this research, it was hoped there would be prevalent genetic variants contributing to common diseases and that GWAS would find them. Hence, the moderate heritability of these traits would be explained in terms of actual genes. However, a typical result of many GWAS was that very few SNPs produced significant associations with the phenotype being studied, and those few combined only accounted for a small proportion (at most 1–3%) of the variance in the phenotype. This result was found not only for numerous common diseases, such as autism, schizophrenia, and diabetes, but also for quantitative traits with moderate to high heritabilities, such as IQ, height, and weight.

Since these GWAS were motivated by the fact that normal and abnormal traits being investigated had all demonstrated substantial heritabilities in behavior genetic twin studies, these disappointingly meager results from GWAS posed the puzzle of missing heritability. For instance, twin studies typically find heritability for human height of around .90 and for IQ of around .50. Thus, the missing heritability puzzle was the large gap between the small amount of genetic variance accounted for by GWAS results and the large indirect estimates of this genetic variance based on previous behavior genetics twin studies.

Several explanations were offered to account for this commonly observed phenomenon of missing heritability. These explanations included (1) a very large number genetic variants (i.e., alleles) with very small additive effect sizes (i.e., a highly polygenic etiology); (2) rare variants with large effects that are hard to detect with existing SNP chips utilizing common variants; (3) CNVs, which are deletions or duplications of segments of DNA; (4) high levels of gene–gene interaction (called *epistasis*); (5) G × E interactions; and (6) overestimation of heritability by behavior genetic designs (Manolio et al., 2009).

Possibility 6 posed a serious threat to the validity of many decades of research in behavior genetics, and was embraced by some critics, who asserted that the conclusion of moderate heritability for many human traits and disorders was fundamentally mistaken. As we will see, later empirical results have indicated that possibility 6 is quite unlikely, and that instead possibility 1 appears to hold for continuously distributed individual differences such as those in height and IQ. Possibilities 2 and 3 are more likely mechanisms to explain the missing heritability of severe developmental disorders, such as autism and schizophrenia, and possibility 4 is supported in some recent studies of dyslexia, which are reviewed in Chapter 10.

To understand why current GWAS require enormous samples sizes (tens to hundreds of thousands of individuals) in order to identify common variants affecting human traits such as IQ and height, and common human disorders, it is important to understand the relation between effect size and allele frequency for alleles that affect important aspects of human development. An important model for understanding this relation is called the "mutation–selection" model (Keller, 2008), which was proposed to explain why deleterious disorders such as schizophrenia and autism persist at a fairly high rate (~1%) in the population. Both of these disorders reduce individuals' reproductive success (i.e., how many children they have), so natural selection should quickly eliminate common risk alleles with larger effect sizes. Hence, risk alleles with large effect sizes that persist in the gene pool will necessarily be rare. Thus, we need an explanation for why natural selection has not eliminated the risk alleles for common deleterious conditions such as schizophrenia.

The mutation–selection explanation proposes that new mutations balance the elimination of old risk alleles for such disorders, leading to a fairly stable prevalence of such disorders over time. So the mutation–selection model holds that common variants with large (i.e., detectable with current GWAS) effect sizes on common disorders will not be found. Instead, such deleterious variants will be rare, and there will be an inverse relation between effect size and allele frequency, which are represented on a log scale in Figure 2.1. Effect size means what proportion of the population variance in the phenotype is caused by the risk allele, and allele frequency is the prevalence of the risk allele in the population. As can be seen in Figure 2.1, most genetic variants affecting human traits will fall along the diagonal. Those with big effect sizes, like the genes for Mendelian diseases, such as PKU or HD, are rare (upper left circle in Figure 2.1), whereas common genetic variants affecting common, adaptive traits such as height or IQ will have small effect sizes, and most will fall into the bottom right circle in Figure 2.1. PKU and HD are examples of Mendelian diseases (i.e., caused by a mutation in a single gene, which can be recessive, as in PKU, or dominant, as is true for HD). In the upper right corner of Figure 2.1, there is a circle for *one* of the exceptions to this general pattern: common variants with large effect sizes affecting common diseases. This exception is mostly for diseases with a late onset that consequently escape elimination by natural selection. An example would be the *APOE-4* risk variant, which considerably increases the risk for Alzheimer's disease and is common in the population. Because learning disorders have an early onset, this model predicts there will not be such common variants with large population effect sizes for learning disorders. However, there could be rare variants with large effect sizes in some families (genetic heterogeneity). The other exception, in the lower left corner of Figure 2.1, consists of very rare allelic variants with low effect sizes. Such variants will be extremely difficult to identify.

So the mutation–selection hypothesis explains missing heritability in GWAS of adaptive traits with the first possibility, a highly polygenic etiology. If the mutation–selection hypothesis is true, then most existing GWAS are dramatically underpowered to detect individual alleles with very small effect sizes. GWAS have a very stringent threshold for significance because of the magnitude of the multiple testing problem encountered when testing across the whole genome (e.g., $p < 10^{-8}$), so only SNPs with a relatively large effect size will be detected unless the sample size is in the tens or hundreds of thousands of individuals.

To test whether previous twin studies overestimated heritabilities (i.e., the heritability is missing because it is not really there), different methods of analyzing GWAS data are needed, ones that estimate the cumulative, additive effect size of *all* the SNPs across the genome, not just the ones that cross the stringent threshold for significance. Such methods have been developed, and they exploit the fact that individuals in a GWAS, who are from different families, nonetheless vary in their degree of DNA sharing across all the SNPs in the analysis (Yang, Lee, Goddard,

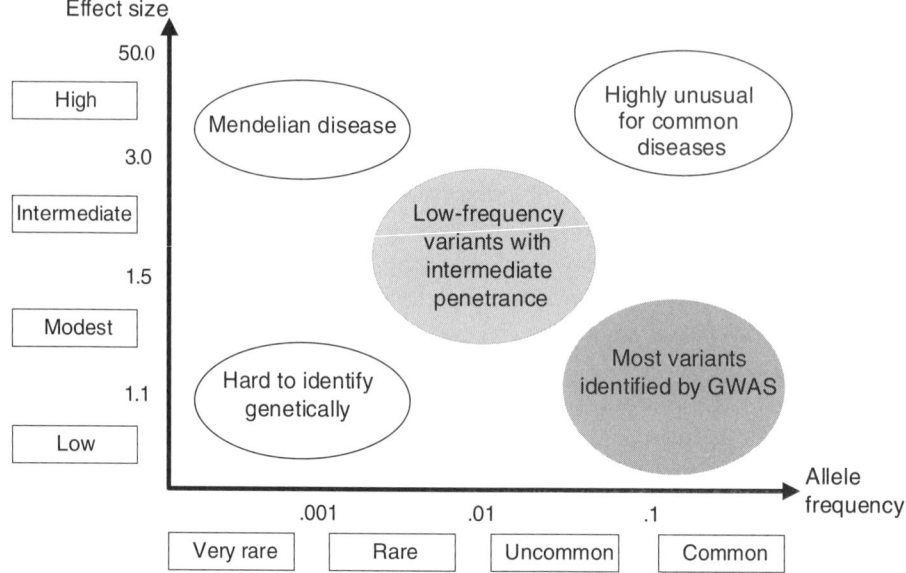

FIGURE 2.1. Feasibility of identifying genetic variants by risk allele frequency and strength of genetic effect. Adapted from Zemunik and Boraska (2011).

& Visscher, 2011). Notice that these unrelated individuals do not share a common family environment (C) and are unlikely to share a unique environment (E), so that any phenotypic similarity is due mainly or exclusively to additive genetic similarity (A). Consequently, the relation between their genetic similarity and their phenotype similarity can be evaluated to give a direct, molecular estimate of heritability. This method is referred to as genomewide complex trait analysis (GCTA).

When the GCTA approach has been applied to GWAS data for height (Yang et al., 2010) and IQ (Chabris et al., 2012; Davies et al., 2011; Plomin, Haworth, et al., 2013), SNP heritability estimates come closer to twin study heritability estimates, but there still is some missing heritability. This small amount of remaining missing heritability could be due to possibilities 2 (rare variants), 3 (CNVs), 4 (epistasis), and 5 (G × E interaction) in the list presented earlier. In summary, the phenomenon of missing heritability does not mean that twin study estimates of genetic influence on many typical and atypical human traits are wrong. It does mean, however, that very many alleles of very many genes may be involved in the etiologies of those traits, and that working out the many developmental pathways may be very difficult.

SUMMARY

Behavioral genetics studies have established contributions of both genes and environments in the etiology of learning disorders. To answer questions about which specific genes are implicated, molecular genetic methods are necessary. Molecular genetics has undergone a revolution in the past decade. Technological innovations have enabled study designs that interrogate the entire genome, and there has been an increasing focus on methodological rigor (i.e., powering studies for realistically small effect sizes), which has led to better replicability of genetic findings. While these efforts have proved fruitful for several adult psychiatric disorders (Psychiatric GWAS Consortium Bipolar Disorder Working Group, 2011; Schizophrenia Working Group of the Psychiatric Genomics Consortium, 2014), many of the childhood disorders (with the exception of autism) are still awaiting their first large-scale, genomewide association studies that can identify statistically significant genetic variants. Based on past findings, we can expect that the effect sizes of any single genetic variant will be quite small (i.e., much less than 1% of the variance), but these gene identifications will still be important for identifying novel biological pathways that increase risk for the disorders.

CHAPTER 3

Brain Mechanisms of Learning Disorders

This chapter is concerned with how the etiologies we just discussed act on brain development. Whereas etiology is concerned with the distal causes of a disorder, brain mechanisms are needed to understand proximal causes of any disorder that affects behavior. In medicine, proximal causes of a disorder are labeled *pathophysiology*. To understand the pathophysiology of learning disorders, we (1) review stages of brain development, including neurodevelopmental disorders that arise at each stage; (2) discuss how brain connectivity develops; (3) consider three models of brain–behavior development; (4) discuss brain plasticity; (5) discuss neuroimaging methods that have been applied to neurodevelopmental disorders; and (6) conclude with a summary of the chapter. Parts of this chapter appeared earlier in Pennington (2015).

It is important to recognize that there is currently a huge gap between the earliest alterations in brain development in these neurodevelopmental disorders, which are mostly unknown, and what we currently know about the brain phenotypes in these disorders from neuroimaging studies, which have mostly been conducted in school-age children or adults. This gap is not only temporal but also empirical and theoretical. Because the brain is plastic and changes with development in many ways we currently do not understand, we can rarely pinpoint which early change in brain development led to a neuroimaging phenotype observed much later in development.

Identifying a gene variant involved in a particular disorder can begin to close this gap if we can determine when this gene is expressed in early brain development and with what other genes it interacts. For instance, as we will discuss in later chapters, the gene responsible for fragile X syndrome is involved in synaptogenesis, as are a number of the genes involved in autism. Hence, it is important to understand the stages of early brain development and what has already been learned about how different etiologies can disrupt them.

STAGES OF BRAIN DEVELOPMENT

Typical brain development is described in detail in Stiles, Brown, Haist, and Jernigan (2015), so we focus here on examples of atypical development that occur at each stage of brain development (Table 3.1).

Although the stages listed in Table 3.1 concern early structural development of the brain, it is important to realize that structural and functional brain development are intertwined throughout development, beginning prenatally. For instance, spontaneous neural activity in the retina of each eye in the fetus is necessary for the immature lateral geniculate nucleus (LGN) of the thalamus to differentiate into layers specific to each eye (Shatz, 1992). This layering of the LGN is clearly innate (present before birth) but not hardwired in the genome, because it depends on activity-driven competitive and cooperative interactions among thalamic neurons. As we discuss later, input from each eye is necessary for the differentiation of ocular dominance columns in the primary visual area of the neocortex. In both cases, a new structure (eye-specific layers or columns) arises because of competitive and collaborative interactions between neurons from each eye.

As can be seen in Table 3.1, several examples of less prevalent cases of atypical development are caused by disruptions of particular stages of brain development. Examples of some of the etiologies of each pathology are given, with genes listed first and environmental risk factors listed second. We now discuss these examples in order. In the first stage of brain development, called *embryogenesis*, the neural tube forms (called *neurulation*). Occasionally the neural tube fails to close completely, leading to neural tube defects such as spina bifida. There are both genetic (e.g., a mutation in the *VANGL1* gene) and environmental (e.g., folic acid deficiency in the mother's diet in pregnancy) causes of neural tube defects. Once the neural tube is formed, the next main stage of brain development is *cytogenesis*, in which billions of neurons and glial cells are generated. Disruptions of the first substage of cytogenesis, called *neuronal proliferation*, can result in too few neuroblasts being formed, resulting in a brain that is *microcephalic* (smaller than normal), or in the worst case, *anencephalic* (largely absent). Mutations in two important genes, *ASPM* and *MCPH1*, that influence brain size by influencing neuronal proliferation, have been identified as etiologies of microcephaly. As we discuss later, microcephaly is also found in genetic syndromes such as Down syndrome and Williams syndrome. On the environmental side, prenatal infections (e.g., Zika virus or cytomegalovirus) or radiation exposure in early pregnancy can also cause microcephaly.

The next substage of brain development is neuronal migration. After being formed in the germinal matrix close to the ventricles, neuroblasts need to transport themselves (migrate) to their appropriate location in the brain. Both gross and subtle changes in brain development can be caused by disruptions of neuronal migration. For instance, *lissencephaly* (smooth brain) is a severe brain defect caused by an extensive failure neuronal migration that results in intellectual disability. More subtle migrational failures are found in *periventricular nodular heterotopia* (PNH). In PNH, some neurons fail to migrate to the neocortex (i.e., ectopic neurons) and stop instead in the white matter adjacent to the lateral ventricles. In PNH, these

TABLE 3.1. Summary of Brain Development

Stage	When	What happens	Pathology	Some etiologies
Prenatal				
I. Embryogenesis	3–5 weeks	Neural tube forms	Spina bifida	VANGL1; lack of folic acid
II. Cytogenesis				
A. Proliferation	1–6 months	Overproduce neurons and glia	Microcephaly	ASPM, MCPH1; cytomegalovirus, Zika virus, radiation
B. Migration	2–6 months	Cells travel to "home"	Lissencephaly, periventricular nodular heterotopia (PNH), dyslexia	RELN; viral infection; FLNA; KIAA0319
III. Growth and differentiation				
A. Axonal formation and guidance	3–7 months	Axons find targets	Agenesis of corpus callosum	Multifactorial
B. Dendrite formation and early synaptogenesis	4–9 months	Early networks	—	—
Postnatal				
C. Experience-expectant synaptogenesis	Birth–2 years, 5 years	Overproduce synapses	Rett syndrome	MECP2
D. Experience-dependent synaptogenesis	Lifelong	Learning	Anti-N-methyl-D-aspartate (NMDA) receptor encephalitis	Ovarian teratoma (Dalmau et al., 2007)
E. Myelination	Lifelong	Insulate axons	Leukodystrophy, demyelination	Krabbe disease (GALC); inhalant abuse (Filley, Heaton, & Rosenberg, 1990)

Note. Key to gene names: *VANGL1* (1p13.1), *VANG-LIKE 1*, codes for a planar cell polarity protein 1 (Kibar et al., 2007); *ASPM* (1q31), abnormal spindle-like microcephaly associated (Pattison et al., 2000); *MCPH1* (8p23.1), microcephalin 1 (Jackson et al., 2002); *RELN* (7q22), reelin (Hong et al., 2000); *FLNA* (X_q28), filamin A (Chang et al., 2005; Fox et al., 1998); *KIAA0319* (6p22.2)(Cope et al., 2005; Paracchini et al., 2006); *MECP2* (Xq28), methyl-CpG-binding protein 2 (Amir et al., 1999); *GALC* (14q31), galactocerebrocidase (Cannizzaro, Chen, Rafi, & Wenger, 1994).

ectopias can be seen on a structural magnetic resonance imaging (MRI) scan, which is otherwise normal. Patients with PNH are at increased risk for adolescent-onset seizures and developmental dyslexia, but are otherwise behaviorally normal (Chang et al., 2005). Interestingly, idiopathic developmental dyslexia may also be caused by subtle, localized variations in neuronal migration, as we discuss later in Chapter 10.

In the next stage of brain development, growth and development, immature neurons need to form axonal and early dendritic connections with other neurons. New axons from migrated neurons sometimes travel long distances to reach targets in the other hemisphere (thus passing through the *corpus callosum*, the white matter fiber bundle connecting the two halves of the brain) or in the same hemisphere (e.g., axonal connections from posterior cortex to prefrontal cortex [PFC]). To achieve their correct destination, complicated molecular mechanisms of axon guidance are needed. A classic example of a pathology of axon guidance is agenesis of the corpus callosum, in which a child is born without a corpus callosum, either completely or partially.

Most of synaptogenesis (substages III-C and III-D) occurs postnatally, first in an experience-expectant and then in an experience-dependent fashion (Greenough, Black, & Wallace, 1987). In experience-expectant synaptogenesis, which occurs in the first few years of postnatal life, the brain produces excess synapses, which are pruned by species-typical, universal experience, to form functional circuits for species-typical behaviors, including *stereopsis* (depth perception), language, social cognition, and executive functions. Pruning leads to grey matter thinning and strengthens local networks.

In experience-dependent synaptogenesis, which occurs throughout the lifespan, we find a brain mechanism for individual differences. Now the relevant experiences are not universal but can vary across individuals. These experiences lead to the formation of new synapses and the pruning of old ones, and are the main mechanism of learning across the lifespan.

Atypical cognitive development may be caused by the alterations in synaptogenesis. Both fragile X syndrome and Rett syndrome are due to single gene mutations that disrupt early synaptogenesis. Some of the candidate genes for autism spectrum disorder also disrupt early synapse formation.

The final process of brain development in Table 3.1 is *myelination*, in which axons are wrapped in a myelin sheath. Myelination of axonal connections within and between local networks contributes to the differentiation and integration of cognitive development. Early demyelination is produced by some genetic syndromes, called *leukodystrophies*, resulting in severe disruptions of motor and cognitive development. An environmental risk factor, inhalant abuse, can result in later demyelination and resulting cognitive deficits.

Although we can trace some forms of atypical development to problems at different stages of early brain development, for many others we do not know when and where early brain development goes awry. The brain necessarily changes in a lifelong way as cognitive development (and devolution) proceeds, and three important mechanisms of later cognitive development are (1) synaptic pruning in interaction with environmental inputs, (2) protracted myelination, and (3) experience-dependent synaptogenesis. This means that examining the changes in brain connectivity that result from these processes will be also important for understanding much of cognitive development. As an example of a later change in brain development that contributes to a neurodevelopmental disorder is the recent discovery that mutations in an immune system gene, *C4A*, contribute to the development of schizophrenia (Sekar et al., 2016). The immune system, including *C4A*, is involved in pruning excess synaptic connections in the brain, in this case in the prefrontal cortex, which is still being pruned in adolescence. Mutations in the *C4A* gene in schizophrenia lead to overpruning in the PFC, a fact that helps explain the late onset of schizophrenia.

CONNECTIVITY ANALYSES

In recent decades, noninvasive methods have been developed to measure structural and functional connectivity in humans, and these methods have provided a new window on typical and atypical cognitive development. Structural connectivity refers to white matter tracts in the brain. These tracts can be measured and reconstructed from a structural MRI scan with a method called *diffusion tensor imaging* (DTI). The Human Connectome Project, a database of DTI results from many studies, allows researchers to generate connectivity maps in typical humans at different ages and in some disorders. *Functional connectivity* refers to patterns of coactivation of voxels in a functional MRI (fMRI) scan. Graph analysis (Sporns & Zwi, 2004) is a useful method for analyzing network structure in both structural and functional connectivity data. In this method, nodes and their connections and connection strength are identified in the data, and an overall brain network is constructed. Several summary statistics can be calculated that quantify network properties, such as the degree of local and global organization.

A basic finding is that human brain networks have a *small-world pattern* of organization, in which small local networks are connected by longer pathways (e.g., between local networks in the posterior cortex and the PFC). Connectivity patterns change with development, are correlated with individual differences in IQ, and differ in some disorders, such as autism (Rippon, Brock, Brown, & Boucher, 2007) and schizophrenia (Van Den Heuvel, Stam, Kahn, & Hulshoff Pol, 2009).

These approaches for studying the development of brain connectivity hold great promise for extending our understanding of brain–behavior relations across the lifespan. For instance, we now know that the longitudinal growth curves for neocortical grey matter and underlying white matter have different slopes and shapes. Frontal and parietal grey matter increases postnatally until around age 12, then decreases because of synaptic pruning. In contrast, white matter volume increases linearly throughout postnatal development until around age 22 or so (Giedd, Shaw, Wallace, Gogtay, & Lenroot, 2006), and there is continued myelination in some fiber pathways throughout adulthood. As discussed earlier, there are individual differences in these trajectories for grey and white matter that relate to individual differences in IQ (Shaw, Greenstein, et al., 2006) and to specific developmental disorders, such as attention-deficit/hyperactivity disorder (ADHD; Shaw et al., 2007).

Patterns of functional connectivity also change with development. These patterns of functional connectivity can be measured by taking activity levels of individual voxels in the brain as inputs, then modeling the correlations among individual voxels and clusters of voxels using graph analysis. The resulting structure of functional connectivity, like structural connectivity, also has a characteristic "small-world" organization, which means that it has many small, richly interconnected local networks and a few long-distance connections between local networks. Such long-distance connections include those between posterior local networks (in the occipital, parietal, and temporal lobes) and anterior local networks in the PFC, as well as interhemispheric connections that pass through the corpus callosum. Development of functional connectivity in childhood and adolescence is characterized by initial development of local networks and slower development of long-distance connections. Using this method, Dosenbach et al. (2010) and T. Brown et al. (2012) were able to reliably predict the chronological age of individual participants using fMRI data. So we now have global metrics of both developmental and individual differences in brain connectivity, and these metrics are being applied to explaining both developmental and individual differences in cognition.

THREE MODELS OF BRAIN–BEHAVIOR DEVELOPMENT

Now that we have reviewed these well-established facts of brain development, we can evaluate three competing theories proposed by psychologists of how cognitive development relates to brain development. These competing theories recapitulate the nativism versus empiricism, or nature–nurture, debate at the level of brain development. As we saw in the chapter on etiology, extreme positions on both sides of this debate proved to be wrong. So the same is very likely to be true with respect to brain development. Brain development is not completely determined by the genome (which is the nativist or nature position) or by the environment (which is the empiricist or nurture position), but by the interplay of the two.

A key theoretical model in this field, interactive specialization (IS), is described in Johnson and de Haan (2011). The IS model contrasts with two competing models, a maturational model (i.e., the nature side of debate) and a skill learning model (i.e., the nurture side of the debate). The maturational and skill learning models correspond respectively to the traditional nativist and empiricist theories of cognitive development, whereas the IS model corresponds to the constructivist model, which was developed by Piaget (1952) to provide a resolution to the competing nativist and empiricist theories of the origins of ideas or concepts. The IS model rejects these deterministic models of brain development and instead posits that brain development proceeds in a probabilistic and emergent fashion.

At the neural level, it is important to be clear about the constraints shared and not shared by all three theories. All three theories have to agree that there are innate neural structures and that there is some prenatal learning, as well as extensive postnatal learning, simply because such structures and learning are well-established empirical findings. All three theories agree that infants have to learn a *particular* language and a *particular* number system, and form representations of *particular* faces, among other things. The three theories disagree on whether deeper levels of processing necessary for *all* languages (e.g., syntactic structures), *all* number systems (number sense or the mental number line), or *all* faces (configurational processing) must be innate because they are unlearnable, or whether they could be acquired in the process of learning. So, in maturational theory, postnatal learning merely fine-tunes innate cognitive representations, whereas in the other two theories, innate cognitive representations are rejected, and their formation must rely instead on postnatal learning. At the end of this section, we examine the constraints posed for all three models by known limits on brain plasticity.

The maturational model assumes *deterministic epigenesis* (the notion that development follows fixed paths that are largely predetermined by biology), and posits that neocortical specializations are evolved and innate. Functions appear in development as the relevant brain areas mature, with some expected environmental input. For example, the maturational model holds that typical humans have an innate brain region for recognizing faces, the fusiform face area (FFA), which matures early in development (e.g., Kanwisher, 2010).

In the skill learning model (Gauthier, Tarr, Anderson, Skudlarski, & Gore, 1999), there are brain regions that are somewhat specialized for a broad class of skill because of their input and output connections, but the particular skill acquired depends crucially on the individual's learning history. For example, the entire fusiform area is part of the ventral visual pathway in the brain that is specialized for visual object recognition, because it is more connected to foveal input from the retina than the dorsal visual pathway (which has more parafoveal connections from the retina). The skill learning model holds that the specializations that develop within the fusiform area are solely a function of the learning history of the individual, even in adulthood. Humans typically develop an FFA because of massive practice looking at human faces, but with similar training, adults can develop similar specializations for other visual objects, whether familiar objects such as sheep or cars, or invented ones for which experience can be controlled experimentally. Gauthier et al. (1999) developed a set of imaginary creatures, called "greebles," which differed in their physical features but lacked facial features. Recognizing individual greebles poses a challenge similar to recognizing individual human faces, but it cannot depend on innate face processing. Increased experience with greebles led to better recognition, and associated with this expertise was increased activation in the fusiform "face area." Thus, this study provided strong evidence against the nativist claim that the FFA is innately programmed to respond only to human faces.

Now, we compare and contrast these three models of brain–behavior development in more detail. One way in which they differ concerns assumptions about brain plasticity. At the outset, it is important to consider two meanings of the term *plasticity* in the field. The first meaning refers to normal changes in the number, development, and connections among neurons, all of which are important for behavioral development. A subset of these normal neuronal changes underlies postnatal learning, which is assumed by all competing theories of brain–behavior development discussed earlier. The second meaning refers to the ability of the brain to compensate for pathological influences, whether they are due to genetic variations, atypical environmental influences, or outright damage. The three theoretical models take different stands on the relation between these two kinds of plasticity.

The IS model takes plasticity as a key premise and assumes that the same brain mechanisms underlie both developmental and lesion-induced plasticity. The skills learning model also assumes shared mechanisms for the two types of plasticity but differs from the IS model with respect to how previous learning affects the scope of later plasticity (i.e., whether there are sensitive periods for plasticity). In the IS model, there are sensitive periods, because previous learning leads to what is called "entrenchment" of representations, which limits later plasticity, whereas the skill learning model assumes fewer limits on adult plasticity. *Entrenchment* simply means that as a neural network tunes its synapses to learn a particular content (e.g., a spoken language), it becomes harder to learn new contents (e.g., a second language), because the synapses in the networks have stabilized their weights for the first content (i.e., the flat, asymptotic final portion of the learning curve). Of course, humans exhibit more plasticity for some contents (e.g., individual faces) than others (e.g., spoken languages), but even in the domain of faces, entrenchment occurs, as demonstrated by the problem posed by cross-racial face recognition. If we are mainly exposed to one race or ethnic group when we are developing face recognition, we will find it harder to distinguish individual faces of people from different racial or ethnic groups. The concept of entrenchment is similar to the concept of "restriction of fate" in embryology: Embryonic stem cells can become part of any organ in the body, but their fate becomes increasingly restricted as the embryo differentiates.

Only the maturational model holds that the two kinds of plasticity have distinct mechanisms: a specialized mechanism that acts after acquired brain injury, and another mechanism for the learning required to tune innate brain specializations. One can readily see that these theories make competing predictions about the ability of the developing brain to acquire concepts after early focal brain lesions, which is discussed in more detail in the next section. For instance, if the brain has innately localized modules that are specialized for number sense, syntax, or faces, as has been claimed by maturational theorists such as Feigenson, Dehaene, and Spelke (2004), Kanwisher (2010), and Pinker (1994), then early damage to those brain locations should gravely impair the development of those specific domains of cognition. In contrast, the other two theories would predict that plasticity permits each of these cognitive domains to develop in other brain regions after early brain damage. The IS and skill learning theories differ on how much the age of injury affects the degree of recovery, with the IS theory holding that plasticity in the face of injury declines with age simply because other brain regions are already entrenched or committed to other functions.

How do each of the three models explain localization of function in the adult human neocortex? As already explained, the maturational model holds that these localizations are innately specified and the skill learning model holds they derive from experience. As we have already discussed, neither of these positions is truly developmental, so it is unsurprising that neither fully accounts for mammalian brain development. Instead, recent evidence demonstrates that the division of the cortex into distinct processing regions emerges from a complex interplay between intrinsic and extrinsic mechanisms (Sur & Rubenstein, 2005).

The constructivist IS model is consistent with Sur and Rubenstein (2005) in that it holds that localizations emerge. In the IS view, localized functions found in the typical adult brain arise from a developmental process in which interactions and competition among connected neocortical regions lead to increases in the specialization of the computations performed by a particular region. Hence, the specialization of a given neocortical region is not fixed in advance by the genome and prenatal brain development, but instead depends mainly on this postnatal developmental process. This developmental process depends in turn on the environmental inputs available to the developing brain, and relies on both experience-expectant and experience-dependent synaptogenesis (Greenough et al., 1987). Environmental inputs strengthen some synapses (or create new ones) and eliminate others, thus allowing neural networks to learn the regularities that exist in different domains of the environment. Specialization arises because of competitive interactions (involving in some cases both local excitation and more distant inhibition, as occurs in the formation of ocular dominance columns). Thus, neocortical specializations emerge through a self-organizing process.

Of course, if every part of neocortex were equally able to process every kind of information, functional brain architecture would vary considerably across individuals based on their different learning histories (even though there is much more individual variability than the standard brain maps imply). To avoid complete equipotentiality of neocortex, the IS theory needs some innate constraints. Indeed, different neocortical regions already have different genetically influenced inputs and outputs at birth. The eyes are connected to occipital cortex, the ears are connected to temporal cortex, and so on, although these connections continue to develop after birth.

If sensory inputs are missing in early development, then neocortical specializations can change dramatically, which contradicts the maturational model. Congenital deafness leads to a drastic remapping of visual functions onto auditory cortex (Bavelier & Neville, 2002). In congenital blindness, another dramatic remapping occurs: Language functions are mapped onto visual cortex (Bedny & Saxe, 2012). These are both examples of plasticity, and each requires that there typically be cross-modal connections between sensory visual inputs and auditory cortex, and vice versa, allowing the nature of the input to determine postnatally a different specialization of a posterior neocortical region. Both of these examples are consistent with the IS and skill learning models but are very problematic for a maturational model, in which the specialization of visual or auditory cortex is determined prenatally, and experience only acts to allow that region to mature.

The IS model also depends on some biases to explain why some specializations are universally human (language and faces) and others are not (calendrical calculation), even though all can be learned by human children. Edelman (1987) found in simulating neonatal brain development that his model would not work unless it had some innate valences or preferences, so it may be that innate subcortical motivational structures in the brain, discussed below, are important inputs to neocortical development. Early or innate attentional biases explain why human neonates focus more on some parts of the environmental input (e.g., human faces and human speech) and less on others. We know from children with autism that the *absence* of these attentional biases for social stimuli can lead to very different and unusual specializations, or savant skills, not all of which could possibly be innate. For instance, why does a Colorado child with autism, who lived in the mountains, become an expert on varieties of ski lifts, whereas another Colorado child from the Front Range becomes an expert on the trees found in the Front Range but not in the mountains?

The IS model thus depends on brain plasticity, especially during early development. In the IS model, plasticity of a given neocortical region *decreases* as development proceeds, which is called *entrenchment*, as explained earlier. As that region becomes increasingly committed through learning to computing a particular set of input–output mappings, it becomes less able to learn a different set of such mappings. So, for instance, decreased ability for second language learning with age is not explained by an external cause, like the closing of a maturational "window," as it would be explained in a maturational theory, but simply by the specialization that has already developed.

Finally, the IS model also critically depends on the *principle of probabilistic epigenesis* formulated by Gottlieb (1991), in which two-way interactions among genes, brain, and behavior lead to emergent functional properties in development. Probabilistic epigenesis contrasts with *deterministic epigenesis*, in which the direction of causality is unidirectional from genes to brain to behavior, and functional specializations of neocortical regions are largely predetermined or innate.

One could ask why these three models are important for research on atypical cognitive development. They are important because they make fundamentally different predictions about why and how neurodevelopmental disorders happen. So, here is a clear case of the reciprocal relation between research on typical and atypical development. Each neurodevelopmental disorder is a test case for each of these three theories of typical functional brain development. If the maturational theory is true, then the brain structure needed for a particular aspect of cognition, such as syntax or face processing, should already be different at birth, and that specific function should be *selectively* deficient once the child reaches the age when that function typically matures. From then on, development in that domain remains selectively impaired. So phenotypic development will be homotypic (i.e., the same cognitive deficits are persistent across development). If the IS theory is true, then the mapping between brain structure differences and functional deficits will be less transparent, and phenotypic development may be heterotypic: Different cognitive deficits will be apparent at different ages. It is less clear how the skills learning theory would explain a neurodevelopmental disorder caused by an inherited brain difference, but it could certainly be relevant for explaining an environmentally caused cognitive disorder. It would explain such a disorder as resulting from deprivation of the necessary experience. If disorders are examined only in later childhood or adulthood, it is more difficult to distinguish among these models, as Karmiloff-Smith and Thomas (2003) and others have made clear. That is because the three theories may predict similar outcomes in later development but differ in their early predictions. So, to use neurodevelopmental disorders to test these three competing theories, we have to study the early development of children with these disorders.

Brain Plasticity Following Acquired Lesions

As discussed earlier, recent findings about human brain plasticity provide a test of these three models, and we now evaluate each model with these recent findings. The discovery of considerable brain plasticity in both animals and humans (see Stiles, Reilly, Levine, & Trauner, 2012, for a review) was a major breakthrough in the field of neuroscience and has had a considerable impact on the emerging field of developmental cognitive neuroscience.

How are these three models (i.e., IS, maturational, and skill learning) of functional development of the human brain constrained by *limits* on its plasticity? This issue is particularly important for atypical cognitive development, because it is well known that plasticity does not compensate for all perturbations in early brain development. Otherwise, we would not be writing this book!

How the developing brain fares in the face of early damage depends on numerous factors, including the extent, timing, location of the lesion, and the particular functional outcome (e.g., language vs. spatial cognition). Easy generalizations about the *timing* of brain lesions are too simple. One of these is mislabeled the Kennard (1936) principle, which holds that earlier lesions produce less serious functional effects than later ones, because the younger brain is more plastic. Another such simple generalization is the opposite of the Kennard principle, namely, the early vulnerability hypothesis (Hebb, 1949), which holds that earlier lesions produce more serious functional consequences, because there is less normal brain to develop. Incidentally, the so-called "Kennard principle" is "neither Kennard's nor a principle" (Dennis, 2010). This is because Margaret A. Kennard, an early pioneer in developmental neuroscience who anticipated many more recent findings, had a much more nuanced view of the effects of early lesions, and the simplistic principle is incorrectly attributed to her. We have since learned that for global intellectual outcomes (i.e., psychometric IQ and academic skills), focal lesions acquired before age 2 years produce worse deficits than later lesions, consistent with the early vulnerability hypothesis and contrary to the Kennard principle. For more specific cognitive outcomes, the story is more complicated, as we discuss below.

What else has been learned since Kennard's time about the effects of early lesions on cognitive development? Although there is still much to be understood, here is a list of generalizations that reflect current evidence:

1. *Mechanisms.* There are multiple neural mechanisms of plasticity following a lesion, including unmasking of function in adjacent cortex, sprouting of new axonal and dendritic connections, and actual formation of new neurons, called neurogenesis (Galaburda & Pascual-Leone, 2003).
2. *Extent.* The functional effects of early bilateral or diffuse lesions are worse than the effects of focal lesions (Stiles et al., 2012).
3. *Loss of cognitive reserve.* Early lesions make the individual more vulnerable to later brain injury or disease.

The last generalization reflects the fact that any loss of brain tissue affects the later adaptability of the brain. For instance, earlier severe traumatic brain injuries are known to increase the risk for the later onset of Alzheimer's dementia, because there is less healthy brain tissue remaining to compensate (Van Den Heuvel, Thornton, & Vink, 2007).

The role of *lesion location* merits a longer discussion because of the challenges it poses for the IS model. As stated earlier, the IS model is proposed for neocortical functions, and it is evident that plasticity is greatest in the neocortex, which in humans supports extensive learning through cultural transmission. The neocortex needs to be plastic because human children live in many different environments and in many different cultures, despite being one species with one evolved brain. We know this must be the case, because human children can develop quite normally when adopted from one culture into another.

But the existing evidence does not support equal plasticity across the whole neocortex or across all cortically mediated functions, which poses a potential challenge for the IS model. Early focal lesions to the primary motor and somatosensory areas cause lasting functional deficits, partly because the axonal connections of these areas myelinate early (Stiles et al., 2012). Instead, the IS model appears to hold best for language development, which relies on the integrated function of multiple secondary and tertiary cortical regions in both hemispheres (Stiles et al., 2012).

In contrast, the IS model seems less valid for the PFC, which has a unique function based on its extensive connectivity with all the rest of the brain, and a distinct form of neurocomputation (active maintenance of limited amounts of information). So, the PFC is an important and unique convergence zone in the brain, and it follows that it may be difficult, if not impossible, to transfer its functions to some other neocortical region. The results of acquired lesions to the PFC in adults and children are consistent with this view because there is less recovery of function from PFC lesions than from other neocortical lesions (Grattan & Eslinger, 1991). Echoing Kennard's (1936) pioneering conclusions, however, functional recovery of prefrontal lesions in both animals and humans is influenced by multiple factors, including age at injury, age at assessment, lesion size, sex, and nature of the behavioral assessment (Kolb, Gibb, & Gorny, 2000). Indeed, as first discovered by Kennard (1936), the full effects of early frontal lesions in children and monkeys may not be evident until later in development, when these individuals "grow into deficit" (Dennis, 2010; Grattan & Eslinger, 1991). This "sleeper" effect demonstrates that both age at injury and time since injury are important developmental factors that must be separately considered, though in practice, they are often difficult to disentangle. Furthermore, the relation between age and injury and extent of recovery for PFC lesions is nonlinear. In humans, the poorest outcomes for such lesions are tied to prenatal insults; these children show global cognitive and IQ decrements, as well as poor performance on more specific frontal tasks (i.e., executive function [EF] measures). The best outcomes, at least for most laboratory-based EF tasks, appear to be for PFC lesions sustained in middle childhood. Lesions acquired at age 10 years or older tend to produce an adult-like profile, with a relatively (though not completely) specific deficit pattern (Jacobs, Harvey, & Anderson, 2007). This phenomenon likely relates to the developmental timing of various processes, including neurogenesis and synaptogenesis. Although we have a relatively well-developed theory of how the neuronal-level changes map onto behaviorally observed "critical periods" for functional recovery in rats (Kolb et al., 2000), the connections across these levels of analysis are currently less clear for humans (Jacobs et al., 2007).

A second challenge for the IS model is that cortical structures outside the six-layered neocortex proper (i.e., isocortex) show markedly less functional plasticity in the face of early lesions than does the neocortex itself. Such structures include the simplest type of cortex, corticoid cortex (in which there is a mix of cortical and nuclear features), and the more layered allocortex (Mesulam, 1997). The amygdala is one example of corticoid cortex, and the hippocampus is an example of allocortex. Both are convergence zones, as is the PFC. The amygdala integrates higher and lower inputs important for emotional and autonomic functions. Early amygdala lesions in both monkeys (reviewed in Stiles et al., 2012) and humans (Adolphs, 2003) produce lasting deficits. The hippocampus integrates inputs from multiple neocortical sites and from motivational structures such as the amygdala to form new episodic memories. Again, acquired lesions in the hippocampal formation in both young monkeys (Bachevalier, 2008) and human children (Vargha-Khadem et al., 1997) lead to lasting deficits in the ability to form new episodic memories, just as they do in adults (Squire, 1987). In both cases, age at lesion (childhood vs. adult) results in some differences in the profile of deficits, but the important point here is other structures cannot take on the functions served by the amygdala and hippocampus.

Turning to subcortical structures, there is even less evidence for plasticity, again because the relevant structures have fairly unique connectivity. The basal ganglia do not recover function after early lesions. This fact is relevant for the procedural learning deficit hypothesis of some learning disorders, such as language impairment (LI) and dyslexia. The hypothalamus is the central portion of the autonomic nervous system, which is an important part of the peripheral nervous system. Similar to the amygdala, lesions to the hypothalamus have lasting and sometimes devastating effects.

In summary, because the brain added layers in its evolution, we may need different answers to which of these three models (IS, maturational, and skill learning) best describe functional brain development for different layers of the brain. It is clear that the IS model has the strongest support for a number of neocortical functions, including language. In contrast, some human brain functions are undoubtedly innate (i.e., present at birth or before) and not very plastic in the face of injury, such as many of the functions mediated by the autonomic nervous system, or those mediated by the amygdala. So a maturational model might best describe functional development for these brain structures. It is less clear whether the skill learning model is the best fit for some other functions.

What can we extrapolate from the developmental effects of early acquired brain lesions to possible brain mechanisms for idiopathic neurodevelopmental disorders? First, because of plasticity of neocortex, focal congenital changes in neocortical grey matter associated with high levels of plasticity (e.g., unilateral posterior lesions) are unlikely to lead to a lasting disorder with a relatively specific neuropsychological profile. Second, widespread changes in the number of neurons or in white matter will lead to lasting (relatively global) deficits, as is demonstrated in cases of microcephaly, macrocephaly, and congenital white matter disorders (leukodystrophies). Third, an early change in the mechanisms of brain plasticity themselves, such as the mechanisms of synaptic stabilization and pruning, should also produce global deficits. Fragile X (discussed later) and Rett syndrome provide demonstrations of this principle. Fourth, neurotransmitter depletion or excess should also have lasting consequences, as in the case of early-treated phenylketonuria (PKU) and more subtly in ADHD. Fifth, given the previously discussed importance of the development of structural (white matter) and functional connectivity for the development of intelligence, alterations in the development of this connectivity should have lasting consequences for behavioral development. Such alterations in connectivity have been demonstrated in schizophrenia (Van Den Heuvel et al., 2009) and autism (Piven, 2001). Sixth, and finally, anything that changes basic learning mechanisms, such as statistical learning mediated by the basal ganglia, should have lasting effects. As we have seen, plasticity is limited for early basal ganglia lesions.

INTEGRATING BRAIN AND COGNITIVE DEVELOPMENT

The model embraced here also depends on a connectionist view of how the brain learns and processes information (O'Reilly & Munakata, 2000). *Connectionist models* are computer programs that simulate learning and cognitive processing with layers of neuron-like elements that have adjustable connections between elements. Each learning trial adjusts the connections according to a learning rule. O'Reilly and Munakata (2000) identified three different kinds of processing performed by the real neural networks in the human brain and have simulated each kind of processing with computational neural networks. These three kinds of processing are (1) the slow learning of overlapping distributed representations of the environment performed by the posterior cortex, (2) active maintenance by the PFC of limited amounts of information over short time intervals to enable problem solving, and (3) rapid acquisition of unique conjunctions of novel information by the hippocampus and related structures. The first kind of processing corresponds to semantic memory, the second corresponds to working memory, and the last, to episodic memory. In later work, O'Reilly and colleagues (Frank, Seeberger, & O'Reilly, 2004) simulated a fourth kind of processing, procedural memory, which is mediated by the basal ganglia. Although these four kinds of processing have been simulated separately, in a real brain, they must interact. In what follows, we provide an account of that interaction.

How can we combine this connectionist view with other ideas presented in this chapter to sketch out a theory of how brain and cognition might codevelop? To do this we need the additional concepts of (1) novelty and relevance detection, (2) the transition from effortful to automatic processing, and (3) the hierarchical nature of cognitive skills and representations. Learners at all ages, from infancy to old age, first need to select which new things to learn, then transition from effortful to automatic processing of the new content or skill, and finally use this new knowledge to facilitate processing and learning at the next level of the knowledge or skill hierarchy.

To explain this developmental process, consider what happens when a child learns a new spoken or written word. First of all, the child has to detect that the new word is both novel and relevant (i.e., worth learning); that is, the new word has to fall into what Vygotsy (1979) called the child's "zone of proximal development." For the child learning to speak, that means he or she already has a prelinguistic semantic representation for what the new word means, and that concept has to be important enough to the child to make it worth learning. For the child learning to read a new word, a similar process needs to occur; that is, the new written word is either already part of the child's spoken vocabulary or has a meaning that is already present in the child's semantic system *and* crosses the relevance threshold. Otherwise, the new word will be ignored or just assimilated into the child's existing vocabulary.

A new word that passes this initial test will become the focus of attention and effortful processing. The child will repeat the new spoken word to him- or herself or practice reading the new written word. The child will also be primed to notice the new word subsequently, so that it will seem to occur frequently after it is first encountered. In this model, both the frontal lobes and the salience system interact to facilitate effortful processing of the new word. Eventually, processing of the new word will become automatic and be incorporated into the existing lexicon, which is diffusely represented in other parts of the brain, including posterior neocortex.

For newly automated skills and procedures, subcortical structures such as the basal ganglia and cerebellum are involved. So, once the executive system masters a new skill or knowledge, it "delegates" it to other brain systems that do not require effortful processing. This transition is also called the *transition from reflective to reflexive processing,* or *from declarative to procedural memory,* and frees up the limited capacity of the executive system for new tasks.

The newly acquired knowledge or skill is incorporated into the hierarchical structure of prior knowledge and skills, thus permitting the learner to take on the next task in the sequence of development. The concept of resource allocation is relevant here. If a child cannot automatically process the words in a spoken or written discourse, he or she will have fewer cognitive resources left for the task of comprehending the discourse. Similarly, if a child cannot automatically process grammatical relation in a discourse, he or she will also have trouble comprehending it. Or if the child has not automated a basic motor skill, he or she will have trouble executing a sequence of movements that includes that basic motor skill.

We can relate this developmental process of learning something new to three previously discussed aspects of brain development: (1) the interactive specialization model, (2) the emergence of functional networks, and (3) developmental changes in grey and white matter. The interactive specialization model holds that when the brain is learning something new, more of the brain will be activated, including the frontal lobes. Incidentally, this would explain an apparent paradox in the fMRI literature, namely, why better behavioral performance on a task is sometimes associated with *less* brain activity on an fMRI scan of the whole brain. If the task is less automatic for some participants than for others, it will result in more widespread activation in those participants. Conversely, if the region of interest (ROI) in the fMRI scan is a part of neocortex becoming specialized for a given knowledge representation (e.g., written words or faces), then participants with less well-developed representations will have *less* activity in that ROI.

Regarding functional networks, their small world hubs would become specialized for automated representations of knowledge and skills, and the long-distance connections would correspond to white matter tracts connecting those hubs. As a given hub develops its representations under the influence of environmental input, it would prune it connections, leading to thinning of the neocortex. As it develops its long-distance connections, myelination of those connections will increase, resulting in increases in white matter with age.

The foregoing accounts predicts that each learning disorder described in this book will have both localized and distributed features of its neuroimaging phenotype, and that many of the localized features, but perhaps not all, will be a product of development rather than an innate difference. Table 3.2 provides a summary of localized and distributed neuroimaging features for the learning disorders described in this book. As can be seen, these disorders have both specific and shared neuroimaging features. Clearly the specific alteration in the activity of the fusiform word area in dyslexia is a product of development, since this specialization emerges with reading acquisition in typical readers. Other, earlier developing neuroimaging features of dyslexia, such as disruption of left-hemisphere white matter tract, may somehow lead to the fusiform phenotype found in dyslexia. Likewise, number-sensitive processing in the left inferior parietal sulcus (LIPS) is a product of development, and this neuroimaging difference in math disability (MD) is the product of a developmental process. In contrast, the imbalance in synaptic homeostasis found in intellectual disability (ID) likely emerges much earlier in development and results in both structural and functional differences in the hippocampus in ID syndromes. In summary, the neuroimaging phenotypes of learning disorders are obviously not static, but instead change with development. Much remains to be learned about the causal relations between earlier and later brain changes in these disorders.

SUMMARY

What have we learned in this chapter about how etiologies act on brain development, and how malleable developmental outcome are? We have seen that there are specific genes influencing different stages of early brain development, such as neurulation (formation of the neuronal tube), proliferation and migration of neurons, and experience-dependent synaptogenesis. Mutations in these genes can lead to major neurodevelopmental disorders such as spina bifida, microcephaly, lissencephaly, and Rett syndrome. In contrast, changes in the expression levels of these genes, produced by mutations outside of their coding regions (called *exons*), can produce more subtle neurodevelopmental disorders, such as dyslexia.

But even in fetal life, genes are not the only factors shaping brain development. The activity of neurons is also important in prenatal brain development (Shatz, 1992), and the mother's nutrition and stress levels can produce fairly permanent epigenetic changes in gene expression in the fetus, so brain development is interactive and fits the principle of probabilistic epigenesis. As described, postnatal

TABLE 3.2. Key Neuroimaging Phenotypes of Learning Disorders

Disorder	Localized	Distributed
Dyslexia	Fusiform word area	Left-hemisphere WM tracts
ADHD	RIFG, frontal–striatal	Abnormal interaction between executive, default, and salience networks
LI	LIFG?	Language networks
MD	LIPS	Salience and executive networks
DCD	Parietal, cerebellum	?
SSD	Speech circuit?	?
ASD	Medial PFC	Network connectivity
ID	Hippocampus	Microcephaly, macrocephaly, PFC

Note. ASD, autism spectrum disorder; DCD, developmental coordination disorder; WM, white matter; RIFG, right inferior frontal gyrus; LIFG, left inferior frontal gyrus; LIPS, left inferior parietal sulcus; PFC, prefrontal cortex.

experience interacts with synaptogenesis and synaptic pruning to partly shape both typical and atypical cognitive development. Different neocortical regions have different timetables for the peak of early synaptogenesis and subsequent pruning, with PFC having the latest peak and most protracted period of pruning, whereas posterior cortical areas reach their peaks and stabilize their synaptic number earlier (Huttenlocher & Dabholchar, 1997). These different timetables map roughly onto different stages of cognitive development and are also consistent with developmental changes in patterns of structural and functional connectivity, which have been demonstrated to relate to typical and atypical cognitive development, as discussed earlier. There are likely many currently unknown genes that contribute to these processes in interaction with various environmental influences, so much remains to be discovered.

With regard to the fundamental issue of nativism versus empiricism or nature versus nurture, what we know about brain–behavior development challenges both nativism and empiricism. The interactive specialization model fits existing data best, but not perfectly, because plasticity varies across different brain regions. Early hippocampal or prefrontal lesions have lasting effects, as do subcortical lesions to the basal ganglia, amygdala, and hypothalamus. So some parts of the brain may fit a maturational or nativist model better than either the interactive specialization or skill learning models. In contrast, the dramatic examples of neocortical plasticity strongly contradict the maturational model. Finally, much of brain–behavior development is malleable, because much of the neocortex has considerable plasticity, but there are definite limits to this plasticity.

CHAPTER 4

Neuropsychological Constructs

We come now to neuropsychology, which is the third level of analysis in the model (Figure 1.1) of how learning disorders develop. Neuropsychology is also part of the pathophysiology of learning disorders and is therefore a proximal cause of learning disorders.

One could reasonably ask why we need a neuropsychological level in our multilevel model of how learning (and all other behavioral) disorders develop. Why not just etiology, brain mechanisms, and behavior? Both performance on neuropsychological tests and the symptoms that define disorders are behavior, and it is the brain that causes behavior. The answer is that neuropsychological constructs can provide a parsimonious explanation of why a set of seemingly diverse symptoms co-occur, thus providing a theoretical bridge between brain mechanisms and behavioral symptoms.

Indeed, the greatest progress so far in understanding learning disorders has come from psychological studies, whose methods are still developing rapidly. The considerable progress in understanding cognition and how it develops has come from behavioral experiments and neural network models. This progress has led to and benefited from a very fruitful interaction between studies of normal and abnormal cognition, including typical and atypical cognitive development (the subject of this book).

We do not attempt to summarize this progress in this chapter, but examples of this rich interplay are provided in Chapters 9–14, which deal with specific disorders. For instance, we have a fairly mature understanding of the cognitive mechanisms underlying dyslexia, because there is a well-developed cognitive psychology of mature reading and reading development, which studies of acquired and developmental dyslexia have advanced in turn. The same is true for language impairment. In the case of autism, the abnormal social cognition found in this disorder has been the leading edge of this reciprocal interaction, because it has stimulated very productive research on the typical development of social cognition, much in the way amnesia found in patient H. M. opened a whole new paradigm in the cognitive psychology of memory.

Neuropsychology is the study of brain–behavior relations. The guiding assumption is that the neuropsychological phenotype of a given disorder can help us understand which brain processes cause the behavioral symptoms that define the disorder, but going from the neuropsychology of a given disorder to its neurological *causes,* the brain mechanisms underlying that disorder, is theoretically and methodologically challenging, to say the least.

Studies of the neuropsychology of learning disorders usually begin with case–control designs in school-age children and adults, often employing both chronological age (CA) and developmental-level control groups (e.g., mental [MA] controls for a study of intellectual disability [ID] or autism spectrum disorder [ASD], language controls for a study of language impairment [LI] or speech sound disorder [SSD], and reading age [RA] controls for a study of dyslexia). Developmental-level control groups such as these can help eliminate neuropsychological correlates that are not actually causes of the disorder (e.g., they may instead be *results* of the disorder). But additional methods are needed to help establish whether a neuropsychological deficit found with these two kinds of case–control designs is actually a cause of the disorders. These additional methods include early longitudinal studies and (rarely) treatment studies, but firmly establishing cause also requires the other levels of analysis covered in Chapters 2 and 3. For most of the disorders covered in this book, both cross-sectional and longitudinal behavioral studies have been used to identify potential neuropsychological causes of the disorder in question, and these have been further tested with behavioral genetics and neuroimaging methods. One overall conclusion from this work is that multiple rather than single neuropsychological deficits are needed to cause each learning disorder considered here.

However, firmly establishing causal links from the second level of analysis of brain mechanisms to the neuropsychological level of analysis requires closing an enormous theoretical and empirical gap. Closing this theoretical gap requires solving the formidable brain–behavior problem, which depends in part on closing at least three empirical gaps: (1) identifying the early brain changes in the disorder, (2) determining how those early brain changes lead to the later neuroimaging phenotypes that characterize a particular disorder, and (3) determining how those neuroimaging phenotypes produce the neuropsychology of the disorder. As discussed in Chapters 1 and 3, the neurocomputational level of analysis can help close the second gap. At this point in our science, we have very few relevant data for closing the first two gaps.

Since the second edition of this book (Pennington, 2009), there have been several important advances in our understanding of the developmental neuropsychology of learning disorders. As we discussed briefly in Chapters 1 and 3, we now have a much better understanding of what kinds of early learning are impaired in different learning disorders. A second important advance is that we now have a better understanding of how brain structure and function change as learning and development proceeds, as discussed in Chapter 3. Finally, we now have a better understanding of what psychometric *g* (intelligence) is and the different ways that learning disorders impact the development of *g*. We turn now to a discussion of the first advance, which is identifying what kinds of early learning are impaired in these learning disorders.

WHAT IS THE EARLY LEARNING DEFICIT IN LEARNING DISORDERS?

In the first edition of this book, Pennington (1991) made the incorrect assumption that explicit long-term memory (LTM) is not impaired in learning disorders. By the second edition (Pennington, 2009), we reviewed emerging evidence that explicit LTM is impaired in Down syndrome (DS), consistent with the reduced size of the hippocampus in that disorder. In neither edition of this book did we consider the role that *implicit* LTM might play in learning disorders. What has changed since 2009 is (1) accumulating evidence that explicit LTM is a shared deficit in other ID syndromes besides DS, namely, in both Williams syndrome (WS) and fragile X syndrome (FXS), and (2) accumulating evidence that implicit LTM is impaired in both LI and dyslexia (or reading disability [RD]).

These discoveries have led to a new theoretical framework for classifying learning disorders based on explicit versus implicit LTM. In this new framework, whether or not explicit LTM is impaired distinguishes ID from other learning disorders such as LI and RD, which have impairments only in implicit LTM. For instance, explicit LTM is impaired below MA level in DS, WS, and FXS (Lee, Maiman, & Godfrey, 2016), whereas intact explicit LTM appears to play a compensatory role in learning disorders such as LI and RD (Ullman & Pullman, 2015). Krishnan, Watkins, and Bishop (2016) reviewed evidence consistent with the view that subcortically mediated implicit or procedural LTM is impaired in LI and RD. Although evidence for a procedural deficit in LI had been recognized for some time (e.g., Ullman & Pierpont, 2005), the evidence for a such a deficit in RD is more recent and includes a meta-analysis of several studies of a serial reaction time task in RD (Lum, Ullman, & Conti-Ramsden, 2013) and a study of statistical learning in RD (Gabay, Thiessen, & Holt, 2015). In LI, a procedural deficit contributes to the key deficit in the acquisition of syntax, whereas in RD, one can speculate that it contributes to the key deficit in the development of phonological representations. This new framework is theoretically appealing because of its parsimony, and because it provides an account of what kinds of early learning is impaired in different learning disorders. It makes sense that an impairment in explicit LTM would slow the rate of cognitive development and thus lead to ID, whereas more specific impairments in implicit LTM could affect early learning of specific aspects of language. Obviously, more research is needed to test this new framework. One critical issue that needs to be addressed in future work is the poor reliability of current procedural learning measures (West et al., 2018). If this important methodological issue can be resolved, this implicit/explicit framework may hold promise as a new way of understanding how early learning goes awry in different learning disorders.

One could ask, what about implicit LTM in ID syndromes? There are fewer relevant data on this question. Vicari (2004) studied both explicit and implicit LTM in DS, WS, and MA-matched controls, and found that the DS group was impaired relative to MA-matched controls on explicit LTM, but not implicit LTM, whereas the WS group had the opposite profile. However, subsequent studies reviewed by Lee et al. (2016) have found explicit LTM deficits in WS. Even if implicit LTM is at the MA level in DS or other syndromes, it is still not totally normal, and we would expect it to contribute to impaired cognitive development, but perhaps not as much as the deficit in explicit LTM. However, we also know that early hippocampal lesions impair explicit LTM, especially episodic LTM, but do not produce ID (Vargha-Khadem et al., 1997). In addition, executive functions are also notably impaired across ID syndromes, as reviewed in Chapter 14, and also contribute to impaired cognitive development. As we discuss later, there is accumulating evidence that long-term potentiation (LTP) is impaired across ID syndromes. Such an impairment would likely lead to impairments in both explicit and implicit LTM, as well as working memory. Hence, it would be a mistake to interpret this new framework as postulating a single cognitive deficit for either ID or other learning disorders, as there are notable complexities that rule out simple, single-deficit explanations.

What about ASD? Its LTM profile is mostly distinct from both ID syndromes and other learning disorders, such as LI and RD. Explicit LTM is impaired only in ASD with comorbid ID, not ASD without ID (Boucher, Mayes, & Bigham, 2012), whereas implicit LTM is not impaired in ASD (for a meta-analysis, see Foti, De Crescenzo, Vivanti, Menghini, & Vicari, 2015). Hence, neither form of LTM appears to account for the defining symptoms of ASD.

Although implicit and explicit LTM are distinct neuropsychological constructs, this does not mean they do not interact in novel learning. As we discussed in Chapter 3, initial learning of a new fact or skill requires effortful processing, but gradually the new fact or skill becomes automatic. This development of automaticity depends on a transition from explicit to implicit learning. For instance, in adults who are learning a new, non-native speech category, both LTM systems are involved, with participants initially relying more on explicit LTM, then transitioning to implicit LTM (Maddox & Chandrasekaran, 2014). In this and other studies discussed in Chapter 9, both humans and rodents that were able to transition faster from explicit to implicit learning performed better on the task. Consistent with its known role in basal ganglia development, variants of the *FOXP2* gene influence how quickly this transition from explicit to implicit learning occurs. In the following sections, we discuss the third advance, namely, the relation of psychometric cognitive constructs to learning disorders.

PSYCHOMETRIC COGNITIVE CONSTRUCTS

Psychometric cognitive constructs come from hierarchical models of intelligence, such as Carroll's (1993) three-stratum model. Figure 4.1 illustrates the hierarchical model of intelligence applied to the Wechsler Intelligence Scale for Children—Fifth

Edition (WISC-V; Wechsler, 2014). At the top of the hierarchy is psychometric intelligence, the thing that is measured by IQ tests and, arguably, by other tests of mental ability, such as the Scholastic Aptitude Test (SAT), American College Testing (ACT), and the Graduate Record Examination (GRE). The next level of the hierarchy has five broad constructs: crystallized intelligence, fluid intelligence, visual–spatial intelligence, working memory, and processing speed.

The lowest level of the hierarchy consists of more specific constructs, which are represented in Figure 4.1 as specific subtests, with the subtests standing for constructs such as spatial reasoning (Block Design), vocabulary knowledge (Vocabulary) or verbal short-term memory (Digit Span). However, in Carroll's (1993) model, the lowest level constructs are more than just individual tasks. Instead, they are narrow latent traits that capture what is common across multiple measures of that particular construct.

In the standardization of the previous version of the WISC, the WISC-IV, a hierarchical four-factor structure was well supported by both exploratory and confirmatory factor analyses (Wechsler, 2003). We first focus on the broad constructs of fluid and crystallized intelligence, then consider working memory and processing speed. Unlike the WISC-IV, which had four Index scores, the WISC-V has five Index scores. It split the Perceptual Reasoning Index score into Fluid and Visual Spatial Index scores. This split is controversial. Recent factor analyses of the WISC-V did not support the notion of five second-level factors, because the Fluid and Visual Spatial factors were not distinct (Canivez, Watkins, & Dombrowski, 2016, 2017). These results should remind us not to reify the results of factor analysis. The number of factors that are found can vary across datasets, and the name given

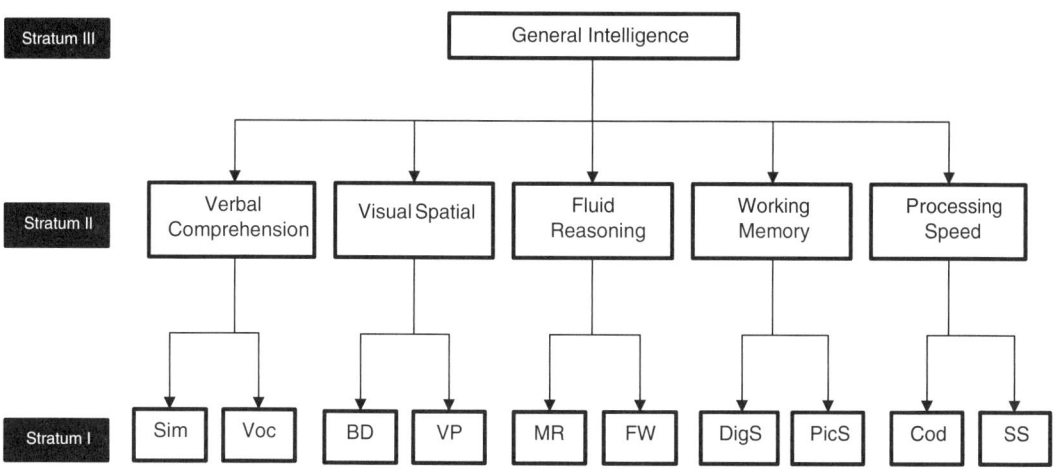

FIGURE 4.1. Carroll's (1993) hierarchical model of intelligence illustrated by the WISC-V. Sim, Similarities; Voc, Vocabulary; BD, Block Design; VP, Visual Puzzles; MR, Matrix Reasoning; FW, Figure Weights; DigS, Digit Span; PicS, Picture Span; Cod, Coding; SS, Symbol Search. In the calculation of the WISC-V Full Scale IQ, only seven subtests are included: Sim, Voc, BD, MR, FW, DS, and Cod.

to a factor is hypothetical. Most importantly, the underlying multivariate data distribution from which factors derive is continuous, with no sharp boundaries.

The psychometric theory of fluid and crystallized intelligence was proposed and tested by Spearman's student, Cattell (1943, 1963), and elaborated by Cattell's student, Horn (Cattell & Horn, 1978; Horn & Noll, 1997). The distinction between the concepts of fluid and crystallized intelligence has been made by numerous psychologists both before and after Cattell's work using many different but conceptually similar labels for these constructs. Some of these psychologists were attempting to understand the cognitive deficits associated with acquired brain damage or aging.

Hence, these constructs have a long history in psychology and have been extensively validated by psychometric, developmental, and neuropsychological studies. These two constructs also correspond to two widespread intuitive notions of what it means for someone to be "smart," namely, by either being good at solving new problems (fluid intelligence) or knowing a lot (crystallized intelligence). The paradigmatic fluid intelligence task is a matrix reasoning task, and the paradigmatic crystallized intelligence task is a vocabulary test. So, simply put, fluid intelligence is novel problem-solving ability, and crystallized intelligence is accumulated, mostly verbal, knowledge. Each of these two kinds of intelligence has a distinct developmental course. Fluid intelligence reaches a lifetime peak in late adolescence and slowly declines thereafter (e.g., WAIS-IV norms for Matrix Reasoning show that the highest average raw score is attained by 16- to 29-year-olds), whereas crystallized intelligence keeps increasing until at least middle age (e.g., WAIS-IV norms for Vocabulary show that the highest average score is attained by 45- to 64-year-olds (Wechsler, 1997a, 1997b, 2008). Fluid intelligence is also much more vulnerable to acquired brain damage than is crystallized intelligence.

The WISC-V has three factors that correspond closely to these two constructs. The Verbal Comprehension factor corresponds to crystallized intelligence and is measured by two subtests that tap accumulated verbal knowledge (Similarities and Vocabulary). As already mentioned, the separate Fluid Reasoning (measured by the Matrix Reasoning and Figure Weights subtests) and Visual Spatial (measured by the Block Design and Visual Puzzles subtests) composites are now provided, but recent factor analyses have not confirmed the validity of this split, and both factors heavily emphasize fluid intelligence. While difficulties with specific aspects of visual–spatial processing are relevant to understanding some acquired neurological problems, visual–spatial deficits are less important for most developmentally based learning disorders.

Next we consider working memory and processing speed. *Working memory* refers to the transient storage and processing of information, so it is essentially the same thing as active memory in the O'Reilly and Munakata (2000) model. The construct of working memory is closely related to the construct of short-term memory. Of the four cognitive constructs considered here, working memory is the most "respectable" from the point of view of cognitive theory. Much current research in cognitive neuroscience is focused on understanding working memory. Indeed, the inclusion of a working memory factor on the WISC-IV and the WISC-V represents a positive trend toward the gradual integration of the psychometric and cognitive approaches.

One might say, in contrast to working memory, that the construct of processing speed is the least "respectable" from the point of view of cognitive theory. But it is a very robust psychometric factor, and it is useful for understanding both cognitive development and cognitive disorders, including learning disorders. The reason it is less respectable is that measures of processing speed are seen as having more "impurity" than other neuropsychological constructs, because any measure of speed necessarily involves speed of doing a specific task, which introduces task-specific variance that is not of primary interest. Nonetheless, reduced processing speed is a pervasive finding across both developmental and acquired cognitive disorders, as well as in aging (Salthouse, 1991). Moreover, there are marked developmental changes in processing speed that help explain cognitive development (Kail, 1991). This pervasive role of processing speed in both individual and developmental differences in cognitive skill may arise because processing speed actually requires the integrated activity of the whole brain, which depends on white matter connections. Lifespan developmental increases and eventual decreases in white matter may help explain the rise and later fall of processing speed in typical development. As we discuss later, reduced white matter development is found in several learning disorders. Although some processing speed measures, such as choice reaction time, are deceptively simple, performing consistently well on them requires the concerted activity of brain networks involved in perception, attention, motivation, and action selection (as well as inhibition). Furthermore, processing speed may affect the efficiency of cognitive components, such as working memory, necessary for complex problem solving.

For instance, Fry and Hale (1996) used path analyses to test relations among age, processing speed, working memory, and fluid intelligence. They found that working memory mediated 41% of the total relation between age and fluid intelligence, and that processing speed mediated 71% of the relation between age and working memory. In other words, their results support a developmental cascade in which age-related increases in processing speed lead to age-related increases in working memory, which in turn lead to age-related increases in fluid intelligence. Although this was a cross-sectional correlational study, which cannot establish the direction of causality, these authors were able to reject an alternative, top-down model in which fluid intelligence mediates the developmental relation between age and speed. So, this study, and other related work, gives us a view of how one key aspect of intelligence, fluid reasoning, may develop. We have already considered how crystalized intelligence develops in our discussion of explicit memory. In summary, we have covered four psychometric constructs that are important for understanding developmental and individual cognitive differences, including the learning disorders covered in this book, and related those to key cognitive neuroscience constructs. Table 4.1 summarizes the relation between these psychometric and cognitive neuroscience constructs. As can be seen, there are more cognitive neuroscience constructs than psychometric constructs. Hence, some cognitive neuroscience constructs, such as explicit and implicit LTM, are not directly tapped by IQ tests.

TABLE 4.1. Relation between Psychometric and Cognitive Neuroscience Constructs

Psychometric	Cognitive neuroscience
Crystallized intelligence	Language
Fluid intelligence	Cold EFs
Verbal working memory	Verbal working memory
Spatial reasoning	Spatial reasoning
Processing speed	—
—	Explicit LTM
—	Implicit LTM
—	Error monitoring
—	Hot EFs
—	Reward processing
—	Default mode processing
—	Perception

Note. EF, executive function; LTM, long-term memory.

GENERAL VERSUS SPECIFIC COGNITIVE DEFICITS IN LEARNING DISORDERS

Although we tend to view learning disabilities such as dyslexia and mathematics disorder as being more on the specific end of the spectrum that runs from specific to general cognitive deficits, which we discussed in Chapter 1, few studies have directly tested this hypothesis. Just as for cognitive tasks, virtually all individual academic tests are positively correlated with each other and with Full Scale IQ, raising questions about how "specific" are learning disabilities defined by poor academic skills development. The most relevant published data rely on factor analyses of the norming samples of standardized academic batteries, such as the Woodcock–Johnson Tests of Achievement and the Kaufman Tests of Educational Achievement (Kaufman, Reynolds, Liu, Kaufman, & McGrew, 2012; McGrew & Woodcock, 2001; Shrank, McGrew, & Mather, 2014). Overall, the structure of academic skills appears to mirror that for intelligence and to be well described by the hierarchical Cattell–Horn–Carroll (CHC) model (McGrew et al., 2014). Much variance is shared across all academic measures and can be conceptualized as an academic g (Kaufman et al., 2012). This academic g is highly correlated with cognitive g (around .8) but not identical to it (Deary, Strand, Smith, & Fernandes, 2007; Kaufman et al., 2012). At the middle level of the academic model, math and literacy constructs can be identified (Kaufman et al., 2012; Shrank et al., 2014), and these in turn can be further subdivided into more specific skills such as word reading and reading comprehension or calculation and math problem solving. Although it is easy to imagine a direct mapping from a single cognitive construct to a single academic construct (e.g., language to literacy and fluid intelligence to math), the truth appears to be more complicated. For instance, language and processing speed contribute to both reading and math outcomes (Peterson et al., 2017).

As we mentioned previously, some children with academic difficulties may be well described by a specific, circumscribed deficit at the lowest level of the hierarchy, such a child with "classic" developmental dyslexia who struggles markedly with word reading but not in other areas. These individuals with uneven profiles have historically received much attention from researchers, as well as clinicians and educators. But there are also many children whose educational difficulties are better understood at higher levels of the hierarchy, and who show generally low but even performance across most, if not all, academic and cognitive tasks. Although some children have such severe learning disabilities that they qualify for a diagnosis of ID, many more fall into a grey area. Whether, when, and how to diagnose and intervene with such children remains controversial and is discussed further in later chapters. Clearly, g is important for understanding learning disorders, but what is g? We next turn to that topic.

WHAT IS THE NEUROPSYCHOLOGY OF g?

The g factor, first discovered by Spearman, is a robust empirical phenomenon that emerges when virtually any battery of cognitive tests is factor-analyzed, and often accounts for up to around 40% of the total variance in the test battery. Hence, the existence of psychometric g is an important empirical fact, but this does not necessarily mean there is a single psychological or neural cause of g. Some researchers have tried to reduce psychometric g to a single psychological or neural or (even genetic) cause, but so far these efforts have not succeeded. For instance, researchers have found that psychometric g is not reducible to reaction time, inspection time, processing speed, working memory, or executive functions, although each of these psychological constructs is correlated with g. The brain correlates of g are distributed rather than localized, and its etiology is multifactorial and highly polygenic, similar to other biologically important quantitative traits such as height and weight.

Two main theoretical alternatives to a single psychological g have been proposed, namely *sampling* theory (Thompson, 1917) and *mutualism* (van der Maas et al., 2006), both of which have been tested through simulations. Sampling theory holds that each cognitive task has multiple subcomponents (e.g., perception, attention, working memory, and response selection), some of which overlap across many or all cognitive tasks. These overlapping subcomponents produce a psychometric g in a simple additive fashion. This theory was tested with simulations by Bartholomew, Deary, and Lawn (2009), who demonstrated that factor analysis cannot distinguish between sampling theory and a single psychological g. In contrast to sampling theory, mutualism (van der Maas et al., 2006) holds that reciprocal interactions among a small set of cognitive components lead to an emergent g factor. Again, simulations supported this theory. In summary, both theories, sampling and mutualism, hold that the g factor arises from multiple rather than single cognitive components, but they differ in their account of the relation among these cognitive components, one being additive and the other being interactive. Hence, the existence of psychometric *g* has alternative psychological explanations, and factor analysis alone cannot decide between.

One can use data from learning disorders to help resolve the question of whether there is a single psychological *g*, because the cognitive phenotype of each learning disorder includes some reduction in Full Scale IQ (and hence *g*), as we discuss in later chapters. However, the cognitive reason for this reduction vary across disorders. For instance, as discussed earlier in this chapter, a deficit in explicit LTM contributes to the IQ deficit in ID syndromes, but not in other disorders, such as like dyslexia and LI. This pattern suggests that psychometric *g* has multiple cognitive components, since it can be lowered for different reasons in different disorders.

Another source of data bearing on this question comes from neuroimaging studies of psychometric IQ, which we discussed briefly in Chapter 3. A relevant neuroimaging study was conducted by Hampshire, Highfield, Parkin, and Owen (2012), using factor analyses of both cognitive tasks and functional magnetic resonance imaging (fMRI) data. They found a distributed set of "multiple demand" brain regions in the prefrontal, parietal, anterior cingulate, and insular cortices that changed their activity level in response to a difficulty manipulation across different cognitive tasks. Activity in these multiple demand regions was correlated with IQ, but so was activity in some nondemand regions, specifically the left inferior frontal gyrus and bilateral temporal lobes, which are associated with language skills. One interpretation of their results would be that they found neural correlates of both fluid intelligence (demand regions) and crystallized intelligence (nondemand language regions). Hence, multiple interacting cognitive processes and associated brain regions appear to underlie psychometric *g*.

COGNITIVE NEUROSCIENCE CONSTRUCTS

While psychometric constructs grew out of applied research aimed at predicting individual differences in educational and occupational settings, cognitive neuroscience constructs come from basic research aimed at developing a universal theory of human cognition and understanding how it is mediated by the human brain. So, developing and testing competing theories of cognitive processes are at the heart of this enterprise. Like the psychometric approach, the cognitive neuroscience approach has both broad and narrow constructs that may be arranged hierarchically. But the critical difference is that the subordinate constructs are based on an analysis of the cognitive components necessary to perform a given task, whether it is pronouncing a printed word, solving the Tower of Hanoi puzzle, or encoding a new memory. Increasingly, as discussed earlier, this theoretical analysis is implemented as a functioning computational model. In other words, a satisfactory cognitive theory would enumerate the underlying processing mechanisms used by real humans in sufficient detail, so that human performance can be simulated by a machine. From a cognitive theorist's point of view, all the lowest level, stratum I constructs in the psychometric model (Figure 4.1) require further analysis into cognitive components, and the relations across strata require a theoretical explanation in terms of shared cognitive processes. So, for a cognitive theorist, it is not enough to say that measures of numerical analogies and Piagetian reasoning both load on a fluid factor. What is required is an empirically tested cognitive explanation of why they do so framed in terms of shared cognitive processes.

Some of the broad constructs in cognitive neuroscience are things such as perception, language, memory, executive functions, and social cognition, but each of these domains is divided into subtypes (e.g., memory is divided into short-term memory, long-term memory, and implicit memory) that are then subjected to a componential analysis. So, for a cognitive scientist, it is not very meaningful to talk about individual differences in global constructs such as language or memory. Nonetheless, cognitive analysis is proving very useful for understanding the broad individual differences described by psychometricians.

In addition to LTM, the three broad cognitive constructs that are most relevant for understanding the learning disorders covered in this book are (1) *language* (which is important for understanding speech, language, and reading disorders, as well as autism and intellectual disability); (2) *attention and executive functions* (which are important for understanding attention-deficit/hyperactivity disorder [ADHD], autism, and ID), and (3) *social cognition* (which is important for autism). A cognitive analysis of these broad domains is provided in later chapters.

Table 4.2 lists the key cognitive risk factors for learning disorders, divided into those that are shared and not shared with other learning disorders. As discussed in more detail in later chapters, the shared cognitive risk factors help explain the high rate of comorbidity among these learning disorders.

BEYOND NEUROPSYCHOLOGY?

One may ask how a neuroscience explanation (as diagrammed in Figure 1.1) differs from a psychological explanation. The simple answer is that a neuroscience explanation has more levels of analysis. In most of the history of psychology,

TABLE 4.2. Key Cognitive Risk Factors for Learning Disorders

Disorder	Nonshared	Shared
RD	Letter knowledge	PA, PS, implicit LTM
LI	Syntactic knowledge	PA, PS, implicit LTM
SSD	Oral–motor praxis	PA
ADHD	Inhibition	PS, EFs
MD	Number sense, counting	PS, verbal WM
ID	Explicit LTM	PS, EFs, implicit LTM
ASD	Intersubjectivity	EFs

Note. PA, phoneme awareness; PS, processing speed; LTM, long-term memory; EF, executive function; verbal WM, verbal working memory.

explanations had only two levels of analysis: (1) observed behaviors and (2) psychological constructs. These two levels essentially correspond to the two levels on the right side of Figure 1.1. Hence, the goal of most psychological explanation has been to use a single psychological construct (e.g., intelligence, attachment, or emotion regulation) to predict a wide range of observed behaviors. Such psychological explanations were thus parsimonious, insofar as the list of explanatory constructs was much shorter than the list of behaviors to be explained. Predictive relations were tested cross-sectionally, sometimes longitudinally, and more rarely, experimentally. But explanation usually stopped at the level of the psychological constructs themselves.

The field of neuropsychology, for much of its history, operated in much the same way, but it made the additional requirement that its explanatory constructs be grounded in brain function. But the operationalization of this requirement was not very strict. A candidate brain function was a function that had been observed to be impaired by brain damage. But if one is a materialist (i.e., believes that mind has a physical basis in the brain), then any human function could be a neuropsychological construct: Language and memory could be, but so could theory of mind and personality. This strategy for dissecting brain functions was also inherently unparsimonious. Finer and finer divisions of cognitive functions could be justified by patients with contrasting lesions and contrasting deficits, so the list of cognitive functions continually expanded.

So, how is a neuroscience explanation different from a neuropsychological or psychological explanation? The basic answer is that it makes a much more explicit and detailed commitment to materialism. One needs to explain how interactions among neurons produce behaviors. Presumably, psychological or neuropsychological functions are an intervening step in the causal chain that runs from interacting neurons to behaviors. But it is a strong assumption that those psychological functions map onto the dynamics of neuronal processing in a simple or direct way. In other words, some of our favorite neuropsychological constructs, such as working memory or executive function, may not actually exist in the brain in the traditional neuropsychological sense of localization! Instead, they may correspond only roughly to stages of processing in the computations that networks of neurons are performing. Another way of making this point is to say that familiar psychological and neuropsychological constructs are reifications, just like g, which is to say they are simplified placeholders for processes we do not yet understand. So do things such as intelligence, working memory, or personality actually exist? "Yes," insofar as they are reliable and valid psychological constructs, but "no," in the sense that there is not yet any simple or transparent mapping of such constructs onto brain. In other words, the neuropsychological level of explanation may eventually be replaced by a neurocomputational level of analysis that is very closely tied to actual networks in the brain.

But a neuroscience explanation does not stop there. As discussed in Chapter 3, one next has to ask how those interacting neurons developed (and how they evolved), and to answer those questions takes us down to the level of cells, to molecules and genes. Hence, a complete neuroscience explanation of an individual difference in behavior, such as skill in reading or math, must begin with genes and how their interplay with the environment produces a developing brain. This is a tall order indeed, and one could argue that reaching this goal is either impossible or very far in the future. On the other hand, the progress that has been made in just a few decades is truly amazing, and we now have at least a preliminary sketch of a complete neuroscience explanation for several disorders. In the second half of the book, we present such sketches for disorders like dyslexia and autism.

SUMMARY

Neuropsychology is the third level of analysis in our multilevel framework for understanding how learning disorders develop. Neuropsychology is part of the pathophysiology of learning disorders, with the other part being abnormal brain development. Neuropsychology, including neural network models, provides a crucial bridge between brain development and the symptoms that define learning disorders. For instance, the constructs of explicit and implicit learning and memory are helping us understand what kind of learning is impaired in different learning disorders. Clinicians use both psychometric and cognitive neuroscience constructs to understand learning disorders, and research is bringing these two ways of understanding individual differences in cognition much closer together. For instance, our neuropsychological understanding of Spearman's g is developing rapidly. Neuropsychological constructs themselves will continue to evolve as we gain a better understanding of the brain mechanisms in increasingly realistic neural network models of brain development.

CHAPTER 5

Comorbidity

Comorbidity, the co-occurrence of two or more disorders in the same child, is pervasive in developmental psychopathology. Epidemiological studies indicate that at least one in three children with one disorder also meet criteria for one or more additional disorders (Costello et al., 1996; Kessler et al., 2012), and rates of comorbidity are even higher in clinically referred samples. For children with learning disabilities, approximately half show evidence of learning problems that impact multiple academic domains (Moll, Göbel, Gooch, Landerl, & Snowling, 2014). Such children with multiple comorbidities tend to be less responsive to interventions (Aro, Ahonen, Tolvanen, Lyytinen, & de Barra, 1999; Hinshaw, 2007; A. Miller et al., 2014; R. Nelson, Benner, & Gonzalez, 2003; Rabiner, Malone, & Conduct Problems Prevention Research Group, 2004) and are more likely to experience serious functional impairment, including school failure and criminality (Connor, Steeber, & McBurnett, 2010; Larson, Russ, Kahn, & Halfon, 2011; Sexton, Gelhorn, Bell, & Classi, 2012; Waschbusch, 2002) compared to children with an isolated disorder. Despite the pressing clinical importance and pervasiveness of the problem, we still know very little about the cognitive and neural mechanisms that increase a child's risk for multiple disorders.

Fortunately, there is an increasing focus in the scientific literature on the challenges that comorbidities pose for assessment and treatment of children with learning disorders. As in the rest of this book, we adopt a multiple-deficit framework for understanding the prevalence and predictors of comorbidity. As detailed in Chapter 1, the multiple-deficit model initially arose out of research on comorbidity. This model stipulates that there are multiple, probabilistic predictors of learning disorders across levels of analysis, and that comorbidity arises because of predictors that are shared by disorders (Pennington, 2006). This multiple-deficit framework has been useful for advancing the science of comorbidity. However, as we discuss next, additional challenges are hindering progress toward a broad understanding of comorbidity across the spectrum of developmental disorders.

Analytically, the prevailing research designs and statistical techniques are not optimal for directly testing shared risk factors that could give rise to comorbidity. For example, the bulk of studies on developmental disorders employ one of three designs: (1) recruiting "pure" groups without comorbidities, (2) forming separate groups based on comorbidity status (i.e., reading disability [RD], attention-deficit/hyperactivity disorder [ADHD], RD + ADHD), or (3) analyzing one disorder while statistically controlling for the other. While each of these strategies is useful for specific research questions, none of them directly addresses why the disorders co-occur in the first place. In fact, (2) and (3) address the question of what *distinguishes* one disorder from the other. Although this question is undeniably important, it is also necessary to ask what is *shared* by both disorders (Caron & Rutter, 1991). We have strong evidence across levels of analysis (discussed further below) that shared etiological, brain, and neuropsychological mechanisms are contributing to comorbidity. Our group has been addressing these analytic challenges by using structural equation modeling approaches that enable one to predict multiple disorders/symptom dimensions and their relationship (McGrath et al., 2011; Peterson et al., 2017; Willcutt et al., 2010). The novel aspect of this approach is the focus on predicting the relationship between symptoms of each disorder, or their covariance, rather than variance in a single disorder. We propose that this analytic framework represents an important shift from prediction of variance to prediction of *covariance*, which could yield important insights about the causes of comorbidity across levels of analysis.

A second challenge results from the complex clustering of comorbidities. Studies typically focus on two disorders at a time, but even this important step forward is still insufficient to account for the full spectrum of neurodevelopmental comorbidities. In the learning disabilities literature, increasing recognition of this challenge has resulted in more sophisticated statistical models to deal with multiple outcomes and their covariance (i.e., Moll et al., 2014; Peterson et al., 2017). For example, studies are more frequently considering several academic skills and ADHD symptoms in the same statistical models in order to disentangle shared versus specific neuropsychological factors (Moll et al., 2014; Peterson et al., 2017). Nevertheless, such studies are still the exception rather than the rule. Still, such innovations are necessary to continue pushing the science of comorbidity beyond consideration of one or two disorders at a time.

A third challenge for this field is the greater focus on homotypic comorbidities compared to heterotypic comorbidities. *Homotypic comorbidity* refers to co-occurring disorders that are in the same diagnostic class, such as learning disabilities with other learning disabilities, or anxiety disorders with other internalizing disorders (Angold, Costello, & Erkanli, 1999). *Heterotypic comorbidity*[1] refers to co-occurring

---

[1] Note that the term *heterotypic* comorbidity implies comorbidity of disorders from distinct diagnostic classes at a specific time point, whereas the term *heterotypic continuity*, discussed in Chapter 1, refers to the changing developmental manifestations of an underlying risk factor.

disorders that span broad diagnostic classes, such as learning disabilities with internalizing or externalizing disorders (Angold et al., 1999). It is not surprising that homotypic comorbidities are better studied, because these comorbidities are typically more prevalent and fall within a similar area of expertise of the researcher. Unfortunately, this has led to a splintering of the literatures for developmental disorders into separate categories for learning disabilities and developmental psychopathologies, such that they are rarely studied together. This splintering is reflected at many levels of the scientific process, including conferences, journals, and grant review committees. Nevertheless, heterotypic comorbidities are still common and can be quite informative for discerning unexpected shared risk factors for two disorders. In fact, such heterotypic comorbidities might be *more* informative for advancing theoretical models of comorbidity, since they require explanations of common mechanisms that can lead to quite distinct disorders. Thus, this artificial splintering of the field is detrimental for a comprehensive understanding of comorbidity. In fact, a notable exception to the focus on homotypic comorbidities in the learning disorders field, the RD + ADHD comorbidity, has illustrated the value of pursuing mechanisms underlying heterotypic comorbidities across levels of analysis.

RD (also known as *dyslexia*) and ADHD are both highly prevalent disorders (5–10%) with a high comorbidity rate (25–40%) (DuPaul, Gormley, & Laracy, 2013; Willcutt & Pennington, 2000a). Several theoretical models of comorbidity (M. Neale & Kendler, 1995; Caron & Rutter, 1991; Rhee, Hewitt, Corley, Willcutt, & Pennington, 2005) have been tested in RD and ADHD (Pennington, Willcutt, Rhee, 2005; Willcutt, 2014), including ruling out artifactual explanations attributable to referral biases (Semrud-Clikeman et al., 1992; Willcutt & Pennington, 2000a) and rater biases (Willcutt et al., 2010). Alternative explanations for the RD + ADHD comorbidity, such as simple causal explanations that reading problems cause attention problems or vice versa, have not been strongly supported by neuropsychological (Willcutt et al., 2005) or longitudinal behavioral genetic studies (Ebejer et al., 2010; Wadsworth, DeFries, Willcutt, Pennington, & Olson, 2015), though some behavioral studies have yielded mixed results on this important question (i.e., A. Miller et al., 2014). DSM-5 identifies three subtypes of ADHD: inattentive, hyperactive–impulsive (HI), and combined. Previous research has consistently found that inattention, rather than HI, is most strongly related to reading both phenotypically (Sims & Lonigan, 2013) and genetically (Willcutt, Pennington, & DeFries, 2000; Willcutt, Pennington, Olson, & DeFries, 2007). Thus, here we focus on the relationship between reading and inattention, with the latter measured by behavioral ratings of symptoms underlying the inattentive dimension of ADHD.

The reading–inattention comorbidity is one of the most well-studied comorbidities across the genetic, cognitive, and behavioral levels of analysis (Willcutt et al., 2010), so we use the example of RD + ADHD comorbidity throughout this chapter to illustrate methods that could be applied more generally across the learning disorders.

DEVELOPMENTAL NEUROPSYCHOLOGY

The focus we are advocating on shared risk factors between comorbid disorders carries across the genetic, brain, and neuropsychological levels of analysis. We start here at the neuropsychological level of analysis. As described, the multiple-deficit model holds that shared cognitive risk factors are responsible for the frequent comorbidities seen among developmental disorders (Pennington, 2006). Thus, documenting shared cognitive deficits that account for the covariance between comorbid traits is one critical test of the multiple-deficit model. The first comorbidity to be explored with the multiple-deficit model was the RD + ADHD comorbidity, so we turn now to that particular pairing for an illustration of a neuropsychological analysis of comorbidity.

Neuropsychology of RD and ADHD

Neuropsychological research on comorbidity between RD and ADHD has typically focused on the extent to which the comorbid group is merely an additive combination of deficits found in each disorder individually, or a distinct subtype with a unique neuropsychological profile (for a review, see Germano, Gagliano, & Curatolo, 2010). Results so far have been mixed, but there has been reasonable consistency about cognitive deficits associated with both RD and ADHD individually, such as processing speed (PS) (Caravolas, Volín, & Hulme, 2005; Catts, Gillispie, Leonard, Kail, & Miller, 2002; Kail & Hall, 1994; Kalff et al., 2005; McGrath et al., 2011; Peterson et al., 2017; Shanahan et al., 2006; Weiler, Bernstein, Bellinger, & Waber, 2000; Willcutt et al., 2005), rapid naming (Arnett et al., 2012; Norton & Wolf, 2012; Rucklidge & Tannock, 2002; Tannock, Martinussen, & Frijters, 2000), and specific domains of executive function (EF): working memory (WM) (Cheung et al., 2014; Martinussen, Hayden, Hogg-Johnson, & Tannock, 2005; Roodenrys, Koloski, & Grainger, 2001; Rucklidge & Tannock, 2002; Swanson, Mink, & Bocian, 1999; Tiffin-Richards, Hasselhorn, Woerner, Rothenberger, & Banaschewski, 2008; Willcutt et al., 2001, 2005), inhibition (de Jong et al., 2009; Purvis & Tannock, 2000; Willcutt et al., 2001, 2005), and sustained attention (Purvis & Tannock, 2000; Willcutt et al., 2005). A limitation of this body of research is that studies varied in the extent to which they accounted for clinical and subclinical comorbidities, so it is difficult to tease out the extent to which associations are due to the primary disorder versus clinical and subclinical comorbidities. Perhaps most importantly, these studies focused on predicting variance in the individual disorders, rather than the relationship (or covariance) between RD and ADHD. Thus, these studies provide a list of potential shared cognitive deficits to test in further modeling, but a different analytic approach focused on predicting covariance is needed to address the question of whether these shared cognitive deficits explain why the disorders co-occur. Note that just because a cognitive factor is associated with both outcomes does not mean that this cognitive factor is associated with the covariance of the traits. This is because the cognitive factor may predict *unique* variance in both reading and attention and therefore none of their covariance. In other words, a given cognitive weakness might be associated with two different disorders for two different reasons and might not contribute to their overlap. Thus, further modeling is required to clarify the relationships.

Despite strong evidence for multifactorial contributions, very few studies have directly tested a multiple-deficit model of comorbidity. Our group was the first to do so (McGrath et al., 2011). In this study, we tested the contribution of a range of cognitive variables to reading, inattention, and their covariance in a population-based sample (McGrath et al., 2011). Key results showed that phonological awareness (PA), rapid automatized naming (RAN), and PS predicted untimed single-word reading, whereas inhibition and PS predicted inattention. The most compelling result was that PS (measured by a latent factor composed of coding and two experimental PS tasks) predicted *both* reading and inattention, and accounted for 75% of the correlation between these skills (McGrath et al., 2011). These findings suggest that PS is a shared cognitive deficit that explains a portion of the RD + ADHD comorbidity (McGrath et al., 2011; Peterson et al., 2017; Shanahan et al., 2006; Willcutt et al., 2005).

It is important to highlight here that the reading measures were untimed and the inattention measures were from mother, father, and teacher-report, so the associations with PS were not due to method variance. In an expanded sample, we were able to find the same association between PS and reading–attention using the same latent constructs (Peterson et al., 2017). Additionally, an independent group has conducted similar analyses with partially overlapping constructs. Moura et al. (2017) reported that naming speed (numbers and alternating shapes/colors) was a shared cognitive deficit between RD and ADHD. Although not a direct replication, their findings do point to the potential role of speeded measures in the comorbidity of RD and ADHD, and suggest that further development and characterization of PS measures will be needed to determine which speeded tasks are most strongly associated with RD, ADHD, and their comorbidity.

None of the other cognitive factors included in the multiple-deficit model emerged as potential shared cognitive deficits, but this does not mean that others will not be found in future research. The multiple-deficit model specifies that shared cognitive risk factors will exist but does not limit the number of these shared neuropsychological predictors.

We highlight these analyses of RD and ADHD as a proof of concept that an analytic focus on covariance can bring a new understanding to developmental comorbidities, in this case implicating a generalized cognitive deficit (PS) in the mechanisms of comorbidity. This multiple-deficit approach to comorbidity has also been fruitful beyond RD + ADHD. In a study of the comorbidity between RD and math disability (MD), Slot, van Viersen, de Bree, and Kroesbergen (2016) found that PA, a risk factor thought to be specific to reading, was actually shared between reading and math and therefore might contribute to their comorbidity. This surprising finding further emphasizes the utility of a multiple-deficit analytic approach to comorbidity (Slot et al., 2016).

ETIOLOGY

Behavioral Genetics

Behavioral genetic analyses can make an important contribution to an etiological understanding of comorbidity. Although behavioral genetic methods are most frequently invoked to establish the heritability of a single disorder, they may also be used to establish the extent of genetic sharing between two different traits or disorders, such as two frequently comorbid disorders (Knopik, Neiderhiser, DeFries, & Plomin, 2017). In this chapter, we rely on a statistic, the *genetic correlation*, that is used to describe the genetic relationship between two different traits or disorders. The genetic correlation refers to the extent to which genetic influences on one trait overlap with genetic influences on the second trait. A genetic correlation of 0 means that completely different genes affect the two traits. A genetic correlation of 1.0 means that all of the genetic influences on one trait also influence the second trait (Plomin & Kovas, 2005). One way to interpret the genetic correlation is that it expresses the probability that a gene associated with one trait will also be associated with the second trait (Plomin & Kovas, 2005).

The multiple-deficit model proposes that shared genetic influences contribute to shared brain and cognitive influences that lead to comorbidity (Pennington, 2006). This proposal can be tested directly through bivariate (and multivariate) extensions of heritability analyses. A broad view of the bivariate heritability analyses across learning disorders and developmental psychopathology leads to the general conclusion that there is a high degree of genetic sharing (Lichtenstein, Carlstrom, Rastam, Gillberg, & Anckarsater, 2010; Plomin & Kovas, 2005). Estimates vary based on the pairing of disorders studied, but most frequently comorbid disorders share some degree of genetic influence. For cognitive and academic traits, the pervasiveness and extent of the genetic sharing has led to the *generalist genes hypothesis* proposed by Plomin and Kovas (Kovas & Plomin, 2007; Plomin & Kovas, 2005). This hypothesis holds that most (but not all) genes are "generalists," which means that they impact a wide range of learning and cognitive traits. Across studies, the average genetic correlation between academic traits is approximately .70 (Kovas & Plomin, 2007). Overlaps between cognitive and academic traits are slightly lower but usually still greater than .50 (Plomin & Kovas, 2005). The generalist genes hypothesis also applies to the full range of the distribution, which means that substantially similar genes influence the high and low tails of academic and cognitive traits (Haworth et al., 2009; Plomin & Kovas, 2005). Taken together, the bulk of the findings point to substantial genetic sharing between academic and cognitive traits across the full range of the distribution. This sharing means that it will be difficult to distinguish learning disorders from a genetic perspective (Haworth et al., 2009).

With the generalist genes' emphasis on genetic sharing, one might wonder how "specific" learning disorders develop. Such specific cases do exist, although they are not the norm in clinical practice. There are at least two etiological explanations for how these "specific" or "pure" learning disorders may develop. First, the generalist genes hypothesis indicates that most, but not all genes, are generalist.

When genetic correlations are less than 1, as we have seen in this chapter, there are "specialist" genes influencing each trait, which increase risk for one learning disorder but not others. Second, nonshared environments, the portions of the environment that serve to make twins different from each other, are primarily specialists. For example, the nonshared environmental correlation was .39 between reading and math (Kovas & Plomin, 2007) and .24 between different components of math (Kovas & Plomin, 2007). These estimates are much lower than the genetic correlations and indicate that nonshared environments are primarily specific to academic skills. Thus, a combination of a small portion of specialist genes and a larger portion of specialist environments could explain the fact that specific learning disorders do exist.

Taken together, behavioral genetic analyses find a high degree of genetic sharing between academic and cognitive traits underlying the learning disorders discussed in this book. Behavioral genetic analyses give estimates of the portions of variance accounted for by genetic and environmental influences, but they cannot identify the specific genes involved. For that, molecular genetic methods are necessary.

Molecular Genetics

Molecular genetic methods have advanced considerably in the past decade, moving from candidate gene approaches that yielded largely unreplicated findings (Duncan, Pollastri, & Smoller, 2014) to comprehensive genomewide methods that have been more fruitful (Ripke et al., 2014; P. Sullivan, Daly, & O'Donovan, 2012). Separate methods are used to detect genetic variants that are common in the population (i.e., > 5% of individuals) and those that are rare (i.e., < 1% of the population). In the case of both common and rare genetic variants, molecular genetic studies have uncovered a surprising degree of genetic sharing among the disorders that have received the most attention so far: schizophrenia, bipolar disorder, major depression, autism, and ADHD (Cross-Disorder Group of the Psychiatric Genomic Consortium et al., 2013; Smoller, 2013b). These findings are consistent with the generalist genes hypothesis, but they extend the reach of this hypothesis to psychiatric disorders. This extension is important, because the generalist genes idea emerged from behavioral genetic studies of cognitive and academic traits. In parallel, a greater appreciation of cross-disorder findings is simultaneously emerging from molecular genetic studies of psychiatric disorders. Hence, there is convergence across phenotypes and methods for the generalist effects of genes. What has not yet been systematically investigated is whether the generalist genes for cognitive and academic traits are overlapping with the generalist genes for psychiatric disorders.

We turn now to a consideration of the learning disorders covered in this book and start with research examining common genetic variation. At this point, only autism and ADHD have sample sizes large enough to reliably estimate cross-disorder effects for common genetic variants (Demontis et al., 2017; Grove et al., 2017). One recent study currently in prepublication reported the genetic correlation of autism and ADHD to be .36 using molecular genetic methods (Grove et al., 2017). These results are in line with estimates derived from behavioral genetic methods, though behavioral genetic methods have tended to find slightly higher genetic correlations that exceed .5 (Rommelse, Franke, Geurts, Hartman, & Buitelaar, 2010). We discussed this question of the discrepancy between behavioral genetic and molecular genetic methods, also termed the "missing heritability" problem, in Chapter 2. For our purposes here, we emphasize that both molecular genetic and behavioral genetic methods are finding significant evidence of cross-disorder genetic effects for ASD and autism, which may partly explain their high rates of comorbidity.

Rare genetic variants have also shown a surprising degree of cross-disorder genetic sharing. Here, we focus on copy number variations (CNVs), which are deletions or duplications in the genome. These deletions and duplications can be varying sizes, but larger events (i.e., > 100 kilobases) tend to be rarer in the population and more pathogenic. In CNV studies of individual disorders, there has emerged a striking consistency in the CNVs that increase risk for a multitude of neurodevelopmental disorders, including autism, intellectual disability (ID), epilepsy, ADHD, schizophrenia, Tourette syndrome, and obsessive–compulsive disorder (OCD) (for reviews, see Malhotra & Sebat, 2012; McGrath et al., 2014; E. Morrow, 2010). Recurrent CNVs in specific regions throughout the genome have been associated with several different neurodevelopmental disorders with wide-ranging odds ratios (i.e., typically in the range of 3–30), indicating highly variable risk profiles for each disorder depending on the genetic locus (Malhotra & Sebat, 2012). Taken together, it is surprising to see specific CNVs associated with such diagnostically distinct disorders. These findings underscore that behavioral diagnoses do not necessarily reflect underlying etiological processes (Smoller, 2013a). Interestingly, many of these CNVs are sometimes seen in unaffected controls as well. These findings underscore the *probabilistic,* rather than deterministic, nature of the risk and the complexity of the risk factors in the learning disorders.

Thus, there is evidence from molecular genetics that genes might be largely generalists for neurodevelopmental disorders, as we saw in the behavioral genetic analyses. Next steps for these molecular genetic designs are to directly test whether individual genetic risk factors increase the risk for specific comorbidity patterns in individuals. Right now, we know that the same genetic risk factors are associated with different disorders in different samples, but we do not yet have the large-scale phenotypic information on comorbidity to test whether these same genetic risk factors are found more often in people with versus without specific comorbidities. When these study designs become feasible, we will have a better understanding of how shared genetic risk may contribute to comorbidity.

Cross-Disorder Genetic Sharing in RD and ADHD

We now turn to the specific comorbidity of RD and ADHD to illustrate how behavioral and molecular genetic methods have been applied to this specific comorbidity. The comorbidity of RD and ADHD has been well-studied with bivariate behavioral genetics methods. The *correlated liabilities model* (Willcutt, 2014) is most strongly supported by behavioral genetic (Ebejer et al., 2010; Greven, Rijsdijk, Asherson, &

Plomin, 2012; Wadsworth et al., 2015) and neuropsychological (Willcutt et al., 2005) evidence. This model posits that shared genetic influences between RD and ADHD cause both disorders to manifest in the same child more often than expected by chance (Pennington, 2006; Willcutt, 2014). Estimates of the genetic correlation are approximately .70 (Willcutt et al., 2010). Longitudinal behavioral genetic twin studies also show that these shared genetic influences are stable across childhood and adolescence (Ebejer et al., 2010; Greven et al., 2012; Wadsworth et al., 2015). In other words, the genetic factors that are shared between reading and attention remain stable over time, even despite new genetic influences on each phenotype that can arise over time (Ebejer et al., 2010; Greven et al., 2012; Wadsworth et al., 2015).

We mentioned earlier that our neuropsychological studies of the RD + ADHD comorbidity have identified PS as a potential shared cognitive deficit (McGrath et al., 2011; Peterson et al., 2017; Willcutt et al., 2010). In a genetic follow-up study to these findings, we utilized twin modeling to show that *all* of shared genetic influences between reading and inattention were also shared with PS (Willcutt et al., 2010), which indicates that PS may be a marker of the correlated liability of the two disorders. This study design illustrates how neuropsychological predictors can be integrated into behavioral genetic designs to begin constructing a multilevel explanation of comorbidity.

Molecular genetic studies have not yet identified consensus, replicated, shared risk genes for reading and attention although some early studies pointed to genetic neighborhoods where these genes might be found (Willcutt et al., 2002). Currently, molecular genetic studies are limited by the massive sample sizes required for cutting-edge, genomewide analyses. Although sample collection efforts are ongoing, sample sizes in RD and ADHD, along with several of the other learning disorders, have lagged behind the thresholds needed to find replicated genetic effects in other psychiatric disorders (i.e., schizophrenia, $N = 36,000$ cases; Ripke et al., 2014). In the meantime, while sample collections are proceeding for the learning disorders, the generalist genes hypothesis implies that many of the genes found for one learning disorder will also be associated with others. This powerful concept means that genetic advances in one disorder will likely be relevant to other learning disorders. This is good news given that amassing sample sizes in the tens of thousands for each learning disorder would be prohibitively expensive. Instead, the generalist genes hypothesis can guide the judicious use of resources to benefit genetic advances for the learning disorders collectively.

Brain

The generalist genes hypothesis also has implications for cognitive neuroscience (Kovas & Plomin, 2006). Embedded in this hypothesis is the possibility that generalist genes will manifest in "generalist brains" by influencing distributed brain networks, which in turn impact multiple cognitive functions (Kovas & Plomin, 2006). This conceptualization is somewhat at odds with the more traditional cognitive neuroscience framework that seeks to identify specific brain regions that are linked to specific cognitive functions. However, Kovas and Plomin (2006) point out that as the body of cognitive neuroscience findings is growing, it is rare to find 1:1 mappings between a cognitive task and a specific brain area. Most cognitive tasks activate multiple brain areas and, similarly, many brain areas respond to different types of cognitive tasks (Kovas & Plomin, 2006). These emerging patterns have led to an increasing focus on functional networks in the brain rather than specific brain regions. This emphasis corresponds with a generalist pattern at the brain level that mirrors the findings at the genetic level. Similarly, the multiple-deficit model (Pennington, 2006) predicts that shared neural risk factors will contribute to comorbidities across the developmental spectrum. Hence, both the generalist genes hypothesis and the multiple-deficit model highlight the importance of searching for generalized neural risk factors underlying comorbid developmental disorders.

In line with the broader cognitive neuroscience literature, neuroimaging studies of learning disorders have mainly focused on differences in brain structure and function between persons with a single disorder and typically developing controls (reviewed in Chapters 9–14). However, despite high rates of comorbidity, it is relatively rare for neuroimaging studies to directly study these comorbidities. Of the learning disorders, two comorbidities that have garnered early interest from a neuroimaging perspective are RD + ADHD (i.e., Kibby, Kroese, Krebbs, Hill, & Hynd, 2009) and ASD + ADHD (Gargaro, Rinehart, Bradshaw, Tonge, & Sheppard, 2011). These studies most commonly use a group-based design in which they compare, for example, ASD only versus ADHD only versus ASD + ADHD versus controls to determine whether the comorbid group shows the additive effects of each individual disorder or a unique pattern characteristic of comorbidity. To date, sample sizes have been small, and there is no clear consensus on this question for the RD + ADHD and ASD + ADHD comorbidities.

Neuroimaging studies of comorbidities in learning disorders are rare, but it is rarer still to consider transdiagnostic neural correlates that are common to a broader range of disorders. Yet these studies are the ones that most directly test the implications of the generalist genes hypothesis and the multiple-deficit model. In a recent meta-analysis, Goodkind et al. (2015) took such a transdiagnostic approach to identify shared neural correlates of a broad spectrum of adult psychiatric disorders. We review these findings because, to our knowledge, such a whole-brain analysis has not been undertaken for learning disorders (for a cross-disorder analysis of the cerebellum, see Stoodley, 2015), yet the method and approach are clearly relevant.

In the Goodkind et al. (2015) meta-analysis, the authors focused on structural neuroimaging findings, specifically voxel-based morphometry studies of clinical disorders versus controls. The disorders covered a broad range of adult psychiatric disorders (i.e., schizophrenia, bipolar disorder, major depressive disorder, substance use disorders, OCD, and anxiety disorders). The authors meta-analyzed the existing studies of each disorder, then conducted a conjunction analysis to identify regions of overlap that were common across disorders. Results pointed to the dorsal anterior cingulate cortex and the bilateral insula as regions with less grey matter across clinical disorders. Furthermore, the authors showed in follow-up analyses in datasets of healthy adult controls that these two regions are tightly coupled when the brain is at rest and during task performance, and that less grey matter in these regions is correlated with poorer executive functioning on behavioral tasks. Additional analyses ruled out medication use as an explanation for the structural commonalities across disorders.

Recent studies provide additional context for the regions of interest identified by Goodkind et al. (2015): the dorsal anterior cingulate cortex and the bilateral insula. These areas are core nodes in an important brain network termed the *salience network*. The salience network is hypothesized to play a role in cognitive control by guiding attention to motivationally salient stimuli. Consistent with Goodkind et al., structural and functional alterations in the salience network have been implicated in a diverse range of psychiatric disorders (for a review, see Peters, Dunlop, & Downar, 2016). These findings are notable for identifying a transdiagnostic neural signature that is common across a diverse array of adult psychiatric disorders (Goodkind et al., 2015).

One lesson from Goodkind et al. (2015) is that the predominant approach to clinical neuroimaging studies, which involves contrasting those with a single disorder and controls, will lead to an underappreciation of the commonalities across disorders. Although this study focused on adult psychiatric disorders, it is relevant that the findings implicate brain regions associated with executive dysfunction. These findings coincide with the literature in child-onset disorders, which has similarly reported executive dysfunction and other aspects of higher-order cognition as cross-disorder deficits (McGrath et al., 2016; Willcutt, Sonuga-Barke, Nigg, & Sergeant, 2008). Thus, it is reasonable to predict that similar analyses conducted with child samples might uncover brain commonalities across learning disorders that are associated with executive dysfunction, though this hypothesis awaits empirical confirmation.

These kinds of transdiagnostic studies align well with the current National Institute of Mental Health (NIMH) initiative called the Research Domain Criteria (RDoC), which aims to provide a new, cross-disciplinary research framework for mental health disorders (Insel et al., 2010). The goal of the RDoC is to encourage research in the pathophysiology of disorders, especially genomics and neuroscience, that is not constrained by current diagnostic boundaries. The hope is that this transdiagnostic framework will guide future classifications systems that are better aligned with the pathophysiology of disorders (Insel et al., 2010). While the RDoC initiative is emerging out of the NIMH, it is still clearly relevant for the learning disorders as well.

Neuroimaging of RD and ADHD

There are robust neuroimaging literatures for RD and ADHD, but despite high levels of comorbidity, research designs are just beginning to examine the comorbid group (i.e., Kibby et al., 2009). As noted earlier, there is not yet a consensus on whether the comorbid group is an additive combination of the deficits associated with each of the single disorders, or whether it is a qualitative or quantitative departure from an additive combination. Nevertheless, this study design, which compares the comorbid group to the single-disorder groups, is not optimized for identifying shared neural correlates between RD and ADHD. For instance, a contrast of RD only versus RD + ADHD typically focuses on regions in which the comorbid group differs from the single-disorder group, not regions where they have similar abnormalities compared to controls. Yet this latter analysis is the most relevant one for identifying shared risk factors and potential contributions to comorbidity.

It is clear from the existing neuroimaging literatures of RD and ADHD that there are not obvious points of overlap in the brain regions classically associated with each disorder. For RD, the most commonly implicated neural correlates involve a reading network that comprises left occipitotemporal regions, left temporoparietal regions, and the left inferior frontal gyrus. For ADHD, the prefrontal cortex and striatum tend to be the most common associations. Without an obvious candidate region of overlap, studies will have to be powered for discovery of new associations common to both disorders.

Although there is not a specific region of the brain that is consistently associated with both RD and ADHD, previous work on the neuropsychological correlates of RD and ADHD can guide hypotheses. For example, we previously discussed our finding that PS is a shared cognitive deficit of both RD and ADHD. The most consistent neural correlate of PS is white matter volume and integrity, with broad involvement from frontal, parietal, and temporal regions (Turken et al., 2008). These associations lead to the hypothesis that compromised white matter integrity may jointly increase risk for reading and attention problems via processing speed impairments. This hypothesis illustrates how the multiple-deficit model can make predictions across levels of analysis to elucidate mechanisms underlying comorbidity.

As these hypotheses indicate, there is much more work to be done toward identifying shared neural correlates for RD and ADHD specifically, and learning disorders more generally. As in the genetics work, advances in comorbidity science at the brain level of analysis will require large samples that are well-characterized across a full spectrum of developmental phenotypes, so that associations with brain regions can be properly attributed to a single disorder versus a comorbid state. In addition, a methodological focus on *shared* neural correlates for comorbid disorders rather than the prevailing emphasis on neural *distinctions* between disorders will be most relevant for testing the multiple-deficit model and identifying neural factors that increase risk for multiple disorders simultaneously.

SUMMARY

The multiple-deficit framework for this book seeks to identify mechanistic explanations for learning disorders across levels of analysis. It is increasingly clear that the same multilevel approach to comorbidities is needed. This kind of research is inherently complex, involving multiple levels of analysis, as well as covariances within each level of analysis (see Figure 5.1).

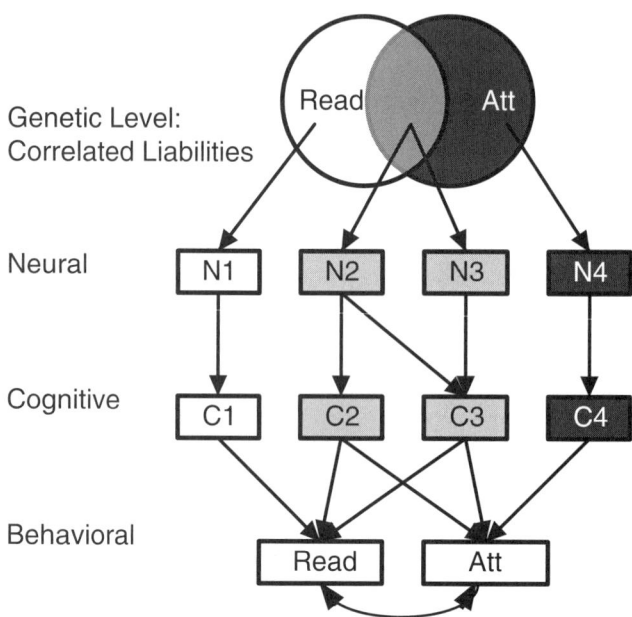

FIGURE 5.1. Hypothetical, multilevel multiple-deficit model depicting shared (grey) and unique (black and white) cognitive and neural predictors of the reading–attention comorbidity.

This research will benefit from research designs that directly focus on predicting covariance between comorbid disorders. As described earlier, typical statistical methods focus on variance (rather than covariance) and unique predictive power (rather than shared predictors). Thus, the research that will advance comorbidity science most effectively will require a departure from the typical methods in the learning disorders field. Comorbidity science could also benefit from developmental research designs to map a clearer understanding of causal pathways between disorders over time (i.e., to what extent does RD predict ADHD, ADHD predict RD, and/or both are attributable to a third factor?) By drawing on statistical and developmental methods already available and deploying them in the context of the multiple-deficit framework, comorbidity science is poised to make considerable gains in the coming years.

Clinical Implications

One clinical implication from this chapter is that some comorbidities are so prevalent that an assessment for one disorder necessitates an assessment for the other. This is certainly the case for RD and ADHD. In fact, ADHD is comorbid with all of the other learning disorders discussed in this book and should therefore be screened as part of these assessments. Similarly, a referral for one learning disability should often be accompanied by at least a screening assessment of a broad range of academic and language skills because of the frequent comorbidities of RD, mathematics disability, and language impairment. Furthermore, learning disorders are frequently accompanied by socioemotional challenges at such high rates that we recommend a broadband screening questionnaire for general psychological concerns even when these issues are not part of the referral question.

A related clinical implication is that we should expect and even plan for comorbidities in children with learning disorders. The child with a "pure" disorder is the anomaly, not the child with comorbidity. Such a lens on our clinical work can lead us to look for resilience factors in children with the "pure" disorders that may have prevented the onset of comorbidity. Such insights could lead to new research ideas about interventions that might prevent the onset of comorbidity.

As clinicians, we seek to understand the developmental unfolding of these disorders and even to infer causal precedence to one disorder over another. In the case of learning disorders, this inference can be difficult to make. In many cases, we do not have the research data from longitudinal studies to guide these inferences. A common example of such an inference is the idea that a child's ADHD is secondary to reading problems or that his or her reading problems are secondary to ADHD. We see both of these interpretations commonly in our clinical work, yet such a causal argument can lead to reduced services for children who truly struggle with symptoms of both RD and ADHD. For clinicians, we would like to highlight the explanation that is most consistent with the genetic and neuropsychological evidence that children with comorbid RD and ADHD have "true" forms of both disorders that arise from shared genetic and neuropsychological risk factors for both disorders. With this interpretation, the default assumption is that a child would need supports for both of these symptom dimensions rather than assuming that ADHD symptoms will improve when reading improves or that reading will improve when ADHD improves. Although these latter possibilities would be excellent outcomes, we believe the evidence argues that we should not wait for these optimal outcomes but instead plan for meeting the child's educational and behavioral needs related to both RD and ADHD.

The inevitability of comorbidity also encourages us to have strong interdisciplinary collaborations in our clinical work. Gillberg (2010) coined the acronym ESSENCE (Early Symptomatic Syndromes Eliciting Neurodevelopmental Clinical Evaluations) to describe the generalized neurodevelopmental symptoms that often present in children by ages 3–5 years. These early symptoms often progress to full-blown learning and developmental disorders in later years. He notes that these children may have their first point of clinical contact with any one of a host of medical and mental health providers (special educators, social workers, pediatricians, speech and language pathologists, neurologists, child psychiatrists, child psychologists, geneticists, occupational therapists, physical therapists). Yet because of the diffuseness of the children's symptoms, they often need consultation and services from several of these professionals but do not receive them, especially during these early critical years for intervention (Gillberg, 2010). As clinicians, we need to plan for the inevitability of comorbidities that will require a broad range of services.

In this chapter, we have highlighted the prevalence and breadth of symptoms that should be expected for children who present with learning disorders. The research indicates that these children are some of the most vulnerable in terms of response to treatment and functional outcomes. Fortunately, important advances are being made in comorbidity research that should yield more promising assessment and treatment protocols for these children.

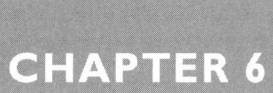

CHAPTER 6

Specific Learning Disorder
DSM-5 and Beyond

This chapter brings us to the final level of analysis in our multilevel model, namely, the level of behavioral symptoms that define disorder. It provides an overview of the DSM-5 diagnosis specific learning disorder, including the strengths and weaknesses of the DSM-5 approach. The biggest changes from the DSM-IV to DSM-5 are the use of a single "umbrella" diagnosis of specific learning disorder, with specifiers to indicate which academic skills are impacted as opposed to distinct diagnoses for specific learning disorder in reading, writing, or math; and a shift in the type of discrepancy that is required for diagnosis. DSM-IV required that a child's achievement be below expectations for both age *and* intelligence, whereas DSM-5 requires only age discrepancy. The specific academic skills domains considered by the DSM have also been updated, with the current manual including specifiers related to basic reading (word reading or decoding), complex reading (reading comprehension), basic math (calculation or number sense), complex math (problem solving), basic writing (spelling), and complex writing (composition). The main strengths of the new approach are (1) recognition of the high rate of comorbidity among learning disorders and (2) the distinction between what we call "simple" and "complex" learning disorders. The main weakness is the failure to appreciate that some of the six possible diagnoses are not empirically validated. A second weakness is that some very bright individuals with clinically impairing academic difficulties no longer qualify for diagnosis. In what follows, we present the DSM-5 approach and its strengths and weaknesses in more detail.

To understand how academic skills develop through formal schooling, it helps to consider what it takes to become an expert in some nonacademic skills, such as painting, musical composition, tennis, or fly-fishing. Any expert in these domains has spent many years mastering basic skills (drawing skill, instrumental music skill, basic tennis strokes, or casting skills, respectively) before he or she can deploy those basic skills strategically and creatively. Therefore, an expert has to have developed *automatic* basic skills, then be able to combine these with higher-level thinking skills. The same is true for the three complex academic skills listed earlier (reading comprehension, math problem solving, and written composition). They depend on automatic and highly specific basic skills (i.e., in single-word reading, handwriting and spelling, and basic number concepts and calculation skills, respectively) coupled with more general higher-level cognitive or language skills. We call these latter skills "complex *non*academic skills" (Table 6.1). They are *complex* because they have more cognitive components than basic academic skills; they are nonacademic (at least in part) because they develop without formal instruction, although formal instruction definitely strengthens them.

Thus, just as a visual artist cannot become an expert without highly developed drawing skills, a child cannot become an expert in reading comprehension without automatic basic reading skills. Similarly, becoming an expert in written composition requires automaticity in the basic academic skills of handwriting and spelling (which we call *transcription*). Becoming an expert in mathematical problem solving requires automaticity in the basic number concepts and calculation skills. Despite considerable practice, some individuals find it much harder to develop automaticity in some of these basic skills, and they may have a specific learning disorder in that basic academic skill (i.e., what is sometimes called *dyslexia, dysgraphia,* or *dyscalculia,* respectively). Other individuals may develop automaticity in a basic skill, say single-word reading, but still struggle to use that skill to understand what they read (sometimes called *poor comprehenders*). This view of the development of expertise in academic skills embodies a simple but powerful theoretical concept, the *resource allocation hypothesis* (Perfetti, 1998), which holds that cognitive resources are limited, so performance in a given complex academic skill depends on one's overall level of cognitive resources and on how many of those resources have to be devoted to basic skills that are not yet automatic. Hence, any complex academic skill is limited by the level of basic academic skill the person has. As a result, even a very bright child with a basic skill deficit will perform more poorly at the complex level than would otherwise be expected, because too much of the child's attention and processing resources are being devoted to a basic academic skill. Consequently, a child with a problem in single-word reading (i.e., dyslexia) will have poorer reading comprehension than his or her oral language comprehension skill would predict, because too many cognitive resources are being devoted to decoding individual words, which are not recognized automatically. Similarly, a child with poor handwriting and spelling (poor transcription skills) will have poorer written composition than his or her oral language composition skill (which we call "narration") would predict, for the same reason. And, a child with poor basic math skills (in basic number concepts and calculation skills) will have poorer mathematical problem-solving skills than his or her general ability to solve novel problems (fluid intelligence) would predict.

This resource allocation hypothesis is captured in so-called "simple" models of reading comprehension and written composition; a similar model could be proposed for mathematical problem solving. Gough and Tunmer's (1986) simple model of reading comprehension proposes that the complex academic skill of

TABLE 6.1. Generalized Simple Model of Academic Skills

Basic academic skill	+	Complex nonacademic skill	=	Complex academic skill
1. Single-word reading	+	Listening comprehension	=	Reading comprehension[a]
2. Transcription (spelling and handwriting)	+	Narration	=	Written composition[b]
3. Basic number concepts and calculation skills	+	Novel problem solving	=	Math problem solving

[a]Gough and Tunmer (1986).
[b]Berninger et al. (2002).

reading comprehension depends on two subskills, single-word reading skill (a basic academic skill) and listening comprehension (a higher-level nonacademic skill). Research indicates that automaticity in single-word reading sets a limit on reading comprehension, even in adults, providing strong support for this model (García & Cain, 2014). A "simple model" of writing skills has been proposed (e.g., Berninger et al., 2002), paralleling the simple model of reading comprehension. In the simple model of writing skill, the two subskills are transcription (i.e., handwriting fluency and spelling) and narration. Empirical studies reveal that the higher-level skill of written composition is limited by degree of skill in the basic or lower-level skill (transcription). The empirical results for each simple model (of reading comprehension and written composition) are consistent with the resource allocation hypothesis (Perfetti, 1998) discussed earlier. As mentioned earlier, one could also formulate a simple model of skill in mathematical reasoning or problem solving.

Table 6.1 presents these three simple models of complex academic skills we have been discussing. In each case, a complex academic skill, such as reading comprehension, is predicted by the sum of a basic academic skill and a complex nonacademic skill. The domains of academic skills listed in DSM-5 diagnostic criteria (see Table 6.2) map closely onto the basic and complex academic skills listed here. Of these three, the simple model of reading comprehension has been tested most extensively. Future research will refine this overall model by (1) testing which basic academic and complex nonacademic skills are key in each of the three domains, (2) examining the degree of etiological and cognitive overlap across the three domains, and (3) testing how specific learning disorders relate to other developmental disorders, such as attention-deficit/hyperactivity disorder (ADHD), speech sound disorder (SSD), and language impairment (LI), as well as to other internalizing and externalizing childhood psychopathologies. As we noted earlier, some of the six specific learning disorders are not yet well validated, so future research may result in some diagnoses being "lumped" into existing categories (e.g., language disorder). Future studies will also continue to wrestle with the question of how "specific" learning disorders have to be, and whether a child with generally low and even performance across numerous cognitive and academic domains should be said to have a learning disability.

TABLE 6.2. Synopsis of DSM-5 Criteria for Specific Learning Disorder

A. Persistent difficulties in one or more of these six academic skills:
   1. *Basic*: Single-word-reading accuracy and fluency (defining symptom of *dyslexia*).
   2. *Complex*: Reading comprehension ("poor comprehenders" have this defining symptom).
   3. *Basic*: Spelling (nearly always found in dyslexia; does not define a separate disorder).
   4. *Complex*: Written expression.
   5. *Basic*: Number sense, math facts, and calculation skills (defining symptom of *dyscalculia*).
   6. *Complex*: Mathematical reasoning.

B. The score on a test of the academic skill is substantially below the mean score for the patient's chronological age[a] and causes functional impairment.

C. Problems begin in early school years, but complex learning disorders only become clinically significant in later academic years.

D. Not due to intellectual disability (ID); peripheral sensory disorders; other mental or neurological disorders; psychosocial adversity; lack of proficiency in the second language used for instruction (e.g., child is a native Spanish speaker in the United States and is not yet proficient in English); or inadequate educational instruction.

[a]The penultimate draft included the phrase "or IQ," which is important for identifying gifted children with learning disorders (see text).

DSM-5, unlike DSM-IV, incorporates this important distinction between basic and complex academic skills. Some children have a specific learning disorder only in a simple skill, others only in a complex skill, and still other children have problems in both. Differential diagnosis among these three alternative possibilities is important for treatment. A child whose reading problem is restricted to reading comprehension, called a "poor comprehender" in the research literature (Cain, Oakhill, & Lemmon, 2004; Nation, 2005) needs a different intervention than a child whose reading problem is mainly at the level of single-word reading accuracy and fluency. The same can be said for children with handwriting versus written composition problems or math fact/calculation problems versus problems with mathematical reasoning.

Hence, as we discuss later, current research provides some support for six specific learning disorders: two each in reading, writing, and mathematics, although the research support for this distinction between a basic and complex learning disorder is much stronger in the domain of reading than in the domains of writing and mathematics. These six learning disorders correspond closely, but not perfectly, to the six specifiers in DSM-5. The six specifiers do not include handwriting skill, which, when combined with spelling, makes up the basic academic skill of transcription. There is not empirical support for an isolated learning disorder in spelling.

DSM-5 also marks a major and controversial change over DSM-IV in putting all specific learning disorders under one heading ("lumping" instead of "splitting"). In DSM-IV, there were four specific learning disorders (i.e., reading disorder, mathematics disorder, disorder of written expression, and learning disorder not otherwise specified [LD-NOS]), and each disorder was described separately from the others. In contrast, in DSM-5, there is now *one* diagnosis, specific learning disorder, with different specifiers to indicate which domains of academic skills are affected. This shift to one umbrella diagnosis is consistent with considerable research (reviewed in Chapter 5) demonstrating substantial comorbidity among specific learning disorders. However, the change also introduces two new problems. First, it risks neglecting the fact that some specific learning disorders (including dyslexia, which is also called *reading disability* [RD], and mathematics disorder [MD], which is sometimes called *dyscalculia*) have much more evidence to support their diagnostic validity than others. The practitioner should not assume that all the possible specific learning disorders that can be generated by the six descriptive feature specifiers (see Table 6.2) are valid disorders, as discussed earlier, and this will be made clearer in what follows. Second, differential diagnosis among specific learning disorders is still important, because different treatments are needed for different specific learning disorders.

Another major change in DSM-5 over DSM-IV is the criteria for determining what makes the learning disorder *specific*. As spelled out in Section D in DSM-5 criteria (Table 6.2), the word *specific* in this context is meant to contrast with general learning problems that would generally be expected in cases of intellectual disability and other more severe diagnoses. So, the notion of a specific learning disorder means that the child's profile of academic skills is significantly uneven, such that only one or just a few academic skills are well below most other academic skills, which are at the level expected for a child's age or IQ, or both. In DSM-IV, the deficit in a specific academic skill had to be "substantially below that expected given the person's chronological age, measured intelligence, and age-appropriate education." The last of these three criteria meant that a child could not be given a specific learning disorder diagnosis if he or she had never been to school, had inadequate exposure or teaching, or had learning problems related to learning English as a second language. How to determine whether the learning problems were due instructional, contextual, or language factors was not spelled out and remains an active area of research.

With regard to the first two criteria, DSM-IV required that the deficit in an academic skill be significantly discrepant from both age *and* IQ expectation; that is, the diagnosis required *both* an age discrepancy and an IQ discrepancy. For instance, if a child's standard score on a reading achievement test was 70 (mean = 100, SD = 15) and his or her IQ was 100, then the child would meet the DSM-IV discrepancy criteria, because the child's reading was two SDs below both the mean for age (100 on the reading test) and his or her IQ (100).

This requirement of needing *both* and an age discrepancy and an IQ discrepancy for diagnosis was the focus of considerable subsequent research and public policy debate. Subsequent research found little external validity for the distinction between age-discrepant and IQ-discrepant RD (Francis, Shaywitz, Stuebing, Shaywitz, & Fletcher, 1996; Hoskyn & Swanson, 2000; Stuebing, Barth, Molfese, Weiss, & Fletcher, 2009; Stuebing et al., 2002). Children identified as RD by either discrepancy (age or IQ) appear similar in terms of their underlying neuropsychology and the types of treatments that are helpful.

Since the distinction between age and IQ discrepancy is therefore not clinically useful, DSM-5 *should* use an "or" criterion rather than an "and" criterion with respect to these two criteria. Instead, DSM-5 utilizes only an age-discrepancy criterion but acknowledges that "specific learning disorder may also occur in individuals identified as intellectually 'gifted'" (American Psychiatric Association, 2013, p. 69), which is typically defined as an IQ of 130 or greater (at least 2 *SD*s above the mean IQ of 100). But requiring a significant age discrepancy in such a child (e.g., the suggested cutoff of a standard score of 78 in some academic skill) makes it much harder for a gifted child to meet diagnostic criteria than a nongifted child, because the child must perform at least 3.5 *SD*s below his or her IQ level, whereas a child with an average IQ of 100 need only perform 1.5 *SD*s below his or her IQ level! A very bright child might be only IQ discrepant in a specific academic skill such as reading accuracy or fluency, whereas a child with an average or lower IQ might be only age discrepant. We argue that *both* these children should receive a diagnosis of specific learning disorder if their problems are clinically impairing, whereas *neither* child would have met DSM-IV criteria, and only the second child meets DSM-5 criteria.

In DSM-IV, defining learning disorders was based primarily on performance on individually administered standardized tests. A positive change in DSM-5 is its emphasis on the full clinical picture—including history and observations, in addition to specific test scores. Nonetheless, standardized test scores remain very important in diagnosis and, according to DSM-5, are required in individuals ages 17 and younger.

In later chapters, we provide more detailed information on the two best-validated learning disorders, dyslexia and mathematics disorder. Less research has been done on writing disorders. We were only able to identify two epidemiological studies of writing disorders, each using a single sample (Katusic, Colligan, Weaver, & Barbaresi, 2009; Yoshimasu et al., 2011). Results included (1) the school-age population prevalence of DSM-IV disorder of written expression was 6.9–14.7%, depending on the exact definition; (2) there was a male predominance in the gender ratio (two to three males per female); (3) the comorbidity with RD or dyslexia was very high (75%); and (4) of the remaining 25% without dyslexia, nearly 30% had ADHD. This high comorbidity with RD indicates that a clinician evaluating writing problems in a child should always evaluate for dyslexia and, conversely, a clinician evaluating reading problems in a child should always consider whether the child also has writing problems.

Wagner et al. (2011) modeled the development of written language skill and found results broadly consistent with the simple model of writing explained earlier: The simple skill of handwriting fluency and the complex skill of productivity (i.e., number of words produced) each had a median effect size of over 2.0 (Cohen's *d*) in explaining developmental differences between first and fourth graders in written composition skill. Hence, this study demonstrated that the development of written composition skill requires both automaticity in handwriting and the ability to generate words to express ideas. Consequently, in evaluating a child with a writing problem, these two components should be assessed, along with the child's reading skill (because of the high comorbidity between reading and writing problems). ADHD should also be assessed, because it not only can affect the ability to organize a written or oral discourse but it also shows high comorbidity with all learning disabilities.

Unfortunately, assessing writing skills in children has turned out to present some practical challenges. We have found in our research and clinical practice that different measures of writing, particularly those assessing higher-level aspects of writing, are not highly correlated, which raises questions about how reliable they are and whether they are assessing the same underlying construct. For example, in a sample of approximately 100 children ages 8–16 that consisted of children with learning disabilities, ADHD, and controls, we found a correlation of just $r = .10$ for the Story Composition score on the Test of Written Language, Fourth Edition (TOWL-4), and the Thematic score on the essay of the Wechsler Individual Achievement Test–Third Edition (WIAT-III). This relationship was smaller than virtually all other correlations among a wide variety of cognitive and academic tasks, including some that were designed to measure theoretically distinct constructs. In contrast, writing tasks that focus on some of the more basic aspects of writing, such as the Woodcock–Johnson Writing Fluency and Writing Samples tasks showed a stronger correlation, $r = .49$, in our sample. These results highlight the need for more reliable measures of higher-level writing skills in order to assess this important domain, which is frequently impaired in children with learning disabilities and/or ADHD.

How should clinicians implement the framework provided by DSM-5 for diagnosing learning disabilities? Chapter 7 provides an overview of the general evaluation approach that we recommend and also tackles some common questions and issues that may arise. Here, we briefly critique two approaches that have been recognized by U.S. law (the Individuals with Disabilities Education Act [IDEA], 2004) as appropriate for identification of learning disabilities in educational settings. Although the definition of specific learning disability is not identical in DSM-5 and IDEA, they are quite similar. Both have at their core poor academic skills development in the absence of a few exclusionary conditions. Both posit that the academic difficulties must cause clinically significant problems but do not specify precisely a cutoff that should be used. IDEA, however, does identify two general approaches that may be used to diagnose specific learning disability: the patterns of strengths and weaknesses model (PSW) and the response-to-intervention model (RTI).

As its name implies, the idea behind PSW is to identify meaningful clusters of strength and difficulty in the child's profile. Such an approach seems appealing because it considers the child's academic weaknesses in the context of other cognitive and academic skills, and aligns with our intuitive sense that there must be something *specific* about a specific learning disability. However, we have already seen the challenges inherent in trying to set even *one* cutoff point on a continuous distribution of any single academic or cognitive skill. Operationalizing a PSW definition necessarily requires setting cutoff points on multiple continuous measures, which just magnifies this difficulty. The result is that the majority of students with clinically impairing literacy problems do not meet PSW criteria, and even a relatively small change in diagnostic criteria results in a large shift in which specific children are identified (Miciak, Fletcher, Stuebing, Vaughn, & Tolar, 2014; Stuebing, Fletcher, Branum-Martin, & Francis, 2012). These problems make using the PSW for individual diagnosis impractical and potentially harmful.

The RTI model attempts to address many of problems inherent in other diagnostic approaches. It is increasingly used in schools and is recognized by both by IDEA and DSM-5 as an acceptable method to identify specific learning disabilities. The idea behind RTI is that all children should be provided with evidence-based instruction, and the progress of all students should be monitored. Children who are not making expected progress then participate in some additional instruction (e.g., increased attention from the classroom teacher or more work in small groups) but do not initially go through a lengthy evaluation progress or receive a diagnosis or individualized education program (IEP). Some of these children respond well to instruction and may not need further intervention. Children who fail to respond adequately progress to a higher level of intervention. Eventually, more detailed evaluation, such as that required for IEP eligibility, is considered, though schools vary in how many "tiers" of initial intervention the child must pass through first.

The RTI model has many notable strengths. First, it should go without saying that *all* schools should provide *all* children with core academic instruction that is based on the best available evidence. Second, RTI attempts to address the problems inherent in setting a single diagnostic threshold on a continuum by providing for more fluid movement in and out of intervention than has historically been the case with special education eligibility. Third, RTI emphasizes early intervention, which is known to be more effective than waiting until children have experienced years of academic failure, and can almost certainly help prevent some cases of learning disabilities.

The RTI model is not without challenges either, however. In practice, it can sometimes mean that more comprehensive evaluation and intensive intervention are delayed, because a child with difficulties must pass through several levels of intervention first, each of which takes time. Further evaluation with an appropriate expert may be especially important for a student whose academic difficulties are not due solely to an isolated learning disability, but who might have an undiagnosed autism spectrum disorder, intellectual disability, language disorder, psychiatric disorder, or ADHD. As we have already seen, comorbidity among learning disorders is the rule rather than the exception, but the RTI model emphasizes limited assessment of academic domains, typically by individuals who do not have the appropriate training to evaluate for these comorbid disorders.

SUMMARY

As this chapter has illustrated, the conceptualization of learning disabilities has evolved with the iteration of DSM-IV to DSM-5. Simultaneously, the dialogue between psychology and education about best practices for learning disorder identification in schools continues. At this point, there continue to be important unresolved issues. Some that we have highlighted in this chapter are the questionable validity of some of the specific learning disorder specifiers, challenges in diagnosing gifted children, and questions about the best implementation of RTI for children with varying levels of severity of learning challenges.

CHAPTER 7

Evidence-Based Practice in Assessment

In Chapters 1–6 we have described the multilevel, multiple-deficit model that guides our understanding of learning disorders and provided evidence for that model across levels of analysis. Our goal in this chapter is to help clinicians apply the theoretical model to diagnostic decision making in individual cases. Toward that end, we provide a general overview of our approach to the assessment of learning disorders, then discuss some specific issues that diagnosticians frequently face. First, however, we discuss the important reservations many adults have about "labeling" children and the question of whether behavioral diagnoses are appropriate at all.

Teachers, parents, and even clinicians are frequently suspicious of behavioral diagnoses for children. Many have seen examples of the diagnostic process gone awry: a child mislabeled or a diagnosis improperly conveyed. Furthermore, some children change so much in such a short amount of time that it may not be appropriate to label them. Adults may understandably be unsure about applying a "medical model" approach to diagnosis out of concern that it does not capture the individuality of the child's problems. Robin Morris (1984) has said, "Every child is like all other children, like some other children, and like no other children." In other words, some characteristics are species-typical, others are typical of groups within the species, and still others are unique to individuals. As diagnosticians and therapists, it is important to have a good handle on which characteristics fall into which category. Some patients have symptoms that they feel are unique to them but that are in fact virtually species-typical. Other symptoms are fairly specific to a particular diagnosis, and still others are unique to a given patient. Although a good clinician must be aware of and make use of a patient's unique attributes, scientific progress in understanding and treating mental disorders (including all the learning disorders included in this book) depends on there being "middle-level" variation—differentiating characteristics of groups within our species. If not, mental health work reduces either to just treating the life problems everyone faces or to re-creating the field for each unique individual. On the one hand, we say there are no mental disorders, because everyone is "in the same boat." On the other hand, we say there are no mental disorders, because everyone is different. A science of mental health is not tenable at either extreme. Although there is much confusion and many limitations in the current state of knowledge about developmental disorders in children, this state of affairs hardly means that a science of developmental psychopathology or developmental neuropsychology is impossible.

Another important point to remember is that the patient has the diagnosis rather than the diagnosis having the patient (e.g., Achenbach, 1982). In other words, diagnoses do not provide an explanation for every aspect of the patient's being. Furthermore, nosologies classify disorders, not people. It is easy to fall into the shorthand of talking about "dyslexics," "autistics," or "schizophrenics," but these labels can be just as stereotyping and potentially stigmatizing as other labels based on ethnicity, religion, or certain medical illnesses. So many mental health practitioners and advocates prefer "people-friendly" language, which holds that a person with autism is not reducible to an *autistic*. Perhaps not surprisingly given the historical stigma associated with disabilities and the power of words to impact attitudes, this question remains controversial, and some in the disability community have more recently expressed a preference for "identity-first" language, because it emphasizes the disability as an inherent part of who the person is (e.g., "an autistic woman" rather than "a woman with autism"). We emphasize person-first language throughout this book but recognize that many factors influence which terminology might feel preferable to an individual person. We strongly support the idea that people with disabilities should be able to make their own choices about what language feels right and best conveys a sense of dignity.

Although diagnoses have limitations, they are important for several reasons. Diagnoses permit efficient identification and treatment, and facilitate communication among professionals caring for a child. Diagnosis itself can be therapeutic for parents and children, because an accurate diagnosis provides an explanation for troubling symptoms and a focus for the efforts the parents and child patient are already making to alleviate the symptoms. In many cases, access to appropriate educational or therapeutic supports is dependent on having a particular diagnosis. From a public health standpoint, research on a given diagnosis can lead to early identification/prevention. Finally, studies of diagnostic groups can contribute to basic research on human development.

OVERALL APPROACH TO ASSESSMENT

The assessment process begins when a child is referred by a particular source. For most of the learning disorders considered in this book, children are usually referred by parents, teachers, pediatricians, or other professionals because of concerns about their progress in school, although for disorders with relatively more general effects on development (e.g., intellectual disability, and autism), concerns typically arise before formal schooling. Clear understanding of the referral question is a critical first step in any evaluation. The evaluator should first ensure that answering the question falls within his or her boundaries of competence, and if so, should use the information provided to begin tailoring his or her approach. Referral questions can provide early clues about potential diagnoses, neuropsychological domains most likely to be impacted, and which people or institutions in the child's life may need guidance in supporting the child.

The overall approach should be holistic in three ways. First, it should consider the developing child in the context of his family, school, and broader community. Indeed, one way of understanding the reason a child is referred for evaluation is because of a mismatch between his skills and abilities at a given point in his development and the environmental demands being placed on him, rather than a deficit that resides within the child alone (Bernstein & Waber, 1990). The focus on a growing brain—rather than an already mature system—is a fundamental difference between child and adult assessment, and means that professionals who evaluate children must have specialized knowledge regarding typical and atypical child development.

Second, the assessment should include careful evaluation of multiple domains of functioning. These will include not only the neuropsychological domains discussed in Chapter 4, but also social, emotional, and behavioral adjustment. Third, the competent professional uses multiple streams of information to understand the full clinical picture. The HOT (History, Observations, Test results) mnemonic (Bernstein & Waber, 1990; Bernstein & Weiler, 2000) is a useful way to remember the three main streams of information to be analyzed in the evaluation process. In our experience, most professionals who perform learning disorder evaluations do gather and report information from all three streams. However, common errors include failing to integrate across the three or overemphasizing individual data points in decision making. Diagnostic errors can easily occur when clinicians base their conclusions on limited data, such as assuming that a child who hand flaps must have autism, or that a child with intact phoneme awareness cannot have dyslexia. Competent diagnosis arises not from a single symptom or test score, but from a balanced integration of all the data from three streams of information in the HOT mnemonic. Below, we briefly review considerations related to each of these information sources.

HISTORY

For children, history is provided largely by the parents or guardians. In our clinics, we use structured background parent questionnaires to gather information about the referral problem, the family history, pregnancy and birth, relevant medical history, the child's early development, school history, and psychosocial history. This information is clarified through follow-up clinical interview with parents or other primary caregivers. Older children and adolescents may often provide some of the relevant history themselves. Parents and children vary in the accuracy of their reports, and errors are not uncommon. Thus, it is valuable also to gather more objective historical data such as educational records and any previous evaluation reports. For children whose learning or developmental problems may be linked to an underlying medical condition, review of medical records is also important. Evaluation of such children should only be undertaken by a professional with appropriate background knowledge and training related to the medical diagnosis, such as a pediatric neuropsychologist.

Several aspects of a child's history are particularly relevant for accurate diagnosis of learning disorders. First, the clinician should have a clear understanding of the history of the referral problem. As discussed previously, more global neurodevelopmental disorders such as intellectual disability or autism typically onset early in development, well before school entry, whereas a relatively more specific learning disability typically is evident relatively soon after formal schooling begins. An individual who made good educational progress for many years before the emergence of school difficulties is unlikely to have a traditional learning disability. Of course, the child's context will also help determine the extent to which problems are evident. For example, some symptoms related to attention-deficit/hyperactivity disorder (ADHD) (e.g., difficulties with organization) may become evident only when environmental demands increase. Clinical concern often arises once the child reaches a new academic "stress point," such as the transition from elementary school to middle school, when a much higher level of independent organization is expected. Typically, in these cases, careful history taking will reveal subtle weaknesses that have been present for a long time but were not necessarily clinically impairing in a different environment. Sudden onset of new learning or developmental problems in a previously typically developing child is rare and generally inconsistent with the learning disorders covered in this book. Such a presentation is concerning and would warrant a referral to the primary care physician and/or specialist to determine what further medical and psychiatric workup may be needed.

As should already be clear, it is always important to gather the child's early developmental and educational histories. Did the child achieve early motor, language, and social milestones within the expected time frames? Did he or she participate in any early physical, occupational, or speech–language therapies? When did teachers first become concerned? How do teachers typically describe the child? Has he or she gotten extra help in school, and if so, what kind? The astute diagnostician should be aware that parents and professionals more frequently observe some kinds of developmental problems than others that may go unnoticed. For example, delayed acquisition of early language skills is a hallmark of a language disorder, but these delays may be missed unless the child also has a comorbid speech sound disorder (D. Bishop & Hayiou-Thomas, 2008). Once again, these issues interact with the child's context, and a child from a lower socioeconomic status (SES) family is particularly at risk for not coming to clinical attention (D. Bishop, McDonald, Bird, & Hayiou-Thomas, 2009).

Since all of the disorders considered in this book are partly heritable, biological family history is highly relevant to the evaluation. This, of course, includes any history of diagnosed learning disorders, especially in those closely genetically related to the referred child. However, because some family members may not have been formally evaluated or diagnosed, it can be helpful to ask more general questions about any relatives who may have had trouble in school or with learning or behavior. More guidance around these issues is provided in Chapters 9–14 on specific disorders.

For the majority of children with developmentally based learning disorders, pregnancy, birth, and medical histories are either unremarkable or noncontributory, but some children have risk factors (e.g., significant prematurity, prenatal alcohol exposure, or congenital heart disease, to name just a few) that might help to explain their current difficulties. A review of these factors and their expected effects on brain and cognitive development is beyond the scope of this book; for an overview, see Yeates (2010). We do recommend gathering information about sleep on all children presenting for evaluation. Inadequate quality or quantity of sleep can cause problems with attention, behavior, and/or learning that are best treated with sleep-related interventions (e.g., Ali, Pitson, & Stradling, 1996). Furthermore, children with a variety of neurodevelopmental disorders are at increased risk for sleep problems. Even when sleep problems are not the primary cause of a child's developmental problems, there is growing evidence that sleep may moderate the outcomes and thus be an important potential treatment target (e.g., Breslin et al., 2014).

A thorough understanding of the whole child also entails taking a good psychosocial history. In some cases, psychosocial adversity may be all or part of the etiology of the child's problems and may potentially even help to clarify the diagnosis and drive treatment (as in the example of a previously typically developing child who develops symptoms of inattention only after exposure to a traumatic event). Furthermore, because of the comorbidity between learning disorders and other developmental psychopathologies (e.g., depression, anxiety, or oppositional defiant disorder), all children referred for learning concerns should be considered to be at elevated risk for emotional and behavioral difficulties, and should at least be screened for concerns in these areas.

OBSERVATIONS

Behavioral observations can provide a rich source of information about a child's functioning across diverse neuropsychological domains, including social skills, emotion and behavior regulation, attention, language and communication, motor skills, and even aspects of nonverbal skills and memory. The chance to gather this information begins with the clinician's first contact with the child and continues throughout the evaluation process. Accumulated clinical experience with a diverse clientele eventually allows a thoughtful practitioner to develop "internal norms" about what sorts of behaviors are especially notable or meaningful in the evaluation environment. Of course, these norms should be sensitive to factors such as the child's age, gender, family background, and other contextual considerations. In addition to these relatively general behavioral observations, structured observations on objective tests (e.g., regarding problem-solving approach, error type) can be very important. As we discuss in more detail in the specific disorder chapters, such observations can be part of the accumulation of evidence for or against a particular diagnosis.

Thus, behavioral observations provide their own source of data that must be integrated with the child's history and objective test scores in developing a holistic picture of the individual. No psychological test provides a "pure" measure of a single domain of cognitive functioning; instead, good performance relies on many factors. Thus, behavioral observations are also important to ensure appropriate interpretation of various test scores. For example, a child might earn a low score on a design copying test because of problems in visual–spatial judgment, motor coordination, impulse control, attention, or even language comprehension if he or she is confused about the directions. Thus, automatically interpreting a low score as indicative of a problem in "visual–motor integration" or as a "constructional deficit" would be inaccurate in many cases, and careful behavioral observations may help clarify the true reason or reasons for the difficulty.

Clinicians generally collect behavior samples in standardized and semistandardized contexts. These offer a number of advantages, as we discussed earlier, because over time, the clinician develops a good sense of common versus unusual reactions to different testing conditions, as well as which of those reactions correlate with the "middle-level" variation so important to accurate diagnosis. However, the testing environment has limits as well, and usually does not give a realistic picture of many important aspects of children's functioning. How do the children interact with peers? How do they regulate their behavior in a busy classroom environment filled with distractions? Some professionals schedule outside observations of children in the school setting to address this limitation. We prefer to rely on vicarious observations provided by parents, teachers, and other professionals through interviews and behavior rating scales. We find this approach more efficient and cost-effective, as well as more accurate, because people who know the child well have a much larger sample of behavior on which to draw.

TEST RESULTS

As the foregoing discussion should make clear, the evaluation process is about more than just tests. Accurate diagnosis and optimal treatment planning do not simply flow from a mechanical interpretation of even the most thoughtfully selected or comprehensive test battery. However, standardized, objective tests can be quite powerful and help us understand a particular child and answer the referral question at hand. Below we discuss a few issues for consideration in the development and interpretation of a test battery for learning disorders.

Performance Validity

Before interpreting a child's performance on any test, the evaluator will want to be reasonably confident that the score provides a valid estimate of the child's functioning. In other words, if a child gets a low score, we want to know that it is because the child truly had difficulty with the task and not because he or she was not paying attention, refused to follow directions, was falling asleep, or pretended to have more significant difficulties than he or she really has (to name just a few possibilities). Historically, evaluators working with children have relied primarily on their clinical judgment to ensure the child is optimally engaged with the task and thus to infer that the results were valid. However, a growing body of literature highlights the fact that clinical judgment alone is inadequate to make this determination, and that inclusion of objective performance validity tests is an important component of evaluation with children. For an in-depth review of this topic, see Kirkwood (2015).

Objective measurement of performance validity has long been recognized as important in adult assessment, but only more recently has it received attention in the child/pediatric realm. This is likely because many practitioners have assumed that children would not intentionally exaggerate difficulties in front of a clear adult authority figure. However, we now know that children can deceive adults, that under some circumstances, children do feign a variety of medical, psychiatric, and cognitive problems, and that adults do not consistently detect children's deceptions. Thus, just as good clinicians do not rely on judgment alone to assess a child's intelligence, language functioning, memory, or any other cognitive skill, they should also routinely include objective measurement of performance validity in psychological testing batteries.

Several performance validity tests have now been validated for use with children or developed specifically for pediatric use (for a review, see Kirkwood, 2015). In general, these tests are quick and easy to administer. They are designed to look difficult but are actually easy and relatively insensitive to ability-based cognitive problems. In most cases, school-age children with true learning or developmental problems can readily pass these tests as long as they exert adequate effort. Validity test failure has substantial implications for interpreting the remainder of a psychological test battery. For example, one study indicated that validity test performance accounted for nearly 40% of the variance in ability-based test performance (Kirkwood, Yeates, Randolph, & Kirk, 2012).

Because the importance of objective validity testing in children has only recently been recognized in the research and clinical realms, the rates of validity test failure in various populations are largely unknown. The rate of exaggerating or feigning cognitive problems is thought to be quite high (>50%) in some forensic or compensation-seeking contexts, such as children referred for independent evaluation for Social Security Disability evaluation (Chafetz, 2008). In clinically referred samples, rates appear to vary by population. Children referred with persistent problems following a mild head injury are thought to have the highest rate of invalid or "noncredible" presentations among those seeking clinical evaluation, roughly around 15% (Kirkwood, 2015). The rate of noncredible presentations among children and adolescents referred clinically for learning concerns is most likely lower but not zero. Consider the substantial potential for secondary gain depending on the evaluation results, such as access to accommodations for high-stakes testing or to stimulant medication (Harrison, Flaro, & Armstrong, 2015).

Some clinicians may be reluctant to include formal validity tests in their assessment batteries, because they are understandably uncertain about how to handle failures. What becomes of the rest of the assessment, and what sort of feedback should be given to the family under these circumstances? The answers, of course, will vary depending on clinical context. On any single test, false positives and false negatives can certainly occur, so inclusion of multiple measures is recommended. In addition, considering whether the overall pattern of test results is consistent with the child's history and presenting concerns is important. In cases in which the evaluator becomes reasonably confident that the child has put forth suboptimal or inconsistent effort, this by itself becomes a clinically important finding. The next step is to attempt to determine what the child's motivation might be, so that appropriate interventions or responses can be designed. A model exists for how to handle suspected noncredible effort with adult patients (Carone, Iverson, & Bush, 2010) and fortunately, a related model has been developed for use in pediatric settings (Connery & Suchy, 2015). Preliminary evidence suggests that use of this model relates to positive outcomes, including high levels of parent satisfaction with the evaluation process (Connery, Peterson, Baker, & Kirkwood, 2016).

For example, one of us (RLP) previously evaluated Jake, a 16-year-old boy who was a junior in high school. Jake had done very well throughout elementary and middle school, but his grades had dropped a bit in the previous year (from all As to a mix of As and Bs). He told his parents that he felt he "couldn't focus" in class or on homework and thought he had ADHD, so they brought him for evaluation. Review of educational records revealed no attentional or behavioral concerns from teachers early on. His performance on multiple performance validity tests was indicative of suboptimal effort. In addition, scores on some additional measures in the battery were far below average and inconsistent with Jake's educational and developmental histories. Careful clinical interview revealed that he felt considerable pressure to excel in school and thought that he "had" to attend one of a few highly competitive colleges. Jake was overwhelmed by his current schedule, which included multiple extracurricular commitments. On most nights, he did not start his homework until after 9:00 P.M. and did not fall asleep until midnight. He had a close friend who had been prescribed stimulant medication and found it helpful. Jake seemed to think that an ADHD diagnosis would lead to a similar prescription for himself, which he hoped would allow him to study harder and perform better in his courses and on high-stakes testing.

At the feedback session, Jake's suboptimal effort was explained to his parents and potential reasons were explored. They were at first surprised that he would not have tried his best on all the tests, since he was typically a very hardworking young man. However, they did acknowledge that he was likely overwhelmed and overscheduled, and were open to the possibility that he may have thought stimulant medication would offer him an "out." No ADHD diagnosis was rendered. The clinician explained that while Jake might be having difficulties focusing at times, these were more likely related to stress or inadequate sleep than to a developmental disorder. In feedback with Jake, he did not openly admit to poor effort, but he did agree that he felt stressed about school and wanted help. Jake was referred to psychotherapy to help him clarify his own goals for school and activities, and to promote healthy coping and stress management skills.

In summary, since the previous edition of this book was published, it has become increasingly clear that objective performance validity tests play an important role in the assessment of school-age children and adolescents referred for learning or developmental concerns. These tests are quick and easy to administer, are fairly insensitive to ability-based problems, and have substantial implications for both interpretation of the rest of the evaluation data and clinical management.

Battery Selection

We advocate a flexible battery approach that is tailored to address the referral question and guide clinical management. For diagnosis of the disorders considered in this book, objective test results are helpful and in many cases necessary. However, information from a well-chosen test battery provides more than just diagnostic clarification. If we cared only about arriving at the correct diagnostic decisions, the test battery could sometimes be quite brief. On one extreme, consider the case of ADHD, which primary care and mental health providers routinely diagnose on the basis of clinical interviews and behavior rating scales alone. However, even in this case, more comprehensive neuropsychological or psychoeducational testing can help identify comorbid learning disorders or weaknesses that may be contributing to the observed problems (Pritchard, Nigro, Jacobson, & Mahone, 2012).

We discussed in Chapter 4 the neuropsychological constructs that are most relevant to understanding learning disorders, including crystallized and fluid intelligence; attention, executive functions, and processing speed; and language/communication. In most cases, the test battery should at least touch on each of these domains, although the depth of assessment needed will vary depending on clinical presentation. As previously discussed, declarative learning/long-term memory is less relevant to most of the disorders considered in this book, with the exception of intellectual disability. Thus, detailed objective assessment of this domain is often not critical, but it may still be valuable to provide information to parents and teachers, including help answering referral questions related to memory concerns. Academic skills are not considered a neuropsychological domain per se, but objective assessment in this area is critical to rule specific learning disabilities in or out. Finally, as discussed in the "History" section, every child referred for school or attention concerns should be screened for emotional and behavioral problems (i.e., through parent and/or self-report rating scales and clinical interviews) because of the comorbidity between learning disorders and other childhood psychopathologies.

In most cases, appropriate measurement of all these domains involves a fairly comprehensive test battery. However, in some cases, a more abbreviated approach is also reasonable, while being more cost-effective and efficient. For example, consider a child who has a clear history of fairly isolated difficulty with literacy acquisition in the context of otherwise normal development and school performance. In this case, careful assessment of literacy skills, along with a brief cognitive/language screening, may suffice for the clinician to provide diagnostic clarification and treatment guidance. Of course, even in such a case, the examiner should remain attentive to any evidence of possible comorbid conditions.

Table 7.1 provides a (nonexhaustive) summary of psychological tests and rating scales appropriate to measure the neuropsychological and academic domains most relevant to the assessment of learning disorders. In addition, Chapters 9–14 on specific disorders include case examples with sample test batteries.

Base-Rate Variability

Interpretation of standardized psychological test performance is typically performed by determining where an individual's score falls in the population, based on the normal curve. For example, consider a child who earns a scaled score of 5 on a particular test, which corresponds to a standard score of 75 and falls 1.67 SDs below the mean, at the 5th percentile. This score is "below average," so it may be considered to be indicative of some degree of impairment. However, the meaning of a low score can vary depending on how many tests have been administered. While it is true that only 5% of the population scores at or below a scaled score of 5 on that particular test, no psychological evaluation includes only a single test. How many children earn one low score out of 10, 20, or even more subtests, as would typically be included in a testing battery? The answer turns out to be quite a lot. For example, 31% of children earned one or more scores at or below the 5th percentile on the 10-subtest Wechsler Intelligence Scale for Children, Fourth Edition (WISC-IV; Brooks, 2010). Furthermore, although some clinicians interpret subtest scatter as itself being indicative of learning problems, this approach is misguided, because such variability is also common among typically developing children. Again considering the WISC-IV, 73% of healthy children had at least a 2 SDs (6 scaled score points) spread between their highest and lowest subtest score, while 23% had at least a 3 standard deviation (9 scaled score points) spread (Brooks & Iverson, 2012; Wechsler, 2003). Frequency of scatter varies with performance level, with greater scatter being even more common among overall higher-performing children.

Both of the preceding examples are based on the WISC-IV, but the presence of some low scores and scatter within a battery of tests is common regardless of the specific tests used. The issues arise because, with each subtest, the clinician is really testing a statistical hypothesis on a single individual. Just as researchers must adjust the threshold for statistical significance when making multiple statistical comparisons, savvy clinicians must do the same thing. To aid clinicians and researchers attempting to make meaning out of multiple test scores, an empirically derived definition of "neuropsychological impairment" has recently been proposed using the National Institutes of Health (NIH) Pediatric Sample (Beauchamp et al., 2015). These researchers found that performance at or below 1.5 SDs below the mean on at least two out of a battery of eight subtests identified approximately 5% of the sample and was considered abnormal, or indicative of neuropsychological impairment. Of course, most clinical batteries include substantially more than eight subtests, so this empirical criterion will need to be adjusted accordingly (i.e., more than two scores would need to be low in a larger battery to be considered abnormal). In addition, as previously noted, it is always very important for evaluators to

TABLE 7.1. Psychological Tests Commonly Used in the Assessment of Learning Disorders in Children and Adolescents

Construct	Test	Reference
Performance validity	Medical Symptom Validity Test (MSVT)	P. Green (2004)
	Test of Memory Malingering (TOMM)	Tombaugh (1996)
	Memory Validity Profile (MVP)	Sherman & Brooks (2015)
	Word Memory Test (WMT)	P. Green (2003)
Crystallized and fluid intelligence[a]	Wechsler Intelligence Scale for Children—Fifth Edition (WISC-V)	Wechsler (2014)
	Wechsler Preschool and Primary Scale of Intelligence—Fourth Edition (WPPSI-IV)	Wechsler (2012)
	Wechsler Adult Intelligence Scale—Fourth Edition (WAIS-IV)	Wechsler (2008)
	Wechsler Abbreviated Scale of Intelligence—Second Edition (WASI-II)	Wechsler (2011)
	Differential Ability Scales—Second Edition (DAS-II)	Elliott (2007)
	Kaufman Brief Intelligence Test—Second Edition (KBIT-2)	Kaufman & Kaufman (2004/2014)
	Woodcock–Johnson—Fourth Edition (WJ-IV) Tests of Cognitive Abilities	Schrank, McGrew, & Mather (2014c)
Language[b]	Comprehensive Test of Phonological Processing—Second Edition (CTOPP-2)	Wagner, Torgesen, Rashotte, & Pearson (2013)
	Clinical Evaluation of Language Fundamentals—Fifth Edition (CELF-5)	Wiig, Semel, & Secord (2013)
	Clinical Evaluation of Language Fundamentals—Preschool—Second Edition (CELF-Preschool-2)	Semel, Wiig, & Secord (2003)
	Peabody Picture Vocabulary Test—Fourth Edition (PPVT-4)	Dunn & Dunn (2007)
	Test of Language Development—Fourth Edition (TOLD-4)	Newcomer & Hammill (2008)
	Expressive Vocabulary Test—Second Edition (EVT-2)	Williams (2007)
	Woodcock–Johnson—Fourth Edition (WJ-IV) Tests of Oral Language	Schrank, McGrew, & Mather (2014b)
Attention, processing speed,[c] and executive functions	*Performance-based measures*	
	Conners Continuous Performance Test Third Edition (Conners CPT 3)	Conners (2014a)
	Conners Kiddie Continuous Performance Test Second Edition (K-CPT 2)	Conners 2014b)

(continued)

TABLE 7.1. *(continued)*

	Gordon Diagnostic System	Gordon, McClure, & Aylward (1996)
	Test of Everyday Attention for Children—Second Edition (TEA-Ch2)	Manly, Anderson, Crawford, George, & Robertson (2016)
	Delis–Kaplan Executive Function System (D-KEFS)	Delis, Kaplan, & Kramer (2001)
	Tower of London—Drexel University—Second Edition (ToLDX-2)	Culbertson & Zillmer (2005)
	Selected subtests, NEPSY—Second Edition (NEPSY-II)	Korkman, Kirk, & Kemp (2007)
	Wisconsin Card Sorting Test (WCST)	Grant & Berg (1948); Heaton, Chelune, Talley, Kay, & Curtiss (1981)
	Rey Complex Figure Test (RCFT)	Rey (1941); Osterrieth (1944); Meyers & Meyers (1995)
	Questionnaire measures	
	ADHD Rating Scale–5 (ADHD-RS-5)	DuPaul, Power, Anastopoulos, & Reid (2016)
	NICHQ Vanderbilt Assessment	National Institute for Children's Health Quality (2002)
	Conners—Third Edition (Conners 3)	Conners (2008)
	Behavior Rating Inventory of Executive Function—Second Edition (BRIEF-2)	Gioia, Isquith, Guy, & Kenworthy (2015)
Academic skills	*Performance-based measures*	
	Woodcock–Johnson—Fourth Edition (WJ-IV) Tests of Academic Achievement	Schrank, McGrew, & Mather (2014a)
	Wechsler Individual Achievement Test—Third Edition (WIAT-III)	Breaux (2009)
	Wide Range Achievement Test—Fourth Edition (WRAT-4)	Wilkinson & Robertson (2006)
	Kaufman Test of Educational Achievement—Third Edition (KTEA-3)	Kaufman & Kaufman (2014)
	Gray Oral Reading Tests—Fifth Edition (GORT-5)	Wiederholt & Bryant (2013)
	Test of Word Reading Efficiency—Second Edition (TOWRE-2)	Torgesen, Wagner, & Rashotte (2012)
	Nelson–Denny Reading Test	Nelson & Denny (1929); J. Brown, Fishco, & Hanna (1993)
	Questionnaire measure	
	Colorado Learning Difficulties Questionnaire (CLDQ)	Willcutt et al. (2011)

(continued)

TABLE 7.1. (continued)

Social, emotional, and adaptive functioning		
	Observation-based measure	
	Autism Diagnostic Observation Schedule—Second Edition (ADOS-2)	Lord, Rutter, et al. (2012)
	Questionnaire measures	
	Behavior Assessment System for Children—Third Edition (BASC-3)	Reynolds & Kamphaus (2015)
	Achenbach System of Empirically Based Assessment (e.g., Child Behavior Checklist)	Achenbach (1991)
	Social Communication Questionnaire	Rutter, Bailey, & Lord (2003)
	Social Responsiveness Scale—Second Edition (SRS-2)	Constantino & Gruber (2012)
	Autism Diagnostic Interview—Revised (ADI-R)	Rutter & Le Couteur (2003)
	Adaptive Behavior Assessment System—Third Edition (ABAS-3)	Harrison & Oakland (2015)
	Vineland Adaptive Behavior Scales—Third Edition (Vineland-3)	Sparrow, Cicchetti, & Saulnier (2016)

[a]Several of these tests include measures of processing speed, working memory, and attention.
[b]As discussed in Chapter 4, there is considerable overlap between many language measures and measures of crystallized intelligence.
[c]Many speeded measures in other areas of this table correlate highly with processing speed (e.g., rapid naming, math fluency).

seek convergent evidence in the child's history, behavior observations, and patterns of test results, to prevent the misinterpretation of a single test score.

COMMON QUANDARIES AND CONFUSIONS

In this section, we discuss a few questions that commonly arise when trying to apply what we know about diagnostic categories to individual patients. Diagnostic decision making generally requires practitioners to make a yes-or-no decision, but many cases fall in a grey area. Anyone who has participated in case conferences to decide whether particular children have the learning disorders we discuss in this book has likely experienced some heated discussions related to the issues below!

Etiology

Definitions of learning disorders are generally defined by symptoms or behaviors regardless of the root causes, or *etiology*, of the difficulties. We know that in terms of understanding variation at the population level, all the disorders in this book are partly genetic and partly environmental. However, these population estimates tell us nothing about etiology in any individual case. There are individuals whose learning disorders are almost entirely genetic and others whose learning disorders are almost entirely environmental. (Imagine two hypothetical boys, one with intellectual disability related to fragile X syndrome, the other with intellectual disability related to fetal alcohol exposure.) Knowing about the etiology of a given child's problems is often meaningful to caregivers and is in some cases relevant to clinical management. However, etiology by itself does not rule behavioral diagnoses in or out.

For some of the disorders included in this book, DSM-5 explicitly excludes children whose problems are due solely to environmental disadvantage. Thus, a child who cannot read or solve math problems only because he or she has had no access to formal education does not have a specific learning disability. Extreme cases such as this are rare among children referred for clinical evaluation, however. For most children, the presenting concerns are the end result of a complex developmental process that has included multiple genetic and environmental risk factors interacting over many years. Some practitioners assume that if a child's learning difficulties appear to be of (partly or fully) environmental etiology, then a "medical model" diagnosis is necessarily inappropriate. We disagree and, in fact, think that this misconception can lead to denial of services that could legitimately benefit children who are already disadvantaged disproportionately.

For example, one of us (RLP) recently evaluated an adolescent girl with longstanding and broad-based learning and cognitive concerns. She was medically healthy, without recent concerns or changes. On objective testing, her intellectual and adaptive functioning scores fell below the cutoff for a mild intellectual disability, and her current clinical difficulties were also quite consistent with this diagnosis. However, previous estimates of some of her cognitive skills many years earlier had been somewhat stronger. She had also experienced several historical environmental disadvantages, including attendance at poor-performing schools (based on the state's rating system), many years of frequent school absences, and significant family stress.

The neuropsychologist diagnosed mild intellectual disability, explained the basis for the diagnosis, and advocated for access to related school-based and community resources. However, the school psychologist questioned the diagnosis, arguing that many of the current learning difficulties were likely a result of environmental disadvantage. It is indeed possible or even likely that under more enriched environmental conditions, this young woman could have developed differently, and ultimately had a relatively higher IQ and adaptive skills. Unfortunately, however, at this point, the clock cannot simply be turned back on the many years of brain development that led to this outcome. In other words, the school psychologist's assumptions about etiology could well have been correct; education does lead to higher intelligence scores. Behavioral diagnosis is not dependent on etiology, however, and in this case, the label of intellectual disability served the meaningful purposes of explaining the clinical presentation and guiding intervention.

Severity

As previously discussed, all the disorders considered in this book are continuous disorders, in which the diagnostic category is thought to capture individuals falling in the low tail of an approximately normal distribution. Although the diagnostic threshold is not completely arbitrary (it would never make sense to say that an individual whose math skills were above the population mean had a math disability, for example), it is also not absolute. For some diagnoses (e.g., intellectual disability), current convention provides fairly concrete guidance about where the threshold should be set, although it is important to recognize that these conventions are determined in a particular sociopolitical context and have changed historically. For most diagnoses, considerable clinical judgment is required, as existing definitions provide only general guidance such as skills that are "substantially below" expectations and cause clinically meaningful problems. Diagnosis should not be based on low scores alone in the absence of evidence for functional impairment, although, of course, impairment also falls on a continuum. Thus, no matter which precise cutoff is used, there will *always* be individuals who fall into a grey area near the threshold and about whom reasonable professionals could disagree.

In these cases, it is especially important to consider the possible functions of a diagnosis discussed earlier. Does diagnosing the child provide a clear benefit by (1) helping to explain clinically significant problems, (2) guiding intervention, or (3) providing access to services or resources that otherwise would not be available? We can imagine two children with identical test scores for whom the answers to these questions might differ, impacting the decision about whether to render a diagnosis.

Practitioners are not obligated to make a black-and-white determination in every case. For some children, it is most appropriate to convey to parents and schools that the child does indeed fall somewhere in a grey area. In such cases, we include language in our written reports along these lines:

> "Johnny demonstrates weaknesses in [reading, math, attention, etc.] similar to those seen in children with [dyslexia, math disability, ADHD, etc.]. However, his difficulties do not currently appear to be severe or impairing enough to warrant a formal diagnosis. He can still be expected to benefit from a few relatively straightforward supports related to these weaknesses. In addition, because the picture may change as he gets older and academic demands increase, he should be monitored closely, and will likely benefit from reevaluation in the future [specific guidance around time frame should be tailored to clinical context]."

Specificity

The following discussion is probably most relevant to "specific" learning disabilities (dyslexia and math disability) and language disorder, though it has implications for nearly all the disorders considered in this book, with the possible exception of intellectual disability. For many disorders, there has historically been an emphasis on children who present with extreme discrepancies in their cognitive profiles, such as poor literacy development despite strong math skills, or weak language development despite good nonverbal problem solving. These cases are so striking to families, educators, clinicians, and researchers that it makes sense they would have come to attention first. However, increasingly, we are learning that they are likely the exception rather than the rule.

We discussed in Chapter 6 the problems of requiring an IQ discrepancy for diagnosis of a learning disability. Although most diagnosticians now recognize this shift in the field, many are still uncomfortable diagnosing learning disorders in the absence of an uneven profile. Consider a hypothetical 10-year-old girl who has long-standing difficulties with academic progress across the curriculum. Objective testing reveals generally low but even performance across multiple domains, including crystallized and fluid intelligence, basic literacy, math calculation, math problem solving, reading comprehension, and writing. Imagine that standard scores on all these measures cluster about a standard deviation and a half below the mean, or roughly between the 5th and 10th percentiles. Does she have a learning disability? In our experience, most clinicians say she does not, since there is clearly nothing very specific about her profile.

Although it makes intuitive sense to look for discrepancies when considering learning disorder diagnoses, there are both practical and theoretical problems with doing so. Many of the practical problems were discussed in Chapter 6. From a theoretical standpoint, we know that a great deal of variance is shared across all academic domains, and that the shared variance is very highly correlated with general intelligence, or g (Deary et al., 2007). Although we can identify individual children who are outliers in the multidimensional space of various academic and cognitive skills, many children who have difficulty in one area can be expected to have weaknesses in other areas as well. Furthermore, they are likely to respond best to the same kinds of evidence-based remediation as are children with a more specific profile (Stanovich, 2005). To us, it seems illogical to deny services (often made available through a learning disability diagnosis) to children on the basis of the fact that they have more widespread problems than children who do qualify for services!

SUMMARY

We have provided in this chapter a general framework for learning disorder evaluations and have discussed some issues that commonly arise in the process. No diagnosis can capture the totality of an individual person. When properly used, however, learning disorder diagnoses can be powerful tools to help us understand, explain, and predict a child's behavior; to guide effective intervention; and to help us provide access to needed services and resources. Disagreement about whether a particular child has a learning disorder frequently occurs, because any system of individual diagnosis that requires imposing a dichotomy on a continuum will be imperfect. However, because humans tend to think categorically, this remains a source of confusion and frustration for many, who continue to wonder if we could just come up with more accurate formulas for who "really" has the disorders. Such a solution is not logically possible, so clinical judgment about whether a diagnosis will be clinically meaningful remains important in diagnostic decisions.

CHAPTER 8

Understanding Achievement Gaps

The learning disorders considered in this book are an example of *individual* differences found within all groups. *Group* differences in cognitive or academic skills, whether groups are defined by country, sex, socioeconomic status, or race/ethnicity, can have a completely different explanation and require different methods of analysis. Because group differences in cognitive and academic skills almost inevitably invite simplistic explanations and considerable controversy, in this chapter we attempt to provide a balanced and nuanced review of this topic based on several recent reviews (Hunt, 2011; Loehlin, 2000; Nisbett, 2009).

Group differences in academic achievement are called *achievement gaps*. Such gaps are disturbing because they contradict our deeply held values about equal opportunity for all. Hence, when we first hear about achievement gaps, one immediate reaction may be to assume the tests must be biased. If the tests are biased, we can blame the test makers and those who use the tests and quickly move on. But what if there are similar gaps in wealth and health? Then it is not so easy to blame the tests. For these latter issues, we are more likely to say there are inequities in our broader society that lead to unequal outcomes. To be clear, it is important to rigorously evaluate the psychometric properties of a test for bias, a topic we will discuss later in the chapter. However, in the absence of data supporting test bias, blaming the tests themselves for achievement gaps can be an ineffective and overly simplistic solution to a complex problem. Like health and wealth gaps, achievement gaps are likely pointing to inequities embedded in our society. If we are committed to equal opportunity and social justice, we must try to close achievement gaps, just as we try to eliminate other inequities in our society.

In this chapter, we will show how we can use science to determine whether achievement gaps are real, and if they are real, how to close them. Our main conclusions are that achievement gaps *are* real, are caused mainly by social inequities, and that we already know a lot about how to remedy them. Given this scientific knowledge, it is incumbent upon all of us to work to change public policy to help close these achievement gaps.

In what follows, we (1) explain the distinction between individual and group differences; (2) present a framework for analyzing group differences; (3) apply it to different examples of group differences in IQ or academic achievement; (4) provide an example of implications for practice, research, and policy; and (5) conclude with a summary. By doing this in a careful, balanced way, we hope both to resolve some of the controversies and point to important implications for clinical practice, research, and public policy. Some decades ago, the National Institutes of Health (NIH) realized that medical research based exclusively on white males may not generalize either to white females or to other racial/ethnic groups. The same point applies to research and practice in the field of learning disorders. Hence, it is important for both scientists and practitioners in this field to evaluate whether what we know about learning disorders generalizes to other populations.

INDIVIDUAL VERSUS GROUP DIFFERENCES

To understand average differences between groups, it is necessary to understand some fundamental conceptual differences between individual and group differences. First of all, individual differences are measured by the *variance* within a group, whereas one measures a group difference mainly by comparing the *means* of the two groups. The variance and mean of a distribution are distinct constructs and are thus not causally related to each other. Hence, it is very important to understand that the etiology of a mean difference between groups tells you nothing about the etiology of individual differences within a group, or vice versa. One could be entirely due to the environment and the other could be entirely due to genes. For instance, a given trait such as height has very high heritability within groups, but many groups differ in height because of environmental differences in things like nutrition and health care. Like all human traits, height is malleable to an extent (i.e., it has an evolutionarily defined reaction range for our species). Because it is malleable, the mean height of groups can change over time as relevant aspects of the environment change. The mean height of the population in many European countries has increased considerably over the last 100 years or so, whereas the mean height of some developing countries has gone down. The etiology of these changes in group height almost certainly has to be due to the environment, because evolution does not happen fast enough to produce such changes. Thus, as the mean height in these countries was changing, the etiology of individual differences within each country remained the same (i.e., mostly due to genes). Height provides a real example of how we could change the environment to reduce group differences. Later, we consider how we might change the environment to *prevent* achievement gaps.

Hence, it is a logical fallacy to conclude that the reason for achievement gaps between groups *must* be genetic, if the etiology of individual differences within each group is largely genetic. That *could* be the case (consider the mean height differences between males and females), but it certainly does not have to be. In the history of the debate about IQ differences among racial groups, some researchers have fallen prey to this fallacy that the etiology of individual differences must be the same as group differences.

FRAMEWORK FOR ANALYZING GROUP DIFFERENCES

Our framework is presented in Figures 8.1 and 8.2. It first addresses the key question of whether the group difference is valid (Figure 8.1). Answering this question requires us to make sure the group difference is not due to a sampling bias and, if it is not, then to make sure the difference is not due to a measurement artifact. In other words, we want to know whether an observed group difference is actually in the *groups* (i.e., valid) and not in the *methods* that found the group difference. Finding the causes of a valid group difference requires the additional methods in Figure 8.2, which we discuss later.

Some of the group differences that have been found for learning disorders are at least partly invalid, because they are due to sampling biases or measurement artifacts. For instance, the often-cited large sex difference in dyslexia (three to four males for every female, abbreviated as 3–4 M:F) was first questioned in Hallgren's (1950) family study more than 60 years ago, but it remains in the literature many decades later. Hallgren demonstrated that this large sex difference was found only in probands (i.e., index cases) referred to his family study, whereas the sex difference in dyslexia among nonreferred relatives was much smaller, about 1.5 M:F. This referral artifact for dyslexia has been replicated numerous times (DeFries, Olson, Pennington, & Smith, 1991; Shaywitz, Shaywitz, Fletcher, & Escobar, 1990). The reasons for the smaller valid sex difference (1.5 M:F) in dyslexia are discussed in Chapter 10.

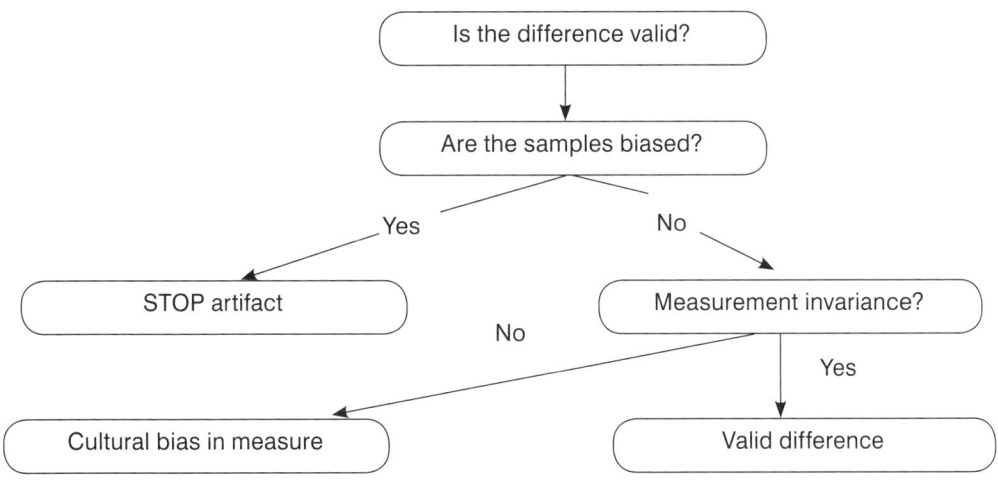

FIGURE 8.1. Framework for determining validity of group differences.

The method for examining a possible sampling artifact is to test whether the group difference replicates in a random population sample. But how do we test for a possible measurement artifact? There are well-established psychometric methods for evaluating test bias, or a deviation from measurement equivalence (Horn & McArdle, 1992; Reise, Widaman, & Pugh, 1993). Establishing measurement equivalence across groups is a multistep process that requires testing whether the internal and external validity of the measure is invariant across groups. With regard to internal validity, if the reliability of the measure, or its rank order of item difficulty, or its factor structure differs between groups, then that means the measure works differently in each group; thus, there is a measurement artifact. However, the most important test of measurement equivalence involves external validity, which requires that the test equally predict relevant outcomes across groups. For instance, an IQ test needs to predict academic achievement similarly across groups. If it does not, it is a biased measure. However, some deviations from perfect measurement equivalence may not completely invalidate a finding of a group difference. For instance, some items on a test may function differentially across groups, but the group difference can still have considerable external validity. Thus, there can be degrees of measurement equivalence across groups.

As we see in Figure 8.1, the issue of test bias is an empirical question. In the case of achievement gaps found in the United States, the results are derived from population samples with academic and cognitive tests that have been systematically examined for measurement artifacts. The results leave us to grapple with the causes of achievement gaps in the absence of strong evidence for test bias. Nevertheless, it is a common assumption in thinking about achievement gaps that any test that finds group differences is *necessarily* biased. However, in the case of the achievement gaps we will be discussing below, this is a less defensible position based on available data. It is also the case that a posture of blaming the tests for being biased, in the absence of supporting data, could stall efforts to make meaningful progress on reducing achievement gaps. If sample artifacts and measurement bias are not the primary explanations, then it is important to identify and address the underlying factors that may be contributing to achievement gaps.

If the group difference is largely valid, how can we determine its cause, that is, its etiology? As we discussed in Chapter 2, etiology consists of genes, environments, and their interplay. As already discussed, it is of fundamental importance to recognize that the etiology of individual differences within groups tells us nothing about the etiology of a difference between groups. As shown in Figure 8.2, an important first step in exploring the etiology of a group difference is to test how persistent it is, either across generations or across development. If the group difference changes across generations or only emerges later in development, then that result suggests the environment may be playing a role in causing the group difference, because evolution does not happen fast enough to produce genetic differences between generations, and because many (but not all) of the genes influencing cognitive development are expressed early in brain development, as discussed in Chapter 3. Hence, if the group difference changes in these ways (across generations and across development), it makes sense to first test environmental risk factors for the group

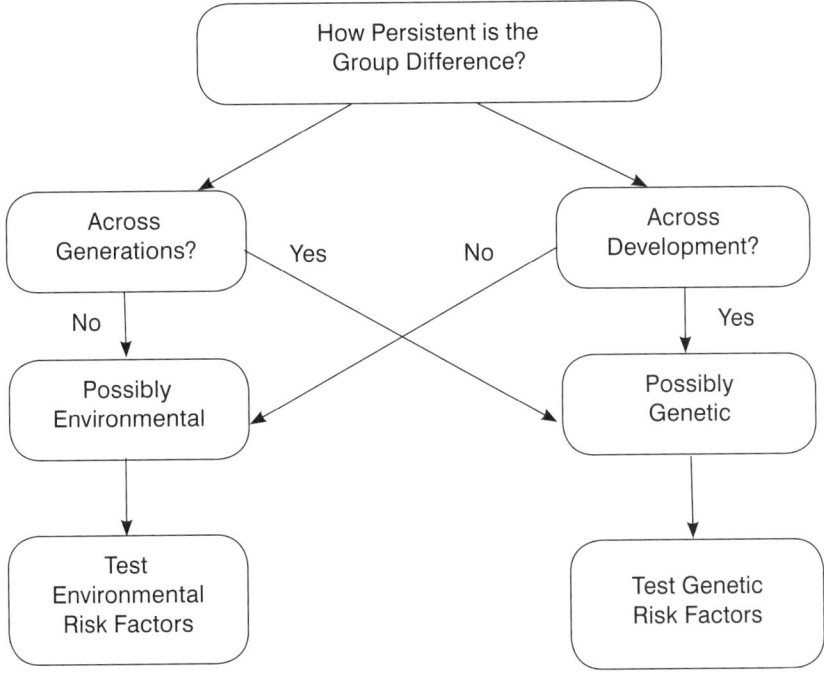

FIGURE 8.2. Analyzing the etiology of a valid group difference.

difference. On the other hand, if the group difference persists across both generations and development, it could still have an environmental etiology, such as one that is invariant across generations and exerts its effects in early development. For instance, lead exposure could work in this way. It could differ between two groups in a persistent way across generations, and it is known to affect early brain development. Testing for genetic risk factors that differ between groups requires knowing what the relevant genes are for the outcome being studied, in this case, cognitive and academic outcomes, then testing whether the frequency of risk alleles for those outcomes differs between groups. Because cognitive and academic outcomes are highly polygenic and most of the risk alleles are unknown, this approach is currently not very feasible. In contrast, for some etiologically simpler health outcomes, such as sickle-cell anemia or phenylketonuria (PKU), there are known ethnic group differences in the frequency of risk alleles that explain group differences in the prevalence of the disorder.

COUNTRY DIFFERENCES: THE WEALTH OF NATIONS REVISITED

Now we apply the framework in Figures 8.1 and 8.2, beginning with country differences. This section draws on an excellent review of this topic by Hunt (2011).

There are well-replicated country differences in average cognitive skills, whether measured by IQ tests or academic achievement tests (Rindermann, 2007). What makes these country differences in cognitive skills important is that they reliably predict country differences in important outcomes such as average income, adult literacy, life expectancy, and democratization. In other words, these country differences in mean IQ have considerable external validity.

To understand country differences in cognitive skills, we apply the analytic frameworks in Figures 8.1 and 8.2 to determine whether these group differences are valid, and if they are, what their causes are. Concerning validity, there are many more concerns about sampling biases and measurement equivalence in the international IQ dataset collected by Lynn and Vanhanen (2006) than in the international achievement dataset used by Rindermann (2007). A random population sample for IQ testing is much harder to obtain in lower-income countries, and in many cases, when data were lacking, Lynn and Vanhanen (2006) estimated a country's average IQ from its neighbor! In addition, measurement equivalence for IQ tests across countries has not been established. Finally, Lynn and Vanhanen (2006) advocated a genetic explanation for country differences in IQ, a claim that could well be fallacious given these threats to validity and the logical problems in extrapolating genetic findings for individual difference in IQ to groups, in this case, country differences.

Given all these problems in the Lynn and Vanhanen study (2006), many readers may be tempted to dismiss the whole topic of average country differences in cognitive skills. And so would we, were it not for the fact that average country differences in IQ reported by Lynn and Vanhanen strongly predicted average country differences in academic achievement (on the Program for International Student Assessment [PISA]) in Rindermann (2007). Sampling biases and measurement equivalence have been thoroughly investigated for the PISA, and indicate that average country differences in academic achievement found in Rindermann (2007) are valid. Because the country differences in IQ predict country differences on the PISA, we cannot so easily dismiss Lynn and Vanhanen's (2006) finding of country differences in average IQ, even though we can certainly disagree about their etiology.

Specifically, Rindermann (2007) found near-perfect convergence between average IQ and average achievement scores across countries. Note here that datapoints represent country means rather than individuals. Both IQ and achievement measures loaded between .97 and 1 on a general cognitive factor. Similar to results discussed in Chapter 4, Rindermann's (2007) results mean that the g of academic achievement is very similar, if not identical, to cognitive g. That this is true of both individual and group differences is an important result, but it is key to remember that despite this similarity in factor loading, the underlying causes may differ in the two cases. For instance, the cause of country differences could be entirely environmental, whereas we already know that the cause of individual differences in IQ and academic achievement has substantial genetic and environmental contributions.

Because he had longitudinal data, Rindermann (2007) was able to do a cross-lagged analysis, which can begin to disentangle the developmental relations among correlated variables, such as cognitive skill and average income. Country averages for both cognitive skill and average income changed over the decades covered by the dataset, indicating malleability. Earlier average cognitive ability of individual countries predicted later average income, but the reverse was also true, indicating reciprocal causation (i.e., a positive feedback loop). Further analyses demonstrated that this virtuous cycle was mediated by adult education level and the country's investment in early education.

In summary, Rindermann (2007) replicated many of the cross-sectional correlations between countries' average cognitive skill and important national outcomes found by Lynn and Vanhanen (2006), but he took the important next step of testing *directional* relations among these variables. He found that both the average cognitive skill and important national outcomes were malleable and reciprocally related to each other. Hence, the policy implications of Rindermann's (2007) results are quite different from the hereditarian perspective provided by Lynn and Vanhanen (2006).

Might there be an environmental explanation for country differences in cognitive skills? Rindermann's (2007) analysis points to the influence of factors such as the country's investment in early education. However, one important, overlooked reason for such differences in cognitive skill is health, particularly the health of children; we consider this topic next.

Eppig, Fincher, and Thornhill (2010) found that an environmental risk factor, namely, parasite prevalence, accounted for about 80% of the variance in country differences in average IQ. Emphasizing the point we made earlier, this finding does not tell us about the etiology of individual differences in IQ *within* each country, which we know are moderately heritable, at least in developed countries. These researchers replicated this result across the 50 states in the United States (Eppig, Fincher, & Thornhill, 2011).

These results have enormous potential public health significance, because they suggest that reducing worldwide parasite prevalence would undoubtedly improve children's health, and could also possibly increase their IQs and, potentially, their economic productivity! However, we first need to rigorously test the causal relation between parasite prevalence and average IQ in an experimental treatment study before we conclude that eliminating parasites will help close country and state gaps in IQ.

SEX DIFFERENCES

Now we turn to group differences whose etiology has been shown to be partly genetic (see Halpern, 2012 for a review of sex differences in cognitive skills). Sex, as opposed to gender identification, is defined chromosomally: Females have two X chromosomes and males have an X and a Y chromosome. Genes on the Y chromosome determine male sex partly by increasing prenatal androgens, which in turn influence the development of the fetus. A male in whom these genes are disrupted will be phenotypically female, despite an XY genotype. A female exposed to extra androgens *in utero* will have more masculine behaviors on average.

Although there are not sex differences in IQ, there are sex differences in some components of IQ (Halpern, 2012; Hunt, 2011). Males have an advantage on measures of spatial reasoning, whereas females have an advantage on measures of language and on processing speed. The male spatial advantage has been linked to prenatal androgens in part. Nonetheless, the male advantage in spatial skill is not invariant across generations, but instead has *decreased*. For instance, to test for generational differences in cognitive skills, DeFries, Corley, Johnson, Vandenberg, and Wilson (1982) examined both parent and offspring scores on g and four broad cognitive skills: verbal, spatial, processing speed, and visual memory, and found different patterns of change across generations. For spatial skill, with the largest sex difference favoring males, the sex difference decreased from about 1.0 SD to about 0.6 SD in one generation. In contrast, females doubled their advantage for processing speed (to about 0.7 SD) in the second generation. The explanation for female gains in both cognitive domains is almost certainly cultural (e.g., increased educational opportunities for females in Hawaii, where this study was conducted). In contrast, the explanation of the contrasting and persistent sex differences in spatial skill (M > F) and processing speed (F > M) may be at least partly biological. As we discuss in later chapters, there are valid sex differences in the prevalence of learning disorders that are partly explained by sex differences in cognitive predictors such as processing speed.

SOCIOECONOMIC STATUS AND RACIAL/ETHNIC DIFFERENCES

We now turn to perhaps the most controversial examples of group differences, those between socioeconomic status (SES) and racial/ethnic groups. Again, we hope to dispel some of the confusion by systematically evaluating existing data. Disparities in IQ or academic achievement across SES or racial/ethnic groups are called *achievement gaps*. There are also well-documented health and wealth disparities across SES and racial/ethnic groups, and the logic and methods illustrated here are also relevant for understanding group differences in health and wealth. Why there are these achievement gaps across groups and how to close them are very important scientific and public health questions that have generated a number of policy initiatives, some of which were well-intentioned but not scientifically realistic.

As an example of an unrealistic policy initiative, one only need to think of the No Child Left Behind Act of 2001 (NCLB) federal policy, which aimed to have every child reading at grade level by 2014. While application of the science of reading to educational practice can certainly raise children's reading levels, some of the causes of reading problems arise much earlier in development and are therefore more difficult to remediate once a child reaches school age. In addition, there will always be individual differences in cognitive skills, and just as we cannot accomplish the Lake Woebegone wish that all children will be above average (a mathematical impossibility), it is very unlikely that we can make all children read (or write or do math) at or above *grade level* (which is typically defined as the average achievement level for a representative group of children in that grade), though intensive evidence-based intervention can certainly promote skill growth in individual children. Importantly, however, this fact about the normal curve of individual differences in academic achievement does *not* mean we cannot help close achievement gaps between groups, as already illustrated by what has been learned about country and sex differences.

In what follows, we (1) document achievement and IQ gaps; (2) review what is known and not known about why they occur, which includes examining how similar the causes of learning problems are across SES and race/ethnicity; and (3) apply our scientific understanding to what can be done to close these gaps.

ROBUST EVIDENCE FOR ACHIEVEMENT GAPS

The data documenting achievement gaps in academic skills come from multiple sources, including federally and state-mandated testing of academic achievement and carefully designed national studies such as the National Assessment of Educational Progress (NAEP) and the National Longitudinal Survey of Youth (NLSY). Anyone who reads a newspaper knows that his or her state's testing repeatedly finds (1) SES achievement gaps, with lower parental SES associated with lower achievement, and (2) racial/ethnic group achievement gaps. Specifically, on state-mandated academic tests, white children score better than black and Hispanic children on average, and Asian children sometimes perform better than white children or equal them. These same patterns have been repeatedly found in carefully designed national research studies such as NAEP and NLSY.

Typical effect sizes (Cohen's d) for these gaps are about 0.7, which means the gap is about seven-tenths of a standard deviation, and that child's ethnicity or SES accounts for 10% or less of the variance in academic skills. As we discuss later, the etiology of the SES gaps is more likely to have both environmental and genetic contributions as compared to racial/ethnic gaps where the evidence strongly points to an environmental etiology. This follows from the fact that individuals can change their own adult SES relative to their parents' SES (social mobility).

Two other conclusions follow from these data on achievement gaps. The achievement gaps are not as big as many people think, and individual differences within these groups account for much more of the variance in academic achievement than group differences. Because the distributions of academic skills across SES and racial/ethnic groups largely overlap, we can find individuals in every group who meet any cutoff for selection (for either good or poor performance). In terms of public policy, it is very clear that it would be empirically *and* morally wrong to use a person's SES, race, or ethnicity to infer qualifications for different academic or employment placements. To do so would be a blatant example of stereotyping or discrimination (Loehlin, 2000). Achievement and IQ gaps are an important public health and social justice issue. For instance, they contribute to income inequality across racial/ethnic and SES groups when these children grow up. To try to close them, we need science to understand why they occur, so that we can design effective prevention and intervention strategies.

WHY ARE THERE ACHIEVEMENT GAPS?

We first consider SES gaps, then turn to racial/ethnic gaps. Although SES and racial/ethnic gaps are correlated in the United States, these two types of achievement gaps could and probably do have different etiologies. It is often assumed that differences in child outcomes associated with parent SES are *caused* by SES acting environmentally. This could be an incorrect determination if we wrongly infer cause from an observed correlation, yet many journalists, educators, and psychologists conclude that SES acting environmentally *caused* the observed gaps in IQ or achievement in groups of children whose parents differ in SES. Psychologists are usually very careful to not infer cause from correlation, but the inference in this case is tempting, because two possible explanations of this correlation can be ruled out as implausible.

To understand this point, recall that there are four competing explanations of a correlation: (1) A causes B, (2) B causes A, (3) a third variable accounts for the relation between A and B, and (4) there is a reciprocal relation between A and B (where A stands for parent SES and B stands for a child's cognitive outcome). Because of temporal order (time's "arrow"), explanations (2) and (4) are impossible in this case. That is because parent SES precedes conception and the development of the child's cognitive skills. But that still leaves us with two competing explanations, namely, (1) parent SES causes the achievement gap and (2) a third variable causes both parent SES and the achievement gap. Moreover, the link between parent SES and child outcome does not have to be 100% environmental. It could result from a complex interplay of genetic and environmental factors.

In the case of SES, we have solid theoretical and empirical evidence that the SES of an individual adult is partly genetic, at least in countries with some degree of social mobility (i.e., it is possible for a child to grow up to have a different SES than his or her parents' SES). In considering potential genetic contributions to SES, it is important to dispel myths associated with genetic determinism. Genetic determinism is the idea that if something is "genetic" then it is fixed and preordained. This is an incorrect and overly simplistic understanding of genetic etiologies (see Chapter 2). While the genetic code cannot be changed, the manifestation of genetic differences can be changed by environmental interventions. Behavior genetic studies, which we discuss next, tell us about the contributions of genetic influences to a trait at a single time point, but they do not tell us about how the weight of genetic influences might change in different environmental circumstances. So, even if SES has a genetic component, it does not indicate that SES is fixed. Indeed, in the most simplistic example, a large sum of money gifted to an individual of lower SES would certainly change, at least in the short term, one dimension of SES measurement, the income-to-needs ratio, regardless of the genetic and environmental influences that contributed to the person's SES in the first place. This simple example illustrates that even traits with genetic influences can be modified through environmental interventions. We turn now to a theoretical exploration of the potential role of genetic influences on SES.

Let us imagine a behavior genetic study of adult SES using the ACE model described in Chapter 2. Recall that in this model, the A refers to the proportion of variance due to additive genetic influences, C refers to the proportion of variance due to shared environmental influences (i.e., shared by siblings in the same family but differing across families), and E refers to nonshared environmental influences (i.e., not shared by siblings in the same family). Given these definitions, which of these three causal factors could lead to social mobility? Clearly, if the etiology of SES were all due to C, there would be no social mobility, because a child's eventual SES would be entirely due to his or her parents' SES. Hence, SES acting environmentally is *conservative* (i.e., it promotes intergenerational consistency) with respect to a child's later SES. Having eliminated C as a possible cause of social mobility, we are left with A and E. If the etiology of SES were entirely due to E, then, by definition, there would be no family resemblance (familiality) for SES, either between parents and children or between siblings in the same family, but we know this is not the case. In summary, the fact that there is social mobility contradicts the possibility that the etiology of SES is all C, and the fact that there is familiality of SES contradicts the possibility that the etiology of SES is all E.

That leaves A: additive genetic influences. You might think A is conservative also, because children inherit their genes from their parents. But A is not entirely conservative, because each child in a family gets *half* their segregating genes from each parent and shares on average half their segregating genes with their siblings. This genetic variability between siblings means that, to the extent that social mobility has some genetic influence, siblings can have different SES outcomes that diverge from their parents.

In summary, innovative influences on SES permit social mobility. Conservative influences on SES account for its familiality. Hence, from this theoretical analysis, we can infer that the etiology of SES must be partly innovative (either A or some combination of A and E) and partly conservative (either A or C or some combination of the two). Do empirical data support this theoretical analysis? We provide one example of a study that supports this conclusion, but there are many others. This example is the now classic cross-fostering study by Capron and Duyme (1989) in France. Using a 2 × 2 design, they examined IQ outcomes for adopted children in four groups created by crossing the biological mother's SES (high vs. low) with the adoptive parents' SES (high vs. low). They found large main effects of *both* factors, biological mother's SES ($d = 1.0$) and adoptive parents' SES ($d = 0.75$), but no interaction. Returning to the ACE model, the main effect of the biological mother's SES reflects A (additive genetic influences), and the main effect of adoptive parents' SES reflects C (shared environment provided by adoptive parents). Since child

IQ predicts adult SES, we can infer that the eventual etiology of adult SES in these adopted children will be partly genetic and partly environmental.

As discussed earlier, it is a common error in thinking about achievement gaps based on SES and race/ethnicity that each has the *same* cause, or that one derives from the other. But that is not necessarily the case. Using the framework in Figure 8.2, we can ask whether these two kinds of achievement gaps have a similar trajectory, either across cohorts or longitudinally, in the same children. The basic answer is "no." For instance, Reardon and Portilla (2016) documented *opposite* trends in the size of SES and racial/ethnic achievement gaps across cohorts from the 1970s to the 1990s. The SES gap widened significantly, while the racial/ethnic gap declined significantly. Hence, the two gaps must have partly different causes, although both gaps are malleable. Reardon and Portilla (2016) then tested whether these trends have persisted into the current century by using kindergarten readiness measures in a nationally representative sample. They found that the SES gap narrowed from 1998 to 2010, as did the white–Hispanic gap, but the white–black gap remained the same. Since similar trends in preschool enrollment occurred over the same period, they speculated that these may have contributed to the narrowing of achievement gaps.

What is most relevant here is that SES and racial/ethnic gaps have different trajectories across cohorts, emphasizing that they are *not* the same phenomenon. It would be interesting to test how these cohort changes relate to the size of family income gaps over the same period. It is well known that the income and wealth gap between SES groups has widened over the last several decades, while the racial/ethnic gap has narrowed.

In our previous discussion, we focused on the SES gap for cognitive and academic achievement. Now we turn to possible explanations for racial/ethnic achievement and IQ gaps. Again, we can ask questions about the developmental trajectory of this gap. Only recently have good-quality longitudinal data emerged in the early development of IQ gaps. Fryer and Levitt (2013) found that the black–white IQ gap was negligible in infancy. They examined data from two large, carefully designed longitudinal studies that began at birth: the U.S. Collaborative Perinatal Project (CPP) conducted in the 1970s and the more recent Early Childhood Longitudinal Study–Birth Cohort (ECLS-B). At 8–12 months, the raw IQ gap between black and white babies on the Bayley Scales was only 0.8 IQ points (0.055 SD). This tiny gap disappeared when obvious confounders such as parental SES, home environment, and prenatal care were controlled statistically. The well-documented IQ gap emerged later, by age 2 years (raw gap = 0.3–0.4 SD; corrected gap = 0.2–0.3 SD) and widened by age 4 years (raw gap = 0.7 SD; corrected gap = 0.3 SD). Even though the Bayley Scales are only modestly related to later IQ ($r \sim .3$), the absence of a discrepancy in infancy argues strongly against a difference between black and white children in early cognitive development. It is important to note that the IQ measures at the two later time points depend much more on language development than the infant Bayley skills. This suggests a possible mediator of the emerging IQ gap, namely, differences in the early language environment that parents provide to their young children. Consistent with this hypothesis, Farkas and Beron (2004) found that the black–white vocabulary gap develops around 36 months.

We do know there are differences in the number of words heard by young children as a function of both parent SES and race/ethnicity (B. Hart & Risley, 1995), as well as differences in the kind of language children hear (more directive and less expository language). Fernald, Marchman, and Weisleder (2013) conducted an important study of the SES language gap. They followed high- and low-SES children from ages 18–24 months and measured their language processing efficiency (with the "looking-while-listening" [LWL] task) and expressive vocabulary at both time points. The LWL task measured language processing efficiency by how quickly children looked at the correct picture of a word being said (when presented with two pictures). They found the expected main effects of both age and SES on vocabulary size across time points (i.e., the older group and the higher SES group had bigger vocabularies). Most interestingly, there was a significant age × SES interaction, such that the higher SES group had a higher rate of vocabulary growth than the lower SES group (i.e., a widening gap). The LWL task also exhibited similar main effects of age and SES group (but not an interaction) and was moderately correlated with the expressive vocabulary measure.

Although more research is needed that more clearly separates SES and race/ethnicity, we can draw a few conclusions from the foregoing. First, the black–white IQ gap develops after the first year of life and widens across the preschool years, arguing against an innate group difference in IQ. Second, both a black–white and an SES gap in language development emerge early and widen across the preschool years, and are predicted by how much and how parents talk to their children. Since language skills are a strong predictor of later academic skills, it seems reasonable to conclude that at least a part of IQ and achievement gaps may be due to differences in early language experience.

AN ILLUSTRATION OF POLICY IMPLICATIONS

To illustrate the policy implications of group differences, let us consider the controversy over whether children from lower SES or racial/ethnic minority groups are over- or underrepresented in special education classrooms. As described in Morgan et al. (2015), apparent evidence for minority disproportionate representation (MDR) has already resulted in changes in federal law requiring school districts to take measures to reduce MDR. While we agree that science should inform practice, we need to ask: How solid is the evidence for MDR?

MDR means that minority groups are overrepresented in special education relative to their proportion in the population, after researchers correct for confounding variables such as parent SES and child birth risks (e.g., prematurity). Researchers vary in which confounding variables they correct for; hence, some of the controversy about whether there actually is MDR hinges on these methodological differences. More fundamentally, studies that find MDR and argue that it represents discrimination may fail to consider how the well-validated achievement gaps, which we have just discussed, relate to rates of special education placement.

To understand this relation, it is important to understand a basic statistical point. If there is a small group difference in the means of a cognitive skill, that difference will be magnified at the tails of the distribution, assuming equal variances in each group. For instance, a 0.5 *SD* difference in the means will result in a 3:1 ratio of the groups in the lower 5% of the distribution and 1:3 distribution in the upper 5% of the distribution, all other things being equal. Hence, belonging to the group with the lower mean increases the probability that a child will fall below the cognitive cutoff for a learning disability or intellectual disability. Hence, given real achievement gaps, children from lower-performing groups will have higher rates of identification for special education services than children from higher-performing groups, assuming that such identification is based on cognitive test scores. In summary, MDR is inevitable given that there are IQ and achievement gaps, all other things being equal.

Are such groups actually over- or underrepresented in special education placements, relative to their proportion of school-age children? Some researchers have presented data that shows they are overrepresented and have argued that this overrepresentation is due to discrimination (e.g., Losen & Orfield, 2002). In a more recent study with better longitudinal data, Morgan et al. (2015) actually found that such groups were *underrepresented* in special education classrooms, with or without covariance adjustment for confounding variables. Hence, there was no MDR, despite valid achievement gaps. Assuming special education helps children with learning disorders, then it is discriminatory to *underdiagnose* children from at-risk groups with learning disorders. The correct test for over- or underrepresentation should correct for mean differences in cognitive or academic performance. If, after such correction, there is still a finding of over- or underrepresentation, then that should be a cause for concern.

As American society becomes increasingly diverse, it is essential that clinicians, researchers, and policymakers have a sophisticated understanding of group differences and how they may be reduced. As we discussed in Chapter 6, clinicians and educators are sometimes wary of diagnosing a learning disorder in a child who is a member of a minority group, because they fear that doing so might seem biased. On the other hand, avoiding a valid diagnosis because of the child's group status may deprive that child of the very services he or she needs! Hence, clinicians should recognize that a child's group status is not a reason to avoid making a diagnosis. Similarly, researchers and policymakers should focus on how to close achievement gaps.

SUMMARY

Understanding achievement gaps is important for all those who work in the field of learning disorders: educators, policymakers, clinicians, and researchers. Achievement gaps are examples of adverse group differences, also called *disparities*. It is important to understand that the etiology of group differences is logically distinct from the etiology of *individual* differences within a group. In this chapter, we have discussed methods for determining whether group differences are valid, and if they are, what their etiology is. One broad conclusion of this chapter is that while individual differences in cognitive and academic skills are known to be moderately heritable, existing evidence supports that many group differences in such skills are substantially environmental in origin. For instance, this appears to be the case for country and racial/ethnic differences in such skills. Understanding the cause of the SES achievement gap is more complicated, because the fact of social mobility means that genetic and environmental influences can work in innovative and conservative ways to contribute to mobility. Social justice demands that we work to eliminate the environmental risk factors that are contributing to achievement gaps. To the extent that the etiology of an achievement gap is environmental, we can improve the early environment of children in the low-achieving group to partly or even wholly *prevent* a later achievement gap.

PART II
REVIEWS OF DISORDERS

CHAPTER 9

Speech and Language Disorders

CHAPTER SUMMARY

Speech and language are the oldest topics in the history of neuropsychology, going back to classic case reports by Gall, Dax, Broca, Wernicke, and others in the 19th century. Language is one of the most well-researched domains in cognitive neuroscience, along with vision. Furthermore, speech and language development are arguably the most relevant domains of neuropsychology for understanding virtually all the learning disorders in this book. The traditional learning disabilities in reading, mathematics, and writing all have their origins in earlier speech and language development. Hence, one can make a strong case that early speech and language development is the key target for early identification and preventive treatment of learning disabilities.

Going beyond the traditional learning disabilities to the other learning disorders considered here, speech and language development are also centrally important for understanding intellectual disability (ID), autism spectrum disorder (ASD), and even attention-deficit/hyperactivity disorder (ADHD). So it is critical for child psychologists and neuropsychologists to be knowledgeable about speech and language development. Since language skill is a major component of psychometric intelligence, every case of ID, whether syndromic or idiopathic, necessarily includes delayed language development. ASD disrupts speech and language development, and the best predictor of long-term outcome in ASD is language development at age 5 (Nordin & Gillberg, 1998). Since verbal mediation is a key mechanism for self-regulation, language development is also relevant to ADHD. ADHD has also been linked to difficulties with *pragmatics*, or the social use of language (Westby & Cutler, 1994). Hence, if we can get the science of speech and language development right, we will take a big step toward understanding and treating all the learning disorders in this book.

In this chapter, we review two speech disorders, childhood apraxia of speech (CAS) and speech sound disorder (SSD), and two language disorders, language impairment (LI) and pragmatic language impairment (PLI; also known as social [pragmatic] communication disorder [SCD] in DSM-5). Much more is known about SSD and LI than about CAS and PLI, and debate remains about whether CAS and PLI are valid disorders. In particular, CAS overlaps substantially with SSD, and PLI overlaps with ASD.

Consistent with the overall theme of this book, both general and specific risk factors influence the development of SSD and LI at all levels of analysis considered in this book. At the symptom level, there are comorbidities between LI and SSD, as well as between LI and ADHD, and reading disability (RD) and math disability (MD), indicating that general risk factors must be operative.

At the neuropsychological level, shared cognitive risk factors include deficits in processing speed and phonological memory. As we discussed in Chapter 3, there is also growing attention to the idea that deficits in procedural learning are common to many of the learning disorders in this book (Duda, Casey, & McNevin, 2015; Lum, Conti-Ramsden, Morgan, & Ullman, 2014; Lum et al., 2013). Developmental precursors are also shared across speech and language disorders. Babbling is a key early foundation for the development of speech and language, and delays in babbling are found in SSD, CAS, LI, and RD. There are also delays in babbling in ASD for a different reason, namely, reduced reciprocal face-to-face communication. Since babbling is the mechanism for learning speech perception and production, these delays in babbling may explain the deficits in phonological development found in CAS, SSD, RD, and some, but not all cases of LI.

At the level of brain mechanisms, Hickok and Poeppel's (2007) *dual-stream model* of speech perception and production provides a useful framework for understanding neuroimaging results in SSD and LI, although more work is needed. Briefly, this model is based on the well-established dual-stream model of visual processing (i.e., the "what" ventral visual pathway and the "how" dorsal visual pathway). In Hickock and Poeppel's model, a ventral "what" speech stream is responsible for mapping speech to objects, while a dorsal "how" speech stream is responsible for planning how to produce new words. Compared to the classic Wernicke–Lichtheim–Geschwind model, which emphasized three discrete left-hemisphere regions and their connections, Hickok and Poppel's model includes more widely distributed, bilateral areas. Neuroimaging results of LI have produced variable results but do implicate fairly distributed bilateral networks, more consistent with Hickok and Poppel than with the classic model. Some neuroimaging studies of SSD also fit within the Hickok and Poppel framework and show that the disorder is associated with a developmental delay in both left lateralization and in a shift from the dorsal to the ventral stream for speech processing.

At the level of etiology, there is a rare, dominant single-gene mutation in the *FOXP2* gene that causes some cases of familial CAS. Affected individuals have basal ganglia abnormalities and deficits in procedural learning. Studies of the *FOXP2* gene across species have been very revealing about the evolution of vocal communication. However, most cases of CAS and the other speech and language disorders (SSD, LI, and PLI) have a multifactorial etiology and are influenced by multiple genes. There are genetic correlations among these comorbid disorders, and several candidate genes are shared by these disorders.

HISTORY

Leonard (2000) has provided a history of specific language impairment (SLI) that we briefly summarize here. The first case report of a child with limited speech was published by Gall in 1822, and many case reports followed, spurred in part by advances in understanding acquired aphasia (hence, the term *congenital aphasia* for such developmental cases) (Gall, 1835). The children in these case reports had extremely limited speech output despite normal hearing, and apparently normal language comprehension and nonverbal intelligence. One term for such children in the early literature was *hearing mutism*, which focused on the deficit in speech output despite normal hearing. One can see that these early cases did not distinguish speech production from language, nor did they include children who, despite having speech that developed typically, were still impaired in language comprehension.

Later labels for these children included *developmental aphasia* and *developmental dysphasia*. Eventually, this neurological terminology was dropped in favor of terms such as *developmental language disorder* or *specific language impairment* (SLI). In addition, a clearer distinction was drawn between problems with speech development and language development, and subtypes in each domain were proposed. The two main subtypes of speech problems are SSD, which, as the name implies, is defined by difficulties pronouncing certain speech sounds, and CAS, which is defined by slow, effortful, and imprecise speech potentially related to a motor planning disorder (i.e., an apraxia). The two main subtypes of problems in language development distinguish problems in structural language, including grammar (SLI), from problems in the social use of language (PLI), both of which we define later. Eventually, the term SLI began to be replaced by *language impairment* (LI), the term used here, because, consistent with the overall theme of this book, for many children with language problems, the difficulties are not very specific. DSM-5 uses the term *language disorder* for the same reason, and also recognizes SSD, as well as PLI (which is called SCD in DSM-5). The definitions of these categories exclude children who have an acquired aphasia or other identifiable cause for their language problem. Thus, these definitions focus on children with an *idiopathic* problem in language development, including speech production.

Our understanding of these disorders has benefited enormously from basic science research on both mature language and language development across the fields of linguistics and psychology. Conversely, the study of children with SSD, CAS, LI, and PLI has addressed fundamental theoretical issues about typical language development. In what follows, we discuss this rich interplay between basic and clinical science.

DEFINITION

As the previous paragraphs indicate, there are two speech disorders and two language disorders that we need to define. The two speech disorders are SSD and CAS, and the two language disorders are LI (which is called "language disorder" in DSM-5), and PLI (which is called "social communication disorder" in DSM-5). As discussed in more detail below, LI involves impairment in structural language, especially measures of vocabulary and syntax, and PLI involves impairment in the social use of both structural language and nonverbal communication. The DSM-5 definition of PLI excludes LI, ASD, and ID. Gibson, Adams, Lockton, and Green (2013) used external validators and found that PLI is distinct from both LI and high-functioning ASD, which are distinct from each other. The external validators were peer interaction, restricted and repetitive behaviors (other than the ones used in the ASD diagnosis), and language profile (expressive vs. receptive language). Specifically, they found that PLI is distinguished from LI by worse peer interaction difficulties but *better* expressive language. PLI was distinguished from ASD by fewer peer interaction difficulties, better expressive language, and fewer restricted and repetitive behaviors. Some of these differences among PLI, LI, and ASD are inevitable given their diagnostic definitions, so questions remain about the external validity of the distinction between PLI and ASD, especially since some relatives of ASD probands have PLI. Hence, more research is needed to determine whether PLI is just a milder portion of the autism spectrum.

Although DSM-5 includes CAS as a type of SSD, partly because there is poor reliability among speech–language clinicians in the diagnosis of CAS, we think it is important to distinguish CAS from SSD, because much of the research literature treats them as distinct and supports partly different mechanisms underlying each disorder. To put it simply, children with SSD generally speak fluently but consistently substitute or omit sounds from words more than do same-age peers. The speech errors are often seen for the later-developing speech sounds, such as the "late eight" speech sounds (/l/, /r/, /s/, /z/, /th/, /ch/, /dzh/, and /zh/). The errors of children with SSD interfere with the intelligibility of their speech. In total, a diagnosis of SSD requires that the speech errors are atypical developmentally and cause impairment. In contrast, in CAS, speech is slow, effortful, and imprecise, as if the child cannot find the correct position of their articulators to produce the intended sound. Hence, children with CAS inconsistently produce most speech sounds, and lengthen and distort co-articulatory transitions between speech sounds and syllables. The result of these speech errors in children with CAS is that their speech is even less intelligible than the speech of a child with SSD. The problems with speech movements also affect *prosody* (intonation) in CAS.

As we see later, a computational model of infant speech development (Terband, Maassen, Guenther, & Brumberg, 2014) supports the hypothesis that CAS and SSD arise at different stages of early speech development. According to this model, CAS arises earlier than SSD, when the infant is trying to learn the systematic, bidirectional mappings between acoustic and somatosensory features, and the articulatory gestures that produce those features through babbling. Children with CAS cannot learn these basic mappings because of noise in both sensory and motor representations. In contrast, this model postulates that children with SSD only have noisy motor representations, but intact sensory ones, and can learn basic mappings fairly normally but have trouble learning some phonemic distinctions in the later stage of speech imitation.

As is the case for most of the disorders considered in this book, current definitions of SSD and LI all have three parts: (1) a diagnostic threshold, (2) a requirement of functional impairment, and (3) a list of exclusionary conditions, which usually include a peripheral sensory impairment (e.g., deafness), a peripheral deficit in the vocal apparatus, acquired neurological insults, environmental deprivation, and other, more severe developmental disorders (e.g., ID and ASD). Setting a diagnostic threshold for these disorders on what are essentially continua is inevitably somewhat arbitrary, as we have discussed repeatedly in other chapters. It is not completely arbitrary, as is sometimes claimed, because, in the case of speech and language disorders, the diagnostic threshold chosen can affect the longitudinal stability of the diagnosis. It turns out that some diagnostic cutoffs identify too many children who will grow out of their speech or language delay. In this way, low longitudinal stability undermines the important requirement of functional impairment. For instance, approximately 75% of children who receive a diagnosis of SSD at age 3 have clinically normal speech by age 6. Does this high rate of recovery mean that speech therapy is remarkably effective or that some children diagnosed at age 3 did not really have a disorder? We do not have a clear answer to this question. Similarly, not every late talker goes on to have persisting LI, although the recovery rate is lower than is the case for SSD. Hence, if we had a perfect predictor of prognosis for late takers or children with early speech delay, we would know better which children should receive early clinical intervention. For LI, but not SSD, a further issue is whether the diagnostic threshold should be relative to age or IQ expectations for the particular ability involved.

Traditional definitions of LI have required that the language deficit be significantly below the child's nonverbal IQ level, which means that many children with early language problems will not fit the diagnostic definition, especially children with lower than average intellectual functioning who do not qualify for a diagnosis of ID. These children with nondiscrepant poor language abilities may not meet traditional diagnostic criteria for LI even though their language is significantly below age expectations, significantly interferes with everyday functioning, and responds to treatment. As we discuss in Chapters 6, 7, and 10, discrepancy definitions face practical, empirical, and theoretical problems, and ultimately exclude from services children who clearly need them, so the field has moved away from such definitions.

Recently, Norbury et al. (2016) tested the validity of the IQ-discrepancy versus age-discrepancy distinction for LI in a large, population-based sample of 4- to 5-year-old children in the United Kingdom. Using a battery of language tests that yielded five composite scores, they applied the widely used Tomblin, Smith, and Zhang (1997) criteria for LI, which require a score of at least −1.25 SD on two of the five language composite measures, and exclude peripheral confounding conditions, as well as ID and ASD. Unlike Tomblin, Smith, et al., but consistent with DSM-5, Norbury et al. (2016) did *not* require a nonverbal IQ (NVIQ) of 85 or greater. They found that 7.58% of the sample met this definition of idiopathic LI, and an additional 2.34% of children met this language deficit criterion but were not idiopathic, because they had ID or a medical diagnosis, which was usually ASD. To test the validity of the NVIQ discrepancy criterion, they divided their idiopathic LI sample into those with a NVIQ of 85 or greater (63.3% of their LI cases) and those with NVIQ < 85 but > 70, (36.7% of their LI cases). They then compared these two subgroups of children with LI on language, social, emotional, behavioral, and academic measures of impairment, and found virtually no differences (the lower NVIQ group did perform worse on the expressive language composite score.) In contrast, both LI subgroups were significantly more impaired than typically developing children in this sample. These results do not support the external validity of NVIQ discrepancy definition of SLI, but do validate the DSM-5 definition of LI.

In summary, there is some empirical support for the validity of the four diagnoses considered in this chapter, all of which require a significant age discrepancy in either speech or language development. In contrast, there is not empirical support for an IQ-discrepancy definition of any of these diagnoses. Considerably more research is needed on the validity of PLI. More research is also needed on the validity of CAS, and on which early cases of SSD and which late talkers need clinical intervention. Later in this chapter, we review the external validity of these diagnoses, except PLI, at three deeper levels of analysis. We next consider the epidemiology and comorbidities of these four diagnoses.

PREVALENCE AND EPIDEMIOLOGY

Prevalence rates for LI range from about 5 to 8%. In Tomblin, Smith, et al.'s (1997) study, the prevalence was 8.1%, with a gender ratio of 1.25. Just as was true for RD and SSD, the gender ratio is higher in referred samples, about 3:1 (S. Smith, Gilger, & Pennington, 2001). Besides its comorbidities with RD and SSD, LI is also comorbid with ADHD (Beitchman, Hood, & Inglis, 1990). The prevalence of PLI is not well established. In one Dutch study, Ketelaars, Cuperus, Jansonius, and Verhoven (2010) found a prevalence of roughly 8% in a population-based sample, with a M/F ratio of roughly 2:1.

The prevalence of SSD in two epidemiological samples from the United States and Australia was very similar. In the U.S. sample, the prevalence was 3.8%, with a M/F sex ratio of 1.5:1 (Shriberg, Tomblin, & McSweeny, 1999). In the Australian sample (Eadie et al., 2015), the prevalence was 3.4% at age 4, and the M/F sex ratio was 1:1. The rate of comorbid LI was 41%, and 21% of the sample had poor preliteracy skills. In five earlier epidemiological samples reviewed by Shriberg et al. (1999), prevalence ranged from 2 to 13% (mean = 8.2%) and the M/F gender ratio ranged from 1.5 to 2.4 (mean = 1.8). As is the case for several other learning disorders, gender ratios for SSD are higher in referred samples (more males are referred for treatment). These authors also found that about one-third of children with SSD had LI, consistent with the results of Eadie et al. (2015). In contrast to

SSD, the prevalence of CAS is not well established, partly because of disagreements about the definition of CAS. Based on a clinical sample, Shriberg, Aram, and Kwiatkowski (1997) estimated the prevalence of CAS to be just 0.2% (i.e., 2 children per 1,000), much lower than most learning disorders.

Interestingly, in epidemiological samples, the prevalence of LI increases as parent SES decreases (Tomblin, Records, et al., 1997), consistent with well-established SES differences in how much (and how) parents talk to their children (e.g., B. Hart & Risley, 1995). In contrast, the prevalence of SSD has not been found to vary as a function of parent SES (Dodd, Holm, Hua, & Crosbie, 2003; McKinnon, McLeod, & Reilly, 2007). It seems that individual differences in early speech development are less related to variability in environmental input than are individual differences in early language development. Indeed, as we discuss later, SSD is more heritable than LI, with one study indicating little or no heritability for LI without comorbid SSD. Also, as we discuss later, the onset of babbling is quite robust across parent SES.

DEVELOPMENTAL NEUROPSYCHOLOGY

In this section, we first provide a brief overview of what mature human language is, including the linguistic description of its components. Then we turn to how it develops typically, and how that development goes awry in the four disorders reviewed in this chapter (LI, PLI, SSD, and CAS).

What is *human language*? As discussed in Pennington (2014), it is a unique, evolved audio–vocal communication system that builds on specialized human social cognition (joint attention and intersubjectivity), and is flexible and generative enough to make virtually any conscious cognitive representation in the mind of a speaker accessible to the mind of a listener, and that requires a degree of fine motor control, working memory, and possibly other cognitive processes that are found only in humans. As far as we know, human language is unique among animal communication systems, because it uses symbols, exhibits compositionality, and is recursive. *Compositionality* means that parts of a human utterance can be manipulated independently from other parts by a human language user, and *recursive* means that the embedding of one clause within another (e.g., "This is the dog that chased the cat that lived in the house that faced the street that ran to the river . . . ") can generate a potentially infinite number of possible human utterances.

The late Elizabeth Bates and her colleague Brian MacWhinney (1988) said that human language is a new machine made out of old parts. The foregoing definition of human language makes clear what some of those old parts are. Two key old parts found in many other species are representation and communication. G. Miller (1963) argued that human language allows the most extensive convergence of representation and communication seen in any species. Any species with a central nervous system can and *must* represent aspects of the external world and use these representations to guide future behavior. A subset of these nonhuman species, including other primates, cetaceans, birds, and even prairie dogs, have impressive communication systems, but the range of what can be communicated is much more limited than is the case for humans. Human language must be served by a distributed neural system that overlaps and interacts with virtually all of cognition: perception, attention, memory, social cognition, executive control, and emotion/motivation. So, language cannot be discretely localized in the brain, although some components of language may be more localized than others. It is obvious that at least some aspects of language must be learned from experience (feral children who are not exposed to language do not learn to speak), and we see in the next section on the brain mechanisms of language that its neural substrates change as it is learned, consistent with the interactive specialization theory, and contrary to the notion of an innate language module.

Whether or not there is a language module has been and continues to be a very controversial issue in the psychology of language, with followers of the linguist Noam Chomsky (Chomskyians) providing theoretical arguments and evidence for such a module, and connectionists countering with demonstrations of how language can be learned using generic cognitive architectures. We return to this debate when we review what we know about typical and atypical language development. But first we discuss the components of mature human language. Linguists define human language in terms of these components (Table 9.1).

The structure of language is hierarchical: Smaller units (*phonemes*) are combined into units of meaning (*morphemes*) that alone or in combination form words in the *lexicon,* which are combined into phrases and sentences in a lawful way (*syntax*), and have meaning (*semantics*). These five components (phonemes, morphemes, lexicon, syntax, and semantics) comprise what is called *structural* language, and, as mentioned earlier, LI involves deficits in structural language, mainly in syntax and the lexicon. The chief deficit in SSD and CAS is at the phonological level of language.

Structural language is distinguished from *discourse* and *prosody,* which are concerned with the social use of language, or *pragmatics*. Hence, impairments in these two components of language characterize PLI. Linguistics has traditionally focused on structural language, and, in particular, the kinds of representations needed at each level of structural language. In contrast, many developmental psychologists have been more concerned with how communication develops in human infants; hence, they begin their account of human language development well before infants can speak. However, as soon as we require that the meanings of structural language be intersubjective, which they are in all typical language use, the distinction between structural language and its social use gets blurred. In other words, because the phrases and sentences of a language allow the speaker to refer to a present, past, or imagined state of affairs that can be *shared* with a listener, successful communication always requires that the speaker monitor whether the listener knows what the speaker is referring to, which is called *securing reference*. How infants learn about securing reference is an important question in the development of language, one to which we return later.

These linguistic definitions have often been taken to imply that each component of structural language is cognitively separate from the others when language is processed in a real human brain, and some linguistic theories make that claim. But recent behavioral, neuroimaging, and computational evidence indicates these

TABLE 9.1. Components of a Sound-Based Language

- *Phonemes.* The individual sound units whose concatenation, in a particular order, produces morphemes.
- *Morphemes.* The smallest meaningful units of a word. (In sign languages the equivalent of a morpheme is a visual–motor sign.)
- *Syntax.* The rules governing how words in phrases and sentences can be combined (called *grammar* in popular usage).
- *Lexicon.* The collection of all words in a given language. Each lexical entry includes all information with morphological or syntactic ramifications but does not include conceptual knowledge.
- *Semantics.* Meanings of words and sentences.
- *Discourse.* The linking of sentences such that they constitute a narrative.
- *Prosody.* The vocal intonation that can modify the literal meaning of words and sentences.

components interact extensively and bidirectionally in language processing. We can readily grasp the importance of interactive and bidirectional processing if we compare our ability to perceive familiar versus unfamiliar spoken words in sentences in a noisy background. Our top-down lexical semantic and syntactic expectations help to rescue a familiar word from noise, but not an unfamiliar one. Because of this bidirectional interactivity, we should not expect clean dissociations in either typical language processing or in disorders, either developmental or acquired. For instance, research has shown developmental links between grammar and the lexicon (Bates & Goodman, 1997), and between grammatical morphology and speech perception (Joanisse, 2007). Close links have also been demonstrated between phonological and lexical development. Hence, the emerging picture is that there are dependencies among the five components of structural language in Table 9.1 in both typical and atypical development.

Combinations of sentences into a narrative or exposition constitute a *discourse*. Discourse processing encompasses both the production and the comprehension of discourses, and requires additional general cognitive processes not required by the comprehension of single sentences or phrases. These additional cognitive processes include making inferences and linking the elements of the discourse into a coherent mental representation. Discourse processing places additional demands on attention and working memory, beyond what is required for processing single sentences, and also depend more heavily on the listener's store of prior knowledge relevant to the topic of the discourse (see Kintsch, 1994). Discourse processing makes it very clear that language and other aspects of cognition cannot be totally separate from each other. In our real, everyday use of language, we are nearly always processing discourses. Because of the additional cognitive demands of discourse processing, its development takes much longer than the development of basic structural language and depends in modern societies on formal education. Much of formal education is devoted to learning a *written* language and learning to produce and comprehend it, a task that continues through college, graduate school, and beyond in "knowledge" workers. Thus, we should expect to find individuals who have difficulties in discourse processing in the absence of deficits in basic structural language.

Finally, we come to prosody, which is considered a paralinguistic or pragmatic aspect of language, which means that it is added to structural language and discourse. *Prosody* is the intonation with which a word or sentence is uttered. Think of at least three different meanings that you can impart to this sentence by changing your prosody: "What is this thing called love?" (*Hint*: It is fine to change the punctuation, even substituting an "!" for "?") Other aspects of pragmatic language are gestures, postures, and facial expressions. We know from our own everyday experiences and from professional mimes that these nonverbal, pragmatic features of language are richly communicative by themselves. Given appropriate social cognition (intersubjectivity) and pragmatics, a lot can be communicated without words, perhaps giving us a glimpse of what human communication was like before the evolution of structural language. In both ASD (see Chapter 13) and in the DSM-5 diagnosis of SCD, there are marked impairments in prosody and other aspects of pragmatic language.

Typical Development

As discussed in Pennington (2014), clearly, children do not speak at birth (the word *infant* literally means "without speech"), so speech and language must develop somehow. How they develop has been a focus of intense investigation and debate in the fields of linguistics and psychology for many decades. The paradigm of behaviorism that dominated academic psychology for most of the first half of the 20th century held that language is acquired like all behavior; that is, it is acquired through learning stimulus–response (S-R) associations. This empiricist approach to language acquisition was severely challenged by Noam Chomsky's (1959) long review of B. F. Skinner's (1957) book *Verbal Behavior*. Chomsky identified several aspects of human language that, he argued, are unlearnable not only by means of S-R associations but also by any purely inductive process. So Chomsky argued that there must be innate language structures that cannot be learned from experience.

There are several key parts of Chomsky's unlearnability argument. First, he argued that the real-world languages infants actually encounter are not rich enough to support the language structures they actually acquire (this is the "poverty of the stimulus" argument). Second, he argued that S-R associations would not support two key properties of human language, namely, its generativity and the already-discussed *recursive* property (i.e., the ability to embed phrases within phrases to generate new utterances). Speakers of a human language, given unlimited time, could generate an unlimited number of grammatical sentences, including many that they have never heard before, and some of which do not make sense. Recursion requires dependencies among nonadjacent words in a phrase or sentence, and it is not clear how S-R associations could capture such dependencies. Third, he argued that human language is unlearnable with any extant computational mechanism. This argument holds that learning grammatical rules is analogous to trying to learn a concept from only positive instances, not from a mix of positive and negative instances, with clear feedback about which instances are incorrect. Infants generally hear only grammatical speech; they are not exposed to instances of ungrammatical speech that are clearly marked as such. Without such negative feedback, it is much harder to constrain the space of possible hypotheses (see discussion in Bishop, 1997). Since language was evidently unlearnable, Chomsky argued that there must be innate and universal language structures (which he called an innate *language acquisition device* [LAD]) that guide an infant's language learning. Regardless of which human language an infant was exposed to, the LAD would permit its acquisition. So Chomsky's theory posits an innate, modular, and maturational view of language acquisition, a view that would seem to require an innate LAD in the brain.

Chomsky was very influential in launching the cognitive revolution in psychology. His view dominated the field of language development for several decades and also stimulated a whole new field of research into children's language development (e.g., R. Brown, 1973). As is often the case in scientific research, eventually stubborn facts about children's language development emerged that challenged Chomsky's highly influential theory (or, one could even say *paradigm*). Two key discoveries were (1) that connectionist networks *could* learn linguistic regularities and exhibit rule-like linguistic behavior, without having the explicit linguistic rules postulated by Chomsky's theory, and (2) that actual human infants were shown to be capable of statistical learning of linguistic regularities (Saffran, Aslin, & Newport, 1996). These discoveries directly contradicted Chomksy's unlearnability argument: The stimulus was actually rich enough to support learning, and the learning mechanism was powerful enough to accomplish that learning. Much of this work with connectionist models and statistical learning focused on the acquisition of syntax (Elman et al., 1996; Marchman, Plunkett, & Goodman, 1997), partly because syntax was so central to Chomsky's theory, but there are also connectionist models of speech and reading development.

To begin our discussion of how normal human infants actually learn a spoken language, it is useful to consider the order in which they learn the components of language in Table 9.1. Basically, the elaborate hierarchy of language in Table 9.1 is built on three early foundations: (1) prelinguistic semantics (early conceptual development), (2) nonverbal communication, and (3) babbling. All three, even babbling, have analogues in nonhuman species (e.g., baby songbirds babble) and hence qualify as "old parts." The first two correspond to G. Miller's (1963) definition of language; infants must first develop representations of things in the world and learn to communicate nonverbally. Then they use babbling to learn to produce and perceive speech sounds, combinations of which form spoken words, the symbols that refer to representations and permit a vastly expanded range of communication. A problem in any one of these three foundational skills will interfere with speech and language development.

First of all, infants must develop a prelexical semantics *before* they can possibly understand the meaning of a spoken word, and this prelexical experience derives from their embodied experience of the world. Otherwise, there is no concept to which a verbal label can be attached. Of course, once *lexical* semantics gets started in development, it helps the child to discover/learn new semantic distinctions in the world, facilitating the acquisition of new concepts. Hence, any risk factor that limited a child's semantics learning would necessarily limit language development. Therefore, an intellectual disability, which slows the development of concepts, should inevitably limit vocabulary development, apart from any speech or language deficits. A similar argument can be made about grammatical development. Children cannot understand a grammatical relation without first understanding the corresponding conceptual relation.

Second, human spoken language builds on earlier nonverbal communication between an infant and a caretaker, starting at birth, or even before. The development of prosody actually begins in the womb in the third trimester. This prenatal learning affects babies' early vocal productions, such that the prosody of crying in neonates differs as a function of the language they heard *in utero*! Mampe, Friederici, Christophe, and Wermke (2009) found that the prosody of neonatal crying is different in French versus German babies, with the neonates in each group matching their crying to the prosody of the language they heard in the womb. This influence of the ambient language continues as infants develop babbling.

Hence, even though prosody is last on the list in Table 9.1, prosody and pragmatics are the earliest components of language to develop. Nonverbal communication necessarily precedes verbal communication in development, a point made by several developmental theorists, including Bruner (1981), Trevarthen (1979), Bates (1998), and Tomasello and Brooks (1999). Parents and other caretakers copy the prosody of infant vocalizations, and infants copy the prosody of the adult vocalizations directed toward them. Early in life, infants and caretakers engage in rich, repetitive "conversational" exchanges of what Stern (1985) calls "vitality affects": sounds, motions, and facial expressions related to basic bodily states like hunger, satiety, elimination, sleepiness, and awakening. Infants make grunts, squeals, cries, and coos when in these bodily states and mothers and other caretakers can imitate these vocalizations and accompanying facial expressions. In these early exchanges, infants are beginning to learn about the pragmatics of communication. Most profoundly, infants learn that there *are* communicative partners in the world that are like them, and with whom they can share experiences, what Trevarthen (1979) calls "primary intersubjectivity." They also learn that conversations involve turn taking and have a basic topic–comment structure.

A baby is born with a preference for its mother's voice, built on its experiences hearing her in the womb, and also an innate preference for face-like perceptual configurations. So, human babies are evolutionarily prepared to orient to human voices and faces. Neonates are also evolutionarily prepared to imitate (Meltzoff & Moore, 1977), especially facial gestures. In their early imitative exchanges with caretakers, neither infants nor caretakers rigidly copy each other. Instead, they improvise. It is as if both partners are saying, "See if you can do this."

Eventually, these protoconversations make reference to objects in the world, in addition to the infant's internal states. Babies learn to request objects through what are called *protoimperatives*, then learn to refer to objects through what are called *protodeclaratives*. The advent of protodeclaratives in the second half of the first year of life marks the beginning of joint attention, a triadic relation between the infant, the caretaker, and an object in the world. Joint attention marks the beginning of what is called *secondary intersubjectivity*, and is viewed by many theorists as the beginning of a child's theory of mind.

In summary, well before children attempt a spoken language, they have rich experiences with nonverbal communications that begin to teach them about the pragmatics of communication. Key questions for understanding ASD and PLI include just when, why, and how this early development of nonverbal pragmatic skills goes awry. Does something interfere with these early affective exchanges, or do such children start out normally but later lose these skills for some reason? We do not know the answer to these questions, but longitudinal research on infants at high risk for later autism is beginning to provide some answers, as discussed in Chapter 13.

After this early development of nonverbal communication, the first component of spoken language to develop is phonology. Because all the other components of structural language in Table 9.1 (morphemes, syntax, and lexical semantics) rest on the foundation of phonology, it is important to understand how children learn the phonology of their native language and how that learning can go wrong. First, we consider how Chomsky's theory accounted for how an infant acquires phonology, discuss the problems with that account, then see how an infant actually learns phonology by babbling.

In the Chomskyan paradigm, knowledge of phonemes is considered innate, so a newborn possesses, in some sense, *all* the phonemes in *all* the world's languages (otherwise Chomsky's theory would have no way of accounting for the fact that any human infant can learn any human language, as is seen in the case of international adoptees). Hence, in Chomsky's view, "learning" the phonology of the infant's native language is simply a process of selection of some innate phonemes and deselection of others. According to this theory, babbling by infants was not considered to be important to the infant's phonological development, because they needed no practice to learn the phonemes of their native language (see review in Mareschal et al., 2007). In Jakobson's (1941) classical work on phonological development, phonology was viewed as independent from babbling, in part because there appeared to be a discontinuity between the end of babbling and the appearance of speech. A second argument for the independence of babbling and phonology is found in Lenneberg's (1967) influential book on language development. Lenneberg reasoned that since babbling appears to be similar in both deaf and hearing infants, it could not be important for their spoken word productions, which differ markedly. (But if phonemes are innate, why would deaf infants have trouble producing them?)

As discussed in Mareschal et al. (2007), more careful observations undermined both Jakobson's (1941) and Lenneberg's (1967) arguments. It turns out that there is continuity between babbling and the development of speech, and babbling in deaf infants is actually delayed in its onset and different from typical babbling once it appears. These discredited arguments for the independence of babbling from phonology may be seen as examples of how one's theoretical paradigm can influence how data are interpreted.

Empirical studies of infants' and children's phonological development have seriously questioned (1) whether phonemes are innate, (2) whether learning phonology is simply a process of deletion, and (3) whether babbling is unimportant in that learning (Mareschal et al., 2007). Instead, research supports the view that infants learn to produce the phonology of their native language through statistical learning. In this learning process, babbling is a self-teaching device through which the child learns the very complex mapping between acoustic and somatosensory features and articulatory gestures, a feat that at first blush *does* seem truly unlearnable. Children clearly imitate the speech they hear, just as they learn many other things by imitation, but in imitating speech, they must copy many articulatory gestures that they cannot see (i.e., those that occur inside the mouth and vocal tract). How can they work around this seemingly insuperable barrier? They do this by imitating ambient language sounds, then practicing them by imitating *themselves* in babbling. Even if they cannot watch their own articulatory gestures, each gesture has a distinct somatosensory and motor "signature." Through repetitive babbling with slight variations, the infant slowly learns the complex mapping between acoustic and somatosensory features and articulatory gestures appropriate for their native language. In this process, perception and production of speech sounds are tightly coupled, and speech sounds the infant masters become more specific to the native language.

Production in babbling changes in the first year of life, and begins with *cooing*, production of isolated vowel sounds before 6 months of age. At around 6 months, canonical babbling appears, with infants producing long strings of repeated consonant–vowel (CV) syllables (e.g., "gagagaga . . . "). Similar to perceptual development, the vowel space of babbling productions is gradually assimilated into the ambient language, a process that has been linked to the increasing ability for vocal imitation (Kuhl & Meltzoff, 1996).

Regarding the infant's development of speech *perception*, between 6 and 12 months of age, infants gradually lose the ability to discriminate non-native phonemes (Werker & Tees, 1984). However, this loss is not simply one of deselection of non-native contrasts, as the Chomskyan selectionist theory would suggest. First of all, that theory has the impossible requirement that all possible speech contrasts are part of any human infant's innate endowment. Since languages evolve and new languages emerge, it is very hard to imagine how evolution could have provided every human infant all possible human speech contrasts as an innate endowment. Moreover, if the deselection theory were correct, infants should lose the ability to make *all* non-native contrasts. Instead, researchers have shown that there is a gradient of performance with non-native contrasts, depending on how they map onto native contrasts (C. T. Best, McRoberts, & Goodell, 2001). So rather than selecting and deselecting from an innate, universal set of phonemes, developing infants assimilate their babbling to match the ambient language, losing some, but not all, non-native contrasts in the process. Kuhl (1991) has demonstrated a similar phenomenon in vowel perception, such that infants exposed to different languages develop different vowel contrasts, with different attractors or prototypes. So perception and production of speech sounds change in tandem in the first year of life to match the ambient native language, and babbling appears to be a crucial self-teaching device in this developmental process.

There are several computational models of the development of speech production based on similar underlying principles (Guenther, 1995; Joanisse, 2000; Joanisse, 2004; Joanisse, 2007; Joanisse & Seidenberg, 2003; Kröger, Kannampuzha, & Neuschaefer-Rube, 2009; Markey, 1994; Menn, Markey, Mozer, & Lewis, 1993; Plaut & Kello, 1999; Westermann & Miranda, 2004). These models are presented schematically in Figures 9.1 and 9.2. The actual models have layers of artificial neurons that are connected by pathways with adjustable "synapses." Through gradual, error-driven learning, these models learn the complex mapping functions between acoustic and somatosensory features and articulatory gestures. These abstract mappings encoded by these layers of hidden units are perceptual representations of speech sounds. These perceptual representations exhibit perceptual invariance just as visual object representations do. We recognize a given object, such as a face or a chair, as the same object despite changes in orientation, size, lighting, and so forth. Similarly, we recognize a given speech sound in our language as the same intended sound, despite considerable variability within and across speakers, allowing us to imitate that speech sound. Unlike visual object representations, perceptual representations of speech sounds include a motor plan for imitating that speech sound. Because speech unfolds over time, and because the mapping from acoustics to articulation is many to one (a motor equivalence problem), it presents a difficult computational problem. Motor control theory attempts to solve these problems by using both a "forward model," which predicts how a given articulatory gesture will sound, and an "inverse model," which captures the complex mapping between acoustics and articulatory gestures. The models of speech perception and production cited earlier contain forward and inverse models, and reciprocal connections between them. A child learning to babble can tune these models by listening to whether their actual sound production matches their intention, and use the discrepancy to slowly change connection weights.

The difficult developmental task these models accomplish is how infants learn these complex mappings even when important aspects of the articulatory gestures made by adult models are not observable. For example, it is difficult for children to observe the placement of an adult's tongue while producing the /th/ sound. Hence, babbling has to supplement imitation in learning these mappings.

These recent simulations of babbling, and recent data on the development of babbling in various disorders considered in this book, provide an exciting new perspective on how these disorders develop. To understand this perspective, examine the neural network model in Figure 9.1. Unlike the model in Figure 9.2, this model does not have a semantic layer, because the development of babbling does not require semantic input. Instead, the function of babbling is for the infant to learn the very complex sensory–motor mappings between acoustic and somatosensory features and articulatory gestures. The hidden units in this model, the layer labeled phonetics, is the layer that encodes this complex mapping. We call this layer "phonetics" rather than "phonology" because, by definition, *phonology* refers to contrasts in speech sounds that signal a difference in meaning. For the preverbal infant, adult speech

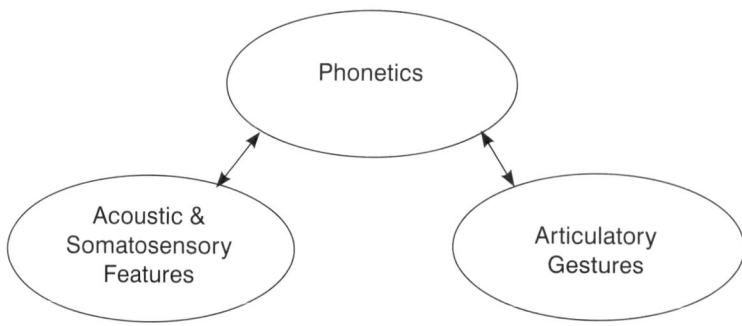

FIGURE 9.1. The development of phonetic mappings.

is beautiful music, which the infant would like to imitate. Using both auditory and somatosensory feedback, the infant is slowly learning to adjust articulatory gestures to correspond to speech sounds that adults make.

An analogy might be someone learning to play a horn with no keys, such as a bugle. To make different sounds with a bugle, one has to learn which different lip configurations and different exhalations produce different sounds from the horn. After that feat has been accomplished, one can learn how to string these sounds together into a melody with a particular meaning. Hence, evolution has provided the infant with an exquisite musical instrument, the human voice, but it has not provided a music teacher. Instead, repetitive babbling allows self-teaching of how to make different sounds with this instrument. Infants have perceptual targets they are trying to match with their articulatory productions. If the production matches the target, the synaptic weights supporting that mapping will be strengthened. On the other hand, if there is a mismatch, then synaptic weights have to be adjusted in proportion to the amount of error. This kind of error-driven learning is readily accomplished by neural networks.

Infants are developing phonological representations through statistical learning in the first year of life, but much more phonological development lies ahead of them as they map phonology onto lexical semantics to acquire a spoken vocabulary in the second year of life and beyond. In this process, there appears to be a reciprocal relation between phonological and vocabulary development. Phonology and phonological memory enable the child to perform "fast mappings" of new names onto already acquired concepts, but the expanding lexicon forces the child to make new phonological distinctions in a process called *lexical restructuring of phonology* (Walley, 1993). Several researchers (e.g., Nittrouer, 1996) have demonstrated the protracted nature of phonological development into toddlerhood and beyond with carefully designed speech perception tasks.

The research presented here is consistent with the view that phonological representations are constructed and change to capture an optimal mapping among acoustic features, the child's vocabulary, and articulatory gestures. So phonological representations change with spoken language development, then change further as a child learns a written language (Morais, Cary, Alegria, & Bertelson, 1979).

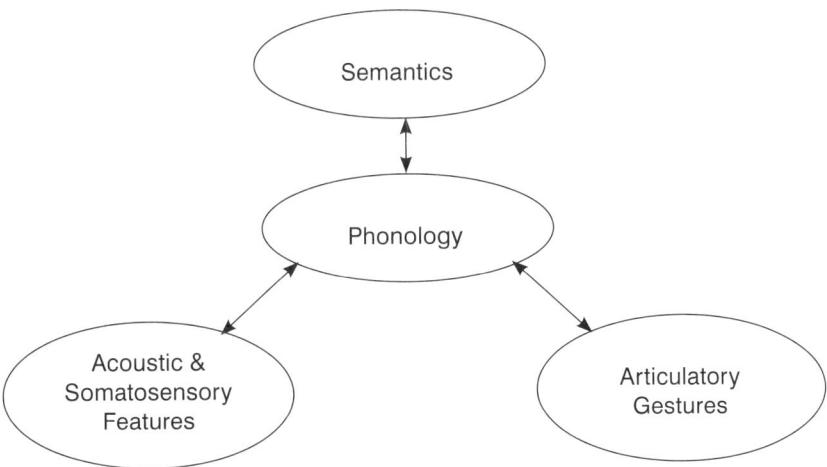

FIGURE 9.2. The development of speech production.

We have now explained how prosody, phonology, and the lexicon develop. What about syntax? As we discussed earlier, in Chomsky's theory, syntactic structures are assumed to be innate, because there is no conceivable way they could be learned. However, the connectionist models of syntax acquisition we mentioned earlier, as well as the discovery of new learning mechanisms in human infants (Saffran et al., 1996; Saffran, Johnson, Aslin, & Newport, 1999) have challenged this innatist view.

In addition to its role in fast mapping and lexical acquisition, phonological memory has a key role to play in syntax acquisition. To assign the correct grammatical role to different words in an utterance, the listener has to maintain a representation of the utterance in short-term memory while its meaning is computed. In addition, sometimes utterances permit more than one parsing, and temporary storage of the utterance is needed to repair parsing errors. Elman et al. (1996) found that their connectionist model could gradually learn syntactic relations only if its short-term memory capacity began small and gradually increased, which corresponds to short-term memory development in human infants and young children. The initial, limited short-term memory capacity served as a kind of filter that limited the syntactic computations the model had to perform initially. Gradually increasing the short-term memory capacity allowed the model to parse longer and longer phrases, eventually including ones with nonadjacent dependencies (the very ones that, according to Chomky's theory, were unlearnable).

In summary, in this review of speech and language development, we have argued that phonological development is the foundation on which the rest of structural language development (the lexicon and syntax) depends, and that phonological development begins with babbling. The development of social communication, including prosody and prelinguistic semantics, begins even earlier in life. Throughout speech and language development, social interaction is crucial, and deprivation of social interaction, either by the environment or because of the child's lack of social engagement, impairs speech and language development, as is seen in ASD.

We next review several other ways, besides social deprivation, that babbling and early speech development can go wrong. These other ways include motor, auditory, and somatosensory impairments, as well as the mappings among motor, auditory, and somatosensory representations. In the next section, we use this understanding to evaluate possible explanations for the four disorders considered here, as well as their comorbidities.

Atypical Development

Speech Disorders

Children with SSD and CAS have delayed onset of babbling, which is less varied once it begins. Furthermore, their vocabulary acquisition in the second year of life is delayed, and their spoken words contain many speech sound substitution errors (Terband, Maassen, et al., 2014; Terband, van Brenk, & van Doornik-van der Zee, 2014). The onset of babbling is also delayed in LI and ID (Patten et al., 2014) and in infants at high family risk for dyslexia (L. Smith, Roberts, Locke, & Tozer, 2010). In contrast, in children from lower-SES families (who, on average, get less language input than children in higher-SES families), the onset of canonical babbling is not delayed, but volubility of babbling is decreased (Patten et al., 2014). Babbling is also somewhat delayed in blind infants (Patten et al., 2014) and in children with congenital deafness, but it emerges once the child receives a hearing prosthesis (either a cochlear implant, hearing aids, or both). In summary, babbling is a robust phenomenon in development, but it can be delayed or reduced by a variety of risk factors, including peripheral sensory deficits, decreased language input from caretakers, and genetic differences that underlie certain neurodevelopmental disorders.

Terbrand, Maassen, et al. (2014) used the computational model developed by Guenther (1995) to simulate babbling in SSD and CAS. Their simulations modeled the effects of two deficits. The first was a motor processing deficit, which was simulated by adding increasing amount of noise in motor and somatosensory state representations in the model. The second was a combined auditory and motor processing deficit, which was simulated similarly but with the addition of increasing amounts of noise to auditory representations. They conceived of these two manipulations as the causes of SSD (motor processing deficit only) and CAS (combined deficit). The outcome measure was the accuracy of speech produced by the model. Interestingly, the SSD model performed fairly normally in the first babbling phase, whereas the CAS model was markedly impaired at learning phonetic representations, with degree of impairment linearly related to the degree of noise. Hence, intact auditory feedback could compensate for noise in the motor and somatosensory state representations. But without intact auditory feedback, the model could not learn phonetic representations of single sounds. In the second, speech imitation phase, both models performed poorly, although for different reasons. Not having learned basic phonetic representations, the CAS model could not learn which phonetic distinctions were phonemic (i.e., meaningfully distinguished speech sounds). In contrast, the SSD model had learned phonetic representations but had trouble implementing the fine articulatory distinctions required to differentiate phonemes because of noisy motor and somatosensory state representations, which means that its phonemic representations were less stable. It would be interesting to test the predictions of this model by examining the development of babbling and speech imitation in infants at family risk for CAS versus SSD.

Terbrand, van Brenk, et al. (2014) performed a different test of their model by examining auditory feedback perturbation in a mixed group of young children with speech disorders, including both SSD and CAS. They used an established experimental paradigm to manipulate auditory feedback. Since models of babbling and speech imitation posit a key role for auditory feedback for successful learning of speech production and perception, they reasoned that children with speech disorders should compensate less well for perturbations in auditory feedback. This is indeed what they found. Moreover, degree of compensation correlated with phonemic accuracy in repeating nonwords and with accuracy of fast sequential oral–motor movements.

In summary, the results of these two studies (Terband, Maassen, et al., 2014; Terband, van Brenk, et al., 2014) provide a developmentally plausible explanation for both SSD and CAS. Poor feedback during babbling and early speech imitation leads to less robust phonetic (in CAS) and phonemic (in both CAS and SSD) representations, thus impairing both speech perception and production, which are necessarily tightly coupled according to the learning account given here.

Language Disorders

The search for a core underlying deficit in LI has led to various, competing single-deficit models. These models can be divided according to whether they posit a deficit in a specific aspect of linguistic *knowledge* versus a specific *processing* deficit that interferes with language development (Leonard, 2014). There are many theories of each type, which are reviewed by Leonard. For our purposes, it is important to point out that knowledge deficit theories all fall within the Chomskyian paradigm, which posits that linguistic knowledge is innate. If that premise is wrong, then we can reject all the knowledge-deficit theories of LI.

An example of a well-known knowledge deficit hypothesis of LI is the extended optional infinitive hypothesis proposed by Mabel Rice and colleagues (Rice, Wexler, & Cleave, 1995). According to this hypothesis, the core deficit in LI lies in the acquisition of a particular aspect of syntax. Evidence for this hypothesis comes from the fact that children with LI make characteristic errors in their expressive language. In English, they most notably have difficulties with the past tense, often substituting an unmarked form for a marked one (e.g., "He walk there" in place of "He walked there"). This kind of error is made by typically developing children early in language acquisition, but children with LI tend to use unmarked (or infinitive) forms much longer than even younger, typically developing children matched for overall language skills. Despite the elegance of this proposal, it faces two major challenges (in addition to positing innate language knowledge). First, it does not adequately explain the cross-linguistic data, which have shown that the syntactic forms causing the most difficulty for children with language impairment vary with their perceptual salience in different languages (Leonard, 2014). Thus, in English, the past tense may be problematic partly because its spoken marker ("-ed") is brief and often unstressed. Second, this proposal fails to explain why children with LI perform poorly on a wide range of language tasks, including those that do not require syntactic competence (Bishop, 1997).

In addition to the extended optional infinitive hypothesis, Leonard (2014) reviews five other knowledge-deficit hypotheses of LI, all of which face the same general difficulties. He also reviews the now very extensive data on the manifestations of LI across languages, even within the same child learning two languages. Evidence from bilingual children with LI is particularly important, because the contrast between languages is a within-subject manipulation. Leonard's broad conclusion is that there does not appear to be a consistent linguistic knowledge deficit across languages in children with LI, even within the same child. Partly based on this evidence, Leonard proposed an alternative "surface account" of LI. Whereas grammatical knowledge deficit theories of LI posit a deficit in the deep structures of grammar, Leonard's account focuses on surface processing of the physical properties of speech, in particular the processing of phonetic portions of the speech stream that are rapid or brief. According to the surface account, the diversity of manifestations of LI across languages derives from which grammatical features of those languages are less salient and harder to process phonetically.

This description of the surface account naturally leads to the question of what cognitive processes are important in both the development of language and its online, real-world processing, and brings us to various processing deficit theories of LI. A relevant processing limitation would both act as a filter on how much of the linguistic signal a developing child could take in and limit how rapidly new linguistic forms could be learned. Four main processing deficit theories of LI have been proposed: (1) the auditory hypothesis, (2) the processing speed hypothesis, (3) the phonological memory hypothesis, and (4) the procedural memory hypothesis. These hypotheses differ importantly in the specificity of the proposed impairment, and each is reviewed very briefly below. We believe that current evidence best supports the last two hypotheses. However, any single core deficit will likely be inadequate to account for the full LI phenotype (Pennington, 2006).

The auditory hypothesis of LI is the least specific of these four hypotheses, because it posits that a nonlinguistic, sensory impairment leads to both phonological and broader language difficulties in LI. This hypothesis was developed in the 1970s by Tallal and colleagues. Early studies demonstrated that children with LI have specific difficulty discriminating rapidly presented nonspeech sounds (Tallal & Piercy, 1973), which presumably led to problems processing certain aspects of the speech stream. However, later studies indicated that despite group differences, many children with LI do not have auditory deficits, while many typically developing children do (Bishop et al., 1999). Furthermore, there is little evidence that the auditory impairments described in these studies are heritable (Bishop et al., 1999), which raises questions, since LI is partly heritable. However, it remains possible that environmentally caused auditory deficits significantly complicate language development in children already at genetic risk for LI (Bishop et al., 1999).

The generalized processing speed hypothesis of LI (Kail, 1994) derives from the well-established empirical finding that LI children have slower reaction times (RTs) than chronological age (CA)-matched controls across a wide range of both linguistic and, crucially, nonlinguistic tasks. Kail proposed that various cognitive processing components were slowed by a constant amount in children with LI; consequently, the slowing on a particular task would be proportional to the number of cognitive components it required. Kail tested this hypothesis by analyzing data from several previous studies of RT in LI and controls across various tasks and found a proportional slowing of about 30% in children with LI relative to controls. As reviewed by Leonard (2014), several subsequent studies have replicated this proportional slowing in groups of children with LI, although some studies have found that the proportion of slowing is more task-specific. In addition, it is not surprising, given the likely heterogeneity of LI, that there are individual differences within LI groups in degree of slowing, with some children with LI performing like controls.

In summary, processing speed (PS) deficits in LI appear to be an important cognitive risk factor, especially given previous research in which we found PS deficits in disorders that are comorbid with LI, such as dyslexia, ADHD, and MD, and with each other. In that previous research, PS deficits helped explained the comorbidity among disorders. Hence, deficits in PS are not specific to LI, but they may be an important general cognitive risk factor that is shared by LI and a number of other disorders reviewed in this book.

The phonological memory hypothesis of LI holds that the core deficit lies in the ability to hold phonological forms in working memory (Gathercole & Baddeley, 1990). Phonological memory is most often measured by asking children to repeat spoken lists of real words, such as numbers (digit span) or individual pseudowords (nonword repetition). This proposal is theoretically attractive, because work with brain-damaged adults, second-language learners, and typically developing children has converged in highlighting a role for phonological memory in language learning, particularly vocabulary acquisition (Baddeley, Gathercole, & Papagno, 1998). Furthermore, a computational model demonstrated that phonological deficits cause impairments in learning syntax (Joanisse & Seidenberg, 2003). Also, phonological memory impairment does appear to be a robust endophenotype for LI. Furthermore, phonological memory deficits are heritable, and correlate significantly with degree of language difficulty in individuals with LI (Bishop et al., 1999). Finally, phonological memory deficits persist even in individuals whose broader language problems have resolved (Stothard, Snowling, Bishop, Chipchase, & Kaplan, 1998). For all these reasons, a deficit in phonological memory appears to be important in many cases of LI.

Last, the procedural memory hypothesis of LI (Ullman & Pierpont, 2005) holds that a deficit in procedural memory explains the symptoms of LI. As we explained in Chapter 4, procedural, or implicit, memory is different from declarative, or explicit, memory, with each type of memory being served by different parts of the brain. Procedural memory relies on subcortical structures such as the basal ganglia and cerebellum, and allows an individual to learn new sequences, including motor sequences and statistical patterns, such as those that characterize human language. Procedural memory is demonstrated in performance gains but cannot be explicitly declared. For instance, if you practice your tennis strokes, you will get better at tennis, but you will not be able to say very much about what changed. In contrast, declarative memory relies on the hippocampal formation to acquire new semantic and episodic knowledge that can be declared. For instance, if you learn the meaning of a new word, you will also be able to give its definition later. Much of what a typical adult knows about phonology or grammar is implicit knowledge, not declarative knowledge. Infants have been shown to use statistical learning, which is a form of procedural learning, to learn patterns in the speech stream (Saffran et al., 1999). According to this hypothesis, learning language is like learning a new motor skill. A child pronounces words and produces grammatical sentences, but he or she certainly cannot tell you how he or she does that. Hence, assuming that procedural learning is an important mechanism for learning language in early development, a deficit in procedural memory is a plausible explanation for LI. As discussed by Leonard (2014), evidence for a procedural learning deficit in LI has been found by several different investigators. A procedural learning deficit provides a plausible explanation for the grammatical deficits found in LI, but it is less plausible as an explanation for the vocabulary deficits found in LI, because vocabulary acquisition depends on semantic memory and not on procedural memory. Lum et al. (2014) conducted a meta-analysis of procedural learning deficits in LI and found that the average effect size was only 0.33. Hence, a deficit in procedural learning cannot account for all cases of LI.

What about a multiple-deficit model of LI? We were only able to find one example in the literature, a study by Conti-Ramsden, Ullman, and Lum (2015). They found that measures of procedural memory, phonological memory, and declarative verbal memory together accounted for 53% of the variance in a measure of receptive grammar. The effect size of differences between the LI group and controls was much larger for phonological memory ($d = 1.79$) and verbal declarative memory ($d = 1.54$) than for procedural memory ($d = 0.63$). As is true for other learning disorders, we are left with the question of whether (1) there are multiple single-deficit subtypes of LI, at one extreme, (2) multiple deficits in all individual cases of LI, or (3) some combination, which is most likely.

BRAIN MECHANISMS

Now we consider possible brain mechanisms for these models of speech and language development, then evaluate whether neuroimaging results in speech and language disorders help us choose between competing models. Can we map the computational models of babbling and word learning in Figures 9.1 and 9.2 onto neural networks in the actual brain? How do these neural networks change with development? If we can at least begin to answer these first two questions, what does that tell us about plausible brain differences in atypical speech, language, and reading development? Do empirical neuroimaging results in the neurodevelopmental disorders considered in this chapter correspond to the results predicted from the answers to the first two questions?

The brain network model of mature spoken language on which most clinical neuropsychologists and neurologists were trained, and which many still use, is over 150 years old. This is the familiar Wernicke–Lichtheim–Geschwind model, which maps adult language processing onto a connected set of left-hemisphere perisylvian structures, and which is sometimes called the articulatory loop (Figure 9.3). In this model, speech perception and comprehension were localized to the left posterior temporal lobe (the left superior temporal gyrus [STG]), and called Wernicke's area. Speech production was localized to left inferior frontal gyrus (IFG), called Broca's area. The connection between these two areas was in a specific set of white-matter tracts, the arcuate fasciculus. To account for problems in language comprehension caused by lesions outside Wernicke's area, Lichtheim added an additional, localized semantics center to this model, as seen in Figure 9.3 (Pennington, 2014). Classical aphasiologists used this model to explain different subtypes of aphasia.

This classical model depicted in Figure 9.3, despite its considerable longevity, can now be considered "dead" (Hickok & Poeppel, 2007; Poeppel, Emmorey, Hickok, & Pylkkänen, 2012). What "killed" it? Several key empirical findings did. As reviewed in Kolb and Whishaw (1990), these include the following: (1) Aphasia may be caused by lesions located outside the perisylvian loop, including lesions to the insula and some subcortical lesions, such as in the thalamus or basal ganglia; (2) similar extraperisylvian disruptions of language are found when direct brain stimulation is done to map language areas before neurosurgery; and (3) there is a lack of independence between classical aphasia subtypes in terms of both predicted language deficits and predicted lesion locations (i.e., poor discriminant validity), as well as poor coverage of all cases of aphasia (about 40% of cases of aphasia do not fit a classical subtype). Additionally, the supposed clean double dissociation between speech perception and production provided by contrasting Wernicke's and Broca's aphasia did not hold up when using modern experimental measures (Hickok & Poeppel, 2007). Nor did the predicted double dissociation between deficits in language comprehension and syntax in Wernicke's and Broca's aphasia, respectively (Shallice, 1988). Taken together, these findings mean that mature human language is both more distributed and more interactive than the classical Wernicke–Lichtheim–Geschwind model predicted. What remains of this classical model? Essentially three things: (1) At least some aspects of mature human language are lateralized to the left hemisphere, including, but not restricted to, the perisylvian loop; (2) consequently, in the large majority of human adults, aphasia is more likely to occur after a focal left- than right-hemisphere brain lesion; and (3) connections between language processing centers are important, but they are not restricted to the arcuate fasciculus.

What is a better model? Hickok and Poeppel (2007) proposed one based on extensive behavioral and neuroimaging research. They call their model the

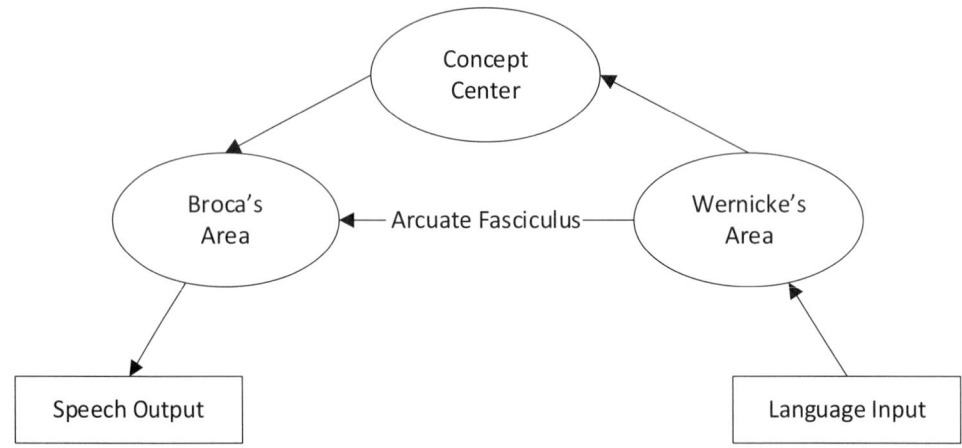

FIGURE 9.3. The Wernicke–Lichtheim–Geschwind model of language processing. From Pennington (2014, p. 118). Copyright © 2014 The Guilford Press. Adapted by permission.

dual-stream model of speech processing, analogous to the well-validated dual-stream model of visual processing. According to this latter model, the two streams in the visual system are the dorsal (how) and ventral (what) streams. We use vision in the dorsal stream (occipital lobe to parietal lobe) to map the location of objects in the world and our physical relation to them, so we can plan how to move in the world. We use vision in the ventral stream (occipital lobe to temporal lobe) to identify objects in the world. Although these two streams accomplish different visual processes, they are not totally independent. For instance, interaction between these two visual streams is necessary when we choose an object to reach for and then pick it up: We have to identify the desired object, then plan how to move our hand to its spatial location. Similarly, in processing speech, we need to both identify the referents of speech we hear and plan new speech movements. As in vision, in the Hickok and Poeppel model, mapping speech to objects is the function of the ventral speech stream, and planning how to produce new words is the function of the dorsal speech stream. The dorsal stream is particularly important in speech development, but it is also needed when adults learn new words in their native language, or when they learn a second language.

Which brain structures are involved in each of the two speech processing streams? The key structures identified by Hickok and Poeppel (2007) include the three left-hemisphere structures contained in the classic Wernicke–Lichtheim–Geschwind model: the dorsal left STG (Wernicke's area), the left posterior IFG (Broca's area), and the connection between them (arcuate fasciculus), as well as a widely distributed conceptual network (in place of Lichtheim's overly localized "concept center"; see Pennington, 2014).

The Hickok and Poeppel (2007) model differs from the classical model in several key respects: (1) It has two streams for processing speech instead of one; (2) the connections between components of the model are bidirectional rather than unidirectional (consistent with recent computational models of speech perception and production); (3) more structures are involved in both speech perception and speech production; and (4) the first two stages of speech processing in the dorsal STG and midposterior superior temporal sulcus (STS) are bilateral, as are the subsequent stages in the ventral speech stream, unlike the left lateralization of all speech processing in the classical model. In the Hickok and Poeppel model, only the last two stages of the dorsal speech stream are strongly left-lateralized, namely, the sensory–motor interface in the posterior sylvian area at the parietal–temporal boundary (called area Spt, for sylvian–parietal–temporal) and the articulatory network.

We can roughly map the correspondence between components of the computational models of babbling and speech imitation in Figures 9.1 and 9.2 and components of the Hickok and Poeppel (2007) model. Besides the obvious correspondences for acoustic and articulatory components across models, the sensorimotor interface (left Spt) is of key interest, because it corresponds roughly to the hidden units in the computational models that perform the crucial mapping between acoustic and somatosensory features and articulatory gestures. In this regard, it is important that area Spt receives input from other sensory modalities beside audition. As discussed earlier, somatosensory information also guides speech perception and production, as does visual information, especially when speech is noisy. We could say that left Spt is a center for amodal perception of speech. The Hickok and Poeppel model represents what is known about brain structures involved in mature speech perception and production. What do we know about what happens in the developing human brain?

Although development typically results by adulthood in a left-hemisphere specialization for structural language (and a right-hemisphere specialization for prosody), these specializations are not present at birth. Indeed, there is remarkable plasticity in the neural substrates for language, which has been demonstrated both by studies of typical development and experiments of nature. By collecting imaging data from sleeping children, Redcay, Haist, and Courchesne (2008) demonstrated bilateral, distributed language processing in younger children (age 2 years) as contrasted with less distributed, more left-lateralized processing in older (age 3 years) children. Xiao, Friederici, Margulies, and Brauer (2016) found continuing connectivity differences between 5- and 6-year-olds that related to increases in sentence comprehension in analyses of resting-state connectivity. Specifically, the only resting-state hub whose internal connectivity increased from 5 to 6 years was the left posterior STG and STS, which are key structures in the Hickok and Poeppel (2007) model, which we discuss later. Children with greater gains in sentence comprehension over the 1-year period also increased their connections between this posterior hub for speech perception and both the left and right inferior frontal cortex. Both the Redcay et al. (2008) and Xiao et al. (2016) results are consistent with an interactive specialization model of language development and inconsistent with an innate or maturational account of the left-hemisphere specialization for language (see Chapter 3 for a fuller discussion of the interactive specialization model of brain development). As discussed in more detail in Johnson and de Haan

(2011), two natural experiments are also pertinent to the question of how the left-hemisphere specialization for language develops: (1) case studies of early unilateral acquired lesions (Bates & Roe, 2001), and (2) visual language in the congenitally deaf (Neville & Bavelier, 2002).

The basic findings from research on infants with early unilateral lesions are (1) that *either* left- *or* right-hemisphere lesions disrupt early language development, but not permanently, as would occur after left-hemisphere acquired lesions in adults, and (2) that early right-hemisphere lesions impair comprehension more than do early left-hemisphere lesions, again in contrast to what is seen in adults. Although these infants with early unilateral lesions do not reach the level of language development (or IQ) of typical controls, their language functioning is still typically within normal limits (i.e., most do not have LI). Turning to the second natural experiment, Neville and Bavelier (2002) have shown that the development of sign language in the congenitally deaf also demonstrates the remarkable plasticity of the developing brain. In this case, visual language processing of signs is mapped onto unused *auditory* cortex. Similarly, in congenitally blind individuals, the visual cortex is involved in processing spoken language, contrary to what is found in sighted individuals.

Blumstein and Amso (2013) reviewed functional magnetic resonance imaging (fMRI) studies of language processing, including the research we just discussed, and concluded that different components are distributed rather than modular, and plastic rather than innately localized. Additional data supporting these conclusions of Blumstein and Amso include the following. First, different components of structural language in Table 9.1, including speech, are subserved by distributed and highly overlapping brain regions. For instance, the IFG is one such overlap area activated by different components of language processing. Second, brain regions that serve language processing also are involved in nonlanguage processing. For example, the STS is involved not only in speech perception but also in biological motion, face processing, and theory of mind. Finally, the plasticity for language localization observed in developing children is also found in adults. In adults learning a second language, the new language is initially processed bilaterally, just as is found in infants learning their first language. In recovery from adult aphasia, the right hemisphere is also recruited as aphasic patients relearn language. Hence, the interactive specialization model of language development extends into adulthood in these cases of adult language learning.

Given these findings about the brain mechanisms subserving language development, we should expect distributed rather than localized changes in brain development in the speech and language disorders reviewed here. Moreover, given the interactive specialization model, we might predict that speech and language processing is more distributed in the brain in children with speech and language disorders than it is in their agemates.

Since the second edition of this book was published in 2009, when we lacked neuroimaging studies of SSD, a few studies have emerged. Preston and colleagues (2012, 2014) conducted an fMRI study followed by a structural MRI study of a sample of 23 school-age children with an earlier diagnosis of SSD without LI, who currently exhibited residual speech errors (mostly on "late 8" speech sounds) and a sample of 54 typically developing, age-matched controls. In their fMRI study, Preston et al. (2012) found that the partly recovered SSD group processed speech more dorsally and more bilaterally than the typically developing group, consistent with a developmental delay. The structural MRI results in the later Preston et al. (2014) study of the same sample also were consistent with this hypothesis. The partly recovered SSD group compared to age-matched controls had more grey matter bilaterally in a key speech hub, the STG, and more white matter in the anterior corpus callosum, which connects frontal articulatory areas on the two sides of the brain. The authors interpreted the grey matter difference as being due to a developmental delay in pruning. The increase in anterior corpus callosum white matter may be consistent with more bilateral processing of speech.

There have been more neuroimaging studies of LI than of SSD. Mayes, Reilly, and Morgan (2015) conducted a systematic review of 18 neuroimaging studies (13 structural and five functional) of LI. The results were quite variable across studies and were not restricted to language regions in the brain, although some of the so-called "nonlanguage" findings, such as those in the insula and premotor cortex, are in structures in the Hickok and Poeppel (2007) dual-stream model of speech and language processing. The most consistent results in this review were volume differences in the caudate nucleus, posterior STG bilaterally (both smaller in the LI groups compared to controls) and in left IFG (in which some studies found smaller volumes in the LI group compared to controls, and others found the opposite). The smaller number of fMRI studies found lower activity in the LI groups in these three structures.

In summary, compared to the sizable neuroimaging literature on speech and language processing in typical adults, neuroimaging studies of SSD and LI are still in their infancy. Future studies could benefit from testing well-established models, like the dual-stream model (Hickok & Poeppel, 2007), and the interactive specialization model, in larger samples of children with SSD and LI.

ETIOLOGY

Familiality

Leonard (2014) reviewed 14 existing family studies of LI. All indicated higher rates of spoken language problems (median of around 35%) in first-degree relatives of a proband with LI than the population prevalence of around 8% that we discussed earlier. Hence, the relative risk of LI for a first-degree relative of a proband with LI is about 4.4. This relative risk is clearly significant but somewhat lower than what is found for the other learning disorders considered in this book. For SSD, B. Lewis et al. (2006) reported a rate of 26% in first-degree relatives of probands with SSD, which is higher than the population prevalence of 3.8% discussed earlier, and yields a relative risk of 6.8, which is higher than that for LI and more similar to that for dyslexia and other learning disorders considered in this book.

There is less research on the familiality of PLI and CAS. We do know that the broader autism phenotype found in relatives of probands with ASD often includes PLI without full ASD, thus establishing that PLI can be familial, but there has not been a family or twin study of PLI itself. Apart from the form of CAS caused by a mutation in the *FOXP2* gene, discussed earlier in Chapter 3 and later in this section on etiology, there are only a few family studies of behaviorally defined CAS, and no twin studies that we could find. For instance, B. Lewis et al. (2004) reported a family study of CAS based on 22 carefully diagnosed probands with CAS out of an initial sample of 42 clinically identified cases of CAS. They compared this group of CAS families with families of SSD-only probands and SSD + LI probands. In the first-degree relatives of these 22 CAS probands, they found a higher rate (86%) of other speech and/or language disorders than in the other two proband groups, consistent with greater family risk for a general verbal deficit in the CAS families. With regard to CAS itself, there were two siblings with CAS out of 27 siblings total (7.4%) in the CAS families and two siblings with CAS in the 143 siblings of SSD only and SSD + LI families (1.4%). Although larger samples are needed for accurately determining the familiality of such a rare disorder, we can make an estimate. Given that the population prevalence of CAS is 2 per 1,000, as discussed earlier, the relative risk for CAS is definitely elevated in both cases (7.4/0.2% = 37 and 1.4/0.2% = 7, respectively). These findings suggest that CAS is highly familial, not only for CAS itself, but also for a general verbal deficit. These results for idiopathic CAS are consistent with what has been found in the KE family, discussed later in this section, which has a rare autosomal dominant form of CAS.

Heritability

We have just seen that SSD is more familial than LI, and this pattern holds when considering their heritabilities. Two twin studies of SSD (B. Lewis & Thompson, 1992; Bishop, 2002), indicated heritabilities for SSD approaching 1.0. Interestingly, the latter study found substantial genetic covariance between SSD and motor problems, with a bivariate heritability of .71. This means that the substantial genetic overlap between SSD and motor problems in general and would be consistent with the Terbrand, van Brenk, et al. (2014) simulation results for SSD discussed earlier, in which SSD could be simulated by adding noise to motor speech representations. In contrast, the heritability for LI is around .45 (B. Lewis et al., 2006), indicating that the environment plays a greater role in the etiology of LI than of SSD.

Since LI and SSD are comorbid, how much does the heritability of one depend on the heritability of the other? Bishop and Hayiou-Thomas (2008) addressed this question in the large Twins Early Development Study (TEDS) sample and found that LI was only heritable when it was comorbid with SSD. This result indicates there are at least two etiological subtypes of LI, one with comorbid SSD that is highly heritable, just as SSD has been found to be, and the other without comorbid SSD that is not substantially heritable.

Gene Locations

One striking example of the role of genes in language development comes from the KE family. About half the members of this family are affected with CAS accompanied by a general speech and language impairment that impacts, most notably, expressive language and articulation. Pedigree analysis revealed that the inheritance pattern was consistent with a single-gene, autosomal-dominant trait (Lai et al., 2001). The gene responsible for this disorder was eventually localized to the long arm of chromosome 7 in the 7q31 region and subsequently identified as the *FOXP2* gene (Lai et al., 2001).

The discovery of the *FOXP2* gene is arguably the most important genetic discovery in the whole field of neurodevelopmental disorders and represents a major breakthrough in our understanding of these disorders. As is often the case in medical genetics, finding a rare gene that produces severe effects in a few families has illuminated how the disorder works in the whole population. For instance, the procedural memory deficit hypothesis of LI (which has since been extended to other learning disorders) derives from neuroimaging findings in the KE family. The discovery of the *FOXP2* gene has also led to important research on the evolution of vocal communication. For instance, a homologue of the *FOXP2* gene is important in birdsong.

The simple Mendelian transmission of this disorder in the KE family is fairly unique and not representative of the larger population of individuals with speech and language disorders (Bartlett et al., 2002). Analysis of LI outside the KE family indicates that though the disorder is significantly heritable, its etiology is typically more consistent with a complex disease model, in which multiple etiological risk factors (genetic and environmental) interact to produce an eventual phenotype. Genomewide scans of multiple families affected by LI have not identified *FOXP2* as a candidate gene. Instead, significant linkage has been reported to 13q21 (using a variety of language phenotypes), 16q (using a phonological memory phenotype), and 19q (again, with a variety of phenotypes) (Bartlett et al., 2002; Specific Language Impairment Consortium, 2002, 2004). Because LI is comorbid with RD, we might expect some genetic overlap. None of these LI loci overlap with those identified for RD, but it is notable that some of the positive linkage results for individuals with LI used reading phenotypes, and also that *FOXP2* has now been associated with RD, although not in a genomewide study (Bartlett et al., 2002; Specific Language Impairment Consortium, 2004). At this point, it is unclear whether the lack of overlap between RD and LI risk loci is due to a lack of power or a true null finding.

The cause of SSD outside the KE family also appears to be consistent with the complex disease model, and we are accumulating knowledge about specific genetic risk factors involved. Again, the *FOXP2* gene does not appear to be implicated in most cases, though mutations in this gene may play a role in the development of SSD in a small minority of cases—notably, among individuals who appear to fit a verbal apraxia subtype (MacDermot et al., 2005). SSD has shown linkage to known dyslexia risk loci, including to chromosomes 3p12–q13 (where *ROBO1* is located), 6p22 (where *DCDC2* and *KIAA0319* are located), and 15q21 (where *DYX1C1* is located) (S. Smith, Pennington, Boada, & Shriberg, 2005; Stein et al., 2004), although not surprisingly given the fairly immature state of this literature, not every study has cleanly replicated these results (Stein et al., 2006). That SSD and RD appear to share genetic risk factors is consistent with the fact that these disorders are comorbid and both are associated with impairments in phonological processing. Existing research has not yet convincingly implicated shared genetic risk factors for LI and RD. However, we expect future studies to do so. These disorders are also comorbid and they overlap at the symptom, neuropsychological, and brain levels. Furthermore, longitudinal studies have demonstrated that children with early language impairments are at much higher risk for later RD than are children with isolated speech sound difficulties, a finding that suggests that the overlap between RD and SSD is partly due to the third variable of LI (Bishop & Adams, 1990). Thus, a goal of future research will be to identify shared etiological risk factors for RD and LI and to clarify the etiological relationship of all three disorders.

Environmental Influences

As discussed earlier, SSD is more heritable than LI overall, and there appear to be etiological subtypes of LI: one comorbid with SSD, which is more genetically influenced, and LI without SSD, which is not substantially heritable. Thus, not surprisingly, more is known about environmental contributions to poor language development than to poor speech development.

It has been clear for decades that there are enormous cross-cultural and subcultural variations in the quantity and quality of language input that parents provide to children, and that these in turn predict children's later language, cognitive, and academic development (Fernald & Weisleder, 2015; B. Hart & Risley, 1992; Heath, 1982). For example, B. Hart and Risley (1992) found that the amount of verbal engagement between parents and children ranged 20-fold in a representative U.S. sample. These differences were associated with various demographic factors (e.g., higher-SES families provided more verbal stimulation to their children than lower-SES families, on average). However, consistent with the broader literature on group differences discussed in Chapter 8, there is also considerable overlap across groups and very significant variability even among families that are demographically similar. What accounts for these striking within-group differences remains largely unknown (Weisleder & Fernald, 2013) and could ultimately become important prevention/intervention targets for LI.

Although these seminal studies produced striking results, they used correlational designs and so did not clearly establish a causal relationship between language input and children's later language ability. It is possible that the observed relationships arise from a third variable, such as genetic influences on language or general intelligence (g) shared by parents and their children. The causal influence could also run largely in the other direction: Perhaps more linguistically or cognitive advanced babies evoke more responses from their caregivers. Several more recent lines of evidence now convincingly demonstrate that quantity and quality of language input do indeed *causally* influence children's language development. First, child-directed speech but not overheard adult-directed speech predicts later language learning (Shneidman, Arroyo, Levine, & Goldin-Meadow, 2013; Shneidman & Goldin-Meadow, 2012; Weisleder & Fernald, 2013). If the relationship between parent and child language were due to shared genes supporting language development, both types of speech should be similarly predictive. Second, the relationship holds even after statistically controlling for the child's earlier language skills (Weisleder & Fernald, 2013), so the causal influence cannot run entirely from child to parent.

Genetically sensitive designs also help establish causality. Rutter and colleagues (Rutter, Thorpe, Greenwood, Northstone, & Golding, 2003; Thorpe, Rutter, & Greenwood, 2003) compared twins to their singleton siblings in a large population sample from the United Kingdom (the Avon Longitudinal Study of Parents and Children [ALSPAC]; Golding, Pembrey, & Jones, 2001). Consistent with previous research, this study indicated that on average, twin children lagged about 3 months behind singletons in language development at age 3 years. This difference could not be attributed to genetic factors, since twins were being compared to other offspring of the same parents. Instead, some twin-specific environmental risk factor must be responsible. Although twins experience more pregnancy and birth complications than do singletons, carefully measured obstetric/perinatal variables were not associated with language outcome in this study (of note, the researchers excluded children with gestational age <33 weeks or other markers of frank neurological injury). However, these twins tended to get less rich communicative input from their mothers compared to singletons, and these differences predicted later language development. Put simply, mothers tended to talk less to each twin child than to a singleton child (perhaps because there were two of them instead of one), and this related to slower language development in the twin group overall.

A final line of evidence supporting a causal relationship between language input to children and their subsequent language skill comes from experimental treatment studies. One small randomized clinical trial in the United States tested an intervention that included eight home visits to low-SES families, designed to increase the amount and diversity of parent talk to their toddlers (Suskind et al., 2016). During the intervention, parents in the treatment group significantly increased quality and quantity of verbal input to their children, and this translated to increased child vocalization during the same period. Gains were not maintained 4 months later, but this small pilot study did demonstrate that language input can cause changes in children's language production. A more recent, large-scale study in rural Senegal demonstrated even more impressive results (Weber, Fernald, & Diop, 2017). In that case, Wolof-speaking caregivers living in some subsistence villages participated in an intervention designed to encourage verbal engagement between caregivers and infants/toddlers. Although practical considerations prevented full random assignment, adults participating in the intervention were compared to well-matched controls in similar villages not participating in the intervention. The intervention led to caregivers nearly doubling the amount of child-directed speech during a play session, as compared to no change for the control group. These group differences predicted parallel changes in children's early language development that were maintained for at least a year afterward.

Since the heritability of SSD is less than 100%, environmental factors must play a role in its etiology as well, but relatively little is known about what these are. Given our earlier discussion regarding the interconnected nature of speech perception/production and broader language development, home language environment is certainly a strong candidate. Indeed, some of the studies on home language environment have included an outcome measure of articulation and found similar results to those reported for language (e.g., Thorpe et al., 2003). Early chronic ear infections (otitis media) have long been hypothesized to contribute to poor speech and language development by reducing available language input, but methodologically rigorous work does not support otitis media as a substantial environmental risk factor for either SSD or LI (Roberts, Rosenfeld, & Zeisel, 2004).

In summary, the quantity and quality of verbal engagement between caregivers and young children causally influences later speech and language development. A relatively impoverished language environment can be a contributing etiological risk factor for LI (although, for a variety of reasons, these may be the very same children who are relatively unlikely to come to clinical attention and hence to receive a formal diagnosis or treatment). In addition to main effects of environment, it is likely that the disorders considered here are influenced by gene × environment interplay.

DIAGNOSIS AND TREATMENT

Diagnosis

Presenting Symptoms

The presenting symptoms in LI vary with the age at which the child comes in for evaluation. In a younger child, concern is more likely to involve language development itself. Parents will note that the child cannot talk or comprehend as well as his peers or siblings. Although symptoms of LI are essentially always present before school entry, parents may not be aware of them unless the child has comorbid SSD or CAS. Preschool children with normal speech but delayed language quite often do not come to clinical attention (Bishop & Hayiou-Thomas, 2008) but may be referred for evaluation after they enter school. In school-age children, academic difficulty is likely to be the key complaint. Because so many children with LI also have an RD, many of the presenting symptoms are likely to be similar to those described in Chapter 10. However, most (but not all) children with LI experience difficulties across the curriculum, because so much teaching and learning depend on linguistic communication. In both older and younger children, adults may comment that the child cannot follow verbal directions, has immature grammar, or will not listen to a story for an appropriate length of time.

As with dyslexia, there will be some cases of LI in which presenting symptoms appear primarily emotional or behavioral. There may be conflict around homework or stomachaches on school mornings. The child may appear "tuned out" in the classroom and may not do what is asked of him or her. In some children, these symptoms reflect the second disorder of ADHD, but other children with LI appear inattentive due to poor language comprehension. Thus, it is important to learn whether the child is also experiencing lapses in attention, difficulties with organization, or hyperactivity that cannot be explained by weak language skills. Some children with LI are extremely frustrated by their difficulty communicating, which in turn may lead to social problems. For example, if the child is teased on the playground and cannot generate a quick verbal retort, the response may well be to hit or shove instead. Some children may present with distress with departures from normal routine. Verbal explanations of what to expect are of limited use to children with significant language difficulties; thus, these children may compensate with overreliance on established routines. Presenting symptoms in PLI overlap to a large extent with those for LI but also include concerns about socialization, such as trouble making and keeping friends or difficulties reading and responding to social cues. Thus, a diagnostic evaluation for PLI should allow the clinician to rule both LI and ASD out or in.

Presenting symptoms in speech disorders, either SSD or CAS, are straightforward and easily observed by parents or other adults in the child's life. The child has difficulty speaking clearly and is not well understood by strangers. In more extreme cases, even siblings or parents may struggle to understand what the child is trying to say. Some children compensate by shortening and simplifying their utterances, so overall expressive language will appear delayed. (Of course, poor expressive language may also reflect comorbid LI). The child may be frustrated by this difficulty, which may be manifest in any number of ways—reluctance to repeat him- or herself, a quiet presentation with strangers, or an attempt to use alternative means of communication (e.g., showing instead of saying). Children with impairing speech problems are more likely to come in for evaluation in preschool or earlier, so school difficulty is unlikely to be a key presenting symptom.

History

The most relevant history for LI concerns early language development. Typically, all language milestones are delayed, particularly for expressive language. Thus, the child is late to produce single words, to combine two words, and to speak in full sentences. Parents and teachers may notice that the child's grammar sounds immature. Errors in verb conjugation, pronouns, and word order persist long after peers have mastered these skills. Often, children with LI have comorbid SSD and therefore a history of articulation difficulty, so it is important to establish whether early language difficulties are limited to articulation or extend to other aspects of language development. Parents often note that strangers understand little of what the child has said. There may be particular difficulty learning terms related to time, sequencing, or directionality (e.g., yesterday–tomorrow, before–after, left–right).

When a child has a history of significant language delay, both autism and ID should be considered for differential diagnosis, so it is important to learn about early social and nonverbal development. Children with LI may develop social problems secondary to communication difficulties, but early social development should have been fairly typical. As a baby or toddler, a child with LI would have shown interest in others, made adequate eye contact, and engaged in spontaneous imitation. Similarly, in a child with LI and not ID, early nonverbal skills should have been reasonably intact, and there would not be a history of major delays in motor milestones or learning to solve puzzles, for example.

The most relevant history for SSD concerns early speech development. Once the child begins talking, he or she is extremely difficult to understand because of the large numbers of sound substitutions and omissions. The child may be perceived as engaging in "baby talk." Expressive language milestones are often delayed, but in a child with isolated SSD, receptive language development should have been fairly typical. This history may be difficult to ascertain, however, since expressive language is much more readily observable by parents. Some children with SSD have broader oral–motor difficulties, which would be evident in the history as early difficulties with feeding, swallowing, or drooling.

As with other disorders we consider in this book, both LI and SSD are partly heritable; thus family history (of the child's biological family) is relevant. Sometimes there is a positive family history that the parents do not believe is genetically based, because the family has developed an alternative explanation. For example, substantial cognitive delays are sometimes attributed to a difficult birth, or speech delays to a physical problem (e.g., a large tongue or tight frenulum, which attaches the tongue to the floor of the mouth). It is important not to accept these explanations at face value but to recognize that they may represent an attempt (partly or fully incorrect) to understand a genetically influenced disorder.

Behavioral Observations

Children with any speech or language disorder often present as quiet or reluctant to speak. Typically, these children have had several years' experience learning that strangers cannot understand them very well and that attempts to communicate will be unsuccessful. It may be helpful to have an initial conversation with the child's parent present to act as "translator," if necessary. The examiner may also select a conversational topic for which there is more likely to be shared understanding, such as objects present in the room or a special logo on the child's shirt or shoes.

Once the child feels comfortable, he or she will provide numerous language samples, so it is important to listen carefully. Does the child speak in full sentences? Does he or she fail to conjugate verbs or make other grammatical errors? Children with LI often make word-finding errors, or have trouble coming up with the specific words they want to say. Such errors may be manifest as "groping" for the word, or the child may simply talk around concepts he or she cannot quite name. Some children make frank paraphasic errors, substituting one word or nonword for another. For example, one young child with LI responded, "Cow" when asked, "What animal goes meow?" This error probably resulted from a combination of a semantic relationship between cat and cow (both are familiar animals) and a phonological similarity to the word the child had most recently heard (*meow*). Behavioral observation may provide rich information about receptive language as well. Some children frequently ask for clarification or appear confused after lengthy directions, or they may repeat directions to themselves while performing the task. Others never ask for repetition but simply act in ways that make clear they have misunderstood the examiner. For any task with complex instructions, it is particularly important to ensure that the child understands what he or she is to do, so that his or her abilities can be accurately assessed.

SSD is easily observed by parents and should be fairly apparent to the examiner as well. In conversational speech, the child makes sound omission and/or substitution errors, and is difficult to understand. The examiner may perceive that the child is talking rapidly, which likely relates to the examiner's own reduced comprehension (just as we often believe people speaking languages other than our own speak very fast). Young children with severely reduced intelligibility often resort to other means of communication, such as getting up out of their chairs to show you what they mean. Children with SSD vary in their willingness to repeat themselves and in their frustration about not being understood. If a child has made multiple attempts to communicate something and you the examiner cannot understand him or her, it may be useful to say, "Let's ask your mom about that at the break."

Case Presentations

Case Presentation 1

Megan is a 9-year-old third grader. Her parents sought the evaluation because they are concerned about her progress in reading, reading comprehension, and math. Homework is very difficult, and often takes Megan more than twice as long as it is supposed to, although she is typically cooperative and attentive to the task at hand. Megan has had particular difficulty with a reading program in which she is required to read a book for homework and answer comprehension questions about it the next day at school. Megan often cannot answer any of the questions accurately, even though she is reading books that are 1–2 years below grade level. Megan herself explained how difficult this task can be, saying, "Sometimes everybody else is on the last question and I'm still on the first one so I just sit there and cry because I'm so frustrated."

The pregnancy with Megan was uncomplicated, but her parents reported that delivery was difficult and required suction and forceps. Although parents did not recall specific Apgar scores, they were thought to be somewhat low, and Megan required supplemental oxygen for several hours. Nonetheless, she was thought to be ready for discharge at 3 days old, at which time she developed a fever. This illness required a weeklong hospitalization with intravenous antibiotic treatment. Early motor milestones were achieved at the expected ages, but language development was somewhat delayed. Megan's parents described how strangers could not understand anything Megan said until she was 3, because her articulation and expressive language were poor. However, she appeared to understand what was said to her. Megan did receive some speech therapy for articulation difficulties when she was in preschool. Although Megan is now quite chatty and is well understood by strangers, her parents continue to have some concerns about her language development. They commented that she cannot follow multistep directions and often has trouble coming up with the specific words she wants to say. Additionally, Megan has a lisp when producing the /s/ sound.

Megan had trouble learning letters in preschool, and she has always been in the weakest reading group. She received extra help from the reading specialist at school in first and second grade, and her parents have also pursued some private tutoring. Her spelling is quite poor, and Megan has always struggled to memorize her math facts. More recently, her parents have become concerned that she is having difficulty mastering new math concepts and solving math word problems.

Megan's father received speech therapy for articulation difficulties when he was ages 3 and 4 but did not report any problems in school. He graduated from college and works as an administrator for a nonprofit organization. Megan's mother did not report any specific speech, language, or reading difficulties, but noted that school was a "struggle," by which she meant that she received B's and C's despite working very hard. She completed a 2-year college degree. Before her children were born, she worked as an administrative assistant. For the last 10 years, she has run a home day care.

Megan's diagnostic testing is summarized in Table 9.2.

DISCUSSION

Megan's history is similar to that of children with a specific RD. However, several aspects of her presentation indicate that her language difficulties are broader than typically seen in children with classic dyslexia alone and are therefore consistent with a diagnosis of LI. Although children with dyslexia alone sometimes have subtle expressive language problems as preschoolers, Megan's difficulties in this area were quite significant, to the point that strangers could not understand her. In addition to early history, current complaints are indicative of a more general language disorder. Her parents have noticed that Megan has substantial difficulty with word finding (coming up with the specific words she wants to say), as well as understanding complex language, such as multistep directions. Many children with language impairments also have articulation weaknesses. Compared to weaknesses in vocabulary or grammar, articulation difficulties are most likely to be noticed by parents or teachers and to result in referral to a speech–language pathologist. Megan likely has had difficulties in all three areas from an early age, though early treatment focused primarily on articulation.

Megan's test results support a diagnosis of LI. Her scores on nearly all language-based tests fall well below age expectations. Although some children with LI also have relatively weak nonverbal skills, Megan shows a large discrepancy. Although her nonverbal reasoning abilities are quite solid, her ability to think and reason using language is only marginally better than that of many children with ID. Furthermore, essentially all aspects of structural language are quite weak, including phonological processing, semantics, syntax, and discourse comprehension (e.g., on the Wide Range Assessment of Memory and Learning, Second Edition [WRAML-2] Story test). Megan did perform relatively better on tests that had lower expressive language demands, including the Peabody Picture Vocabulary Test, Fourth Edition (PPVT-4) and the Semantic Relationships subtest of the Clinical Evaluation of Language Fundamentals—Fifth Edition (CELF-5). The discrepancy between

TABLE 9.2. Test Summary, Case 1

Performance validity

Test of Memory Malingering
- Trial 1 — RS = 42
- Trial 2 — RS = 46 (valid)

General intelligence

WISC-V Full Scale IQ — SS = 84

Crystallized intelligence

WISC-V Verbal Comprehension Index — SS = 76
- Similarities — ss = 6
- Vocabulary — ss = 5

Working memory

WISC-V Working Memory Index — SS = 88
- Digit Span — ss = 6
- Picture Span — ss = 10

Processing speed

WISC-V Processing Speed Index — SS = 100
- Coding — ss = 8
- Symbol Search — ss = 12

Fluid intelligence

WISC-V Fluid Reasoning Index — SS = 100
- Matrix Reasoning — ss = 11
- Figure Weights — ss = 9

WISC-V Visual Spatial Index — SS = 102
- Block Design — ss = 10
- Visual Puzzles — ss = 11

Academic

Reading

History
- CLDQ Reading Scale — 95th %ile

Basic literacy
- WIAT-III Word Reading — SS = 86
- WIAT-III Pseudoword Decoding — SS = 91
- WIAT-III Spelling — SS = 84

Reading fluency
- TOWRE-2 Sight Word Efficiency — SS = 84
- TOWRE-2 Phonemic Decoding Efficiency — SS = 78
- GORT-5 Fluency — ss = 4

Reading comprehension
- GORT-5 Comprehension — ss = 4

Math

History
- CLDQ Math Scale — 91st %ile

Calculation and problem solving
- WIAT-III Numerical Operations — SS = 94
- WIAT-III Math Problem Solving — SS = 83

Math fluency
- WIAT-III Math Fluency — SS = 90

(continued)

TABLE 9.2. (continued)

Oral language

Semantics, syntax, and verbal memory

CELF-5 Core Language	SS = 75
Word Classes	ss = 5
Formulated Sentences	ss = 4
Recalling Sentences	ss = 6
Semantic Relationships	ss = 7
PPVT-4	SS = 90
EVT-2	SS = 77
WRAML-2 Story Memory	ss = 6
WRAML-2 Story Memory Delay	ss = 7

Phonology

CTOPP-2 Elision	ss = 7
CTOPP-2 Phoneme Isolation	ss = 5
CTOPP-2 Nonword Repetition	ss = 3

Verbal processing speed

CTOPP-2 Rapid Symbolic Naming	SS = 94

Attention

Vanderbilt Inattention	
Parent	RS = 0
Teacher	RS = 0
Vanderbilt Hyperactivity/Impulsivity	
Parent	RS = 0
Teacher	RS = 1

Note. SS, standard score with mean = 100 and *SD* = 15; ss = scaled score with mean = 10 and *SD* = 3; RS, raw score; %ile, percentile rank; WISC-V, Wechsler Intelligence Scale for Children—Fifth Edition; CLDQ, Colorado Learning Difficulties Questionnaire; WIAT-III, Wechsler Individual Achievement Test—Third Edition; TOWRE-2, Test of Word Reading Efficiency—Second Edition; GORT-5, Gray Oral Reading Tests—Fifth Edition; CELF-5, Clinical Evaluation of Language Fundamentals—Fifth Edition; EVT-2, Expressive Vocabulary Test—Second Edition; PPVT-4, Peabody Picture Vocabulary Test—Fourth Edition; CTOPP-2, Comprehensive Test of Phonological Processing, Second Edition; WRAML-2: Wide Range Assessment of Memory and Learning, Second Edition; Vanderbilt, NICHQ Vanderbilt Assessment Scales.

her receptive vocabulary on the PPVT-4 and her naming or expressive vocabulary (Expressive Vocabulary Test–Second Edition [EVT-2] and Wechsler Intelligence Scale for Children–Fifth Edition [WISC-V] Vocabulary) is consistent with the word-finding problems her parents describe. Relatively spared receptive vocabulary is common in children with LI, particularly if they have been exposed to good language models in the home. Like most children with LI, Megan has a weakness in verbal short-term memory. This difficulty is evident in her scores on the Digit Span subtest of the WISC-V, the Sentence Repetition subtest of the CELF-5, and the Nonword Repetition subtest of the Comprehensive Test of Phonological Processing, Second Edition (CTOPP-2). Verbal short-term memory impairment likely contributes to her inability to follow multistep directions and can create quite a liability in the classroom setting.

Several qualitative observations also support the LI diagnosis. Megan's verbal responses on the WISC-V were often vague and poorly organized. She demonstrated word-finding difficulties in the testing situation. As one example, she described a woman she knows as "a girl, but she's old." Furthermore, when retelling the WRAML-2 story, Megan made statements such as "The girl had her thing." She often appeared confused when complex directions were presented, and on a few occasions, asked the examiner to "please talk again" (meaning to repeat the instructions).

Like most children with LI, Megan clearly has a very significant reading problem, which merits the additional diagnosis of dyslexia. Megan demonstrates the classic difficulties of a child with dyslexia, including weaknesses in word-level reading and spelling, more pronounced difficulty on timed than untimed reading tests, and difficulty with phonological processing. Her reading comprehension was also poor, resulting from difficulties with both decoding and oral language comprehension. Megan also has difficulties with some aspects of math. Her basic calculation skills are within normal limits for her age, but she struggled with math problem solving on the Wechsler Individual Achievement Test—Third Edition (WIAT-III). Math weaknesses may arise from language difficulties in several ways. First, new math concepts are often explained to children using complex language, which may be hard for Megan to follow. Similarly, she is likely to have difficulty reading and understanding word problems. Verbal memory weaknesses can cause problems memorizing math facts, although in Megan's case, math fact fluency is within normal limits and consistent with other measures of processing speed.

Given Megan's slightly risky birth history, one question is whether her difficulties may result from an acquired brain injury, such as would result from hypoxia. Overall, current results suggest that Megan's learning difficulties are more likely to have a developmental rather than an acquired origin. There is no evidence that Megan demonstrated acute signs of neurological injury in the neonatal period. The base rates of the mild complications she experienced are high, and most children with similar birth histories develop entirely normally. Furthermore, there is at least some family history of speech and language difficulties.

As with all children who visit our clinics, Megan was screened for attentional difficulties. Parent and teacher questionnaire responses were all in the normal range, and neither early history nor observations were consistent with ADHD. In fact, parent report suggests that attention is an area of strength for Megan given that she is able to attend for several hours to homework that must feel extremely difficult and tedious for her.

Case Presentation 2

Gabriel, a 5-year-old boy, will be starting kindergarten in a few months. His pediatrician referred him for this assessment because of concerns about his speech development. Gabriel was a late talker, and his speech has always sounded immature, but his parents had assumed he would grow out of this "baby talk." However, at his 5-year-old well-child visit, Gabriel's pediatrician noted that he continues to struggle with articulation, such that he is difficult to understand, and suggested a more complete evaluation.

Gabriel's prenatal and birth histories are uncomplicated. Early motor milestones were met as expected, but speech–language development was somewhat delayed. He first said single words at 21 months, first combined two words at 2 years, and did not speak in short sentences until he was nearly 3 years old. When Gabriel first began talking, strangers could not comprehend him, and even his parents understood him only about 75% of the time. Despite these delays, his parents always thought his receptive language was fairly good. They remembered that he responded to his name by age 6 months, understood several words by 9 months (e.g., *nose, doggie*) and could follow a simple instruction by the time he began to walk (e.g., "Bring me the book"). Gabriel had a history of regular ear infections as a toddler, which led to placement of tubes at age 2 years, and his parents wonder whether this history relates to his current difficulties. According to his pediatrician, Gabriel's hearing is now normal.

Gabriel has attended preschool for the last 2 years. On the paperwork she filled out for this evaluation, his teacher wrote, "Gabriel is a bright, sweet little boy who is a delight to teach. I hope his speech improves soon because it is difficult for me and the other children to understand him." Gabriel gets along well with his peers and is regularly invited over for playdates.

Gabriel's mother notes that she had some speech difficulties herself and attributed these to having a tongue that was too big for her mouth. She recalled that she said "cimanon" for *cinnamon* and could not pronounce the /r/ sound until she was in third grade. Although her speech has since normalized, she noted that she sometimes has difficulty pronouncing unfamiliar words. She graduated from college and nursing school, and works as a cardiac nurse. Gabriel's father reports no history of speech or learning problems. He has a master's degree and works as a geographer.

Gabriel's diagnostic testing is summarized in Table 9.3.

DISCUSSION

Gabriel's history and current presentation are consistent with SSD. Although children with SSD are at risk for additional disorders of language development, including LI and later RD, Gabriel appears to have an isolated speech disorder. He does not currently have a broader language impairment, and his early literacy skills are developing nicely.

On the Goldman–Fristoe Test of Articulation 3 (GFTA-3), Gabriel consistently distorted the /r/, /l/, and /s/ sounds. In addition, he substituted /f/ for /th/ and had difficulty pronouncing most consonant blends. In conversational speech, Gabriel made multiple sound substitution (e.g., "tat" for *cat*) and omission errors (e.g., "boom" for *broom*), which reduced his intelligibility. Gabriel's scores on the GFTA-3 are clearly discrepant from measures of nearly all his other cognitive/intellectual abilities, most of which are somewhat above age expectations, and warrant a course of speech therapy. In addition to articulation weaknesses, the defining symptom of SSD, Gabriel also demonstrated a relative deficit in verbal short-term

TABLE 9.3. Test Summary, Case 2

Performance validity

Test of Memory Malingering
- Trial 1 — RS = 45
- Trial 2 — RS = 48 (valid)

General intelligence

WPPSI-IV Full Scale IQ — SS = 114

Crystallized intelligence

WPPSI-IV Verbal Comprehension Index — SS = 111
- Information — ss = 13
- Similarities — ss = 11

Working memory

WPPSI-IV Working Memory Index — SS = 116
- Picture Memory — ss = 10
- Zoo Locations — ss = 15

Processing speed

WPPSI-IV Processing Speed Index — SS = 106
- Bug Search — ss = 11
- Cancellation — ss = 11

Fluid intelligence

WPPSI-IV Fluid Reasoning Index — SS = 117
- Matrix Reasoning — ss = 13
- Figure Weights — ss = 13

WPPSI-IV Visual Spatial Index — SS = 118
- Block Design — ss = 14
- Visual Puzzles — ss = 12

Academic

Basic literacy
- WIAT-III Early Reading Skills — SS = 110
- WIAT-III Alphabet Writing Fluency — SS = 106

Math
- WIAT-III Math Problem Solving — SS = 119

Oral language

Speech
- GFTA-3
  - Sounds in Words — SS = 55
  - Sounds in Sentences — SS = 74

Semantics
- WPPSI-IV
  - Receptive Vocabulary — ss = 13
  - Picture Naming — ss = 11

Syntax
- CELF-5
  - Sentence Comprehension — ss = 10
  - Word Structure — ss = 7
  - Formulated Sentences — ss = 9

Phonology
- CTOPP-2 Elision — ss = 11
- CTOPP-2 Blending Words — ss = 10
- CTOPP-2 Nonword Repetition — ss = 5

Verbal processing speed
- CTOPP-2 Rapid Color Naming — ss = 9
- CTOPP-2 Rapid Object Naming — ss = 12

Verbal memory
- WRAML-2 Verbal Learning — ss = 10
- WRAML-2 Verbal Learning Delay — ss = 11
- WRAML-2 Sentence Memory — ss = 6

(continued)

TABLE 9.3. (continued)

Attention

Vanderbilt Inattention	
Parent	RS = 0
Teacher	RS = 0
Vanderbilt Hyperactivity/Impulsivity	
Parent	RS = 0
Teacher	RS = 1

Note. SS, standard score with mean = 100 and *SD* = 15; ss, scaled score with mean = 10 and *SD* = 3; RS, raw score; %ile, percentile rank; WPPSI-IV, Wechsler Preschool and Primary Scale of Intelligence—Fourth Edition; GFTA-3, Goldman–Fristoe Test of Articulation 3. For other abbreviations, see Table 9.2.

memory, a cognitive risk factor for the disorder. Verbal short-term memory difficulties were evident on the CTOPP-2 Nonword Repetition and WRAML-2 Sentence Memory tasks.

Although Gabriel was a late talker, his current broader language skill, as measured by formal testing, is good. It seems likely that his early language delays primarily reflected difficulties with speech development. Children whose early language delays are limited to expressive language have a better prognosis than children with both expressive and receptive delays, and parent report places Gabriel in the former group. Although his parents are concerned about his early ear infections, there is little research to support a causal link to long-lasting speech/language difficulties. Ear infections are quite common in the general population, so many children both with and without SSD are likely to have an early history similar to Gabriel's.

Gabriel is too young to complete an in-depth academic assessment, but a brief screen of his early literacy and math skills was conducted using the WIAT-III. In addition, his phonological awareness and rapid naming abilities were assessed with the CTOPP-2, since these are good predictors of later reading ability. Currently, Gabriel's achievement appears commensurate with his intellectual abilities and is not a cause for concern. His parents can be reassured that the majority of children with SSD do not have unusual difficulty with literacy acquisition, especially when they have strong cognitive abilities. Nonetheless, as mentioned earlier, Gabriel's academic progress, and especially his literacy development, should be monitored carefully, and appropriate intervention should be put in place quickly if difficulties arise. An abbreviated reevaluation at the end of first grade or beginning of second grade was recommended, just to ensure that reading and spelling are developing as expected.

There is a notable family history of speech difficulties through Gabriel's mother. Despite her own account of her difficulties, it is more likely that she had an underlying cognitive–linguistic liability for speech difficulty, just as Gabriel does. Although most outward signs of her early speech difficulty have resolved, the subtle residual of this liability is observable in her current difficulty pronouncing complex unfamiliar words.

Treatment

When the previous edition of this book was published, we concluded that various speech–language therapy-based approaches appeared helpful in treating LI and SSD, but that these interventions did not yet meet all standards for well-established, empirically supported treatments. These same general conclusions hold today. The single, most authoritative summary has been provided by a Cochrane meta-analysis (Law, Garrett, & Nye, 2003).

Specific approaches to treating speech and language disorders include imitation, modeling, focused stimulation, conversational recasts, and milieu teaching, all of which provide the child with LI or SSD targeted exposure to, and practice with, the linguistic forms in which they are deficient. In other words, these therapies provide a more intensive and focused "dose" of some of the things parents and other adults naturally do to stimulate language development. Evaluation of these various approaches reveal gains relative to either untreated controls or untreated linguistic forms in the child's repertoire. Such interventions have also been shown to increase the rate of language development and to transfer to spontaneous speech. In Law et al. (2003), the most reliable treatment effects were for children with speech and expressive vocabulary problems, but not for children with receptive language problems. Much less is known about effect treatment of PLI specifically (Gerber, Brice, Capone, Fujiki, & Timler, 2012), although children with this disorder are likely benefit from treatment approaches used with LI and/or ASD.

Despite these optimistic outcomes from research on the treatment of SSD and LI, there are some caveats. Just as is true in psychotherapy outcome studies, many forms of speech and language therapy appear to work, but all to about an equal extent (Baker & McLeod, 2011; Nye, Foster, & Seaman, 1987). Hence, the treatments provided by clinicians using different approaches may nonetheless share some common elements, but these have not been clearly delineated. Moreover, in the Law et al. (2003) meta-analysis, no significant differences were found between using trained parents versus clinicians to deliver the intervention. Not surprising, including parents in the intervention also makes treatment more cost-effective (Law et al., 2012). A second caveat is that long-term follow-up studies of treated children indicate that initial severity of LI (or SSD) predicts language outcome, but duration of treatment does not (Aram & Nation, 1980; Bishop & Edmundson, 1987). Although these were not treatment studies per se, since the treatments were those that would ordinarily occur in community settings, it is still concerning that there is no evidence of a dose–response relation for duration of treatment. Moreover, since there is a wide range of normal variation in speech and language development in young children, some of those identified as having SSD or LI and given treatment would likely have developed normally anyway. Other children have more persisting problems; the critical question is how much treatment helps those children.

In general, it is difficult for behavioral treatments to meet all standards for empirically supported treatments, but the field would benefit from more studies that meet all of the "gold standards" for treatment evaluation, especially those that include comparison groups receiving equal-intensity intervention. It may also be the case that language disorders are inherently difficult to remediate, making identification of effective treatments even more difficult. We know, in fact, that available treatments do not cure LI or SSD. On average, adults treated for SSD as children still have phoneme awareness deficits and reading problems (Lewis & Freebairn, 1992). Follow-up of children with LI into adolescence (Snowling, Bishop, & Stothard, 2000) or young adulthood (Rutter & Mahwood, 1991) reveals that a sizable proportion have declined in reading, IQ, language, and even social skills compared to how they performed at younger ages. Language skill is so important to development that it is not surprising that a persisting language impairment would exact a greater and greater cost. Just as the social deficit in autism deprives a child of important inputs for development, so does a persisting language impairment.

Table 9.4 provides a summary of current research and evidence-based practice for speech and language disorders.

TABLE 9.4. Summary Table: Speech and Language Disorders

Definition

- Poor structural language (LI), social use of language (PLI), or speech articulation (SSD) skill relative to age expectations. A minority of children with speech articulation problems have a more severe presentation and make certain kind of speech errors that are consistent with a diagnosis of CAS.
- Exclusionary criteria include deafness, peripheral deficit in the vocal apparatus, acquired neurological insults, intellectual disability, and autism.

Prevalence and epidemiology

- LI: 5–8%.
- SSD: 2–13%.
- CAS: < 1%.
- Slightly more males than females are affected (approximately 1.5:1).

Etiology

- Both LI and SSD are partially genetic. LI: linkage to chromosomes 13q, 16q, and 19q. SSD: linkage to chromosomes 3, 6p, and 15q.
- LI without SSD is less heritable than most neurodevelopmental disorders, and there may be an etiological subtype of LI that is of predominantly environmental origin.
- Environmental risk/protective factors include home language environment.

Brain mechanisms

- LI: Neuroimaging results have been variable and have implicated widely distributed bilateral regions. The most consistent findings include structural and functional differences in the caudate nucleus, bilateral superior temporal gyrus, and left inferior frontal gyrus.
- SSD: Little work, but some evidence, suggests that children with SSD process speech more dorsally and bilaterally than their same-age peers, which suggests a developmental delay.

Developmental neuropsychology

- LI: There are many single-deficit neuropsychological theories, none of which can explain all cases of LI. Risk factors that should be tested in future multiple-deficit models include procedural learning, phonological memory, verbal declarative memory, processing speed, and nonlinguistic auditory processing.
- SSD: Phonological processing deficits, including those in phonological awareness and phonological memory. A subset of children have poor oral–motor development.

Diagnosis

- Diagnosis of SSD is typically made by a speech–language pathologist and involves analysis of the child's articulation skills relative to typical developmental expectations.
- Diagnosis of LI can be made by an appropriately trained psychologist or speech–language pathologist and is based on a history of difficulty acquiring language milestones, as well as performance below age expectations on standardized language measures.
- The process of differential diagnosis should consider whether the child's communication difficulties reflect a more severe neurodevelopmental disorder (i.e., ID or ASD).
- In school-age children with LI, rates of specific learning disorders are very high, so assessment should include standardized measures of academic skills. Screening for comorbid ADHD or emotional concerns is also recommended.

Treatment

- Speech–language therapy techniques (e.g., imitation, modeling, focused stimulation, conversational recasts) that provide additional exposure to and practice with the linguistic forms that the child has been slow to develop.
- Training parents to provide therapy at home may be similarly helpful and more cost-effective.

CHAPTER 10

Reading Disability (Dyslexia)

CHAPTER SUMMARY

Reading disability (RD), or dyslexia, is arguably the best understood learning disorder of the six learning disorders covered in this book. We know the most about its developmental neuropsychology, we have converging results regarding its structural and functional brain phenotype, and considerable progress has been made regarding its etiology. The scientific success in our current understanding of dyslexia crucially depended on a mature cognitive science of skilled reading and reading development, but it was also aided by the fact that dyslexia is the most specific of the six disorders covered in this book and has a long research history.

Dyslexia, or RD, is defined as slow and inaccurate single-word reading, and is almost invariably associated with poor spelling. Hence, individuals with dyslexia are slower at learning letter–sound relations and at automating this skill in printed word recognition. Although these basic-level literacy problems often make reading comprehension more difficult, dyslexia is not *primarily* a problem in reading comprehension. There are children who have normal single-word reading skills, but whose reading comprehension is impaired. They are called "poor comprehenders" and almost invariably have broader language processing problems than are observed in dyslexia. Poor comprehenders are discussed briefly in Chapter 6. Dyslexia is found across languages, including logographic languages such as Chinese. Its cognitive predictors (letter knowledge, phoneme awareness, and rapid naming) are fairly universal across alphabetic languages and extend partly to logographic languages as well.

In terms of developmental neuropsychology, dyslexia manifests early in development as problems with speech and language development, but with heterotypic continuity, such that the particular problem with speech and language at a given age is most evident in the newest developmental task (e.g., first speech perception and babbling, then vocabulary and syntax, and eventually phoneme awareness). This developmental course would be consistent with a more general problem in learning language, such as a problem with implicit learning, and not consistent with an exclusively phonological deficit. Because dyslexia first manifests in spoken language, an exclusively visual deficit or an orthographic learning deficit cannot explain dyslexia. However, visual or orthographic deficits may contribute to dyslexia. The best neuropsychological model of dyslexia is one that includes multiple deficits, none of which is both necessary and sufficient to cause dyslexia.

The near universality of the neuropsychological phenotype is mirrored by a near-universal neuroimaging phenotype, in which children and adults with dyslexia have structural and functional differences in a distributed reading network that typically develops in the left hemisphere. This reading network builds on the well-established perisylvian left-hemisphere language network involved in early speech and language development, but adds an occipito-temporal component in the left fusiform gyrus (called the *visual word form area*). This additional component is necessitated by the fact that reading requires mapping visual language (print) onto spoken language.

In terms of etiology, dyslexia is moderately heritable and associated with multiple genes, as is true for all the other disorders discussed in this book. Some of these genes are shared across disorders, thus helping to account for the comorbidity of dyslexia with other disorders such as language impairment (LI), speech sound disorder (SSD), and attention-deficit/hyperactivity disorder (ADHD). The environment is also important in the etiology of dyslexia, and plausible environmental risk factors include a child's spoken language environment and the extent to which parents engage the child in preliteracy activities.

Our well-developed scientific understanding of dyslexia informs best practices for diagnosing and treating it. Because we understand its developmental precursors so well, we can identify children at possible risk for dyslexia by the beginning of kindergarten. We can do this by using not only cognitive predictors of later reading skill, such as letter knowledge and phoneme awareness, but also family history for dyslexia, which make an incremental contribution to predicting later reading development. Kindergarten children at possible risk for dyslexia should receive more intensive scientifically validated literacy instruction, and their progress in learning to read should be monitored more closely than children not at risk.

HISTORY

RD, or dyslexia, was first described more than a century ago by Pringle-Morton (see Pringle-Morgan, 1896) and Kerr (1897), but real advances in our understanding of its cognitive phenotype have only come in the last five decades. These advances have made it much clearer that dyslexia is a type of language disorder and that its underlying neuropsychological deficit partly involves faulty development of phonological representations. Earlier theories of dyslexia postulated a basic deficit in visual processing. These theories focused on the reversal errors made by individuals with dyslexia, such as writing *b* for *d* or *was* for *saw*. Orton (1925, 1937) termed this deficit *strephosymbolia*, which means "twisted symbols," and hypothesized that this visual problem arose because of a failure of hemispheric dominance. According to Orton's hypothesis, mirror images of a visual stimulus in the typically nondominant right hemisphere were not inhibited, thus leading to reversal errors. Vellutino (1979a) demonstrated that such reversal errors in dyslexia were restricted to processing print in one's own language, and were thus really linguistic rather than visual in nature. It is still possible that there may be other sorts of visual processing problems correlated with dyslexia, but any comprehensive theory of dyslexia must account for the well-replicated findings of oral language deficits that precede the onset of reading problems.

DEFINITION

We now consider the similarities and differences across three influential definitions of dyslexia or RD, as well as some implications for individual diagnosis. The three definitions include an expert consensus statement (Lyon, Shaywitz, & Shaywitz, 2003), the legal definition used in the Individuals with Disabilities Education Improvement Act in the United States (known as IDEA 2004), and the definition in the most recent version of the DSM (DSM-5; American Psychiatric Association, 2013). All three definitions center around a core difficulty in basic literacy skills, such as single-word reading, reading fluency, and spelling. All these definitions also include a list of exclusionary conditions, such that the literacy problems cannot be due to inadequate instruction, a primary sensory disability such as blindness or deafness, or a global developmental disorder such as ID, although they vary in how exhaustive the list is. We use the terms *dyslexia* and *reading disability* interchangeably throughout this book. DSM-5 and IDEA 2004 use slightly different terminology (specific learning disorder and specific learning disability, respectively), but as long as the core impairment is in basic literacy skills such as *reading accuracy, reading fluency,* and/or *spelling,* these terms should also be seen as synonymous with dyslexia. It is important to be clear on the fact that these terms are all essentially equivalent to prevent confusion for families. Clinicians and educators can fall into a nominal fallacy of assuming that because the names are different, the underlying disorders and appropriate treatments are different as well. For example, the parents of one boy we previously evaluated told us, "The school team told us he has a learning disability in reading fluency and decoding, but they have not seen any signs of dyslexia!" Although this child was, in fact, receiving an appropriate reading intervention at school, the parents had not sought out useful resources, such as the local branch of the International Dyslexia Association, because they wrongly believed these were inappropriate for their son.

Like all the disorders considered in this book, dyslexia is mainly defined as the low end of a normal distribution of a particular skill or ability, so diagnosis requires setting a somewhat arbitrary cutoff on a continuous variable—in this case, basic literacy (B. Rodgers, 1983; Shaywitz, Escobar, Shaywitz, Fletcher, & Makuch, 1992). The influential definitions do not provide much concrete guidance about where to set that cutoff, other than to say that the difficulties must be severe enough to cause clinical impairment.

The three definitions vary in their assumptions about the underlying neuropsychological deficit that leads to the literacy problem. The consensus definition makes the strongest assumption by stating that problems "typically" result from a problem with phonological processing. The legal definition posits that dyslexia (as well as all other specific learning disabilities) arise from a problem with some aspect of language development. DSM-5 makes no particular assumptions about underlying cognitive deficits. As we see later, there is indeed substantial evidence that dyslexia arises from problems in oral language development and particularly phonological processing in most cases. However, consistent with the multiple-deficit framework that guides this book, it turns out that a single deficit in phonological processing is neither necessary nor sufficient to cause dyslexia (Pennington et al., 2012; Peterson et al., 2009), and the disorder has also been linked to deficits in nonlinguistic skills such as processing speed and visual attention (Lobier, Dubois, & Valdois, 2013; Ruffino, Gori, Boccardi, Molteni, & Facoetti, 2014). Furthermore, the language weaknesses themselves may be the developmental product of an earlier problem in aspects of procedural or statistical learning (Lum et al., 2014).

Many practitioners require evidence of a phonological processing deficit for a diagnosis of dyslexia, on the basis of many decades of group studies showing that phonological deficits appear causal in the disorder. However, it turns out that there is considerable variability at the individual level. For example, in a recent study using a version of the multiple case study approach in two large samples ($N > 800$ each), our group (Pennington et al., 2012) found that less than 15% of children with poor basic literacy skills were best characterized by a single phonological deficit. The remaining children were relatively evenly distributed among the following categories: a single deficit in another area (e.g., naming speed or vocabulary), multiple deficits, or no clear-cut deficits. Thus, requiring a deficit in phonological processing (or any other specific cognitive skill) for diagnosis is inappropriate and would unfairly exclude some individuals with clinically impairing literacy difficulties.

A final point of disagreement concerns how specific the literacy problems must be, with the consensus definition emphasizing specificity relatively more ("often unexpected in relation to other cognitive abilities") and with DSM-5 emphasizing specificity the least. This shift in part reflects broader changes in the field in the decade between these two definitions' publication. Historically, the study of learning disabilities has focused on cases of extreme discrepancies. In fact, the first published case study of dyslexia (Pringle-Morgan, 1896) concerned a 14-year-old boy who seemed "bright and intelligent" in every way, apart from his marked inability to learn to read and spell. It makes sense that children with such an uneven profile would attract more clinical attention initially, simply because they seem more striking and puzzling. As the study of dyslexia progressed in the 20th century, many scientists and practitioners continued to assume that children who showed a gap between IQ and literacy achievement had a true learning disability, while children with relatively low IQ and literacy were "garden variety poor readers" who should be considered separately.

As discussed in Chapter 6, substantial empirical work has now explored the distinction between IQ-discrepancy and age-discrepancy definitions of dyslexia. The two overlap, but some people with clinically significant reading problems meet only IQ-discrepancy criteria (high ability, weaker-than-expected word reading), whereas others meet only age-discrepancy criteria (low ability, poor word reading). There do seem to be some differences at the etiological level for individuals in these two groups. Genetic differences contribute more to high-IQ dyslexia than to low-IQ dyslexia (Wadsworth, Olson, & DeFries, 2010). A related finding is that dyslexia is more genetically based in children from higher socioeconomic status (SES) families than in children from lower SES families, a pattern referred to as a bioecological gene × environment (G × E) interaction (Friend et al., 2009). Together, these results suggest that advantaged children with strong cognitive abilities are likely to be good readers *unless* they have specific genetic risk factors for poor decoding. On the other hand, there are myriad reasons why other children struggle with reading. These include environmental influences associated with low SES, and these account for more of the variance in poor reading in children from lower-SES families than in children from higher-SES families. While the same risk genes are likely important across the range of SES, they contribute less to poor reading in the presence of environmental risk factors. We do not yet know which proximal environmental factors are most likely to contribute to low reading ability, though we discuss some reasonable possibilities later.

Despite this evidence for a different weighting of genetic and environmental risk factors in the etiologies underlying dyslexia in children with high versus low IQ, published work does not support the external validity of the distinction between age-referenced and IQ-referenced definitions in terms of underlying brain bases, neuropsychology, or appropriate treatments. Specifically, poor readers of all general ability levels show dysfunction in left-hemisphere reading and language networks (Tanaka et al., 2011) and have disproportionately poor skills in phonological processing (on average) (Siegel, 1992). As a group, children with dyslexia respond best to treatment emphasizing phonics-based reading instruction. Although there are individual differences in how well individuals with dyslexia respond to such intervention, these differences do not appear to be solely or even primarily a function of IQ (Jiménez, Siegel, O'Shanahan, & Ford, 2009; Stuebing et al., 2009). The implication is that the new DSM-5 definition (which requires age discrepancy in every case) ironically means that fewer children with a stronger genetic etiology will be classified as having dyslexia. Thus, for both research and clinical purposes, we think it is more appropriate to identify children who meet either age- *or* IQ-discrepancy criteria as having dyslexia, as long as their literacy difficulties cause functional impairment.

PREVALENCE AND EPIDEMIOLOGY

As we have seen, prevalence estimates depend on definition. Research studies have set various cutoffs for reading achievement relative to the average for age, including

1.5 *SD*s below, 1.3 *SD*s below, or 1 *SD* below, which identify approximately 7, 10, and 16% of the population, respectively. Some studies have even used the liberal cutoff of 0.7 *SD* below age expectations, which identifies fully 25% of the population! There is a relatively small but significant male predominance (1.5–3.1:1; Rutter et al., 2004) owing to both a slightly lower mean reading score for males and more variability for males than females, especially in the low tail of the distribution (Arnett et al., 2017). The implication of the greater variability is that the difference in prevalence by gender will become greater with more extreme diagnostic cutoffs. Regardless of the cutoff used, the gender difference in referred samples is even higher than what is found in the population (3–6:1; S. Smith et al., 2001). Boys with dyslexia come to clinical attention more often than girls, apparently because they have higher rates of comorbid externalizing disorders, including ADHD (Willcutt & Pennington, 2000b). This suggests that well-behaved girls with clinically meaningful reading difficulties may be underdiagnosed or undertreated.

Socioeconomic Status

As discussed in Chapter 8, SES is associated with reading skill, as with virtually all other measures of achievement. SES effects on literacy are part of the so-called "achievement gap" that has garnered considerable attention in public policy and education circles. For example, in 2011, the overall reading level of a national sample of fourth graders eligible for free lunch was 0.83 *SD* lower than that of students not eligible for free or reduced lunch, a large effect size (National Center for Education Statistics, 2011). Lower SES is associated with both poorer word reading and poorer reading comprehension, though the effect is larger for reading comprehension, particularly at older ages (MacDonald, 2014). The SES–word reading link means that by definition, a disproportionate number of children from lower-SES families will meet diagnostic criteria for developmental dyslexia. Lower SES predicts both poorer early reading skills at the onset of formal literacy instruction, and a slower trajectory of literacy growth over the early school years (Hecht, Burgess, Torgesen, Wagner, & Rashotte, 2000).

Systematic review and meta-analyses have consistently shown that SES accounts for approximately 10% of the variance in reading outcome (Scarborough & Dobrich, 1994; Sirin, 2005; K. White, 1982). While this effect is statistically significant and moderate, of course, it also means that approximately 90% of the variance in reading outcome is independent of SES; thus, many children from disadvantaged backgrounds will be strong readers, while many weak readers will come from advantaged families.

SES probably serves as a proxy for several environmental variables that adversely affect literacy development. However, as discussed in Chapter 8, SES is not solely an environmental construct, at least in societies that allow for a degree of social mobility. Overall, it appears that about 5% of overall reading outcome can be linked to environmental factors that fall under the SES umbrella (Petrill, Deater-Deckard, Schatschneider, & Davis, 2005; Wadsworth, Corley, Hewitt, & DeFries, 2001). Two important caveats are that (1) existing samples may not have included the very low tail of poor environments for reading development, and (2) as discussed earlier, there is evidence for bioecological G × E interaction in reading development, such that the balance of genetic and environmental influences is not constant across SES levels.

What are the specific environmental variables that directly influence reading development? Methodologically rigorous research on this question is still at an early stage of development, but the causal factors are probably many and act at the child, family, neighborhood, school, and broader community levels. In terms of family factors, research indicates that the quality and nature of language interaction between parents and children varies across SES levels (Chazan-Cohen et al., 2009; Hoff, 2003), including around specific preliteracy and literacy activities (Phillips & Lonigan, 2009; S. Robins, Ghosh, Rosales, & Treiman, 2014). As we mentioned in Chapter 8, these findings about the etiology of the SES–reading achievement gap have implications for prevention. If we could lessen or eliminate these environmental risk factors for later literacy skills, we could partly close the SES–achievement gap.

We return to the question of genetic and environmental influences on dyslexia in the "Etiology" section. Importantly, although this research tells us about the distal causes of individual differences in reading, it does not tell us about the extent to which particular environmental treatments (e.g., providing evidence-based reading instruction) can shift the average score for a group with poorer-than-average reading, such as children from lower-SES backgrounds. This issue evokes the Flynn effect that has been demonstrated for IQ, in which the mean IQ of the whole distribution increases over time, and this effect appears to be carried disproportionately by improvements in the low tail of the distribution (perhaps because of basic public health improvements, such as better nutrition; Lynn & Hampson, 1986). Over the last century, there has probably been a Flynn effect for reading as well. Despite these change at the group level driven by environmental factors, the etiology of individual differences may well have remained the same, and may include substantial genetic influence.

Cross-Cultural Findings

Although research on dyslexia initially focused primarily on reading difficulties in English, the nature of dyslexia across languages has recently received a good deal of attention. Here, we briefly summarize what is known about how dyslexia manifests across languages, showing two different types of variability: first, among alphabetic orthographies that vary in the degree of consistency of letter–sound correspondences; and second, in alphabetic versus logographic orthographies.

Children at the low end of the reading ability distribution in languages with more consistent mappings between letters and sounds (e.g., Italian or Finnish) have less severe reading problems than those learning to read less consistent languages (i.e., English), at least in terms of accuracy (Landerl, Wimmer, & Frith, 1997). Difficulties with reading *fluency*, or speed of reading connected text, seem similar across languages (Caravolas et al., 2005). Several studies have noted important universal features in normal and disordered reading across cultures, despite linguistic differences. Cognitive predictors of early reading were similar for five European orthographies (Finnish, Hungarian, Dutch, Portuguese, and French), in agreement with previous results in English. Particularly, phonological awareness was the main predictor of reading in each language, although it had more of an effect in consistent than in less consistent orthographies. Other predictors, such as rapid serial naming, vocabulary knowledge, and verbal short-term memory, made smaller contributions than did phonological awareness, except in Finnish (the most consistent language), in which vocabulary had at least as large an effect on reading (Ziegler et al., 2010).

Cross-cultural similarities appear to extend in large part to logographic languages as well, such as Chinese. By contrast with alphabetic languages, whose letters represent phonemes, the smallest written units in Chinese are characters representing monosyllabic *morphemes* (units of language that convey meaning). However, phonology is not irrelevant to reading in Chinese. Chinese characters have phonological elements, and skilled readers of the language show phonological effects on word recognition (Pollatsek, 2015). Phonological awareness is a key correlate and predictor of reading skill in Chinese, just as in alphabetic orthographies. However, in contrast to alphabetic languages in which awareness of phonemes is critically important, morphological and syllabic awareness play a larger role in learning to read Chinese (McBride-Chang et al., 2005). This finding is not surprising given the differences in how the orthographies represent language.

Comorbidities

Dyslexia is comorbid with most of the other disorders considered in this book, including ADHD (DuPaul et al., 2013); other speech–language disorders, including LI and SSD (Nittrouer & Pennington, 2010); and math disability (Landerl & Moll, 2010; Willcutt et al., 2013). In most cases, evidence indicates that the comorbidity with dyslexia is mediated by shared etiological and neurocognitive risk factors (Pennington & Bishop, 2009; Willcutt et al., 2010). SSD and LI are comorbid themselves, but their relationships with dyslexia are not the same. Perhaps surprisingly, since SSD appears to be a phonologically based problem, children with isolated SSD and no comorbid LI are at fairly low risk for later developing dyslexia. In contrast, the risk for later reading problems (including but not limited to dyslexia) in children with a history of LI is very high (Peterson et al., 2009). These comorbidities are clinically significant, because dyslexia is not diagnosed until after a child has been exposed to formal literacy instruction, but ADHD, SSD, and LI are all likely to be apparent earlier and therefore may indicate a child's risk for later reading problems.

DEVELOPMENTAL NEUROPSYCHOLOGY

Oral language is a human universal. Every culture has a natural language, and essentially all children learn to speak, apart from those with especially severe developmental disabilities. Deaf children may not communicate orally, but they can learn a visually based sign language that is just as rich and complex as other human languages. The process of typical language development is discussed in Chapter 9. Literacy development is different from oral language development, because literacy is a cultural invention and not a human universal. *Homo sapiens* appeared about 200,000 years ago, but the earliest writing system was invented less than 6,000 years ago. Some cultures still do not have a written language. While no healthy adults are without language, many who have never been taught to read are completely illiterate.

One educational philosophy (the "whole-language approach") has posited that children should learn to read as they learn to talk, simply by being surrounded by written language. But as we have already seen, this approach is misguided, because the human brain is not predisposed to acquire written language in the same way that it is built to acquire oral language. Literacy must be explicitly taught, generally through formal education. Literacy development is parasitic on oral language development, which means that children's speaking and listening skills must be well developed before they can begin to read and write.

The ultimate goals of becoming literate include sophisticated reading comprehension and written expression. As discussed in Chapter 6, these skills depend on both basic skills (e.g., decoding, transcribing) and a variety of complex skills (e.g., oral language comprehension, attention, executive functions). The basic skills are most relevant to dyslexia, and their development is the focus here. To read words, children must learn to map particular visual forms (in alphabetic writing systems, spellings) to word pronunciations and their meanings. Below we briefly review typical developmental milestones related to this task.

Milestones in Literacy Development

A detailed review of word reading development is provided by Ehri (2015), who argues that literacy development in an alphabetic language proceeds through four phases. In the first, prealphabetic phase, children have very little letter knowledge and cannot yet segment or manipulate individual sounds (phonemes) in words. They may be able to recognize their own names or some environmental print (e.g., the word *STOP* on a stop sign), but they rely on salient visual or context cues to do so.

True literacy development gets under way in the partial alphabetic phase, which requires children to know most letter names and to begin developing knowledge of letter sounds and phonemic awareness. At this phase, children can begin to recognize some words, but easily confuse similarly spelled words. They attempt to spell some words with "invented spellings" that may reflect one or a few of the sounds in a word (e.g., RLE for *early* or SK for *stick*). Explicit, systematic training in *phonics* (information about how letters and sounds go together) during this phase helps move children to the full alphabetic stage. In the full alphabetic stage, children know most or all letter sounds and are starting to learn about some larger spelling units as well (e.g., *-ing*). They can "sound out" many words based on rules of phonics, with automaticity just beginning to emerge. They have learned spellings for some high-frequency words and can spell unfamiliar words phonetically.

In the final, consolidated alphabetic phase, children have learned a lot about how letters map onto pronunciations. They not only know about how individual letters and sounds go together but also about many larger spelling units (e.g., *-tion*). Such larger units are important in languages such as English, which does not have consistent one-to-one relationships between letters and sounds. Compared to full alphabetic readers, children in the consolidated alphabetic phase show greater automaticity and accuracy in both their reading and spelling. In addition to being able to decode or sound out unfamiliar words, they frequently read unfamiliar words by analogy to known words (e.g., correctly guessing how to pronounce *should* based on knowing how to pronounce *could*).

Of course, there are individual differences in how quickly and well children progress through these phases, which would be expected to result from the genetic and environmental risk and protective etiological factors that contribute to individual differences in reading, including dyslexia. Because literacy development always builds on earlier language development, environmental factors that support early language growth even well before Ehri's first phase could have a significant impact on later literacy. Seminal research documented enormous subcultural variations in how much and how parents talk and read to their children, and these variations in turn predict later cognitive development (B. Hart & Risley, 1992; Heath, 1982). Thus, both quantity and quality of language input throughout children's earliest years would reasonably be expected to impact their later literacy.

Neuropsychology of Dyslexia

The dominant explanation for many years, and the one espoused in the first edition of this book, was that dyslexia is caused by a core deficit in a specific aspect of language development, namely, the ability to process individual sounds in words, or *phonological processing*. In the phonological theory of dyslexia, the ability to attend to and manipulate linguistic sounds is crucial for the establishment and automatization of letter–sound correspondences, which in turn underlie accurate and fluent word recognition through the process of phonological coding. By the time the second edition of this book was published, we knew that although the phonological theory contained a lot of truth, it was an oversimplification, and that multiple interacting risk and protective factors are needed to account for the full heterogeneity of the disorder. The same general view that we advocated in the previous edition continues to characterize our understanding of the neuropsychology of dyslexia today.

We have learned a lot about the neuropsychology of dyslexia from family risk studies, which have allowed researchers to identify developmental precursors of the disorder. These precursors are cognitive or neural differences that are apparent in infants, toddlers, or preschoolers who have not yet been exposed to formal literacy instruction and so cannot yet be diagnosed. The family risk design compares children at high family risk for dyslexia (because they have a parent or sibling with the disorder) to children without close relatives with the disorder and hence at low family risk. Researchers have followed these children longitudinally to determine who eventually developed dyslexia and then retrospectively identified what discriminated children with and without dyslexia even before formal literacy instruction. Importantly, this means that identified differences are not just a consequence of poor reading development. Because dyslexia is familial and heritable, many of the children at high family risk go on to develop this disorder, so this research design allows for identification of reasonable sample sizes of individuals with dyslexia much more efficiently than a general population screening study.

In a seminal family risk study, Hollis Scarborough (1991a, 1991b, 1998) found that a variety of differences in oral language development distinguished young children who later went on to develop dyslexia from those who did not. This pattern is not surprising, since as we discussed earlier, normal literacy development is parasitic on oral language. What was unexpected about Scarborough's work was that the best oral language predictors of later literacy *changed* with developmental level. The constructs that best distinguished children who later did versus did not eventually develop dyslexia included grammar and speech articulation at ages 2–3 years, as well as grammar and vocabulary at ages 3–4 years. Not until age 5 did phonological awareness emerge as one of the strongest predictors.

Since that seminal work, several further longitudinal family risk studies have been completed in multiple countries around the world. A recent meta-analysis of these studies confirmed the general pattern of Scarborough's early work (Snowling & Melby-Lervåg, 2016). These authors concluded that children who go on to develop dyslexia show delayed speech and language development as toddlers. By preschool, differences begin to emerge on various phonological and reading-related tasks, including nonword repetition, verbal short-term memory, phonological awareness, and letter knowledge. By school age, phonological processing problems and vocabulary weaknesses remain evident, but the earlier broader oral language difficulties have otherwise largely resolved (at least at the group level). A subset of small-scale family risk studies has used neurophysiological (mainly event-related potential [ERP]) methods to establish that individuals who will later develop dyslexia show an aberrant neural response to speech stimuli even in infancy (Lyytinen et al., 2005; Zuijen, Plakas, Maassen, Maurits, & Leij, 2013).

Taken together, these studies demonstrate that dyslexia can be conceptualized as a type of subtle language-learning disorder that has its origins very early on, perhaps even prenatally. Whether the learning difficulty is truly specific to language or whether the language problems result from an underlying domain-general problem, such as in implicit learning, remains an open question. Some recent work indicates that individuals with dyslexia have weaknesses in procedural or statistical learning, including for nonlinguistic stimuli (Gabay et al., 2015; Lum et al., 2013).

While early speech and language weaknesses among children who go on to develop dyslexia are robust at the group level, they do not have adequate sensitivity and specificity to permit individual diagnosis prior to formal literacy instruction. In fact, the family risk studies have also demonstrated that the risk for dyslexia is continuous. Children at elevated family risk who do not go onto to develop dyslexia nonetheless perform worse on average than do children at low family risk on early speech and language tasks. Similarly, longitudinal studies of children with early speech–language disorders have found that many children develop normal-range literacy skills despite preschool phonological deficits similar in magnitude to those of children who ultimately develop dyslexia (Bishop et al., 2009; Peterson et al., 2009). Some children with phonological deficits appear to be protected from dyslexia because of relative strengths in other cognitive skills associated with reading, such as processing speed. Conversely, children with multiple cognitive deficits are at much higher risk for dyslexia. Thus, while phonological processing does have a special relationship with basic literacy skill once children reach school age, a single phonological deficit theory of dyslexia is inadequate.

Across countries and languages, many cognitive–linguistic constructs consistently predict later dyslexia. Those most consistently implicated include phonological awareness, rapid serial naming, verbal short-term memory, vocabulary and other aspects of broader oral language skill, and graphomotor processing speed (McGrath et al., 2011; Pennington et al., 2012; Scarborough, 1998; Wolf & Bowers, 1999). Tasks emphasizing speed (i.e., rapid serial naming and processing speed) become increasingly important as literacy development progresses, probably because they are more linked to reading fluency than to single-word reading accuracy (Pennington & Lefly, 2001; Puolakanaho et al., 2008; Scarborough, 1990; Snowling, Gallagher, & Frith, 2003; Torppa, Lyytinen, Erskine, Eklund, & Lyytinen, 2010). Longitudinal research suggests that these various deficits make a causal contribution to reading problems and are not fully accounted for by comorbidities or the cumulative effects of reading difficulties.

Research has made clear for many years that dyslexia does not result from disturbances in basic visual perception (Ramus, 2003; Vellutino, 1979a). However, there has recently been renewed interest in the possible role of visual attentional deficits in reading difficulties (Facoetti, Corradi, Ruffino, Gori, & Zorzi, 2010). Visual attention is measured through serial search, orienting/cueing paradigms, or "crowding" paradigms that require participants to recognize pictures amid varying degrees of visual clutter. Some of these skills likely relate to performance on nonlinguistic processing speed tasks known to be correlated with reading, and may contribute to them. Performance on visual attention tasks in preschool significantly predicted reading ability 2 years later, after accounting for the influence of reading-related phonological processing skills (Franceschini, Gori, Ruffino, Pedroll, & Facoetti, 2012). Initial evidence suggests a similar pattern of results across writing systems with varying degrees of consistency in letter–sound relationships (i.e., Italian and French) (Zorzi et al., 2012). While deficits in visual attention do not easily account for the early speech–language phenotype in predyslexic children, they might represent an additional cognitive deficit that interacts with language problems to cause an RD. Further research is needed on this question.

So the phonological theory of dyslexia is incomplete, because a single phonological deficit is neither necessary nor sufficient to cause the disorder. A second issue for the phonological theory concerns the direction of effect between phonological development and reading (Castles, Wilson, & Coltheart, 2011). Because formal literacy instruction does not begin until children have mastered most of the fundamentals of a spoken language, it seems reasonable that the causal direction should flow from phonology to reading rather than vice versa. Several lines of evidence support this conclusion. First, preschool children who will later develop dyslexia show deficits on various phonological tasks, with phoneme awareness being particularly predictive of later literacy attainment by around kindergarten age (Pennington & Lefly, 2001; Scarborough, 1991b; Snowling et al., 2003). Furthermore, children with dyslexia underperform even younger, typically developing children matched for reading level on phoneme awareness tasks (Wagner & Torgesen, 1987), and these deficits tend to persist in adults with dyslexia who have otherwise compensated well for the disorder (Bruck, 1992; Hatcher, Snowling, & Griffiths, 2002).

However, the conclusion that phoneme awareness deficits have a unidirectional causal link to reading problems is oversimplified for several reasons. Speech scientists complain about the "tyranny of the phoneme" (Greenberg, 2004), because these idealized representations have become reified and likely mislead us about what dimensions in the speech stream are important in development and how those dimensions are flexibly integrated to recover linguistic structures, such as words. There are long-standing controversies about the units of speech perception (Goldinger & Azuma, 2003), and recent evidence demonstrates that speech representations preserve much more than phonemes. This work has led to a proposal that phonemes are not the targets of speech perception, and are mainly important in the context of learning an alphabetic written language (Port, 2007). Work with adult natural illiterates (who are cognitively normal but have no formal schooling) confirms that phoneme-level representations do not arise automatically in language development (Castro-Caldas, Petersson, Reis, Stone-Elander, & Ingvar, 1998; Morais et al., 1979). In other words, as literate adults, we think that individual phonemes exist in the speech signal like beads on a string, but this is an illusion that arises from our extensive experience with an alphabetic script. Thus, difficulties in phonological development in dyslexia are probably not restricted to phonemic or segmental representations and must lie in other dimensions of the speech stream, at least initially. This conclusion is consistent with the family risk studies that indicate early difficulties in several aspects of speech–language development and not just phonological processing. Despite this evidence that learning to read changes phonological development, methodologically rigorous work demonstrates that phoneme awareness training in combination with explicit phonics instruction improves literacy in early school-age children (Hulme, Bowyer-Crane, Carroll, Duff, & Snowling, 2012). The most accurate conclusion therefore appears to be that the relationship between phonology and literacy is bidirectional.

In recent years, there has been burgeoning interest in an orthographic learning account of reading problems, which emphasizes not phonological representations themselves, but the ability to establish mappings between phonemes and graphemes, or letters and sounds (e.g., Aravena, Snellings, Tijms, & van der Molen, 2013). This account has strong face validity to explain dyslexia, which is essentially defined by problems decoding print. Neurophysiological evidence indicates that skilled readers treat letters as single audiovisual objects (Blau et al., 2010), and that individuals with dyslexia show an attenuation in the neural signature for audiovisual integration of letter stimuli (Žarić et al., 2014). The orthographic learning hypothesis states that problems developing such integrated representations interferes with the emergence of fluent reading. Limited behavioral support for this hypothesis comes from research comparing performance of children with and without dyslexia when asked to learn associations between sounds in their native language and an unfamiliar orthography. Although both groups learned the associations, the children with dyslexia performed more poorly than controls under time pressure (Aravena et al., 2013). Furthermore, intensive training in letter–sound relationships improved reading fluency in elementary school children with dyslexia (González et al., 2015).

In addition to its face validity, the orthographic learning hypothesis has a number of strengths. It represents an admirable attempt to integrate across the brain and neuropsychological levels of analysis to explain reading development and difficulties. Furthermore, it avoids some of the reductionistic errors of other accounts that have been put forward as alternatives to the dominant phonological view, such as auditory and visual explanations. However, this account also faces some serious problems. Most critically, it does not account for the early language development of predyslexic children, who (as we have seen) have subtle difficulties with spoken language long before they encounter a written script.

A related point is that it is difficult to test a pure integration account of phoneme–grapheme binding, since we know that children with dyslexia are not equivalent to their typically developing peers in processing phonemes of their native language. So the meaning of the fact that they are slower in learning phoneme–grapheme mappings is ambiguous; it could arise directly from the unimodal phonological deficit. To show that there is an additional contribution of crossmodal letter–sound processing over and above the well-established phonological processing problem in dyslexia, we need behavioral studies that can somehow control for unimodal phonological and orthographic processing across groups. This is an important issue to be addressed by future research.

BRAIN MECHANISMS

Because reading is a linguistic skill, we would expect it to involve activation of brain structures used in oral language processing and some additional structures associated with visual–object processing and establishment of visual–linguistic mappings. Indeed, functional imaging studies have consistently revealed that individuals with dyslexia show abnormal activations of a distributed left-hemisphere language network (Demonet, Taylor, & Chaix, 2004; Richlan, Kronbichler, & Wimmer, 2009). Underactivations have been reported in two posterior left-hemisphere regions: a temporoparietal region believed to be crucial for phonological processing and phoneme–grapheme conversion, and an occipitotemporal region, including the so-called "visual word form area," which is thought to participate in whole-word recognition. Abnormal activation of the left inferior frontal gyrus is also commonly reported. Structural imaging studies have revealed gray matter decreases in this same network. Family risk studies have demonstrated that both structural gray matter decreases and functional underactivations predate literacy instruction and are therefore not just a consequence of reading failure (Raschle, Chang, & Gaab, 2011; Raschle, Zuk, & Gaab, 2012).

That individuals with dyslexia show functional abnormalities in both posterior and anterior language networks has led to the hypothesis that dyslexia is a disconnection syndrome. Accordingly, much research has explored white matter correlates of dyslexia by use of diffusion tensor imaging. The most consistent findings have included local white matter changes (as indexed by fractional anisotropy) in children and adults with dyslexia in white matter tracts connecting the left temporoparietal regions to the left interior frontal gyrus (i.e., arcuate fascicules and the superior longitudinal fascicules) (Deutsch et al., 2005; Klingberg et al., 2000; Rimrodt, Peterson, Denckla, Kaufmann, & Cutting, 2010). Studies have consistently indicated correlations between white matter integrity in these tracts and phonological skills. This work is beginning to be integrated into neuropsychological theories of dyslexia, and this area should be a continued focus of future research. For example, a disconnection between posterior auditory processing areas and anterior motor planning areas is potentially consistent with disrupted development of phonological representations. Because of its emphasis on letter–sound binding, the orthographic learning hypothesis also aligns with a disconnection account.

An interesting new line of inquiry into the brain bases of dyslexia has moved away from looking at individual brain regions and focuses instead on neurophysiological differences in the brains of skilled versus disabled readers. Perrachione and colleagues (2016) used functional magnetic resonance imaging (fMRI) to study *neural adaptation*—defined as reduced brain activation in response to a repeated stimulus—in dyslexia. Compared to unimpaired readers, adults with dyslexia showed reduced adaptation to all stimulus types tested (spoken words, written words, visual objects, and unfamiliar faces). A more limited experiment including only spoken word stimuli was conducted with children and produced equivalent results. An important future question will be to clarify how this neural difference maps onto the neuropsychology of the disorder.

The neural correlates of dyslexia appear remarkably uniform across different alphabetic languages that have varying degrees of consistency in their letter–sound mappings (Paulesu et al., 2001; Silani et al., 2005) and even across alphabetic and logographic orthographies (Hu et al., 2010). However, learners of consistent alphabetic orthographies are less likely to display clinically significant reading problems compared to learners of inconsistent orthographies (probably because those with reading vulnerabilities can still read accurately, even if slowly in consistent languages). In summary, cross-cultural work suggests universality in the neurobiological and neurocognitive causes of dyslexia, but there is cross-cultural specificity in the manifestation of these underpinnings, with the same biological liability more likely to cause substantial impairment in some languages than in others.

ETIOLOGY

Scientific progress concerning the etiology of dyslexia has been built on a fairly mature understanding of its neuropsychology. It turns out that the neuropsychological deficits associated with a developmental disorder are often more stable and heritable than the defining symptom itself, and are frequently present in family members who do not meet full diagnostic criteria for the disorder. In the case of dyslexia, relatives of affected family members can have reading skills in the normal range despite deficits on some specific phonological processing tasks. In other words, neuropsychological constructs can serve as endophenotypes for behaviorally defined disorders. Most of what we know about the genetics of dyslexia has depended on decades of research on its neuropsychology, which has allowed for the use of optimal endophenotypes in etiological studies. The relationship is reciprocal because, as scientists discover links from etiology to pathogenesis, that knowledge will further constrain the neuropsychological level of analysis and will particularly help inform which brain and cognitive changes may be causal in a disorder (as opposed to associated with the disorder for other reasons).

Behavioral Genetics

Main Effects of Genes and Environment

Both dyslexia and normal variations in reading skill are familial and moderately heritable (Christopher et al., 2013; Harlaar et al., 2005; Logan et al., 2013; Pennington & Olson, 2005), with the caveat that the heritability of reading skill changes with age. For instance, Logan et al. (2013) demonstrated that the heritability of individual differences in reading skill steadily increases from .22 at 6 years to .82 at 12 years. These increases in heritability likely reflect (1) a narrowing of environmental influences on reading produced by a fairly standard reading curriculum once children enter formal education, and (2) an increasing correlation between genotype and environment (i.e., gene–environment [G–E] correlation) as children increasingly are able to pick niches that fit their level of reading skills (e.g., good readers read more on their own and become even better readers, while poor readers avoid reading). Both of these explanations are examples of G–E interplay, which we discussed in Chapter 2 and will discuss later for reading. Because these results come from mainly middle-class twin samples in developed countries, it is important to remember that they may not generalize to other populations (but see Hensler et al., 2010, who found moderate heritability, > .50, both for dyslexia and typical reading skill in a more ethnically and economically diverse sample).

G–E Interplay

Going beyond the main effects of genes and environment, we can ask how genetic and environmental risk factors act together in the development of abnormal behavior, including dyslexia. As discussed earlier, Friend et al. (2009) found evidence for a bioecological G × E interaction in dyslexia. Specifically, the heritability of dyslexia increased as parent education increased. This result suggests that the child's literacy environment is, on average, both more favorable and less variable as parent education increases, resulting in genetic risk factors playing a bigger role in a child's dyslexia. Conversely, as parent education decreases, the child's literacy environment is on average less favorable and more variable, resulting in environmental risk factors playing a bigger role in a child's dyslexia. The stability of this bioecological G × E interaction for dyslexia is still being investigated, as a recent study in an Australian sample did not find a similar effect (Grasby, Coventry, Byrne, & Olson, 2017).

There is also increasing evidence for the importance of transactional processes in atypical development, in which the child and environment mutually alter each other over time. G–E correlation is an example of such a transaction. Such transactions occur because children evoke different kinds of reactions from their environments (Scarr & McCartney, 1983), and select different kinds of environments for themselves. Not surprisingly, the individual characteristics that influence such reactions and selections are genetically influenced. There are three subtypes of G–E correlation: passive, evocative, and active (Scarr & McCartney, 1983). In the case of reading development, an example of a passive G–E correlation is the relation between parents' reading skill and the number of books in the home. Parents' reading skill is partly due to genes, and parents who are better readers on average have more books in their homes. Without any action on the part of their biological children, their literacy environment is correlated with their reading genotype on average. In contrast, an evocative G–E correlation occurs when adults in a child's environment notice the child's interests and talents, and seek to foster them. In the case of reading development, an example of an evocative G–E correlation would be a parent or relative taking a child who likes to read to the library. Finally, an active G–E correlation occurs when children on their own initiative seek or avoid environments as a function of their genotype. Dyslexia provides a clear example of an active G–E correlation. Even before formal literacy instruction, children at genetic risk for dyslexia who later develop the disorder avoid being read to and spend less independent playtime looking at books than their siblings who do not develop dyslexia (Scarborough et al., 1991). As they get older, school-age children with dyslexia read dramatically fewer words per year than typically developing children (Cunningham & Stanovich, 1998), such that this reduced reading experience negatively influences both their reading fluency and their oral vocabularies (Torgesen, 2005; Stanovich, 1986).

Molecular Genetics

Using molecular methods, dyslexia has been linked to nine risk loci (which are termed *DYX1–DYX9*, with *DYX* standing for dyslexia and the number indicating the order of discovery) through replicated linkage studies (Fisher & DeFries, 2002; McGrath, Smith, & Pennington, 2006), although not every study has replicated these results (Ludwig et al., 2008; Meaburn, Harlaar, Craig, Schalkwyk, & Plomin, 2008).

More precise mapping methods have led to the identification of six candidate genes that have been replicated in at least one independent sample in some of the nine replicated risk loci (a risk locus is specified by its chromosome number out of the 23 human chromosomes, which of the two arms, short (p) or long (q), the risk locus is on, and an "address" on that arm, indicated by a number). These six candidate genes are *DYX1C1* in the *DYX1* locus on chromosome 15q21; *DCDC2* and *KIAA0319* in the *DYX2* locus on chromosome 6p21; *C2Orf3* and *MRPL19* in the *DYX3* locus on chromosome 2p16–p15; and *ROBO1* in the *DYX5* locus on chromosome 3p12-q12. In addition to these six candidate genes, at least three other genes first implicated in other disorders have since been shown to be associated with reading ability or dyslexia in at least two independent samples (reviewed in Mascheretti et al., 2017). These three include *FOXP2* on chromosome 7q31, *CNTNAP2* on 7q35–q36, and *GRIN2B* on 12p13.

It is important to note that the psychiatric genetics field, generally, has struggled with replication (Duncan et al., 2014). While the genes mentioned above have been replicated in at least one independent sample, there are also notable nonreplications. For example, in a recent set of analyses, including a reevaluation of the existing *DCDC2* literature, Scerri et al. (2017) did not find evidence in support of a specific deletion variant that has been implicated in other studies of dyslexia. While this study does not rule out the role of other mutations in *DCDC2*, it does call into question one of the most well-studied genetic variants in this gene. This example illustrates an overall point that the dyslexia genetics literature is in a relatively early stage compared to that of other complex behavioral disorders, such as schizophrenia and autism. Further studies using large samples and genomewide methods will be necessary to assess whether the literature converges on the existing candidate genes and/or whether different genes emerge as the most likely candidates.

One piece of evidence that potentially speaks to the validity of the existing candidate genes is their role in similar brain developmental processes that are plausibly linked to dyslexia. For example, studies of the role of the dyslexia candidate genes in brain development (Kere, 2011) in rodents has shown that *DYX1C1*, *DCDC2*, *KIAA0319*, and *ROBO1* affect prenatal processes of brain development, including *neuronal migration* (the movement of immature neurons from where they are first formed to their final destination in the brain) and the formation of connections once they reach that destination (e.g., neurite—axon and dendrite—outgrowth and guidance). More generally, these two processes of early brain development are each genetically controlled by a family or network of genes that interact with each other through molecular signals. In contrast, very little is known about the functions of the two *DYX3* candidate genes.

A few genomewide association studies (GWAS) of dyslexia have now been published (Eicher et al., 2013; Field et al., 2013; Gialluisi et al., 2014, 2016; Luciano et al., 2013). Previously identified candidate genes did not reach significance in these studies, possibly because of low power. This pattern has been fairly common in GWAS of other traits, especially with smaller N's. Hence, confirmation of current candidate genes for dyslexia awaits larger samples and testing for their roles in molecular signaling networks. The GWAS did identify new potential candidate genes, but these have not yet been replicated in independent samples (Carrion-Castillo et al., 2016). Even if the most promising current candidate genes are ultimately confirmed to play a role in the etiology of dyslexia, each one will likely explain only a small portion of the variance in eventual reading outcome. Thus, most of the heritability of dyslexia remains unaccounted for and much important work remains.

Exciting new research is beginning to integrate knowledge about the development of dyslexia across the etiological, brain, neurocognitive, and behavioral levels of analysis using animal models. The rat homologue of human dyslexia candidate gene *KIAA0319* is known as *Kiaa0319*, and neuroscientists have created a "knockdown" in the rat model via *in utero* RNA interference, which causes reduced expression of *Kiaa0319*. This knockdown probably yields more severe changes in gene expression those associated with dyslexia in humans, but is hypothesized to lie along the same continuum as the dyslexia risk in humans. Rats with the *Kiaa0319* knockdown are largely developmentally and behaviorally normal, but show subtle changes in brain development and auditory processing of speech sounds (Szalkowski et al., 2013). At a structural level, knockdown leads to focal disruptions of neuronal migration (Platt et al., 2013), similar to those first described in the brains of adult humans with dyslexia many years ago by Galaburda, Sherman, Rosen, Aboitiz, and Geschwind (1985). Furthermore, these rats show an atypical neurophysiological response to speech sounds in auditory cortex (Centanni et al., 2013) and are less effective than typical rats at discriminating phonemes (Centanni et al., 2014). Of most direct clinical relevance, intensive behavioral training using speech sounds normalized the rats' behavioral performance (Centanni et al., 2014). This work has more recently been extended to the rat homologue of *DCDC2* as well (Centanni et al., 2016).

Another strategy for linking candidate dyslexia genes to brain structure and function is a genetic neuroimaging study in humans, in which the association between risk genotypes for dyslexia and established brain phenotypes for dyslexia can be tested. As reviewed earlier, reductions in left-hemisphere white matter volume are a well-replicated brain phenotype in dyslexia. Darki, Peyrard-Janvid, Matsson, Kere, and Klingberg (2012) tested whether this brain phenotype was associated with genetic markers for variants in each of three established risk genes for dyslexia—*DYX1C1*, *DCDC2*, and *KIAA0319*—in a sample of typical adults, and found a significant association for all three risk genes. The fact that these associations were found in a typical population is consistent with the fact that dyslexia is a continuous rather than a categorical disorder, such that individuals without diagnosed dyslexia may nonetheless have some of the risk factors for dyslexia. More work is needed to replicate and extend both the animal and human findings, but the emerging picture is that risk genes for dyslexia alter brain development differentially in the left hemisphere, thereby altering speech and language development so as to make the acquisition of written language more difficult.

More recently, Woo et al. (2016) conducted a genetic neuroimaging study of a dyslexia risk locus at 15q11.2 that contains the *CYF1P1* gene. This locus was chosen because previous studies revealed that copy number variations in this locus were associated with language disorders. (It is important to emphasize that this locus is distinct from the *DYX1C1* locus at 15q21.) In a large sample, Woo et al. (2016) found that a variant single-nucleotide polymorphism (SNP; rs4778298) in the *CYF1P1* gene was associated with a smaller surface area in the left supramarginal gyrus, and they replicated this result in a much larger second sample.

In a review of the molecular genetics of dyslexia, Carrion-Castillo, Franke, and Fisher (2013) discussed the two molecular signaling networks already implicated in the development of dyslexia: neuronal migration and neurite outgrowth and guidance, as well as a third one, ciliary biology. *Cilia* are microscopic hair-like structures on the surface of cells, as in a paramecium, and their rhythmic movement turns out to play a role in the patterning of early brain development. Carrion-Castillo et al. also discussed in detail the sometimes inconsistent evidence found across samples for the various candidate genes for dyslexia. This inconsistency is due partly to the fact that the mutations found in dyslexia are not in the coding regions of genes that directly code for the structure of proteins but in noncoding regions that affect expression levels of structural genes, sometimes with small and subtle effects, and partly to the fact that many of the samples in these studies are too small, as discussed earlier.

Nonetheless, the fact that these candidate genes interact with each other and act on the same molecular signaling pathways is a promising beginning for eventually discovering the likely many more genes involved, and working out the early developmental biology of this disorder.

Environmental Influences

Because the heritability of dyslexia is substantially less than 100%, we know there are environmental factors that contribute to the development of the disorder. However, limited methodologically rigorous work has investigated which specific environments causally influence reading development. Possible candidates include the language and preliteracy environments that parents provide for their children, but unfortunately, much of the research on these topics has used correlational rather than genetically sensitive designs (e.g., twin and adoption studies). Thus, parents with genetic risk for dyslexia may provide less literacy exposure to their children because of the G–E correlations we discussed earlier, so it is not clear that the environment plays a causal role in the child's reading outcome (i.e., van Bergen, van Zuijen, Bishop, & de Jong, 2017). This limitation is avoided in treatment studies that use random assignment. Results of such research suggest that training parents in various home literacy activities promotes young children's vocabulary (a reading precursor; Lonigan & Whitehurst, 1998) and early reading skills (Sénéchal, 2015; Sylva, Scott, Totsika, Ereky-Stevens, & Crook, 2008). This work is broadly consistent with findings from twin studies demonstrating that during the preschool years, individual differences in vocabulary and some other literacy precursors are more influenced by family environment than by genes (Byrne et al., 2009; Hayiou-Thomas, Dale, & Plomin, 2012). However, this work has also shown that over time, the relative importance of etiological influences shifts, and by later school age, genetic influences on oral language and literacy predominate. Thus, further work is needed to know whether the effects of home literacy environment on word reading persist beyond the beginning stages of literacy instruction.

Related research has used randomized controlled trials to study the effects of instructional type on reading development in alphabetic systems. This research has consistently shown that phonics-based instruction, which emphasizes explicit knowledge about letter–sound correspondences, is superior to other forms of literacy instruction that emphasize sight word recognition (e.g., whole-word instruction) or listening comprehension (e.g., whole language) in promoting word-level reading skills, particularly for children who are at risk for reading difficulties (I. Brown & Felton, 1990; Snowling & Hulme, 2011; Vellutino, Scanlon, Small, & Fanuele, 2006). Because literacy curricula vary across and sometimes within countries, instructional type can influence the risk of an individual child meeting standard diagnostic criteria for dyslexia.

DIAGNOSIS AND TREATMENT

Diagnosis

Consistent with the approach we endorsed in Chapter 6, a diagnosis of dyslexia is dependent on convergent data from a child's history, behavior observations, and test results. The key presenting symptom is difficulty learning to read and spell, which is typically apparent from the beginning of formal literacy instruction. Some children with dyslexia have good reading comprehension and like to read, so it is important to ask specifically about reading aloud and learning phonics, two aspects of reading with which virtually all individuals with dyslexia have trouble. Similarly, a report of good performance on weekly spelling tests should be followed by a question to determine the quality of spontaneous spelling, as some children with dyslexia will work hard to memorize the spelling list but not spell even simple words correctly in their usual writing. Parents or teachers may also report slow reading or writing speed, letter and number reversals, problems memorizing basic math facts, and unusual reading and spelling errors. These errors types are discussed below in the section "Behavioral Observations."

Notably, the initial referral may be prompted not by these kinds of cognitive symptoms, but by emotional or somatic symptoms, such as anxiety or depression, reluctance to go to school, or headaches and stomachaches. It is important to find out whether the symptoms occur all the time or only on school days (or even during certain parts of the school day). Even if they occur all the time, the root cause could be dyslexia because of the failures (and fear of failure) of children with dyslexia experience.

History

Most children with dyslexia do not have high-risk events in their prenatal or perinatal histories, nor do they have clear delays in early developmental milestones, although mild speech–language delays are present in some histories. There are three aspects of the history that are particularly informative—family history, school history, and reading and language history.

Because familial risk is substantial in dyslexia, it is important to take a careful history of reading, spelling, and related language problems in the first- and second-degree relatives of the patient. Parents may not necessarily know whether they or their relatives have dyslexia, but they are usually able to report accurately on reading and spelling problems, as well as problems with articulation, word finding, and verbal memory for things such as phone numbers and addresses. Parents with a history of dyslexia often report extreme difficulty learning a foreign language. It is a fairly common clinical experience to discover a parent's or a relative's dyslexia in the course of the child's evaluation.

In terms of school history, literacy difficulties should be evident by first or second grade, and may manifest by kindergarten as problems with learning the alphabet, letter names, or other prereading skills. It is very unlikely that reading problems with an abrupt later onset are due to developmental dyslexia; acquired or psychiatric etiologies need to be considered in this situation.

If the child is an adolescent when first referred, the preschool and early elementary school histories may not be readily available, and the presenting symptoms may have changed. The child may now like to read, though more slowly than other children, and the main complaints may involve poor performance on timed tests or difficulty completing homework.

Behavioral Observations

When evaluating a child for dyslexia, a wealth of information will emerge from the administration of reading and spelling tasks. First, it is important to get a sense of how the child feels about reading. Many children with dyslexia comment that they do not like reading or they appear embarrassed or reluctant when asked to read aloud. Second, pay careful attention to the kinds of reading tasks that are most difficult for the child. Reading weaknesses are often more apparent on timed than on untimed tests, so it is important to include timed tests of word-, nonword-, and paragraph-level reading, which are likely to be most sensitive.

The most important behavioral observations to emerge from testing come from analysis of a child's specific reading and spelling errors. There are four main kinds of reading errors to look for: dysfluency, errors on function words, visual errors (whole-word guesses), and lexicalizations when reading nonwords. We will discuss spelling errors shortly. Children with dyslexia are usually slow and halting in their oral reading, because their automatic decoding skills are weak. However, dysfluency may not be evident in older children with dyslexia who have overlearned a large, automatic reading vocabulary.

By *function word errors,* we mean substitutions on "little" words, such as articles and prepositions. Children with dyslexia frequently interchange *a* and *the,* and misread prepositions. The significance of function word errors is that the child is working hard to properly decode the content words in the sentence and is relying more on context than a typical reader would to identify function words. Function word errors are puzzling to parents and teachers, who remark that if the child can read the big words, why can they not read the little words?

By visual errors, we mean substitutions on content words that are based on a superficial visual similarity to the target word (e.g., *tired* for *tried*). The significance of these errors is that the child is using visual similarity rather than the full phonological code to name the word, so, again, these errors are reflective of a phonological coding or "phonics" problem. Lexicalization errors when reading nonwords refer to misreading a nonword as a real word, usually one that is visually similar to the target (e.g., *clip* for *clup*). The significance of these errors is essentially the same as visual errors: Lacking good phonological coding skills, the child assimilates the target to whatever other schema is available for word recognition.

In terms of spelling errors, we mainly examine the proportion of errors that are not phonetically accurate (i.e., dysphonetic), especially errors in which consonants have been added, omitted, or substituted (e.g., *exetive* for *executive*). Children with dyslexia are also weaker at spelling vowels, but normal developmental acquisition of vowel correspondences is more protracted, so many young typically developing children make vowel errors. In the groups we have studied, the mean rates of phonologically accurate (with regard to consonants) errors have been about 70% for typically developing children ages 8–12 and about 80% for adolescents and adults (Pennington, Lefly, Van Orden, Bookman, & Smith, 1987). As a rough guide, a phonological accuracy rate for consonant sequences lower than 60% in children and 70% in adolescents and adults would be suggestive of dyslexic difficulties.

The final kinds of error to mention are the so-called "reversal" errors in reading and spelling. Although earlier accounts of dyslexia viewed reversal errors as the hallmark of dyslexia, their rate of occurrence in people with dyslexia is actually quite low and many people with dyslexia do not make such errors (Liberman, Shankweiler, Orlando, Harris, & Berti, 1971). Nonetheless, the presence of reversal errors in patients age 9 years and older is of some potential diagnostic significance, as normal readers that age and older virtually never make such errors. By a *reversal error*, we mean substituting a visually similar letter in reading or spelling (e.g., *bog* for *dog*). These errors most typically involve *b* and *d* confusions. Vellutino (1979b) convincingly argued that the primary basis of many such reversal errors is linguistic: *b* and *d* are both phonetically and visually similar. As discussed earlier, reversal errors do not indicate that dyslexia is caused by visual problems. Rather, reversal errors may be better understood as a correlate or consequence of poor reading rather than a cause.

Finally, it is valuable to look for subtle language difficulties that are characteristic of dyslexia. For instance, some children are unusually quiet because they have word-finding and verbal formulation problems. Such difficulties may often be observed on the verbal subtests of the Wechsler or in spontaneous speech.

Case Presentations

Case Presentation 3

Dominic is a 7-year-old second grader. His parents sought an evaluation because his progress in reading and spelling has been slow in spite of extra help. This year, he has become increasingly frustrated with homework. Completing it takes him between 1 and 2 hours a night, although his teacher suggests that the amount of work assigned should take approximately 30 minutes. Dominic's frustration often leads to angry and tearful confrontations with his parents that end with him refusing to do any more work. This fall, he has complained frequently of not wanting to go to school, particularly on days when his homework is not completed, and his parents note that they have had to "bribe him" to get in the car some mornings.

Dominic's prenatal, birth, and early developmental histories are unremarkable. He was a sociable and happy child who was well-liked in preschool. His parents noted that he was slower to learn his letters than his older sister, and that when they asked his kindergarten teacher about it, she said that Dominic was just not "developmentally ready." In first grade, he was placed in the weakest reading group, and part way through the year, his teacher nominated him for extra help. Twice a week, he arrived at school a half-hour early, and a fifth-grade student sat with him to practice reading. Dominic also received private reading tutoring in the summer between first and second grade. Now in second grade, Dominic remains in the weakest reading group; his reading is slow and error-prone, and his spelling seems very poor. His parents have been encouraging Dominic to read at home for practice, but he is reluctant to do so, and they are hesitant to push him and evoke more conflict. Dominic has had trouble learning the days of the week and still gets them confused. Although his math skills seemed strong initially, he is now struggling to memorize basic math facts.

Dominic's father reports no history of school difficulties. He is a college graduate and works in sales. Dominic's mother earned an associate's degree and does not work outside the home. Although she reports that school went well for her overall, she had a sister who repeated first grade because of difficulty learning to read. Dominic's mother notes that her own spelling is "atrocious" and that she had great difficulty with Spanish class in high school.

A summary of Dominic's diagnostic testing is found in Table 10.1.

DISCUSSION

Dominic's history is highly suggestive of dyslexia. Although his early development was normal, problems with reading and spelling were evident from first grade onward, and his parents picked up on subtler reading-related difficulties even when he was in kindergarten. Both the age of onset and the persistence of Dominic's problem are noteworthy. There is a family history of reading difficulty on the mother's side, with the mother's own weaknesses in spelling and learning a foreign language indicating a mild phonological processing deficit. Problems learning math facts and the days of the week suggest weaknesses in rote verbal memory. Dominic's parents' rating of his reading history on the Learning and Behavior Questionnaire does a good job of capturing his dyslexia history. The fact that Dominic's current behavior problems did not emerge until after he had already experienced 2 years of school difficulty suggests that they are secondary to his reading problem rather than symptoms of an additional, comorbid disorder. However, the current

TABLE 10.1. Test Summary, Case 3

Performance validity

Test of Memory Malingering
- Trial 1 — RS = 42
- Trial 2 — RS = 47 (valid)

General intelligence

WISC-V Full Scale IQ — SS = 93

Crystallized intelligence

WISC-V Verbal Comprehension Index — SS = 95
- Similarities — ss = 9
- Vocabulary — ss = 9

Working memory

WISC-V Working Memory Index — SS = 94
- Digit Span — ss = 8
- Picture Span — ss = 10

Processing speed

WISC-V Processing Speed Index — SS = 86
- Coding — ss = 6
- Symbol Search — ss = 9

Fluid intelligence

WISC-V Fluid Reasoning Index — SS = 106
- Matrix Reasoning — ss = 10
- Figure Weights — ss = 12

WISC-V Visual Spatial Index — SS = 100
- Block Design — ss = 9
- Visual Puzzles — ss = 11

Academic

Reading
- *History*
  - CLDQ Reading Scale — 98th %ile
- *Basic literacy*
  - WIAT-III Word Reading — SS = 92
  - WIAT-III Pseudoword Decoding — SS = 87
  - WIAT-III Spelling — SS = 84
- *Reading fluency*
  - TOWRE-2 Sight Word Efficiency — SS = 81
  - TOWRE-2 Phonemic Decoding Efficiency — SS = 76
  - GORT-5 Fluency — ss = 4
- *Reading comprehension*
  - GORT-5 Comprehension — ss = 6

Math
- *History*
  - CLDQ Math Scale — 62nd %ile
- *Calculation and problem solving*
  - WIAT-III Numerical Operations — SS = 104
  - Math Problem Solving — SS = 96
- *Math fluency*
  - WIAT-III Math Fluency — SS = 84

Oral language

Phonology
- CTOPP-2 Elision — ss = 8
- CTOPP-2 Phoneme Isolation — ss = 6

Verbal memory
- CTOPP-2 Nonword Repetition — ss = 5
- WRAML-2 Sentence Memory — ss = 7

TABLE 10.1. (continued)		
	WRAML-2 Story Memory	ss = 9
	WRAML-2 Story Memory Delay	ss = 11
Semantics and syntax		
CELF-5 Core Language	SS = 102	
Verbal processing speed		
CTOPP-2 Rapid Symbolic Naming	SS = 88	
Attention and executive functions		
Vanderbilt Inattention		
Parent	RS = 2	
Teacher	RS = 1	
Vanderbilt Hyperactivity/Impulsivity		
Parent	RS = 1	
Teacher	RS = 2	

Note. SS, standard score with mean = 100 and *SD* = 15; ss, scaled score with mean = 10 and *SD* = 3; RS, raw score; %ile, percentile rank; WISC-V, Wechsler Intelligence Scale for Children—Fifth Edition; CLDQ, Colorado Learning Difficulties Questionnaire; WIAT-III, Wechsler Individual Achievement Test—Third Edition; TOWRE-2, Test of Word Reading Efficiency—Second Edition; GORT-5, Gray Oral Reading Test—Fifth Edition; CTOPP-2, Comprehensive Test of Phonological Processing, Second Edition; CELF-5, Clinical Evaluation of Language Fundamentals—Fifth Edition; WRAML-2, Wide Range Assessment of Memory and Learning, Second Edition; Vanderbilt, NICHQ Vanderbilt Assessment Scales.

evaluation also included an assessment for ADHD, as is appropriate in any case when dyslexia is suspected.

Several aspects of Dominic's pattern of test results support a diagnosis of dyslexia: (1) his very low (2nd percentile) fluency score on the Gray Oral Reading Test, which is discrepantly poor relative to both his age and his verbal IQ; (2) overall weaker scores for reading and spelling than for math (with the exception of Math Fluency, discussed further below); (3) poor performance decoding nonsense words relative to reading real words; (4) weaker scores on timed than on untimed tests of single-word reading; and (5) evidence of phonological processing weaknesses, particularly on the Phoneme Isolation and Nonword Repetition subtests of the Comprehensive Test of Phonological Processes (CTOPP). In addition, Dominic displays a profile on the Wechsler Intelligence Scale for Children—Fifth Edition (WISC-V) that is common to children with dyslexia. Although not diagnostic, many children with dyslexia obtain relatively weaker scores on processing speed or verbal working memory (i.e., Digit Span) subtests. In addition, Dominic's Verbal Comprehension Index was slightly weaker than his Perceptual Reasoning Index, although both fell in the average range. It is important to note that many children with impairing RD can nonetheless obtain average-range scores on some reading measures, particularly untimed tests of single-word reading, and particularly when (like Dominic) they have already received some intervention.

Qualitative observations of Dominic's performance also support the current diagnosis. He made multiple whole-word guesses (e.g., *carried* for *covered* and *bars* for *boards*), as well as lexicalization errors on nonwords (e.g., *few* for *faw* and *bike* for *bice*). He made a number of dysphonetic spelling errors, such as GRAGSU for *garage*. He had difficulty on several tests emphasizing verbal rote memory. On the Wide Range Assessment of Memory and Learning (WRAML) Story Memory test, Dominic earned an average score primarily by remembering the gist of the stories; he had been unable to recall specific details, such as names of people or particular amounts of money. Dominic's low score on Math Fluency probably reflects both a more general processing speed deficit and a weakness memorizing math facts related to his poor verbal memory.

Because of the high comorbidity between dyslexia and ADHD, it is important to assess for difficulties with attention or impulsivity in any child with an RD. Dominic's early history is not indicative of ADHD, current parent and teacher ratings of ADHD symptoms are in the normal range, and behavioral observations during testing are not suggestive of an attentional disorder. Dominic's current conflict with his parents is more likely to be a secondary consequence of his reading failure than symptomatic of a second disorder. Conflict around homework and reading should diminish as appropriate treatment for Dominic's dyslexia is put in place.

Case Presentation 4

Laila, a 10-year-old girl who is entering fifth grade, has been diagnosed with an anxiety disorder, and her parents wonder whether she has a learning disability that is contributing to her anxiety about school. Her parents sought an evaluation because Laila is having trouble in reading, spelling, and math.

Laila's birth and early development were unremarkable. Her father reports that he had problems learning to read, but he is college-educated and has a professional career. Laila's parents first became concerned about her academic progress when her kindergarten teacher reported that she was slow to learn letter sounds and had more difficulty learning to read than other children in the classroom. In first and second grades, Laila's teachers did not express too much concern about her reading, but they noted that her reading fluency continued to be slow and suggested that her parents practice reading with her at home. It was difficult for Laila's parents to follow through on this recommendation, because Laila was resistant to reading. In third and fourth grades, Laila's teachers became more concerned about her reading, because she was continuing to fall behind her peers. She began receiving extra reading tutoring at school. Laila also had difficulty remembering the addition, subtraction, and multiplication math facts. During these years, Laila's mood and anxiety became problematic for the family. She would get angry and upset very easily and scream statements such as "I'm too stupid!" when attempting to complete homework. At the beginning of her fourth-grade year, Laila's parents consulted with a child psychologist, who diagnosed anxiety and initiated cognitive-behavioral therapy. According to her parents, this intervention has improved Laila's sleep, mood, and anxiety, although homework continues to be very frustrating for Laila. Currently, Laila's parents remain concerned about her academic progress, which seems modest despite the fact that she is a bright girl. Her teacher has noted that Laila's academic skills are pretty much at grade level, but she has difficulty getting motivated to do her schoolwork and seems worried and anxious.

A summary of Laila's diagnostic testing is found in Table 10.2.

TABLE 10.2. Test Summary, Case 4

Performance validity
Test of Memory Malingering
    Trial 1   RS = 49
    Trial 2   RS = 50
                          (valid)

General intelligence
WISC-V Full Scale IQ   SS = 109

Crystallized intelligence
WISC-V Verbal Comprehension Index   SS = 116
    Similarities   ss = 15
    Vocabulary   ss = 11

Working memory
WISC-V Working Memory Index   SS = 110
    Digit Span   ss = 11
    Picture Span   ss = 12

Processing speed
WISC-V Processing Speed Index   SS = 83
    Coding   ss = 8
    Symbol Search   ss = 6

Fluid intelligence
WISC-V Fluid Reasoning Index   SS = 118
    Matrix Reasoning   ss = 14
    Figure Weights   ss = 12
WISC-V Visual Spatial Index   SS = 94
    Block Design   ss = 8
    Visual Puzzles   ss = 10

Academic

Reading
History
    CLDQ Reading Scale   94th %ile

Basic literacy
    WIAT-III Word Reading   SS = 90
    WIAT-III Pseudoword Decoding   SS = 92
    WIAT-III Spelling   SS = 87

Reading fluency
    TOWRE-2 Sight Word Efficiency   SS = 86
    TOWRE-2 Phonemic Decoding Efficiency   SS = 84
    GORT-5 Fluency   ss = 7

Reading comprehension
    GORT-5 Comprehension   ss = 9

Math
History
    CLDQ Math Scale   66th %ile

Calculation and problem solving
    WIAT-III Numerical Operations   SS = 111
    Math Problem Solving   SS = 115

Math fluency
    WIAT-III Math Fluency   SS = 90

Oral language
Phonology
    CTOPP-2 Elision   ss = 8
    CTOPP-2 Phoneme Isolation   ss = 7

Verbal processing speed
    CTOPP-2 Rapid Symbolic Naming   SS = 82

Verbal memory
    CTOPP-2 Nonword Repetition   ss = 7
    WRAML-2 Sentence Memory   ss = 10
    WRAML-2 Story Memory   ss = 14
    WRAML-2 Story Memory Delay   ss = 13

(continued)

TABLE 10.2. (continued)

Attention and executive functions

Attention			Executive functions		
Vanderbilt Inattention			D-KEFS Verbal Fluency		
Parent	RS = 3		Letter Fluency	ss = 6	
Teacher	RS = 4		Category Fluency	ss = 9	
Vanderbilt Hyperactivity/Impulsivity			D-KEFS Trail Making Test		
Parent	RS = 0		Visual Scanning	ss = 12	
Teacher	RS = 0		Number Sequencing	ss = 8	
			Letter Sequencing	ss = 7	
Gordon Diagnostic System			Number–Letter Switching	ss = 8	
Vigilance Correct	Z = 0.57				
Vigilance Commissions	Z = −0.78				

Social–emotional functioning

RCADS			RCADS-P		
Social Phobia	T = 69		Social Phobia	T = 73	
Separation Anxiety	T = 67		Separation Anxiety	T = 69	
Otherwise WNL			Generalized Anxiety	T = 68	
			Otherwise WNL		

Note. D-KEFS, Delis–Kaplan Executive Function System; RCADS, Revised Children's Anxiety and Depression Scale; RCADS-P, Revised Children's Anxiety and Depression Scale—Parent Version; WNL, within normal limits. For other abbreviations, see Table 10.1.

DISCUSSION

The diagnostic issues in this case are subtle because of Laila's strong verbal abilities. Children with strong verbal abilities are less likely to be referred, because they may be at or near grade-level performance in reading, even though their reading scores are far below IQ expectations. Also, as we discussed earlier, girls with dyslexia are less likely to be referred for services than boys with dyslexia. It is noteworthy that this referral came following Laila's fourth-grade year, which is about the time when children move from "learning to read" (fluent decoding of words) to "reading to learn" (using reading to gain knowledge). Children with dyslexia whose decoding abilities remain behind grade expectations have difficulty garnering the required information from texts. Children who were not referred at earlier ages may come to clinical attention around fourth grade, because their learning is being hindered by their weak reading skills.

Although Laila has concurrent internalizing symptoms, her difficulties with reading, spelling, and math facts are all suggestive of dyslexia. The fact that Laila has difficulty getting started with schoolwork and is easily frustrated by her work is sometimes indicative of attention difficulties, so these symptoms were also assessed in the evaluation.

In terms of history, family history (her father's self-reported difficulties with learning to read) and reading history (the early onset of Laila's difficulties with learning letter sounds in kindergarten), and the persistence of her difficulties with reading and spelling are notable. The reading questions from the Colorado Learning Difficulties Questionnaire capture Laila's personal history of reading problems; her parents reported more reading difficulties than 94% of the norming sample.

Laila's attention was quite focused in the one-on-one testing setting, and she appeared to be motivated to perform well. Furthermore, her score on an objective performance validity test (Test of Memory Malingering [TOMM]) was well above the threshold indicating adequate effort and engagement. The main behavioral observations of Laila's test performance included dysphonetic spelling errors (e.g., BEILILE for *believe*), lexicalization errors of nonwords (e.g., *snake* for SNIRK) and dysfluencies. All of these errors are consistent with a diagnosis of dyslexia. Parent and teacher reports on the ADHD Rating Scale did not indicate clinically significant difficulties with attention. Similarly, Laila performed well on the Gordon Diagnostic System, which, as a continuous performance test (CPT), shows a modest relationship with ADHD diagnosis. Because CPTs are not very sensitive, good performance does not exclude ADHD, but in Laila's case, it is part of the converging body of evidence suggesting that, overall, her attention is age-appropriate.

The test results confirm a diagnosis of dyslexia via several converging patterns of evidence. Most importantly, Laila's performance on the most sensitive measures of basic literacy skills (timed word reading, timed decoding, timed paragraph-level reading, and spelling) cluster around an *SD* below average for her age and 2 *SDs* below average for verbal ability. Using strict DSM-5 criteria, Laila falls in a "grey area," because, relative to age expectations alone, her reading difficulties are not that pronounced. Laila is a good example of a case in which an IQ-discrepancy definition is more appropriate, because her reading difficulties clearly cause clinical impairment, and because there is a lot of convergent evidence from her history, behavioral observations, and her neuropsychological profile (see Chapter 6 for a fuller discussion of DSM-5 and IQ discrepancy definitions of dyslexia). The other notable patterns to emerge from the data include clusters of weakness impacting processing speed (WISC-V Processing Speed, CTOPP-2 Rapid Naming) and phonological processing (e.g., CTOPP-2 Phoneme Isolation, Nonword Repetition). These are both cognitive risk factors for dyslexia. Although Laila's Math Fluency is within the average range, it is weaker than would be expected given her untimed math performance and likely also reflects this processing speed weakness. Laila's scores were also relatively weak on certain subtests of the Delis–Kaplan Executive Function System (D-KEFS); in her case, these difficulties seem most likely to reflect difficulties with processing speed (all subtests administered were speeded tests), or phonological/orthographic knowledge (Letter Fluency, Letter Sequencing) rather than a primary executive dysfunction.

We screen social–emotional functioning for all referred children, generally using a combination of clinical interviews and broadband behavior rating scales (see Table 7.1 in Chapter 7 for examples). In Laila's case, the assessment also included a more focused evaluation of her current level of depressive and anxious symptomatology using the Revised Children's Anxiety and Depression Scale (RCADS). She and her parents continued to report concerns for some aspects of anxiety, mostly falling in the mild to moderate range (which likely represents some improvement in symptoms she had prior to cognitive-behavioral intervention). Of note, several items that load on the Social Phobia or Separation Anxiety subscales ask specifically about how the child feels about school. Children with dyslexia sometimes experience anxiety and poor self-esteem that result from their frustration with reading. They compare themselves to their peers and feel that they are less bright because of their particular difficulty with reading. In this case, Laila seems to have a particular vulnerability for anxiety that is activated by her learning disability.

Laila's dyslexia diagnosis explains both the referral concerns regarding her progress with reading and spelling, and her difficulties with math. Although dyslexia is a language-based disability, it can affect math performance via verbal short-term memory weaknesses that make it difficult to learn and retrieve basic math facts. The observation that Laila is slow to get started with her work is partly explained by her slow processing speed, but she also has the additional complicating factor of the anxiety she experiences, which may slow her down even further. It will be important for Laila's parents and teachers to understand the nature of her learning disability and its associated cognitive weaknesses, as well as how Laila's learning disability contributes to her anxiety disorder.

Treatment

The development of evidence-based treatments for dyslexia has benefited from our understanding of its neuropsychology, and the best interventions provide intensive, explicit instruction in phoneme awareness, the alphabetic principle and phonics, word analysis, reading fluency, and reading comprehension (McArthur et al., 2012; National Reading Panel, 2000; Snow, Burns, & Griffin, 1998; Vaughn, Denton, & Fletcher, 2010).

The later elementary school years mark an important transition in which the educational emphasis moves from "learning to read" (generally from kindergarten to third grade) to "reading to learn" (generally from fourth grade and on). Thus, children with reading difficulties in the early years typically have problems with the foundational skills implicated in dyslexia, such as decoding and fluency, whereas children whose reading difficulties appear later may have intact decoding but problems with language comprehension or other aspects of cognitive development (Catts, Compton, Tomblin, & Bridges, 2012). Accordingly, the most appropriate type of reading intervention varies somewhat for younger versus older children, though there is also overlap.

Recent work on treatments for reading difficulties in the early grades (Scammacca, Vaughn, Roberts, Wanzek, & Torgeson, 2007) support the following conclusions: (1) Intervention is most effective when provided in a one-to-one or small-group setting (Vaughn et al., 2003); (2) successful interventions heavily emphasize phonics instruction; and (3) other valuable treatment elements include training in phoneme awareness, supported reading of increasingly difficult connected text, writing exercises, and comprehension strategies. Many effective treatments are relatively low-cost, further highlighting the importance for public health of early identification, prevention, and treatment of dyslexia.

Many practitioners and educators know that phoneme awareness difficulties are implicated in dyslexia and make phoneme awareness one target of intervention. This can be appropriate for many students, as long as direct reading instruction is also included. When phoneme awareness training alone is compared to phoneme awareness plus direct reading instruction (e.g., letter–sound training, practice reading connected text), research has consistently found stronger effects for the integrated treatment (e.g., Bradley & Bryant, 1983; Cunningham, 1990; see also National Reading Panel, 2000). Phoneme awareness training can have some additional benefit, which may be specific to children at risk for RD (Hatcher, Hulme, & Snowling, 2004). In that study, young children (ages 4–5 years) at risk for dyslexia responded best to a program that included both letter–sound knowledge training and phoneme awareness training. In contrast, the low-risk children experienced no additional boost of phoneme awareness training over and above the phonics program. Presumably, the phoneme awareness training helped the at-risk children develop the skills they needed to benefit most from reading instruction, while the typically developing children may have been able to infer the necessary skills without explicit instruction. A separate, but related, phenomenon is that compared to eventual good readers, young children who later develop RD not only have deficits in their absolute levels of phoneme awareness skill but also in the slower rate at which they respond to phoneme awareness training (Byrne, Fielding-Barnsley, & Ashley, 2000). It is important to note that the added benefit of phoneme awareness training over and above direct reading instruction may not generalize to older struggling readers (Alexander & Slinger-Constant, 2004; Wise, Ring, & Olson, 2000).

It appears that accuracy problems are easier to treat than fluency problems, perhaps in part because fluency is so dependent on reading experience, which varies dramatically by reading level. It may be nearly impossible for poor readers to "close the gap" in print exposure once they have accumulated several years of reading failure, but there is some evidence that fluency problems can be prevented with appropriate intervention in kindergarten and first grade, at least over the short term (Torgesen, 2005). An important conclusion is that professionals should not wait until children are formally diagnosed with dyslexia or experience repeated failures before implementing reading treatment, when remediation has been shown to be less effective than early intervention (Vaughn et al., 2010).

Interventions that focus solely on foundational reading skills show smaller effect sizes for older versus younger readers on average. Generally speaking, the most effective reading treatments for older children with reading problems emphasize language and cognitive skills such as vocabulary and comprehension strategies. However, even adolescents can benefit from phonics and fluency training to a degree, so a combined approach may be most appropriate for older students with dyslexia (Scammacca, Roberts, Vaughn, & Stuebing, 2015).

There are individual differences in how well individuals with dyslexia respond to treatment, with about half of successfully treated children maintaining gains for at least 1–2 years. It has been challenging to identify individual variables that predict a substantial portion of the variance in treatment response, although the well-documented preschool predictors of later reading skill (i.e., phoneme awareness, letter name and sound knowledge, and rapid serial naming) have shown small effects in some cases (Fletcher et al., 2011; Stuebing et al., 2015). Regarding long-term prognosis independent of treatment, language skill is a known protective factor for both children and adults with dyslexia (Shaywitz, 2003).

There are a growing number of intervention–imaging studies investigating how remediation of dyslexia alters brain activity. Briefly, effective intervention appears to promote normalization of activity in the left-hemispheric reading and language network that has shown reduced activity in dyslexia. There is also some evidence for increased activation in a variety of brain regions, which may reflect compensatory processes (Barquero, Davis, & Cutting, 2014; Gabrieli, 2009).

While there is a solid evidence base for treatments emphasizing direct instruction in reading and phonological training, several alternative therapies that either lack sufficient evidence or have been shown to be ineffective for dyslexia should not be recommended to children and families (for a review, see Pennington, 2011). Most of these therapies are based on sensory–motor theories of dyslexia and include training in rapid auditory processing (e.g., Fast ForWord®), various visual treatments (colored lenses, vision therapy), and exercise/movement-based treatment (e.g., vestibular training).

Table 10.3 provides a summary of current research and evidence-based practice for RD.

TABLE 10.3. Summary Table: Reading Disability (Dyslexia)

Definition

- Poor basic literacy (word reading, reading fluency, spelling) skill relative to age expectations.
- Exclusionary criteria include uncorrected sensory deficits, inadequate instruction, acquired neurological insults, and intellectual disability.

Prevalence and epidemiology

- Approximately 7%, depending on diagnostic cutoff.
- Slightly more males than females are affected (approximately 1.5:1), but many more males are referred for services.
- Comorbid with several other learning disorders, including ADHD, math disability, LI, and SSD.

Developmental neuropsychology

- Even before formal literacy instruction, children who later develop dyslexia show weaknesses in several aspects of speech and language development.
- By school age, phoneme awareness deficits show a strong relationship with dyslexia. The causal relationship between phoneme awareness and literacy is bidirectional.
- No single cognitive deficit explains all the variance in literacy or all individuals with the disorder. Multiple-deficit models including PA, other language skills (e.g., vocabulary, verbal short-term memory), and verbal and nonverbal processing speed are more powerful.
- Although sensory problems (visual, auditory, and other) are found in some individuals with dyslexia, they do not appear to be causal. Visual attention problems may represent an additional risk factor in a multiple-deficit framework.

(continued)

TABLE 10.3. *(continued)*

Brain mechanisms

- There are well-established structural and functional differences in the left-hemisphere reading/language network. The most consistent findings implicate occipitotemporal and temporoparietal regions, as well as the inferior frontal gyrus.
- There is good evidence for reduced white matter connectivity between posterior and anterior left-hemisphere cites, which correlates with reading skill.
- Many of the structural and functional brain differences predate literacy instruction and so are not just a consequence of reading difficulties.

Etiology

- Behavioral genetics work suggests a multifactorial etiology with substantial genetic effects.
- There are nine replicated linkage sites (termed *DYX1–DYX9*).
- Researchers have identified six candidate genes—two on chromosome 2p (*C2Orf2* and *MRPL19*), one on 3 (*ROBO1*), two on 6p (*DCDC2, KIAA0319*), and one on 15q (*DYX1C1*). Four of these genes (all but the two on 2p) are believed to be involved in prenatal brain development processes, such as neural migration and axon path finding.
- Less is known about specific environmental risk factors, but they likely include home language/literacy environment and instructional quality.
- Evidence for G–E interplay includes greater heritability of dyslexia in more favorable environments (a bioecological G × E interaction) and individuals with dyslexia spending less time with books (an active G–E correlation).

Diagnosis

- Diagnosis requires a history of difficulties acquiring basic literacy skills (i.e., learning to read and spell words) that is typically present from the early elementary school years.
- In addition, performance on standardized measures of reading accuracy, fluency, and/or spelling should cluster below age expectations.
- In some intellectually gifted individuals, literacy skills may fall within normal limits for age but well below expectations based on IQ. A diagnosis of dyslexia can still be appropriate if the literacy difficulties cause substantial clinical impairment.
- Associated cognitive difficulties in phonological awareness, rapid naming, nonverbal processing speed, verbal short-term memory, vocabulary, and/or other language skills are common. However, there is great variability across individuals and no particular cognitive deficit or profile can be used to rule diagnosis in or out.
- Assessment should include screening for exclusionary conditions (i.e., sensory deficits) and common comorbid disorders (ADHD, LI, math disability, internalizing difficulties).

Treatment

- Effective treatments provide intensive, explicit instruction in phoneme awareness, phonics, decoding, reading fluency, and reading comprehension strategies.
- Intervention is most effective when provided in a one-on-one or small-group setting on a daily basis (or at least several times per week).
- More is known about treating reading problems in younger children than in older children and adults. Thus, early intervention is an important public health goal.

CHAPTER 11

Mathematics Disorder

CHAPTER SUMMARY

Mathematics disorder (MD) and typical mathematics development nicely illustrate the overall theme of this book, which is that both learning skills and learning disorders result from a developmental process involving a mix of substantial general and more modest specific factors across multiple levels of analysis.

At the neurocognitive level, general cognitive factors outweigh specific ones in predicting variance in math skills. These general cognitive factors include g (intelligence), language, verbal working memory, processing speed, and even phonological awareness, most of which have been shown to be genetically correlated with math skill. An important specific factor in math development is number sense, whose development begins in infancy and is gradually elaborated by the development of counting and eventually by formal instruction. Hence, contrary to Piaget's (1952) theory of number development, a child's gradual developmental understanding of number begins much earlier in life.

An important controversy in the developmental psychology of typical and atypical math development is the relative importance of approximate versus symbolic number sense. The approximate number system allows for estimation of the size of a group without relying on language or symbols, whereas development of a symbolic number system allows the child to represent precise quantities. The current evidence indicates a greater role for the symbolic number sense in predicting later math skill. An important methodological issue for this field is the weak psychometric properties of both kinds of number sense tests, especially compared to the much stronger psychometric properties of measures of general cognitive factors implicated in math development, and math measures themselves. It will be important to examine whether the predominance of general factors in math development is maintained once more robust measures of number sense are utilized.

At the level of brain mechanisms, a widely distributed network subserves the development of math skill, and most hubs in this network are not specific to math (with the one possible exception being the left intraparietal sulcus [IPS]). Moreover, this brain network changes with development, consistent with the interactive specialization model of brain–behavior development. Hence, the left IPS does not appear to be an innate, localized brain module for number sense.

At the etiological level, there is moderate heritability for both MD and the entire range of individual differences in math skill. These genetic influences are more general than specific, because they overlap substantially with genetic influences on g, language, and reading.

Finally, at the symptom level of analysis, MD is substantially comorbid with reading disability (RD), language impairment (LI), and attention-deficit/hyperactivity disorder (ADHD), and these comorbidities are mediated by general cognitive risk factors and by generalist genes. More research is needed to identify precisely the brain mechanisms underlying these comorbidities, but existing research points to some likely candidates.

Our current research understanding of MD and typical math skill has important clinical implications for the diagnosis and treatment of MD. In terms of diagnosis, it is important to carefully assess the different dimensions of math skill itself (number sense, counting, place values, automaticity of math facts, calculations, and word problems), as well as the general cognitive risk factors and comorbidities of MD. Although the hypothesis that there are valid cognitive subtypes of MD has a long history, there is currently little empirical support for such subtypes. Despite being substantially heritable, math skills are malleable, and empirically supported therapies are available. These therapies focus on math skills directly, whereas process-oriented therapies that focus on general cognitive risk factors such as working memory are not empirically supported.

HISTORY

Like reading, mathematics is a relatively recent cultural invention (roughly 8,000 years old) that is grafted onto much older, evolved cognitive skills. Some of these older, evolved cognitive skills are shared with other species (i.e., magnitude estimation, also called the *approximate number system*). But some are uniquely human (i.e., language), the brain mechanisms for which coevolved with human culture. One could speculate that human brain mechanisms continued to coevolve once written numbers and words were invented. However, this seems very unlikely, largely because the survival of the vast majority of humans did not hinge on their being either literate or numerate. Hence, learning disabilities in reading or math only became clinically significant once human culture began providing universal education roughly 100 years ago. For most of human history, there were millions of individuals with undiagnosed learning disorders (i.e., they had the genetic risk factors and brain phenotype of dyslexia or dyscalculia), who were perfectly successful being farmers and craftsmen.

Here we come to an important asymmetry between reading and math. While it was fine for these millions to be illiterate, they still needed some mathematical skills to function in their lives. Lacking any formal training in mathematics, they could still count and rely on physical tallies (e.g., fingers and toes, knots on a string, or notches on a stick) to keep track of their possessions and to trade them. While the majority of the world's languages lack a written form, no one has yet found a human culture without at least some number words and some use of physical tallies (Wilder, 1968). Unlike other animals, virtually all humans learn about exact numbers, which are symbolized by words that allow the items in a set of objects to be precisely counted. While primitive people have a concept of number, many *modern* people lack a clear concept of a phoneme, including many who are literate. Hence, spoken symbols for numbers and a means of counting are presumably quite old in prehuman history, although we do not know exactly when these cultural inventions arose.

Appreciation of *approximate relative numerosity* (the ability to perceptually distinguish a larger set of objects from a smaller one) is much older evolutionarily than the human species, since it is found in many nonhuman animals. The approximate number system has been the focus of considerable research in recent decades, and its role in the development of the exact number system in human children is an important issue for how we understand typical and atypical mathematical development.

Turning now to MD itself, two important strands in its research foundations have only recently come together. One early strand is neuropsychological; the other, later, strand is developmental. We first review the neuropsychological strand.

In 1925, Henschen coined the term *acalculia* to describe acquired deficits in arithmetic (Henschen, 1919/1925). Later, other behavioral neurologists distinguished subtypes of acalculia associated with different lesion locations. These included an aphasic subtype associated with left perisylvian lesions, a spatial subtype associated with right-hemisphere lesions, and a planning and perseveration subtype associated with frontal lesions (H. Levin, 1979; Badian, 1983; Berger, 1926; Hecaen, Angelergues, & Houillier, 1961; Luria, 1966). The three subtypes may be thought of as secondary acalculias, in which deficits in arithmetic are caused by a broader cognitive deficit that also produces other symptoms. In contrast, the fourth subtype, called *semantic dyscalculia* or *primary anarithmia*, is considered to be a primary acalculia. It is characterized by a pure deficit in the understanding of numerical quantity and is associated with lesions of the left IPS, which is dorsal to the angular gyrus (Dehaene, 2003). The conclusion that it is primary and specific is based on performance dissociations across patients with acquired lesions and neuroimaging data of typical individuals performing mathematical tasks (Dehaene, 2003).

As is true for other learning disorders, initial work on developmental problems with arithmetic was heavily based on earlier work with acquired disorders. So the original name for MD was *developmental dyscalculia*. This term was introduced by Kosc (1974), who did the first systematic study of children with arithmetic problems. Similarly, because Dehaene's (2003) view of acquired semantic dyscalculia is localized and modular, he expected there would be analogous cases of *developmental* semantic dyscalculia caused by a localized failure in the development of the left IPS. But, as we discussed in earlier chapters, it is obviously a mistake to expect neurodevelopmental disorders to mirror acquired disorders, because brain–behavior relations change across development. Ansari (2010) provides an excellent discussion of this issue in regard to MD.

This list of acquired subtypes of acalculia makes it clear that there are multiple cognitive components of mature arithmetic operations, and this is likely to be even more true in development. Since mathematics includes a great deal more than arithmetic, there are quite likely to be different kinds of MD beyond arithmetic disorders, but most research on acquired acalculia and on developmental MD has focused on problems with arithmetic. Even when MD is restricted to problems with arithmetic, analyzing it will likely be much more complicated than analyzing a disorder such as dyslexia, in which the impaired skill, printed word recognition, is much simpler. A child learning arithmetic not only has to become automatic at recognizing printed numbers but also has to learn how to perform operations on these numbers to solve problems.

Another important point about the history of MD is that it is largely ignored in developmental psychology research on the typical development of mathematical concepts, the second strand mentioned earlier. That research initially focused on Piaget's (1952) research on the development of conservation of number, the understanding by a child that the number of items in a set remained invariant across physical rearrangements. Piaget made the strong theoretical claim that children could not understand anything about the concept of number or about arithmetic unless they had already mastered conservation of number. Considerable research in the 1970s and 1980s demonstrated that this strong claim was wrong (e.g., Gelman & Gallistel, 1986; Pennington, Wallach, & Wallach, 1980). This research demonstrated that children can have workable partial concepts of number and begin to learn arithmetic *before* they fully master Piaget's conservation of number task. Failures on this task turned out to have more to do with executive dysfunction elicited by a conflict task than with a deficit in numerosity itself (Lubin, Simon, Noude, & De Neys, 2015).

If conservation of number was not the key developmental precursor to later mathematical skill, maybe something else was. Partly inspired by the success of the phonological theory of dyslexia, researchers studying mathematics development and disorder sought the equivalent of phoneme awareness in reading development, namely, a single, early developing, domain-specific, nonacademic cognitive skill that would strongly predict later success or failure in mathematics once formal schooling began. With the discovery of the approximate number system in both human babies and other animals (Halberda & Feigenson, 2008), researchers pursued the hypothesis that the approximate number system is the key developmental precursor to later mathematical skill. As we review later in this chapter, this hypothesis has not been well supported empirically. Instead, both general cognitive skills and mastery of the *exact* number system embodied in counting and written numbers have turned out to be stronger predictors of later mathematical skill, although exact number skills likely require an intact approximate number system.

Since the previous edition of this book was published in 2009, research on mathematics development and MD has accelerated greatly, and the findings of this new research are incorporated into this chapter. Much more now is known about (1) the early development of quantitative skills; (2) the comorbidities of math disorder; (3) the neuroimaging profile of typical and atypical mathematics development; (4) math anxiety; and (5) interventions for MD and math anxiety.

DEFINITION

Any diagnostic definition of MD, or any other learning disorder in this book, requires imposing a somewhat arbitrary cutoff on a continuous symptom dimension. What validates a particular cutoff is that it identifies a minority of children (i.e., the prevalence of the disorder must be somewhat rare to be atypical), who are also functionally impaired by having this disorder. Functional impairment means significant problems in everyday life, which for younger children mainly comprises school. But how rare and how impairing this must be to count as a disorder are still somewhat arbitrary decisions. Researchers can escape this dilemma by studying the entire symptom dimension, then testing whether the same pattern of results is found across different cutoffs on the low tail of the distribution. Clinicians, however, cannot escape this definitional dilemma, because they have to make a categorical decision as to whether *this* particular child needs services or not. So, what diagnostic cutoffs have been chosen by diagnostic manuals, such as the DSM or the ICD? As discussed in Chapter 6 and further below, there was a major change in the cutoff chosen for SLD in the latest edition of the DSM, namely, DSM-5 (American Psychiatric Association, 2013).

The previous DSM edition (DSM-IV-TR; American Psychiatric Association, 2000) defined MD as a substantial discrepancy between a child's performance on individually administered tests of math skills and what is expected based on age, intelligence, and education, that also causes associated functional impairment. The requirement of an education discrepancy was meant to exclude math problems due to inadequate instruction. If a sensory disorder was present, the math problems needed to be greater than what is expected based on the sensory disorder alone.

Hence, this DSM-IV-TR definition, required both age *and* IQ discrepancy. As is the case with many other DSM diagnoses, the degree of discrepancy is not operationally defined, although practitioners and researchers often pick either 1 *SD* below the mean (the bottom 16% of the population) or 1.5 *SD*s below the mean (the bottom 7% of the population). Because there are additional exclusionary criteria in the diagnostic definition, the observed prevalence will be lower than what these cutoffs dictate.

In contrast to DSM-IV-TR (American Psychiatric Association, 2000), DSM-5 (American Psychiatric Association, 2013) only requires a significant *age* discrepancy for a specific learning disability (SLD), whether in mathematics, reading or writing. The rationale for this change came from extensive research on the validity of the distinction between IQ-discrepant and age-discrepant poor reading, as we discussed in Chapter 10. Because this research revealed little, if any, validity for this distinction for dyslexia, and because the requirement of an IQ discrepancy for formal diagnosis discriminated against poor readers who were only age discrepant, the new version of the Federal Individuals with Disabilities Education Act (IDEA) prohibited the exclusive use of an IQ discrepancy for the diagnosis of any SLD.

But DSM-5 went further than the law and completely eliminated the use of an IQ discrepancy, as did some U.S. states (including our home state of Colorado) as well. Unfortunately, this exclusive reliance on an age-discrepancy definition of SLD also leads to a potential social injustice, because many gifted children with only an IQ-discrepant SLD will not qualify for a diagnosis or special education services. As we have argued elsewhere (Pennington & Peterson, 2015), the solution to these social justice issues is to allow either an age *or* IQ discrepancy to qualify a child as having an SLD, as long as there is evidence that the child's learning difficulty causes functional impairment.

This major change from DSM-IV-TR to DSM-5 automatically *increased* the prevalence of MD. This is necessarily so, because some children who have a significant age discrepancy in mathematics will *not* also have a significant IQ discrepancy. In contrast to dyslexia and LI, there has been much less research on the validity of age- versus IQ-discrepancy definitions of MD. As long as the correlation between math achievement measures and IQ is less than 1.0, there will inevitably be children who only meet an IQ-discrepancy definition of MD. Although we lack research on such children, it seems reasonable to think that such children need to be identified and helped.

PREVALENCE AND EPIDEMIOLOGY

Population studies using the DSM-IV-TR requirement of both an age and IQ discrepancy found prevalences of 3–6.5% for MD (reviewed in Shalev & Gross-Tsur, 2001). Further epidemiological work on using DSM-5 criteria is still needed. However, an earlier epidemiological study in an Israeli population comparing age-discrepancy-only criteria to age- and IQ-discrepancy criteria nicely illustrates how DSM-5 has increased the prevalence of MD (Gross-Tsur, Manor, & Shalev, 1996). These authors used a two-stage procedure in the epidemiological study. First, a citywide screening of over 3,000 10- to 11-year-olds identified those scoring in the bottom 20% on a group-administered arithmetic achievement test. This cutoff resulted in an age-discrepant group of roughly 600 children, a large subset of whom would likely meet other DSM-5 criteria for MD. This group of roughly 600 children was then given individual IQ and math assessments. Those obtaining an IQ greater than or equal to 80 and scoring at or below the mean of children two grades younger on the math measure were classified as having developmental dyscalculia (i.e., MD), because they had both the age and IQ discrepancy required by DSM-IV-TR. There were 140 such children (4.6% of the original 3,000), with a nearly equal gender ratio (1.1/1, M/F). Hence, one can see that the DSM-5 criteria identify several times as many children as MD as the DSM-IV-TR criteria (around 20 vs. 5%)! It is also important to point out that Gross-Tsur et al. (1996) did not identify many gifted children with MD, most of whom would not have had the required age discrepancy.

The prevalence of MD in this and other studies (6.3% in Badian, 1983; 3.6% in C. Lewis, Hitch, & Walker, 1994) is higher than the 1% figure cited in the DSM-IV-TR (2000), based on clinical samples. The explanation for this discrepancy may be that children with isolated MD are less likely to be referred. In our clinical experience, it is much rarer for a child with a specific MD than one with a specific RD to come in for assessment.

Comorbidities

Based on the subtypes of acquired acalculia, one would expect cases of MD to be comorbid with language, spatial, or attention problems. Also, as we discussed earlier, because most of the predictors of later math skill are not very specific to math, we would expect MD to be comorbid with most of the learning disorders discussed in this book. Indeed, MD and RD co-occur in 30–70% of individuals with either disorder, a higher-than-chance overlap (Badian, 1999; Kovas & Plomin, 2007; Landerl & Moll, 2010). Less research has investigated the overlap between MD and ADHD, or MD and LI. In a study of 476 children with ADHD, Capano, Minden, Chen, Schachar, and Ickowicz (2008) found a prevalence rate of 18.1% for comorbid MD + ADHD. Furthermore, studies of children with identified LI have revealed group deficits on most mathematical tasks (e.g., Donlan, Cowan, Newton, & Lloyd, 2007; Manor, Shalev, Joseph, & Gross-Tsur, 2001) and suggest that about 25% of children with LI will also have MD. Although exact comorbidity estimates vary across studies for a variety of reasons (e.g., country included, age of sample, specific cutoff used), they all agree on both the comorbidity of MD and other learning disorders and the existence of a substantial portion of children with isolated MD. So specific and possibly primary MD appears to exist, and thus requires an explanation at deeper levels of analysis (neuropsychology, brain bases, etiology).

DEVELOPMENTAL NEUROPSYCHOLOGY

The core issue addressed by this book, general versus specific factors in learning disorders, is useful for organizing what has been learned at the behavioral level about typical and atypical development of skill in mathematics. On the general side, we have found that there is substantial overlapping variance between a latent mathematics factor and g (intelligence; Peterson et al., 2018).

Furthermore, in a test of the multiple-deficit model of mathematics, reading, and inattention (Peterson et al., 2017), we found that 88% of the variance in a latent mathematics factor (defined by both calculation and applied math problem-solving skills) could be accounted for by three general cognitive skills (Peterson et al., 2018). The largest independent contribution was made by verbal ability (standardized path weight of .46), followed by verbal working memory (standardized path weight of .38), and then processing speed (standardized path weight of .13). Processing speed was a shared predictor of all three symptom dimensions, helping to explain the comorbidity among the three related disorders (MD, RD, and ADHD inattentive type [ADHD-I]). Verbal ability was a shared predictor of math and reading, whereas verbal working memory was a specific predictor of mathematics. This last result is consistent with considerable previous theoretical and empirical work on the importance of working memory in mathematics skill (e.g., Fias, Menon, & Szucs, 2013). Although verbal working memory was specific to the math outcome in this particular model, we know, of course, that it is an important contributor to many other academic and cognitive outcomes as well.

Thus, while none of the cognitive predictors of mathematics skill in these studies from our lab (Peterson et al., 2017; Peterson et al., 2018) are truly specific to the domain of mathematics, these results do not mean that children only need these general cognitive skills to learn mathematics. Obviously, they need to be taught about this particular cultural invention, just as they have to be taught to read, and this teaching typically begins with parents, before children go to school. First, parents, and later teachers, teach preschoolers particular precursor skills on which formal instruction later builds. For reading, these precursor skills are nursery rhymes, which teach children about onsets and rimes in words, alphabet knowledge (i.e., not just learning the alphabet song but also knowing both letter names and then letter sounds). For mathematics, the main precursor skill is counting (i.e., not only saying the number sequence but also understanding both 1:1 correspondence and cardinality, as well as other key counting principles we discuss later).

Like RD, studies of MD have benefited from a mature developmental and cognitive science of mathematical skill. Interest in the development of mathematical concepts was stimulated by the seminal studies of Piaget (1952). Research over subsequent decades (e.g., Geary, 1994; Gelman & Gallistel, 1978/1986; Wynn, 1998) has given us a clearer understanding of the roots of mathematical knowledge in infancy and its development through the acquisition of counting skills and calculation strategies.

Milestones in the Development of Mathematics

Developmental research has identified several milestones in the development of mathematical knowledge. The approximate number system is found in early infancy, and subitizing skill develops by 22 months on average (Starkey & Cooper, 1980). *Subitizing* is the ability to discriminate the numerosity of a small set of objects without counting them. The subitizing range in infants is one to three objects, and increases to one to five objects in adults (Starkey & Cooper, 1995). Number name knowledge develops early as children begin to talk in the second and third years of life, but the development of counting is protracted (Wynn, 1992), contrary to Gelman and Gallistel's (1978/1986) proposal that counting principles are innate. Once children have mastered counting, they need to learn to recognize written integer symbols, and then written multidigit numbers. Just as learning letter names and sounds automatically is a protracted process, so too is achieving automaticity in recognizing printed numbers. In addition to really understanding multidigit numbers, children need to understand place value. In first and second grade, children begin to "groupitize." that is, to perceive quickly the numerosity of small sets of objects composed of subitizable subsets (Starkey & McCandliss, 2014). Then children are taught addition and subtraction, and (we hope) they memorize simple math facts for each operation (e.g., 2 + 2 = 4; 5 − 3 = 2). As soon as they move to multidigit calculations, they need to understand place value, which is a specific predictor for growth in arithmetic skill (Moeller, Pixner, Zuber, Kaufmann, & Nuerk, 2011). As we discuss next, these developmental milestones are relevant for understanding where development goes awry in MD. Later we discuss how these milestones may be used in an evaluation for possible MD.

This normative developmental framework has been used to analyze the performance of children with MD (Butterworth, 2005; Geary, Hoard, Byrd-Craven, & DeSoto, 2004). Although children with MD have often learned number names and some aspects of counting procedures, there is evidence that their core understanding of numerosity or cardinality is impaired, which is reminiscent of the deficit found in semantic acalculia (Dehaene, 2003), which we discussed earlier. This evidence includes (1) a study by Koontz and Berch (1996) in which children with MD had a decreased ability to subitize (i.e., automatically recognize the numerosity of small sets of three or fewer items without counting them); (2) a study by Landerl, Bevan, and Butterworth (2004) in which children with MD had slower reaction times on tests of nonsymbolic (dots) and symbolic (digits) magnitude comparison tasks relative to both children with dyslexia and typically developing controls; and (3) a study by Geary, Hamson, and Hoard (2000), in which first graders with MD had small decreases in the accuracy of symbolic number magnitude comparisons.

These results from young, school-age children with MD were interpreted as reflecting an earlier developing deficit in the core understanding of numerosity. Such a deficit would be expected to undermine the later development of counting and calculation strategies. Gelman and Gallistel (1978/1986) described the five implicit principles of counting that typically developing children learn. These principles are *one-to-one correspondence* (also called *itemizing*), *stable order* of counting names, *cardinality* (the last counted number is the cardinal magnitude of the set), *abstraction* (any set of items can be counted), and *order irrelevance* (the same cardinal number is achieved regardless of the order of the count). The abstraction and order irrelevance principles are not necessary for practical success at counting. In addition, young children sometimes deduce two nonessential counting principles that contradict order irrelevance, namely, a *standard direction principle* (e.g., counts have to start at the left side of a set) and an *adjacency principle* (counts must proceed from one contiguous item to the next).

As reviewed by Geary et al. (2004), while first- and second-grade children with either MD + RD or MD only were able to identify violations of the first three counting principles (one-to-one correspondence, stable order, cardinality), they were also more likely than their typical agemates to endorse the nonessential adjacency principle, and in first grade were less likely to detect double counts of the first item.

Importantly, children with RD (but not MD) did not differ from typically developing controls, which means these counting problems in MD were not secondary to RD.

Problems with an understanding of numerosity and counting principles would lead to problems with arithmetic. Typically developing children initially solve simple sums by counting all the items in both addends, then learn to count up from the larger addend, and then start to solve harder sums by reducing them to simpler ones (6 + 5 = 5 + 5 + 1). This sequence reflects an increased understanding of the relations among number facts, as well as increased use of memory-based strategies for remembering. Eventually, typically developing children master all their number facts and do not have to rely on counting.

As reviewed in Geary et al. (2004), it has been found in several countries that children with MD + RD and MD make more counting errors in simple calculations and persist in simpler counting strategies (e.g., counting all) longer than do controls. Most dramatically, both children with MD + RD and MD are much worse than typically developing controls at learning their math facts and applying them automatically, a deficit that is still present at the end of elementary school. While both MD groups perform worse on these skills than an RD-only group, the MD + RD group is more impaired than the MD-only group. So while RD does not appear to cause MD in the comorbid group, it may exacerbate it. Alternatively, comorbidity may simply be a marker for more severe difficulties in general risk factors that influence both reading and math.

It is well known clinically that many children with RD are poor at memorizing math facts, presumably due to their poor phonological skills. De Smedt, Taylor, Archibald, and Ansari (2010) tested this hypothesis by examining whether phonological awareness (PA) is a unique predictor of skill in solving small-size, single-digit arithmetic problems for which memorized math facts would be particularly helpful. Their timed experimental arithmetic verification tasks included 20 small (retrieval-based) and 20 large (procedure-based) problems across three arithmetic operations (addition, subtraction, and multiplication). Their sample included 37 typically developing fourth- and fifth-grade children. PA was measured by the Comprehensive Test of Phonological Processing (CTOPP) Elision task, and control measures included the Nonword Repetition Test (NRT), reading fluency (Test of Word Reading Efficiency [TOWRE]), and calculation accuracy (Woodcock–Johnson III [WJ-III] Calculation). They found that after controlling for grade and reading fluency, the PA task accounted for unique variance in both speed (8%) and accuracy (11%) of performance on small but not large arithmetic problems. In contrast, a related phonological task, NRT, did not predict performance. In summary, the phonological skill of PA specifically and uniquely predicted math fact retrieval. It would be useful for future research to test whether some children with MD have problems with memorizing math facts that cannot be accounted for by problems in phonological skill.

At the level of number, counting, and arithmetic skills, there is considerable empirical support for the typical and atypical developmental trajectories just presented. However, because the data come from different, mainly cross-sectional studies at different ages, we do not have strong longitudinal evidence that early numerosity problems cause inefficient counting, or that both of these undermine mastery of math facts.

Specific versus General Predictors of MD?

In the 2009 edition of this book, we concluded that there was not agreement among MD researchers as to whether MD is caused by a specific core deficit in numerosity per se (e.g., Butterworth, 2005) or by a more general deficit in verbal working memory or spatial cognition (Geary et al., 2004). As we discussed earlier, subsequent research has strongly supported the latter view (see Fias et al., 2013, for a review). Some individual studies have found small effects of the approximate number system predicting early math ability before formal instruction. For example, Libertus, Feigenson, and Halberda (2011) found a unique contribution of approximate number system to early math ability in 3- to 5-year-olds (explaining 6–8% of the variance). However, these results have not always been replicated. Furthermore, in a meta-analysis, De Smedt, Noël, Gilmore, and Ansari (2013) found that the association between symbolic number comparison tasks and math achievement at various ages is stronger and more consistent than the association with approximate number system tasks (i.e., dot comparison task).

Very few studies have directly compared approximate number system and symbolic number system measures as predictors of math achievement. Göbel, Watson, Lervåg, and Hulme (2014) followed 165 first-grade children over the course of a school year. The symbolic number system was assessed with a timed number identification task that emphasized both automaticity of knowledge of Arabic numerals and knowledge of place value. The approximate number system was assessed with a task requiring speeded comparison of sets of boxes. Both tasks were strongly related to arithmetic knowledge nearly a year later (as was letter identification skill). However, only number identification (i.e., the symbolic number system) was *uniquely* associated with later arithmetic skill after researchers accounted for general cognitive factors and all other variables in the model. These authors interpreted this somewhat counterintuitive finding to mean that the early ability to make connections between verbal codes and numeric symbols places constraints on later arithmetic development. Hiniker, Rosenberg-Lee, and Menon (2016) also compared the approximate and symbolic number systems in a study of math skill in both children with autism spectrum disorder (ASD; $N = 36$) and children with typical development (TD = 61), matched on age and Full Scale IQ (FSIQ), and similar in reading ability. After accounting for general predictors (IQ, working memory [WM], and age), they found that neither an approximate number system nor a symbolic number system emerged as a unique predictor of math achievement in the TD group. In contrast, in the ASD group, only the symbolic number system measure was a unique predictor.

In another longitudinal study of the relation between the symbolic number system and later math ability, Fuchs et al. (2010) used a latent change score analysis in 280 first graders followed over a 9-month school year. These investigators tested the specific and general predictors of growth in both calculations and math word problems. Specific predictors included two number sense tasks (Geary, Bailey, & Hoard, 2009; Siegler & Booth, 2004). General predictors included two measures each of four cognitive constructs: verbal WM, processing speed, fluid intelligence, and listening comprehension. By using latent growth scores and more than a single indicator for each construct, this study avoided the psychometric problems found in many studies of the relation between number sense and math development. In addition, another strength of this study is that latent growth scores tap developmental *change*, thereby controlling for autoregression, and avoiding the unreliability of raw difference scores. However, the two number sense measures they chose are not pure measures of either the approximate number system or symbolic number system, but instead combine nonsymbolic and symbolic magnitude comparisons.

Fuchs et al. (2010) found that both general and specific predictors accounted for 33% of the total growth in calculation skill, and 65% of the total growth in solving math problems. The authors then partitioned this explained variance into unique and shared influences for the domain-general and domain-specific abilities. About two-thirds of the explained variance in growth for each math skill was shared by the domain-specific and domain-general abilities, whereas each kind of predictor made smaller unique contributions to total growth. More specifically, for growth in calculation skills, 62% of the explained variance was shared between specific and general predictors, 11% was unique to domain-general abilities, and 27% was unique to domain-specific tasks. Similarly, for growth in math word problems, 71% of the explained variance was shared between specific and general predictors, 15% was unique to domain-general abilities, and 14% was unique to the domain-specific tasks.

Fuchs et al. (2010) argued that their results demonstrated the importance of specific cognitive factors (i.e., number sense) in math development, but one could argue that predictive variance shared by general and specific factors should be counted as general, if the definition of a specific factor is one that does not overlap with general factors. Using this definition, the results of Fuchs et al. study demonstrate that 73% of the explained growth in calculations and 86% of the explained growth in word problems is accounted for by general cognitive predictors.

In summary, these results are consistent with a multiple cognitive predictor model of growth in math skill (and by extension, a multiple cognitive-deficit model of MD).

BRAIN MECHANISMS

Since the second edition of this book was published in 2009, many more neuroimaging studies of MD and mathematics skill have been published, and these new results are consistent with a distributed view of the brain networks underlying mathematics skill, and with a multiple cognitive deficit view of MD. These new neuroimaging results contrast with the consensus view around the time of the previous edition, which is summarized next.

The previous consensus view in 2009 was that the left IPS is an innate, evolved structure specialized for nonsymbolic magnitude comparisons shared by humans and other animals. This view also held that in humans, the left IPS became the substrate for symbolic number comparisons, once humans invented an exact number system represented by spoken, and eventually, by written symbols. Evidence for this view is reviewed in Dehaene (2003) and Shalev and Gross-Tsur (2001). The research base of their reviews included dissociations found among adult patients with acquired brain lesions and neuroimaging studies of normal adult subjects and of patients with dyscalculia, including females with Turner syndrome. Because mathematics can be selectively spared when a lesion impairs reading, language, or semantics for nonmathematical content, these researchers argued for some specificity to the neural structures mediating mathematical performance in adults. As we said in 2009, there are alternative explanations for such seeming content-based dissociations (Farah, 2003; Van Orden et al., 2001). So these dissociations may not actually localize modules for mathematics in general or component mathematical operations.

Dehaene (2003) also argued that the left IPS is a key hub in a bilateral cortical network involving portions of the occipital–parietal and frontal lobes that supported mathematical operations, and that localized lesions in this network are associated with impaired performance on different mathematical tasks. He proposed a triple-code model for this bilateral cortical network. In his triple-code model, the three codes are (1) visual object codes for printed numbers, which are hypothesized to be processed by the bilateral ventral visual stream, much in the same way that printed words are processed by the portions of the fusiform gyrus; (2) a general analogic magnitude code, or mental number line, localized in the left IPS; and (3) a verbal code localized in left perisylvian language areas. According to this triple-code model, when individuals are presented with a symbolic number comparison task, they first perceive the printed numbers, then activate the corresponding verbal and magnitude codes. To extend this model to the task of performing written calculation problems, Dehaene (2003) added a frontal–striatal loop that would accomplish either automatic or effortful arithmetic procedures to arrive at the answer.

According to Dehaene (2003), the centrality of the left IPS in this cortical network is supported by the following findings. First, the left IPS is activated in normal adults performing arithmetic calculations or comprehending the magnitude of a number, regardless of input or output modality, or even awareness of a numerical stimulus. Moreover, this activity in the left IPS is proportional to difficulty, whether indexed by number of calculations, size of numbers involved, or numerical distance between them (in a comparison task). Second, patients with acquired lesions to the left IPS have severe deficits in even simple calculations or numerical comparisons and are said to have *pure semantic acalculia,* which is also called *primary anarithmetia.* Third, the one patient with developmental dyscalculia or MD who had been studied at that time with neuroimaging (magnetic resonance spectroscopy) had a localized abnormal signal overlapping this inferior parietal region in the left hemisphere (Levy, Levy, & Grafman, 1999). Based on all these findings, Dehaene (2003) argued that the left IPS supports the semantic representation and manipulation of numerical quantity, which he labels "numerical intuition" or a "mental number line," although he acknowledged that the right IPS may also be partly involved.

The importance of bilateral parietal structures for arithmetic was also supported by neuroimaging studies of females with Turner syndrome. These studies indicated abnormalities in bilateral parietal–occipital areas, both with structural (Murphy, DeCarli, & Daly, 1993; Reiss et al., 1993; Reiss, Mazzocco, Greenlaw, Freund, & Ross, 1995) and functional (Clark, Klonoff, & Hayden, 1990) scans.

In 2009, we concluded that although this convergence of evidence was impressive, we still needed a computational model of how the left IPS accomplishes these functions and what its inputs and outputs are. In addition, there may be portions of adjacent parietal cortex or other parts of the brain that are also sensitive to numerical quantity, so the "mental number line" may not be as localized as Dehaene (2003) argued.

What new evidence has challenged Dehaene's (2003) view of the brain mechanisms underlying mathematical skill? Two recent quantitative meta-analyses of functional magnetic resonance imaging (fMRI) studies of mathematics, one in adults (Arsalidou & Taylor, 2011) and one in children (L. Kaufmann, Wood, Rubinsten, & Henik, 2011), each document that the brain regions reliably activated by number comparison tasks or by calculations are much more widespread and less task-specific than Dehaene's (2003) model predicts. In addition, comparing the adult and child results makes it clear that the brain locations mediating these mathematical tasks *change* with development. These developmental differences are consistent with the interactive specialization model of brain–behavior development and inconsistent with a maturational model espoused by Dehaene and others, which assumes innate modules in the brain that have the same localization across development.

The Arsalidou and Taylor (2011) meta-analysis specifically tested Dehaene's (2003) triple-code model of the brain regions associated with printed number comparisons and with calculations. In contrast to the triple-code model, Arsalidou and Taylor's (2011) quantitative meta-analysis of 93 fMRI studies found many more consensus brain regions (activated by both printed number comparison tasks and written calculation problems) than the three or four predicted by the triple-code model. The consensus-activated sites did include not only those predicted by the triple-code model but also unexpected sites such as the insula, cingulate gyrus, and cerebellum (all three of which were shared by both the number and calculation tasks).

The second meta-analysis (of 19 fMRI studies) by L. Kauffmann et al. (2011) explicitly tested the maturational assumption of Dehaene's (2003) model that the neural substrates for mathematics will be similar in children and adults. They addressed four questions relevant to this issue, namely, (1) do nonsymbolic (i.e., approximate) and symbolic (i.e., exact) number comparisons activate the *same* brain regions in children as they do in adults, who activate the left IPS for both nonsymbolic and symbolic tasks?; (2) do the brain regions associated with nonsymbolic number processing *change* with age in children?; (3) are there consistent brain activation differences between children with MD and typical children, and are they restricted to the left IPS?; and (4) are the brain regions activated by calculations similar in adults and children? Their quantitative meta-analysis found that answers to these four questions were all contrary to what the mathematical model predicts; that is, the meta-analysis found the following answers to the four questions: (1) no; (2) yes; (3) yes, consistent with but not restricted to the left IPS; and (4) no. Regarding question (3), only three studies were available, and consistent activation differences between MD and typical children included both over- and underactivation differences across both parietal (including right and left IPS), frontal, and other brain structures. In summary, their results disconfirmed the predictions of the Dehaene (2003) model regarding brain–behavior development and instead were compatible with an interactive specialization model.

Summarizing across both meta-analyses, it is now clear that the brain regions associated with mathematics are much more distributed than the Dehaene (2003) triple-code model predicted and include many regions that mediate general cognitive and attentional processes. Consistent with Dehaene's model, the left IPS is a key location for mathematics, but so are other bilateral parietal lobe regions. Rather than being innate, the brain regions subserving the approximate number system change with development.

The other big change in neuroimaging studies of mathematics (and all other brain functions) has been a shift from localization models to large-scale network models. As we discussed earlier in Chapter 3, the brain has several such large-scale networks that interact to perform particular cognitive tasks. In a longitudinal study of math development in young children, researchers applied a large-scale, brain network analysis to neuroimaging data and tested how brain findings related to math outcomes. Increases in functional connectivity within a distributed brain network specialized for math predicted gains in math achievement (Evans et al., 2015).

In summary, research published since 2009 has challenged Dehaene's (2003) triple-code model and a maturational, modular view of the left IPS. Brain activity associated with both magnitude comparison and calculation tasks is more distributed in both children and adults than Dehaene's triple-code model predicts. One key difference not predicted by the triple-code model is the involvement of the salience network, a key hub of which is the anterior insula. New theoretical models involving the interactions between large-scale, distributed brain networks are now being tested to account for individual and developmental differences in mathematical skill.

ETIOLOGY

Research on the etiology of MD has progressed considerably since the previous edition of this book appeared in 2009, particularly in the realm of molecular genetics. By 2009, we already knew that certain genetic syndromes include MD as part of their phenotype, such as Turner syndrome and fragile X syndrome in females. We also knew that nonsyndromal MD is familial and heritable (h^2_g of approximately .4), and that some of the genetic influences on MD are shared with genetic influences on RD (Haworth, Kovas, Petrill, & Plomin, 2007; Light & DeFries, 1995). Moreover, this evidence for genetic influences on MD converged with several studies (Haworth et al., 2007; Knopik & DeFries, 1999; L. Thompson, Detterman, & Plomin, 1991; Wadsworth, DeFries, Fulker, & Plomin, 1995) that found heritability for normal individual differences in mathematics (e.g., .62–.75 in Haworth et al., 2007 and .67 in Knopik & DeFries, 1999). Likewise, there was also evidence of *shared* genetic influences on normal individual differences in mathematics and normal reading skills (Knopik & DeFries, 1999; Light, Defries, & Olson, 1998), similar to what Light and DeFries (1995) found for mathematics and reading scores at the low tail of the distribution. Light et al. (1998) examined which cognitive factors accounted for the covariation between reading and math scores. They found that Verbal IQ and nonword reading ability accounted for most of this covariation, and this relation was genetically mediated in both RD probands and controls. In summary, by 2009, we knew that both MD and individual differences in math across the entire distribution are moderately heritable and share genetic influences with reading and language measures. More recently, these initial findings on the heritability of MD and mathematics skill have been replicated and extended to molecular genetics studies, which we discuss further in the sections that follow.

Generalist Genes

One important hypothesis that has been supported by these more recent studies is the "generalist genes" hypothesis (Plomin & Kovas, 2005), which holds that there are substantial influences of the same genes across a broad range of cognitive and academic skills. S. Hart, Petrill, Thompson, and Plomin (2009) tested this hypothesis by performing a multivariate behavior genetics analysis in the large Western Reserve Reading Project population-based twin sample. They included measures of IQ and multiple measures of reading and mathematics. They found moderate genetic influences shared across all three domains, consistent with generalist genes acting across the whole distribution of individual differences in these three correlated cognitive skills: IQ, reading, and mathematics.

In a related study, Haworth et al. (2009) tested whether generalist genes had similar effects in both the low tail of the distribution and across the entire distribution in a separate very large twin sample (N = 8,000 12-year-olds in the Twins Early Development Study [TEDS] sample). They found quite similar phenotypic and genetic correlations among measures of reading, mathematics, IQ, and language in both the low tail and across the entire distribution. Specifically, the average phenotypic correlation among these four cognitive measures was r = .58 for the low tail and r = .59 for the entire distribution. The average genetic correlations were r = .67 for the low tail and r = .68 for the entire distribution. These correlations mean that these four cognitive skills overlap in about one-third of their variance and that the reason for this overlap is primarily genetic. On average, about two-thirds of the genes that affect any one of these traits are shared with the other traits. These results confirm that generalist genes act quite similarly for both individual differences and for disorders.

S. Hart et al. (2010) tested whether these generalist genes for reading and math also influenced the symptom dimension of ADHD (measured by the Strengths and Weaknesses of ADHD Symptoms and Normal Behavior Rating Scale [SWAN], which also captures variance at the favorable end of the ADHD symptom dimension, unlike the ADHD Rating Scale [ADHD-RS]). Since ADHD is comorbid with both RD and MD, it made sense that there could be genetic influences shared across all three phenotypes. In a Cholesky decomposition, generalist genes (the A_1 factor in the model) loaded at .44 on the continuous ADHD measure (SWAN), .63 on the reading factor, and .33 on the math factor. There were also generalist shared environmental influences (the C_1 factor) that influenced all three traits (.24 for ADHD, .59 for reading, and .90 for math). They found genetic influences that were specific for ADHD but not for reading or math. Hence, both genes and shared environments overlap in the etiology of all three traits.

Harlaar, Kovas, Dale, Petrill, and Plomin (2012) examined whether the genetic overlap between mathematics and reading was stronger for reading comprehension than for reading decoding. This is a plausible hypothesis given that math calculations, math "word" problems, and reading comprehension all place a higher demands on WM and verbal reasoning than does the fairly automatic skill of reading decoding. They found that generalist genes (the A_1 factor) loaded significantly on math (.78), reading decoding, (.46) and reading comprehension (.61). These results confirmed their hypothesis of a greater genetic overlap between math and reading comprehension than with reading decoding only. These generalist genes accounted for *all* the genetic variance in math and 56% of the genetic variance in reading comprehension, but only 25% of the genetic variance in reading decoding.

Heritability of the Approximate Number Sense

Only one published study has examined the heritability of the approximate number system (ANS), while none has examined heritability of the symbolic number system. Tosto et al. (2014) used the Panamath measure of the ANS in adolescents in the large TEDS twin sample and found a surprisingly modest heritability of .32. The other results from their ACE (additive genetic, common, and unique environmental variance) model were that shared environmental influences were null (C = 0), and the largest variance component was nonshared environmental influences (E = .68). In a subset of the sample with genomewide association studies (GWAS) data, the genomewide complex trait analysis (GCTA) estimate of heritability of the ANS was zero. To explain this surprisingly low (or even null) heritability of the ANS, which contrasts markedly with the moderate heritabilities of general cognitive factors such as IQ and language, these authors advanced the speculative hypothesis that the ANS is an evolved, universal fitness trait, like having two arms. Evolution presumably allowed less genetic variation in such universal traits because they were so important to survival.

There are several problems with viewing the ANS as a fitness trait. First, this view requires accepting the null hypothesis that the ANS has virtually zero heritability. But Tosto et al. (2014) did find modest but significant twin heritability of .32. Although the GCTA heritability was null, as discussed in Chapter 2, GCTA or single-nucleotide polymorphism (SNP)-based heritabilities are often lower than twin heritabilities for reasons that do not invalidate the twin heritabilities. Second, a fitness trait, unlike an individual-differences trait, should have little population variance. But ANS demonstrates replicated developmental and individual differences that predict differences in math skill in some studies. Third, as we just discussed, other cognitive predictors of math skill, and math skill itself, are influenced by generalist genes. Hence, it is important not only to test the heritability of ANS itself, but also to examine whether individual difference in ANS are influenced by generalist genes.

A more mundane and parsimonious explanation of the low heritability of the approximate number system measure is unreliability of measurement of the ANS. Examining the bivariate scatter plot for the monozygotic correlation in the Tosto et al. (2014) study for the ANS measure suggests both ceiling effects and considerable noise. Several studies have examined the psychometric properties of ANS and the symbolic number system measures. These studies have found that reliabilities for different versions of both ANS and symbolic number system tend to be lower than the generally agreed upon cutoff (>.65) for the reliability of individual-difference measures (e.g., Gilmore, Attridge, & Inglis, 2011; Inglis & Gilmore, 2014; Maloney, Risko, Ansari, & Fugelsang, 2010; Price, Palmer, Battista, & Ansari, 2012). Even more concerning, the convergent validities among different ANS task versions (Price et al., 2012) were low. The convergence between ANS and symbolic number system measures (Gilmore et al., 2011; Maloney et al., 2010) was also low and typically nonsignificant. Of course, a key developmental prediction for ANS theorists is that the ANS is a critical precursor for later exact number skill. Hence, the lack of convergent validity between ANS and symbolic number system measures poses a major problem for these theorists.

In contrast, the measures of general cognitive predictors of mathematics skill we discussed previously and will again discuss later, such as IQ, language, verbal WM, and processing speed have much stronger reliabilities and convergent validities within construct. Also, studies examining these general predictors often use latent trait models, in which the latent trait has perfect reliability. Until these psychometric problems in ANS and symbolic number system measures are solved, it will be hard to determine how large is the role of these specific cognitive factors in either typical math development or MD.

To replicate and extend the findings of Tosto et al. (2014), we tested the heritability of the Panamath measure (a measure of ANS) in two large twin samples (the Western Reserve Reading Project and the Colorado Learning Disabilities Research Center [CLDRC]) (Lukowski et al., 2017). We also went further and examined whether generalist genes influence the ANS. If the ANS is a species-typical, specific cognitive fitness trait, it should have little genetic overlap with intelligence, which is a classic polygenic trait with moderate genetic influences on individual differences. Consistent with Tosto et al. (2014), we found significant univariate heritability for the Panamath measure (.29 in the Western Reserve sample, but .54

in the CLDRC sample), and large nonshared environmental influences. Contrary to Tosto et al.'s hypothesis that the ANS is a species-typical trait, we found that there were *generalist* genetic influences on the ANS that overlapped with genetic influences on math measures and IQ (Lukowski et al., 2017). Specifically, in both samples, all the genetic influences on ANS were shared with math measures, and a significant proportion of those were shared with IQ. In summary, this evidence does not support the view that ANS is an evolved, universal, and specific cognitive module. Instead, its low heritability is best explained by poor reliability, but the reliable genetic variance it does have overlaps considerably with generalist genes (those that influence both math and IQ).

Molecular Genetics

Twin methods only provide an indirect test of genetic influences, whereas molecular methods provide a direct test by examining DNA variants, usually SNPs (which we explained in Chapter 2). A few studies using such molecular approaches to the genetics of MD have been conducted, but without converging results for candidate genes for MD.

Docherty et al. (2010) used SNPs in the TEDS sample to perform a GWAS of mathematics skill. They found 10 SNPs that were associated with math. None of these SNPs were near previously identified candidate genes for either dyslexia or LI, which is surprising given evidence from the generalist genes hypothesis that most (but not all) genes associated with one academic trait are likely to influence other academic and cognitive traits. These 10 SNPs taken together accounted for 2.9% of the variance in mathematics skill, which is a fairly typical result for GWAS analyses of complex traits.

Marino et al. (2011) used a targeted SNP approach to test whether two dyslexia candidate genes, *DCDC2* on chromosome 6p and *DYX1C1* on chromosome 15q, were pleiotropic for mathematics or language skill in families selected for dyslexia. They found pleiotropic effects of these two candidate dyslexia genes for mathematics skill but not language in their sample.

The most important molecular genetics finding thus far comes from a study by Trzaskowski et al. (2013), which found strong converging molecular and behavior genetic evidence for generalist genes. To test whether there was direct DNA evidence for generalist genes, Trzaskowski et al. (2013) performed a GWAS (explained in Chapter 2) in the large TEDS sample. They used SNP similarity across unrelated individuals (a GCTA analysis) to calculate genetic correlations between general intelligence, g, and composite measures of language, reading, and math. They then compared these genetic correlations with those estimated by the traditional twin method. They found the genetic correlations were quite strong and remarkably convergent across the two methods: for g and language, .81 using GCTA and .80 using the twin method; for g and mathematics, .74 using GCTA and .73 using the twin method; for g and reading, .89 using GCTA and .66 using the twin method. These results validate the existence of generalist genes at the DNA level but, of course, do not identify any specific generalist genes.

Summary

In summary, we have learned that the etiology of MD is similar to that of other learning disorders covered in this book in several important respects. Both individual differences in math skill across the whole distribution and for the low tail of this distribution (i.e., MD), are moderately heritable, polygenic, and have a considerable overlap with genetic influences on reading, ADHD, and basic cognitive skills that predict all learning disorders. In other words, we have learned that math and MD are influenced by generalist genes. As we saw in the section of this chapter on neuropsychology, these genetic results converge nicely with cognitive analyses of both MD and mathematics skill across the whole distribution, which find that the bulk of the variance in each is accounted for by general rather than specific cognitive predictors.

DIAGNOSIS AND TREATMENT

Diagnosis

Diagnosis of MD requires taking a thorough history (to understand the time course of math difficulties and to establish current functional impairment) and individually administered measures of mathematics achievement (see Table 7.1). Given the research discussed earlier, careful observation of the process by which children solve problems, including their use of counting strategies and the automaticity of their math facts, would be helpful. Although a full IQ test is not necessarily required, it is likely to be helpful for a few reasons. The most commonly used IQ tests provide robust measurement of the general cognitive risk factors implicated in MD—not only g but also language, processing speed, and WM. In some cases, an IQ test will also be necessary to rule out ID as the primary explanation for the child's math difficulties.

Since MD is frequently comorbid with LI, RD, and ADHD, it is important to rule these disorders in or out in a child suspected of having MD, since they may modify the severity, nature, and treatment of MD. Shalev and Gross-Tsur (2001) also advise screening for medical illnesses, such as epilepsy, and genetic syndromes, such as Turner syndrome or fragile X syndrome in females.

Case Presentation

Case Presentation 5

Evan, a 13-year-old eighth grader, was referred by his school counselor because of concerns about difficulties with math.

Evan's prenatal, birth, and early developmental histories were unremarkable. He lives at home with his parents and sister. Both parents are college educated and work in office jobs. His mother reports that she struggled in math all through school but never participated in formal evaluation or intervention. There is also an extended family history of depression.

Regarding school history, Evan learned to read and spell early and well, but math was always more difficult for him. In third grade, he was placed on a response-to-intervention (RTI) plan that provided math support. He remained behind his peers in math in fourth grade and was evaluated for an individualized education program (IEP) that year. Results of school-based testing indicated that his intellectual and language skills fell within the average range. Reading accuracy and fluency were above average, reading comprehension was in the average range, and math achievement clustered around the low-average range. He was found not to qualify for an IEP at that time.

His parents remained concerned about Evan's math progress, so they paid for him to participate in tutoring through a large commercial tutoring center when he was in fifth grade. They reported that he did not benefit from the tutoring, because he "could not focus" in the group environment there. On state standardized tests, Evan's scores have consistently fallen in the Proficient range for reading and writing and the Unsatisfactory to Partially Proficient range for math.

Some difficulties with attention and organization were noted by teachers throughout Evan's elementary school years. He needed frequent reminders to persist with challenging tasks and complete his assignments. Organizational difficulties became even more evident and impairing when Evan started middle school, and by the middle of sixth grade, he was failing several classes due to missing assignments. Evaluation through his pediatrician at that point resulted in a diagnosis of ADHD—predominantly inattentive type. Since then, Evan has been prescribed stimulant medication and has participated in an additional organizational/study skills class through his school, which have been helpful. Current grades are mainly B's and C's in core academic classes, with A's in most electives and a D in math. Although homework battles have decreased with ADHD-related supports in place, Evan continues to report that he "hates math" and resists any sort of additional math practice at home.

Evan was described by parents and school counselor as a very likable and well-behaved young man. He plays several sports and has healthy peer friendships. Although his mood on weekends is mostly positive, his mother is concerned that he frequently seems tired and irritated after school. She is also concerned that he lacks confidence, particularly around academics.

Evan's diagnostic testing is summarized in Table 11.1.

DISCUSSION

Evan's history of persistent difficulties with math achievement despite multiple interventions, along with current objective test results, is consistent with a diagnosis of MD. The evaluation also provided ongoing evidence for ADHD-I, although with medical and school supports, these symptoms are better managed than they had been in previous years. In our experience, it is somewhat rare for children with an isolated MD to come to clinical attention. Although Evan did present with one of the common comorbidities of MD, he was really referred because he and his parents were frustrated by his long-standing math difficulties and wanted more help. They were relieved to have an explanation for his struggles and to know that

TABLE 11.1. Test Summary, Case 5

Performance validity
Medical Symptom Validity Test
    Immediate Recognition   RS = 100
    Delayed Recognition   RS = 95
    Consistency   RS = 95
    Paired Associates   RS = 70
    Free Recall   RS = 55
    (valid)

General intelligence		**Fluid intelligence**	
WISC-V Full Scale IQ	SS = 98	WISC-V Fluid Reasoning Index	SS = 97
		Matrix Reasoning	ss = 11
Crystallized intelligence		Figure Weights	ss = 8
WISC-V Verbal Comprehension Index	SS = 106	WISC-V Visual Spatial Index	SS = 102
Similarities	ss = 12	Block Design	ss = 10
Vocabulary	ss = 10	Visual Puzzles	ss = 11
Working memory			
WISC-V Working Memory Index	SS = 82		
Digit Span	ss = 6		
Picture Span	ss = 8		
Processing speed			
WISC-V Processing Speed Index	SS = 100		
Coding	ss = 11		
Symbol Search	ss = 9		

Academic

Reading		Math	
History		*History*	
CLDQ Reading Scale	25th %ile	CLDQ Math Scale	97th %ile
Basic literacy		*Calculation and problem solving*	
WIAT-III Word Reading	SS = 117	WIAT-III Numerical Operations	SS = 73
WIAT-III Spelling	SS = 111	Math Problem Solving	SS = 69
Reading fluency		*Math fluency*	
TOWRE-2 Sight Word Efficiency	SS = 121	WIAT-III Math Fluency	SS = 88
TOWRE-2 Phonemic Decoding Efficiency	SS = 113		

Oral language
CELF-5
    Recalling Sentences   ss = 12
    Understanding Spoken Paragraphs   ss = 10

Attention and executive functions

Attention		*Executive functions*	
Vanderbilt Inattention		D-KEFS Trail Making Test	
Parent	RS = 6	Visual Scanning	ss = 11
Teacher	RS = 7	Number Sequencing	ss = 9

(continued)

212　　　　　　　　　　　II. REVIEWS OF DISORDERS

TABLE 11.1. (continued)			
Vanderbilt Hyperactivity/Impulsivity		Letter Sequencing	ss = 10
Parent	RS = 1	Letter–Number Switching	ss = 6
Teacher	RS = 2	D-KEFS Verbal Fluency	
		Letter Fluency	ss = 11
		Category Fluency	ss = 10

Note. SS, standard score with mean = 100 and *SD* = 15; ss, scaled score with mean = 10 and *SD* = 3; RS, raw score; %ile, percentile rank; WISC-V, Wechsler Intelligence Scale for Children—Fifth Edition; CLDQ, Colorado Learning Difficulties Questionnaire; WIAT-III, Wechsler Individual Achievement Test—Third Edition; TOWRE-2, Test of Word Reading Efficiency—Second Edition; CELF-5, Clinical Evaluation of Language Fundamentals—Fifth Edition; Vanderbilt, NICHQ Vanderbilt Assessment Scales; D-KEFS: Delis–Kaplan Executive Function System.

indeed there was "something more" going on than the ADHD, which had already been diagnosed.

Evan's scores on tests of calculation knowledge and problem solving were well below expected levels for his age, as well as notably weaker than his intelligence, language, and reading skills. As should be clear based on the previous discussion, many children with MD do not show these kinds of striking dissociations. In Evan's case, the clear gap between his math skill and most other cognitive skills was part of what compelled his parents to seek more information about his neuropsychological functioning. In contrast to his weak higher-level math skills, Evan's ability to quickly solve very simple arithmetic problems was within broadly normal limits. His relatively better performance on the Wechsler Individual Achievement Test–Third Edition (WIAT-III) Math Fluency may relate to his intact processing speed. It also appears that his math difficulties are more pronounced for higher-level skills (e.g., problem solving) than for basic arithmetic. This discrepancy may help explain why his current scores on individually administered achievement tests are lower than what he earned on school-based testing in fourth grade, since higher-level skills are increasingly emphasized as children get older. It is also possible that Evan slipped further behind his peers because he has avoided math practice. He understandably dislikes math at this point and likely has developed some math anxiety as well.

Because of the high comorbidity of MD with reading and language problems, Evan was screened for problems in these areas as well. However, consistent with his history and previous test results, no difficulties in these areas were identified; in fact, basic reading appears to be an area of strength for Evan.

Apart from his math difficulties and continuing ADHD symptoms, the other notable pattern to emerge from Evan's testing was a cluster of weakness on some executive functioning tasks (including WM and mental flexibility). Executive functioning weaknesses are implicated in both ADHD and MD, and may represent a shared cognitive risk factor that can help explain the comorbidity between these two conditions.

The main recommendation to come out of the evaluation was for Evan to participate in more intensive, individualized math remediation at school. A course of private one-on-one math tutoring was also suggested, so long as it was logistically and financially feasible for the family, in the hope that this would help improve not only Evan's math skills but also his attitude to math. Overall, it was thought that the relatively mild mood concerns reflected an understandable reaction to the stress of school given Evan's learning disorders. Clinical interviews and responses on broadband rating scales did not indicate concern for significant depressive symptomatology or other psychiatric issues, although ongoing monitoring of his overall adjustment was recommended.

Treatment

In terms of treatment, there has been considerable progress since the previous edition of this book was published in 2009. At that time, we could find only one pilot study (L. Kaufmann, Handl, & Thony, 2003) in which a treatment program focused on basic understanding of the numerical concepts discussed earlier benefited the calculation skills of children with MD. Subsequent research using more rigorous designs has supported the efficacy of treatments for MD. At the time of this writing, a Cochrane Review on interventions for math disabilities was in progress (Furlong, McLoughlin, McGilloway, & Geary, 2016), as was a Campbell Collaboration review on improving math achievement in primary school more generally (Simms, Gilmore, Sloan, & McKeaveney, 2017). Thus, soon we should have systematic information on the best way to teach math to struggling learners, which, we hope, will include good evidentiary support for at least some treatments for MD.

Based on what we have learned from the RD literature, we would expect the most effective math interventions to provide direct, explicit instruction in specific math skills (e.g., counting principles, numerosity, math fact practice, place value understanding, problem-solving strategies). Although it might seem that interventions targeting general cognitive skills implicated in math development, such as processing speed or WM, should be equally helpful, this has generally not proven to be the case. It has been difficult for such intervention programs to demonstrate the kind of "far transfer" they would need to be effective. In other words, while practice with computerized WM or speeded tasks certainly improves performance on those specific tasks, there is much less evidence that those gains transfer to academic growth for math, reading, or other subjects.

There are several commercial programs for MD that have at least an initial track record of peer-reviewed empirical research support (reviewed in Kroeger, Brown, & O'Brien, 2012). All provide direct, explicit mathematics instruction and practice; some are appropriate for younger children, while others are designed for use all the way through the end of high school. Experimental programs emphasizing the same core principles of explicit instruction, skills modeling, practice, and corrective feedback have also been shown to be effective for remediating word problem-solving difficulties in children with MD (Zheng, Flynn, & Swanson, 2013). Math intervention programs generally target multiple component skills, and the principle of limited transfer applies in this context as well. In other words, to improve math fact retrieval, children benefit most from math fact tutoring; to improve estimation, children benefit most from estimation tutoring, and so forth (Fuchs et al., 2008, 2014). Another theme reminiscent of the RD literature is that children with MD do not appear to require a qualitatively different instructional approach from typical learners (Fuchs et al., 2008). Instead, all children benefit from sound, explicit math instruction; children with MD may just need more of it, broken down into smaller steps, and with more opportunities for review compared to their typically developing peers.

A recent intervention–imaging study used fMRI to demonstrate that evidence-based math tutoring changes brain functioning in third-grade students with MD (Iuculano et al., 2015). Prior to intervention, the children with MD showed aberrant overactivation in many parts of the bilateral distributed network implicated in math skill (e.g., bilateral prefrontal cortices, bilateral anterior insular cortices, bilateral parietal cortices, and other regions). Eight weeks of one-on-one tutoring adapted from the Math Wise program normalized the MD group's performance on arithmetic tasks outside the scanner and fully normalized their brain activation patterns as well.

There has recently been interest in combining behaviorally based math interventions with noninvasive brain stimulation techniques, such as transcranial direct current stimulation or transcranial random noise stimulation. Studies in healthy young adults have indicated that compared to a sham condition, stimulating specific brain regions involved in mathematical processing (prefrontal cortices, parietal lobes) during mathematical tasks led to improved behavioral performance (Cohen Kadosh, Soskic, Iuculano, Kanai, & Walsh, 2010; Snowball et al., 2013). There is at least some evidence for transfer to nontrained tasks (Snowball et al., 2013). Existing work suggests that the brain stimulation must be paired with behaviorally based intervention to be helpful. The effectiveness of noninvasive brain stimulation has not been established in children with math disability (Sarkar & Cohen Kadosh, 2016). Furthermore, given the increased financial costs and inconvenience associated with brain stimulation technology, it seems likely that behavioral intervention alone will remain the standard of care for MD for some time to come. However, this work certainly represents an interesting line of inquiry that merits further research.

Since the previous edition of this book was published, we have also learned a lot about the important role that math anxiety plays in math difficulties and their remediation (Maloney & Beilock, 2012). *Math anxiety*—a negative emotional reaction to math tasks—can begin in early elementary school and adversely impacts students' math achievement (Ramirez, Gunderson, Levine, & Beilock, 2013). Math anxiety is negatively correlated with math ability: Children predisposed to having difficulties with math are also more likely to be anxious about it (Rubinsten & Tannock, 2010), potentially setting up a transactional process in which they avoid math tasks, do not progress in their skills, and hence become more anxious and avoidant. But math anxiety is not the same thing as math inability, and it is also influenced by other individual and social factors. A powerful example of the latter is the fact that female elementary school teachers transmit their own math anxiety to many of their female (but not male) students, and that girls who develop more math anxiety subsequently perform worse at math (Beilock, Gunderson, Ramirez, & Levine, 2010). Maloney, Ramirez, Gunderson, Levine, and Beilock (2015) recently explored intergenerational transmission of math anxiety in families. For both boys and girls, children whose parents endorsed more math anxiety were more likely to develop math anxiety and poorer math performance over the course of a school year. However, this relationship only held for parents who spent more time helping their children with homework. For parents who were less engaged with their children in math work at home, there was no relationship between parents' math anxiety and children's math attitudes or achievement. This moderating effect is important, because it makes it much more likely that math difficulties of some children were truly caused by intergenerational transmission of negative attitudes about math rather than by a third variable shared by parents and children with math anxiety (e.g., genetic risk factors for MD).

In both children and adults, the negative relationship between math anxiety and math performance is stronger among individuals with higher WM than those with lower WM. Individuals with strong WM tend to rely on WM-intensive problem-solving strategies, which are vulnerable to being depleted by math anxiety (Ramirez et al., 2013). An fMRI study documented that math anxiety in children even appears to have its own neural signature, involving overactivation in right amygdala regions important for processing negative emotions, as well as reduced activity in widely distributed cortical and subcortical regions implicated in both math reasoning and emotion regulation (Young, Wu, & Menon, 2012). Importantly, in that study, children high and low on math-specific anxiety did not differ on a measure of general trait anxiety, so the math anxiety was not simply a manifestation of a more general psychiatric disorder.

Given the strong link between math anxiety and later math difficulties, math anxiety itself can be an important intervention target. Teaching based on cognitive-behavioral techniques such as regulation of negative math-related emotions, reappraisal of negative thoughts, or reframing of physiological reactions should be helpful for many students (Jamieson, Mendes, Blackstock, & Schmader, 2010; Maloney & Beilock, 2012; Mattarella-Micke, Mateo, Kozak, Foster, & Beilock, 2011). In older students, a surprisingly simple technique for emotion regulation that has been shown to be effective is to have students write freely about their feelings for 10–15 minutes before tackling a stressful event (e.g., a math examination) (Ramirez & Beilock, 2011). A recent downward extension of this technique suggested that keeping math journals helped reduce math anxiety in third graders (Emmert, 2015). Based on the evidence for social transmission of math anxiety reviewed earlier, we would also expect that addressing math anxiety in parents and teachers should help prevent the development of math anxiety in many children and in turn promote stronger math achievement.

Table 11.2 provides a summary of current research and evidence-based practice for MD.

TABLE 11.2. Summary Table: Mathematics Disorder

Definition

- Math skills (i.e., number sense, math fact knowledge, calculation, and/or math problem solving) are substantially below age expectations on objective standardized tests.
- The difficulties cause functional impairment and have been present since relatively early in formal education (although they may become more pronounced as academic demands increase).
- The difficulties are not better accounted for by uncorrected sensory impairment, ID, inadequate instruction, psychosocial adversity, or another mental or neurological disorder.

Prevalence and epidemiology

- For age discrepancy definition, approximately 10%, depending on specific cutoff is used. However, many of these children may not come to clinical attention unless they have other comorbid conditions. Nearly equal gender ratio.
- Comorbid with RD, ADHD, and LI.

Etiology

- A minority of cases are associated with known genetic syndromes including Turner syndrome and fragile X syndrome in females.
- Most cases are due to multiple risk factors, including both moderate genetic and moderate environmental influence.
- Genetic risk factors appear to be largely shared with general cognitive traits such as g, language, WM, and processing speed.
- The field has not yet converged on specific candidate genes for MD.

Brain mechanisms

- The left IPS is one key location for mathematics, but far from the only important location.
- Math skill is also associated with activity of widely distributed bilateral networks, including both parietal lobes, language areas (i.e., left perisylvian regions), the ventral visual stream (i.e., occipital–temporal regions), a salience network centered on the anterior insula, the cingulate gyrus, and the cerebellum.
- The neural basis of math skill changes with development, consistent with an interactive specialization model. Connections among different large-scale brain networks strengthen with age.
- Math disability is associated with aberrant activations of many of the regions just mentioned, including bilateral parietal and frontal sites.

Developmental neuropsychology

- Several different general cognitive risk factors are linked to MD, including g, language skill, WM, and processing speed.
- More specific risk factors for math difficulties include measures of the approximate number system (e.g., subitizing) and measures of the symbolic number system (e.g., place value understanding).
- The symbolic number system is more strongly predictive of later math than is the approximate number system, but research has been limited by somewhat weak psychometric properties of current measures.

Diagnosis

- Diagnosis is made primarily based on a history of clinically impairing difficulties learning math, as well as performance below expected age levels on standardized math measures.
- The evaluation process should include at least a screening for exclusionary conditions, as well as common comorbidities (i.e., dyslexia, ADHD, LI).

Treatment

- Children with MD need direct, explicit instruction in the specific math subskills and problem-solving strategies in which they are weak. Intervention should provide ample opportunities for review and practice, as well as corrective feedback.
- Many children with MD also have math anxiety and could benefit from cognitive behaviorally based approaches to improve their attitude toward math activities. Parents and teachers should be mindful not to communicate their own math anxiety to children.

CHAPTER 12

Attention-Deficit/Hyperactivity Disorder

CHAPTER SUMMARY

Attention-deficit/hyperactivity disorder (ADHD) and the typical development of attention and self-control nicely illustrate the overall theme of this book, which is that both learning disorders and learning skills result from a developmental process involving a mix of substantial general and more modest specific factors across multiple levels of analysis. However, our neuropsychological and developmental understanding of ADHD is less well developed than is the case for all the other disorders covered in this book.

A major puzzle in the neuropsychology of ADHD is that a substantial proportion of children with ADHD lack deficits in the known cognitive predictors of ADHD, although this is a generic problem for behaviorally defined disorders, such as autism, schizophrenia, or depression. Taken together, cognitive predictors only account for around 30% of the variance in ADHD symptoms. One possible solution to this puzzle that needs more study is that emotional lability may help account for this missing variance in ADHD.

At the level of brain mechanisms, both dopaminergic and noradrenergic pathways are implicated, among others. In terms of brain structure and function, widely distributed networks subserve the development of ADHD, including the central executive network and its connections to the basal ganglia, the salience network, and the default mode network. There has been more success in localizing the nonspecific cognitive deficits found in ADHD (e.g., the right inferior frontal gyrus is an important hub for response inhibition, and white matter tracts are important for processing speed and reaction time [RT] variability [expressed as the standard deviation of RT, SDRT]) than localizing ADHD itself. Of course, each of these three networks involved in the development of ADHD are implicated in other disorders, so the specificity of ADHD at the brain level may derive from the dynamic interaction among networks. Moreover, these three brain networks each change with development, consistent with the interactive specialization model of brain–behavior development, so the brain phenotype of ADHD also changes with development, although more research is needed on this topic.

At the etiological level, there is substantial heritability for both ADHD and individual differences in ADHD symptoms. The two correlated symptom dimensions that define ADHD, inattention and hyperactivity–impulsivity, differ considerably in their heritabilities, once the correlation with the other dimension is controlled. The heritability of inattention is similar to that of ADHD itself, whereas the heritability of hyperactivity–impulsivity is much lower. This pattern repeats itself at the levels of neuropsychological risk and comorbidity, with the inattention dimension accounting for most of the risk for neuropsychological impairment and comorbidity in ADHD. Most importantly, the genetic influences on ADHD are partly general, because they partially overlap with genetic influences on all of the other learning disorders considered in this book (with the possible exception of isolated speech sound disorder [SSD]), and with cognitive risk factors shared by these other disorders, including executive functions [EFs], processing speed, and intraindividual variability of RT [SDRT]).

Our current research understanding of ADHD, and gaps therein, has important clinical implications for its diagnosis and treatment. In terms of diagnosis, cognitive risk factors associated with ADHD are less helpful in ruling out ADHD than is the case for dyslexia, mathematics disorder (and, tautologically, LI and ID, which are both defined mainly by cognitive tests). Like the diagnosis of autism spectrum disorder (ASD), the diagnosis of ADHD relies more heavily on carefully evaluating whether there is converging evidence from clinical observations, and the developmental and school histories. Relying on only one source of information inevitably leads to false positives and false negatives. Although DSM-5 describes three presentations of ADHD, there is much less empirical support for the validity of the hyperactivity–impulsivity presentation than the inattentive or combined presentations after the preschool years. Despite being substantially heritable, ADHD is partly treatable, and the best empirically supported treatment is stimulant medication. School accommodations and behavior management training are also useful. Nonetheless, ADHD is a chronic condition accompanied by increased morbidity and mortality in adulthood. Hence, further research is needed to find more effective treatments.

HISTORY

A syndrome involving hyperactivity in children has been in the medical literature as far back as the 1700s (Crichton, 1798). Over 150 years ago, a German physician, Heinrich Hoffmann (1845), wrote a humorous poem describing the antics of "fidgety Phil, who couldn't sit still." Somewhat later, Still (1902) described the main problem in this syndrome as a deficiency in "volitional inhibition" or "a defect in moral control." It may seem odd to us now to think of ADHD as a moral problem, but children with ADHD violate social norms, sometimes in ways that can be quite upsetting for their parents, teachers, peers, and eventually themselves. As we discuss later, research in developmental psychology on the development of self-control and the related construct of effortful control (Rothbart & Bates, 2006) is relevant for understanding ADHD.

Barkley (1996) points out that Still (1902) recognized several features of ADHD that have been validated by contemporary research: (1) It overlaps with oppositional and conduct problems; (2) it is familial; (3) it is co-familial with conduct problems and alcoholism; (4) there is a male predominance of about 3:1; and (5) it may also be caused by an acquired brain injury. As we will also see, problems with inhibition continue to be central to current conceptions of ADHD, although much more is now known about the brain bases of these problems.

Whether there is brain dysfunction in ADHD and how to characterize it have been confusing and controversial issues in the history of ADHD research. The notion that childhood hyperactivity is a brain disorder was also promoted by Strauss and Lehtinen (1947), based on similarities with the behavior of children who had suffered early brain damage. Unfortunately, this analogy led to some muddled terminology, whereby children with hyperactivity were described as having "minimal brain damage" or "minimal brain dysfunction." These terms are misleading for several reasons: (1) The large majority of children with ADHD have a neurodevelopmental disorder, not acquired brain damage; (2) the damage or dysfunction to the brain implied in these labels was not documented directly, but only inferred from behavioral symptoms that could have many different causes; (3) many children with acquired brain damage do not have hyperactivity (Rutter & Quinton, 1977); and (4) these terms were vague and overinclusive, and thus impeded progress in delineating distinct neuropsychological syndromes affecting learning and behavior in childhood.

With advances in neuroimaging, there is now compelling direct evidence that ADHD is a specific kind of brain dysfunction caused mainly by genetic differences between individuals, as established by behavioral genetic studies. Additional supporting evidence for the neurological basis of ADHD derives from the efficacy of stimulant medications (e.g., methylphenidate sold as Ritalin) and norepinephrine agonists (e.g., atomoxetine sold as Strattera) for treating the symptoms of ADHD and normalizing its functional magnetic resonance imaging (fMRI) phenotype, although we still do not know exactly how these medications work. Of all the learning disorders in this book, ADHD is the only one for which there is an effective pharmacological treatment for its main symptoms.

Although ADHD is now more clearly defined and better understood than it once was, it remains a somewhat broad diagnosis. Researchers are making progress testing the validity of subtypes of ADHD, including those in DSM-5 and those defined by comorbidities. As we discuss later, this research supports the validity of two of the three DSM-5 presentations of ADHD (inattentive and combined) but questions the validity of the hyperactive–impulsive presentation.

DEFINITION

DSM-5 (American Psychiatric Association, 2013), like DSM-IV-TR (American Psychiatric Association, 2000), defines ADHD with two distinct but correlated dimensions of symptoms, those involving *inattention* (e.g., making careless mistakes and not paying close attention to details, forgetfulness, difficulty organizing tasks and activities, and failure to begin or complete tasks that require sustained mental effort) and *hyperactivity–impulsivity* (e.g., excessive fidgeting, locomotion, or talking; interrupting or intruding in conversations, games, and other situations). It is important to bear in mind that these two symptom dimensions do not map neatly onto cognitive neuroscience constructs. In cognitive neuroscience, there are several kinds of attention, and which kind, if any, is impaired in ADHD is an important research question. With two dimensions, there are therefore three logically possible presentations of ADHD: inattentive (Inatt.), hyperactive–impulsive (H-I), or combined (C). Someone who meets the diagnostic cutoff (six of nine symptoms) for a single dimension qualifies for that presentation; someone who meets this cutoff on both dimensions qualifies for the C presentation. Because research support for the validity and longitudinal stability of all three subtypes of ADHD in DSM-IV was weak, the DSM-5 committee decided to call these three subgroups of ADHD "presentations" rather than "subtypes" (Tannock, 2013). Research support for this change includes a comprehensive meta-analysis on the validity of ADHD subtypes (Willcutt et al., 2012). Although persistence of an overall diagnosis of ADHD was reasonably high (59%), subtype stability was much lower (35%). This instability of ADHD subtypes partly derives from developmental change. H-I symptoms are more prevalent at younger ages and more likely to resolve as the child gets older, whereas Inatt. symptoms are more stable across age. As discussed earlier, longitudinal instability of behavioral diagnoses is a generic problem, because such diagnoses are not true categories, but are based on cutoff points on a continuous distribution. Because of unreliability of measurement, some diagnosed children inevitably regress across the cutoff on a follow-up assessment and no longer fit diagnostic criteria. Of course, other sources of longitudinal instability could be related to effective treatment and true developmental change.

Additional requirements for the DSM-5 diagnosis of ADHD include the following: (1) the symptoms cause a clinically significant impairment in adaptive functioning; (2) are inconsistent with developmental level (e.g., not just secondary to ID); (3) have been present for at least 6 months, with an onset of some symptoms before age 12; (4) several symptoms are present in two or more settings; and (5) are not better accounted for by another mental disorder (psychosis, or a mood, anxiety, dissociative, or personality disorder).

Unlike DSM-IV-TR, DSM-5 dropped ASD and other pervasive developmental disorders from ADHD's list of exclusionary diagnoses. Hence, according to DSM-5 criteria, children with ASD can also be diagnosed with ADHD if they meet the symptom cutoffs just presented, *with* an adjustment for mental age. This diagnostic decision is based on clinical judgment but could be operationalized by using a regression outlier approach based on the population correlation between IQ and ADHD ratings.

This discussion of ADHD, ASD, and mental age bears on the larger issue of what makes a diagnosis specific. For ADHD, there are two criteria that address the issue of specificity: inconsistency with developmental level (Item 2 in the previous list) and not accounted for by certain other mental disorders (Item 5 in the list). Unlike most of the other learning disorders reviewed in this book, there is no attempt to quantify the age discrepancy or IQ discrepancy implied in Item 2.

In addition to the three presentations of ADHD in DSM-5, clinicians need to be aware of a fourth possible presentation, namely, sluggish cognitive tempo (SCT). SCT symptoms include *sluggish, tired/lethargic, spacey, daydreams, in a fog, lost in thought, slow moving,* and *slow thinking/processing,* among others. Becker et al. (2016) conducted a meta-analysis of studies of SCT. They found strong support for the internal validity of the construct of SCT. For instance, SCT items are reliable and form a factor that is distinct from the two symptom dimensions of ADHD, Inatt. and H-I. Nonetheless, SCT is moderately correlated with Inatt. ($r = .63$ in children and $r = .72$ in adults). There is also evidence for external validity of SCT, in that it is correlated with various measures of impairment. What is less clear is whether it is diagnostically distinct from other established DSM- disorders besides ADHD, especially internalizing disorders.

PREVALENCE AND EPIDEMIOLOGY

ADHD is one of the most common chronic disorders of childhood, and there are world-wide epidemiological studies of its prevalence. For instance, Erskine et al. (2013), who examined data from the Global Burden of Disease study across three time periods and 21 world regions, found an average male prevalence of 2.2% and an average female prevalence of 0.7%. Hence, the M/F ratio was about 3/1, consistent with other studies. They did find some variation in prevalence across countries, and the average world prevalence is lower than the prevalence typically found in the United States. As we discuss later, there is now some research examining the reasons for both sex and country differences in rates of ADHD.

In terms of natural history, earlier research indicated that the age of onset is usually in early childhood, with a peak "age of onset" between ages 3 and 4 (Palfrey, Levine, Walker, & Sullivan, 1985; Report of the Surgeon General, 1999), whereas DSM-IV required an onset before age 7 years for diagnosis. This age cutoff at age 7 has turned out to lack validity, and was changed to age 12 in DSM-5. Vande Voort, He, Jameson, and Merikangas (2014) compared the two age cutoffs in a representative U.S. sample and found prevalences of 7.38%, with an age cutoff of 7 years, and 10.84%, with an age cutoff of 12 years. Children with a later age of onset did not differ in severity of ADHD symptoms or patterns of comorbidity, but they were more likely to come from lower socioeconomic status (SES) or racial/ethnic families.

It is becoming clearer that ADHD is a chronic disorder across the lifespan (Gittleman, Mannuzza, Shenker, & Gonagura, 1985), and many of the tasks of adult development are disrupted by ADHD, because sustained effort, planning, and organization are central to many adult responsibilities. However, controversy remains about adult-onset ADHD. For instance, Moffitt et al. (2015) found virtually no overlap between individuals receiving a child versus adult diagnosis of ADHD in the Dunedin longitudinal study. Faraone and Biederman (2016) argued that a low rate of categorical diagnostic overlap may mask greater continuity at the symptom level. In discussing two recent, large longitudinal studies of ADHD, one from the United Kingdom and the other from Brazil, they pointed out that two-thirds of youth with ADHD continued to have impairing ADHD symptoms in adulthood, even though the full diagnostic overlap was only 15%, consistent with the Moffitt et al. (2015) results.

We tested whether sex differences in cognitive predictors of ADHD help account for the higher rate of ADHD in males (Arnett, Pennington, Willcutt, DeFries, & Olson, 2015). We found that processing speed, inhibition, and verbal working memory together accounted for 14% of the total sex difference in ADHD. The remainder of the sex difference in ADHD is currently unexplained.

ADHD has been found across social classes, racial and ethnic groups, and countries, but with different prevalence. Researchers are beginning to test explanations for these differences in prevalence. There is a negative correlation between parent education and prevalence of ADHD in their children; that is, less educated parents are more likely to have a child with ADHD. We do not know the reason for this negative correlation, but we do know that the heritability of ADHD increases as education decreases, hence, a diathesis–stress gene × environment (G × E) interaction, which we discuss later.

With regard to race, there is a consistently higher level of ADHD symptoms as reported by teachers in African American children than in European American children (T. Miller, Nigg, & Miller, 2009). Yet, paradoxically, the review by T. Miller et al. (2009) found that there is a *lower* rate of actual diagnosis and treatment in African American children than in European American children. This paradoxical finding is reminiscent of the finding we discussed in Chapter 8 that racial–ethnic groups with well-documented achievement gaps are nonetheless *underrepresented* in special education classes. In considering explanations for this paradox of higher ADHD symptom scores but lower rates of diagnosis and treatment in African American children, T. Miller et al. (2009) suggest that racial differences in resources and access to health care may be an explanation, just as we argued in Chapter 8. Although several studies have found factorial invariance for ADHD rating scales across these two races, it remains possible that measurement artifacts may contribute to the group difference in average ADHD scores.

There are also replicated country differences in rates of ADHD that are not well explained. We tested competing explanations for the low prevalence of ADHD in Scandinavia compared to Australia and the United States (MacDonald Wer et al., 2010). We found that there was *not* measurement equivalence across the three countries. Instead, the external validity of ADHD ratings by parents and teachers was stronger in Scandinavia compared to Australia and the United States, suggesting an overdiagnosing tendency in the latter two countries.

Another example of how rates of ADHD can vary by context is provided by the effect of a child's age of entry into elementary school on his or her risk for an ADHD diagnosis. A child's age at entry into kindergarten will typically range from 60 to nearly 72 months. Two studies have found an inverse linear relation between rate of ADHD diagnoses and a child's age at entry into kindergarten (Elder, 2011; R. Morrow et al., 2012). The explanation of this surprising result is as follows: If the school cutoff date is September 1, then children with birthdays just before that date will be the youngest in their class, whereas those with birthdays just after the cutoff date will be the oldest in their class. Since age is a strong predictor of social maturity, and since the teacher's perception of social maturity in a given child is relative to the behavior of their classmates, a child who is young for his or her grade may appear to have ADHD, when in fact the child's behavior is consistent with his or her age. A related issue is whether this finding is actually a season of birth effect, which has been found in schizophrenia and other disorders, in which children born in winter/spring are at increased risk compared to those born in summer/autumn (e.g., Davies, Welham, Chant, Torrey, & McGrath, 2003). However, countering this explanation is the fact that the effect is found in countries with widely differing cutoff dates for entering kindergarten (January vs. September). This effect of age at school entry for ADHD converges with other evidence for cultural and contextual influences on rates of ADHD (Fulton et al., 2009; Nigg, 2006). These findings are important, because they remind us that the prevalence of biologically based neurodevelopmental disorders is not invariant across cultural contexts. Similar cultural influences are found for other learning disorders discussed in this book, such as ASD and dyslexia.

Despite such contextual influences on ADHD diagnosis, existing research supports the conclusion that ADHD is a valid disorder with a higher rate of morbidity (e.g., substance abuse) and even mortality. Dalsgaard, Østergaard, Leckman, Mortensen, and Pedersen (2015) used the national health register in Denmark to follow 32,000 individuals with ADHD. They found a roughly twofold increase in mortality in individuals with earlier ADHD diagnoses compared to those without ADHD diagnoses, and this significant increase in mortality survived correction for comorbid oppositional defiant disorder (ODD), conduct disorder (CD), and substance abuse. Most of the increase in mortality was due to accidents, consistent with other data documenting worse driving records in those with ADHD. Hence, although treatment can alleviate the symptoms of ADHD, it remains a persistent and serious disorder.

Comorbidities

Over half of children who meet diagnostic criteria for ADHD qualify for a comorbid diagnosis (Biederman et al., 1992), and the list of comorbid disorders includes CD, depression, anxiety, Tourette syndrome, dyslexia, LI, and bipolar disorder. In a more recent study, Larson et al. (2011) utilized the 2007 National Survey of Children's Health to examine patterns of comorbidity in ADHD. They found that the U.S. prevalence of ADHD was 8.2% and the rate of comorbidity was 67%, which means that only one-third of children with ADHD had "pure" ADHD.

More research is needed to understand the basis of these many comorbidities and to define purer subtypes of ADHD. In addition, this extensive list of comorbidities suggests that ADHD is likely etiologically heterogeneous, and the research reviewed in the "Etiology" section documents that this is indeed the case.

DEVELOPMENTAL NEUROPSYCHOLOGY

As we discussed in earlier chapters, the goal of identifying a single underlying cognitive deficit that provides a parsimonious causal explanation of the diversity of behavioral symptoms found in learning disorders has proven impossible. (See Morton & Frith, 1995, and Pennington & Welsh, 1995, for discussions of the single-deficit model.) Instead, it has become clear that a single cognitive-deficit model will not suffice for any of these disorders (Pennington, 2006), and this is particularly true for ADHD. Even with multiple cognitive predictors, we can only account for about 30% of the variance in the Inatt. symptom dimension of ADHD, and even less of the variance in the H-I symptom dimension (McGrath et al., 2011). In contrast, our ability to account for symptom variance for specific learning disabilities (SLDs) is much greater, as we discussed earlier. This unexplained symptom variance is a major puzzle for neuropsychological models of ADHD. We consider possible solutions to this puzzle in this section.

One reason for this puzzle is that the developmental neuropsychology of attention and impulsivity is not as well developed theoretically or empirically as is the case for the domains that are relevant for the other learning disorders in this book. We know a lot more about the early development of intelligence, speech, language and reading, mathematical concepts, and even social cognition than we know about the early development of attention and impulsivity. In addition, there are virtually no longitudinal studies of individuals at high risk of developing ADHD, in contrast to what is the case for other learning disorders. Hence, the rich synergy between studies of typical and atypical early development that has benefited our understanding of other learning disorders is just beginning for ADHD. Although developmental psychologists have long been interested in the early development of self-control, that broad field has several different constructs, such as EFs, effortful control, and delay of gratification, which do not always converge with each other or with ADHD. We first review what is known about the early development of both self-control and ADHD, before discussing neuropsychological models of ADHD.

Early Development

One can divide self-control into two interacting components: behavioral regulation and emotion regulation. Most research on ADHD has focused on the former component, behavioral regulation, and there has been much less research on emotion regulation in ADHD, even though increased emotional lability and comorbidity with internalizing disorders are important clinical features of ADHD.

In developmental psychology, Mary Rothbart and colleagues (Posner &

Rothbart, 2000; Rothbart, Derryberry, & Posner, 1994) made a major contribution to research on the early development of self-control by defining and studying what they called *effortful control* (EC). What was novel about their approach was the attempt to integrate research on infant temperament with cognitive neuroscience. They distinguished EC from other dimensions of temperament, such as extraversion and introversion, because EC is active rather than reactive. They postulated that attention is the mechanism of self-control in both children and adults; hence, the development of attention in infancy would enable increasing self-control of both behavior (orienting and reaching to objects) and emotion (recovering from distress).

Subsequent studies by several researchers have examined relations among EC, laboratory measures of attention, and ADHD in early development. For instance, Kochanska and colleagues made a major contribution to the measurement of EC at different ages in preschool by developing behavioral measures of EC to complement parent ratings. Kochanska, Murray, and Harlan (2000) studied the longitudinal relation between the duration of infant sustained attention measured at 9 months and both EC behaviors and EC parent ratings of children at 22 and 33 months of age. Although there were longitudinal relations, they were not as strong as one would expect if a single stable trait were being measured. Interestingly, the sex of the child (females had better EC than males), accounted for more variance in both measures of EC outcome (behavioral and parent ratings) than other predictors, but we do not know what mediates this sex effect. After child sex was accounted for, infant sustained attention at 9 months accounted for 7% of the variance in EC at 22 months, but it was not a significant predictor of EC at 33 months. Maternal responsiveness when the child was 22 months old was an incremental predictor of EC at both 22 months (6% of the variance) and 33 months (5% of the variance). So infant attention does predict toddler EC up to a point, but then other variables become more important. Kochanska and colleagues also found that the convergent validity of the two methods of measuring EC (child behaviors and parent ratings) was weak. Their correlation at the same time point was only .45, and the longitudinal correlation was only .22.

Papageorgiou et al. (2014) also conducted a longitudinal study of the relation between infant attention (measured by fixation duration at 7.7 months) and later EC (measured by parent ratings at 3.5 years). They found a small significant relation. Infant fixation accounted for 2% of the variance in later EC. Interestingly, infant attention was a stronger inverse predictor of a different temperament dimension, *surgency* (i.e., approaching novelty, uninhibited, exuberant), and of ADHD. Surgency is essentially the opposite of the construct of behavioral inhibition, which has been studied by Kagan and Snidman (2009) and others in early development. In the Papageorgiu et al. (2014) study, longer fixations predicted both lower surgency, accounting for 7% of the variance, and lower ADHD, accounting for 6% of the variance. Because infant attention was more strongly related to later surgency than EC, there is less specificity to the attention and EC relation than the Posner and Rothbart (2000) model predicted.

Several other researchers have found a longitudinal relation between behavioral measures of infant attention and later ADHD symptoms. Lawson and Ruff (2004) rated infant attention during play, including play with a challenging toy, and collected maternal ratings of negative emotionality at 1 and 2 years of age. They then tested how well infant attention and negative emotionality predicted ADHD symptoms at age 3.5 years. Consistent with previous research demonstrating that parent education is inversely related to offspring ADHD ratings (i.e., higher parent education predicts lower ADHD in the child), they found that maternal education accounted for 11% of the variance in ADHD ratings at 3.5 years. After accounting for this effect, infant attention and negative emotionality together accounted for an additional 12% of the variance in ADHD ratings at 3.5 years, with the incremental contribution of each of these two predictors being roughly equal. As expected, better infant attention predicted fewer ADHD symptoms, whereas greater negative emotionality predicted more ADHD symptoms. This is one of the very few preschool studies of the early development of ADHD that examined both aspects of self-regulation: behavior regulation and emotion regulation. In this study, both aspects were equally important for predicting later ADHD.

Friedman, Watamura, and Robertson (2005) measured movement–attention coupling in healthy infants at ages 1 and 3 months, then measured ADHD symptoms at age 8 years in a subset ($N = 26$) of the original sample. Less suppression of body movement at the onset of looking (i.e., worse attention) accounted for a surprisingly large proportion (roughly 40%) of the variance in Inatt. symptoms at age 8 years. Unlike some previous infant studies reviewed here, there was no correction for child sex or maternal education.

Arnett, MacDonald, and Pennington (2013) used the large ($N > 1,000$ children) longitudinal National Institute of Child Health and Human Development (NICHD) Early Child Care sample to test for early precursors of ADHD symptoms in third grade. Measures of temperament and activity level in the first year of life were not related to later ADHD. Girls with later ADHD were first detectable at 15 months by their lower score on the Bayley Scales of Infant Development IQ measure, whereas males with later ADHD were first detectable at 24 months by their higher Child Behavior Checklist (CBCL) Externalizing scores. However, the sensitivity and specificity of these early predictors were modest, consistent with most of the research reviewed here.

Language skill is another potential early predictor of later self-regulation (and later ADHD), because the internalization of speech in preschool helps children regulate their actions, as Luria (1961) and Vygotsky (1979) demonstrated long ago. Indeed, ADHD is comorbid with LI. A striking clinical observation in some school-age children with ADHD is that they persist in using overt self-talk to guide their problem solving, whereas typically developing children internalize their self-talk by age 4 or 5 years. I. Petersen, Bates, and Staples (2015) tested a longitudinal mediation model of the relations among early language skill, EC measured behaviorally, and later ADHD symptoms using cross-lag correlations across three time points. They found that language predicted later self-regulation, but not the reverse, and that self-regulation mediated the relation between earlier language skill and later ADHD. As is the case for most of the studies reviewed here, the effect sizes were modest.

Another important method for studying the early precursors of a neurodevelopmental disorder is the family risk design, which has been used extensively in studies of ASD and dyslexia but is notably absent from the ADHD literature. We could find only one, partial example of this approach applied to ADHD. E. Sullivan et al. (2015) oversampled pregnant women for diagnoses of ADHD, then examined emotion regulation in their infants at 6 months. Maternal ADHD was associated with greater anger/irritability in response to physical restraint in their infants, supporting the familiality of problems with emotion regulation in ADHD.

In summary, studies of the early development of ADHD have found modest predictive relations between measures of infant attention and emotion regulation and later ADHD, consistent with the two aspects of EC in the model proposed by Posner and Rothbart (2000). Hence, an important lesson for understanding the neuropsychology of ADHD at later ages emerges from these early development studies, namely, that *both* cognitive control and emotion regulation are important aspects of ADHD. As we see next, most of the research on the neuropsychology of ADHD at later ages has focused on cognitive control, and there has been much less research on emotion regulation.

Despite these successes of the EC model, there are also some empirical challenges. Chief among these are problems with convergent and discriminant validity. With regard to convergent validity, behavioral and questionnaire measures of EC are only weakly related (see also Samyn, Roeyers, Bijttebier, Rosseel, & Wiersema, 2015). This problem is echoed by research on EFs, which found that laboratory measures of EF do not correlate very highly with questionnaire measures of EF, like the BRIEF (Behavior Rating Inventory of Executive Function; Toplak, West, & Stanovich, 2013). With regard to discriminant validity, Papageorgiou et al. (2014) found that infant attention measures were more strongly related to later temperament measures of surgency than to EC. Finally, there are other, more general predictors of later ADHD, such as infant IQ in females (Arnett, MacDonald, et al., 2013) and language skill, which in turn contribute to the development of later self-regulation (I. Petersen et al., 2015). Hence, consistent with the multiple neuropsychological risk factors for ADHD found at later ages, the multiple-deficit model also applies to the early development of ADHD.

Later Development

Most of the research on the neuropsychology of ADHD in school-age children, adolescents, and adults has been dominated by three competing single-deficit theories of ADHD, namely, the executive disinhibition, state dysregulation, and delay aversion theories, but advocates of these theories have all now embraced multiple-deficit models since no single deficit accounts for even close to the majority of ADHD cases.

To understand these three theories, we can somewhat crudely divide them into top-down versus bottom-up theories, or cognitive versus motivational theories. If someone fails to regulate his or her attention or behavior it may be because top-down cognitive control is too weak (as posited by the executive disinhibition theory). But it also may be because his or her bottom-up motivational drives (impulses) are too strong (posited by the delay aversion and state dysregulation theories). Empirically distinguishing these possibilities in ADHD is very difficult, just as it is in disorders of emotion regulation, such as anxiety and depression. Because adaptive action selection always involves an interplay between bottom-up motivations and top-down control, it is probably not too surprising that none of these three single-deficit theories has succeeded in accounting for all of ADHD. Nonetheless, each theory has produced consistent empirical results that any multiple-deficit model of ADHD will need to include.

Each of these three theories is supported by deficits found in ADHD on particular marker tasks. Willcutt et al. (2012), in a comprehensive review of ADHD, included a meta-analysis of cognitive deficits associated with ADHD. Supporting the executive disinhibition theory, they found there were well-replicated correlations between inhibition measures and ADHD ($r = .24$). Such inhibition measures include the stop-signal task and commission errors on continuous performance tasks (CPTs). They also found that the state dysregulation theory is supported by the well-replicated finding of increased variability in RT (longer SDRT, $r = .34$). The delay aversion theory is supported by deficits on choice impulsivity tasks (in which the child picks a smaller immediate reward over a larger, later reward). We review this research next.

Choice impulsivity tasks include (1) delay of gratification tasks (used by Kochanska et al., 2000, and I. Petersen et al., 2015, in their studies of self-control in preschoolers); (2) delay discounting tasks; and (3) a delay aversion task developed by Sonuga-Barke, Taylor, Sembi, and Smith (1992). However, not every study of school-age children with ADHD finds a deficit on the delay aversion task. For instance, in the Willcutt et al. (2012) meta-analysis, the average correlation between the delay aversion task and ADHD symptoms was only .13.

Recently, Patros et al. (2016) conducted a meta-analysis of 26 studies of choice impulsivity in ADHD and found a significant meta-analytic mean group effect of 0.47, which means that groups with ADHD were on average about half a SD worse on choice impulsivity tasks than controls. Since this mean effect of 0.47 is considerably larger than the correlation of 0.13 on the delay aversion task found in the Willcutt et al. (2012), one can infer that other choice impulsivity tasks are more sensitive than the delay aversion task to the deficit in ADHD in older samples. Also, since this effect size was nearly twice as large ($d = 0.83$) in the youngest group (ages 3–8 years) as in the two older groups (Patros et al., 2016), age of the sample may partly explain some of the nonreplications of a delay aversion deficit in ADHD.

In addition to replicated deficits on these three marker tasks, another robust deficit in ADHD is in processing speed (PS; $r = .32$ in Willcutt et al., 2012). Unlike the deficits just discussed, the PS deficit is an empirical finding in search of a theoretical explanation. As one can infer from the average correlation for each of these four deficits, none is large enough to explain all the symptom variance in ADHD, and none is universal in ADHD.

An article by Nigg, Willcutt, Doyle, and Sonuga-Barke (2005) documented this problem for the executive disinhibition theory of ADHD, as well as any EF theory of ADHD. Across three large samples, they found that only around half of children with ADHD in their study had a deficit on the most sensitive inhibition measure (stop-signal reaction time [SSRT]) compared to 10% percent of controls. While nearly 80% of children with ADHD have a deficit on at least one EF measure, the same was true of nearly half of controls. Given these results, Nigg et al. argued that the field should distinguish an EF-deficit subtype of ADHD, since there is also evidence that this subtype is familial, more impairing than ADHD without EF dysfunction, and can be distinguished from other potential subtypes of ADHD (e.g., a delay aversion subtype). So this proposal assumes that we may be able to resolve the heterogeneity of ADHD into a number of different single-deficit subtypes, the EF-deficit subtype being one of these. As far as we know, this heterogeneity theory of ADHD has not been rigorously tested, but it is worth noting that it makes a very strong prediction, namely, that a sample of children with ADHD will contain subgroups, each with one, and only one, single deficit in inhibition, SDRT, delay aversion, or PS.

At the other extreme, a competing theory is a multiple-deficit model in which multiple cognitive risk factors are needed to produce ADHD in every child with ADHD. More plausible is a mixed model, in which some children with ADHD have multiple deficits but others have single deficits. Of course, deciding whether a child has a deficit in some cognitive risk factor is a categorical decision imposed on a continuous distribution until proven otherwise.

We were able to find only one independent test of a multiple-deficit model of ADHD. Sjowall, Roth, Lindqvist, and Thorell (2013) examined multiple predictors of ADHD in a clinic sample of 102 individuals with ADHD and 102 controls matched on age and gender. Appropriately, they did not exclude comorbidity from the ADHD sample, but their clinic sample had a higher rate of comorbid CD or ODD (46%) than would be found in a population sample of ADHD. Their multiple predictors included *both* cognitive (EFs, SDRT, and delay aversion) *and* emotional (a parent rating of emotional regulation and a laboratory measure of the child's emotion recognition) predictors. One main finding was that the cognitive measures alone had weak sensitivity for correctly identifying ADHD cases (65%) but reasonable specificity (84%). Of greater interest was the finding that sensitivity markedly improved when the emotion measures were added as predictors, from 65 to 92%. Specificity increased slightly to 87%, and overall correct classification rate was 90%, considerably higher than previous studies.

If replicated, these findings mean that there may be an emotion dysregulation subtype of ADHD that is not well predicted by cognitive measures. This possibility is supported by the findings of Lawson and Ruff (2004) and E. Sullivan et al. (2015) discussed earlier, both of which found a relation between negative emotionality in infancy and ADHD. It is supported theoretically by the two aspects of EC, behavior and emotion regulation, in the Posner and Rothbart (2000) model.

An important additional question about putative cognitive risk factors for ADHD is whether they are actually *causal*. Nearly all the evidence supporting these cognitive risk factors is cross-sectional instead of longitudinal. Arnett et al.

(2012) used cross-lagged path modeling to test the longitudinal relations between rapid naming speed and ADHD symptoms in a large sample ($N > 1,500$) of young children across four time points. The path from earlier rapid naming to later Inatt. was significant across all time points, whereas the reverse path was only significant at the earliest time point. Although these results do not establish a causal relation, they are consistent with rapid naming being a cognitive risk factor for later ADHD.

Another possible approach for addressing this question about the causal status of cognitive correlates of ADHD is to ask whether medication treatment for ADHD also remediates its cognitive deficits, although this test is not definitive, since the medication could act on a third variable that is correlated with the putative cognitive cause. The short answer is that it does, but not as much as it changes ADHD symptoms. Coghill et al. (2014) conducted a meta-analysis of 36 studies of the effects of methylphenidate (MPH) on both ADHD symptoms and various cognitive risk factors found in ADHD. They found that the effect size of improvements in ADHD symptoms ranged from 0.8 to 1.0, whereas the average effect size of improvements in risk factors was smaller ($d = 0.24$ for RT, $d = 0.26$ for working memory, $d = 0.41$ for inhibition, $d = 0.60$ for short-term memory [STM], and $d = 0.62$ for SDRT). As discussed later, Bedard et al. (2015) likewise found that MPH produced improvements in both ADHD symptoms and CPT performance, but the changes in these two domains were not correlated. This latter result questions the role of cognitive risk factors as causes of ADHD. Instead, it suggests that cognitive risk factors found in ADHD are just pleiotropic manifestations of the underlying etiology and not causal intermediates (i.e., endophenotypes).

Consistent with this latter possibility, van Lieshout, Luman, Buitelaar, Rommelse, and Oosterlaan (2013) examined 18 longitudinal studies that examined the predictive value of cognitive risk factors for ADHD persistence. In this meta-analysis, they found that cognitive risk factors for ADHD do not predict ADHD persistence except in young children (similar to the Arnett et al., 2012, results).

In summary, research in both preschool- and school-age children supports several conclusions about the neuropsychology of ADHD: (1) Multiple deficits are needed to explain ADHD; (2) even with multiple deficits, the majority of symptom variance in ADHD remains unexplained; (3) there may be an emotion dysregulation subtype of ADHD, which would help account for this missing variance; and (4) our theoretical models of the development of ADHD are less adequate than are our theoretical models of some of the other learning disorders reviewed in this book (i.e., dyslexia and LI).

BRAIN MECHANISMS

Since publication of the second edition of this book in 2009, our understanding of brain mechanisms in ADHD has advanced considerably, and this recent progress reflects general trends in neuroimaging research that cut across the learning disorders in this book. The first general trend is a paradigm shift from examining localized to distributed brain mechanisms. A second, more recent trend is an attempt to use dynamic rather than static models of brain function to characterize brain mechanisms in ADHD.

As mentioned earlier, ADHD is the only disorder covered in this book for which there is a well-established medication treatment for the primary symptoms. Because of that distinguishing fact, it is appropriate to begin our discussion of brain mechanisms in ADHD with a section on neurotransmitters implicated in this disorder.

Neurotransmitters

The main stimulant medication to treat ADHD is methylphenidate (MPH, which is sold as Ritalin. MPH was first synthesized in 1944 and was used clinically in adults to treat various conditions, including narcolepsy, for which it was effective (and thus continues to be used for this condition). The use of MPH to treat ADHD began in the 1950s, and its efficacy has been supported by hundreds of randomized clinical trials (RCTs). Despite its well-established efficacy in treating ADHD, exactly how Ritalin and other stimulant medications change brain function is still not well understood. For instance, it has been unclear whether the therapeutic effects of MPH derive from dopamine or norepinephrine increases, or both. Consequently, both dopaminergic (Castellanos & Proal, 2012) and noradrenergic (Biederman & Spencer, 1999) theories of ADHD have been proposed. Moreover, both dopamine and norepinephrine have multiple targets in the brain. Dopamine could act in the striatum or the prefrontal cortex (PFC), or both. Subsequent research has helped answer these two questions. We do know now that MPH is both a dopamine (DA) and a norepinephrine (NE) agonist. It makes extracellular DA more available by inhibiting the dopamine transporter (DAT), which is involved in reuptake of DA by the presynaptic neuron. MPH has similar effects on the NE transporter (NET). In fact, MPH has a higher affinity for NET than for DAT, both *in vitro* and in a human positron emission tomography (PET) binding study (Hannestad et al., 2010).

To understand why the medication effect of MPH is primarily on the PFC, given that there is extensive binding of MPH in the striatum (Volkow, Fowler, Wang, Ding, & Gatley, 2002), one needs to understand a crucial difference between the DA pathways from the substantia nigra (SN) to the striatum and the DA pathways from the ventral tegmental area (VTA) to the PFC, and other related structures. The neurons in the SN pathway have autoreceptors that regulate DA levels, whereas those in the VTA pathway do not. Therefore, an increase in extracellular DA will persist in the PFC but not in the striatum. Consistent with this difference in autoreceptors, Volkow et al. (2012) used neuroimaging to examine DA changes in both the striatum and PFC after short- and long-term treatment with MPH in adults with ADHD. There were only short-term increases in DA in the ventral striatum (which is associated with reward processing), but both short- *and* long-term DA increases in PFC. Both the striatal and PFC DA increases were correlated with long-term improvement in ADHD symptoms.

Based on extensive animal work, Berridge and Devilbiss (2011) have found that DA D1 receptors in the PFC are one main target of prescribed psychostimulants, such as MPH, that calm behavior and enhance cognition. At these low doses these psychostimulants produce somewhat localized increases in both DA and NE in the PFC.

Hence, both animal and human work have established that the long-term therapeutic effects of MPH are mainly mediated by the PFC, not the striatum. In this way, ADHD is distinct from Parkinson's disease (PD). Although both appear to involve DA depletion, the depletion in PD is in the striatum and is caused by extensive degeneration of the SN pathways, so extensive that autoreceptors cannot compensate. Unlike PD, individuals with ADHD can still synthesize DA and adjust striatal DA levels with autoreceptors.

We still need to answer the other question about how stimulants improve ADHD symptoms, whether it is by increasing DA, NE, or both. The striatum, unlike the PFC, mostly lacks NE receptors. Hence, noradrenergic effects of stimulants must be mediated by the PFC or other brain structures with NE receptors.

To answer the question of whether stimulants such as MPH act mainly through DA, NE or both, Overtoom et al. (2003) randomized children with ADHD to medications with a selective effect on NE (desipramine) or DA (L-dopa]), and compared them to a group treated with MPH. Their outcome measure was the stop-signal task. The found *no* treatment effect of L-dopa, in contrast to what is found in PD. The null treatment effect of L-dopa on ADHD replicated two previous studies. In contrast, the selective NE agonist (desipramine) improved one component of performance, the stop signal RT, whereas MPH treatment improved other components of performance (shortened go-signal RTs [Go RTs] and decreased both omission and commission errors). Since previous studies have found that MPH improves all aspects of the stop-signal task, they concluded that the nonadditive combination of both DA and NE increases were important in the medication response in ADHD.

Another important piece of evidence for the role of NE in ADHD comes from the efficacy of atomoxetine (sold as Straterra), a selective NE reuptake inhibitor. Atomoxetine (ATX) has been studied extensively in RCTs for ADHD and is often as effective as MPH, although an extended-release form of MPH, osmotic-release oral system (OROS) MPH sold as Concerta, typically has a larger treatment effect than ATX.

Bedard et al. (2015) conducted a double-blind crossover trial comparing the efficacy of OROS MPH and ATX in treating both ADHD symptoms and a key cognitive deficit in ADHD, performance on a CPT. They studied a large sample of children and adolescents ($N = 102$) with ADHD. Consistent with previous studies, both medications significantly reduced ADHD symptoms, with the effect size for OROS MPH ($d = 1.80$) being greater than that for ATX ($d = 1.33$). In contrast, only MPH improved various dimensions of performance on the CPT, including omissions (but not commissions), RT, and SDRT. Another theoretically important result was that changes in cognitive performance were not correlated with changes in symptoms. These results (1) support the importance of both DA and NE in treating ADHD, and (2) question whether treatment effects on ADHD symptoms act by reducing cognitive deficits in ADHD.

In summary, a single neurotransmitter deficit hypothesis of ADHD, such as DA depletion, is not supported, in contrast to disorders such as PD and early treated phenylketonuria (PKU). Instead, deficits in both DA and NE are implicated in ADHD, and possibly other neurotransmitters, such as serotonin. In addition, medication effects in ADHD are not localized to a single brain structure. While the PFC is an important target for both MPH and ATX, the noradrenergic sites of action are much more widely distributed. Finally, the effects of these medications on ADHD symptoms appear to be dissociable from their effects on cognitive deficits found in ADHD, thus questioning the roles of these cognitive deficits in causing ADHD.

Neuroimaging

As with other learning disorders in this book, neuroimaging research on ADHD initially focused on localized explanations. The most influential of these was the hypothesis of frontal lobe dysfunction in ADHD, which had been advanced for decades by various researchers (Gualtieri & Hicks, 1985; Mattes, 1989; Pontius, 1973; Rosenthal & Allen, 1978; Stamm & Kreder, 1979; Zametkin & Rapoport, 1986), often long before neuroimaging methods were available to test this hypothesis. The frontal lobe dysfunction hypothesis of ADHD was based on the previously discussed efficacy of stimulant medications in treating ADHD and the behavioral effects of frontal lobe lesions. Frontal lesions in both experimental animals and human patients sometimes produce hyperactivity, distractibility, or impulsivity, alone or in combination (Fuster, 1989; Levin, Eisenberg, & Benton, 1991; Stuss & Benson, 1986). Of course, lesions in other parts of the brain can also produce these symptoms.

Because there is a close interaction between the frontal lobes and the basal ganglia (which include the caudate and putamen, called the striatum, and the globus pallidus), the frontal dysfunction hypothesis of ADHD is more accurately described as the frontal–striatal dysfunction hypothesis. As reviewed in the second edition of this book, there is structural neuroimaging support for the frontal–striatal hypothesis of ADHD. Hynd et al. (1990) found absence of the usual right > left frontal asymmetry in children with ADHD children using MRI. They contrasted participants with ADHD, participants with dyslexia, and controls; frontal symmetry was present in both clinical groups, but did not differentiate between the clinical groups even though the group with dyslexia was selected to be non-ADHD. This lack of frontal asymmetry in ADHD has been replicated in two other studies (Castellanos et al.,1996; Filipek et al., 1997). Abnormalities of caudate volume have also been found across numerous studies of ADHD (Castellanos et al., 1996; Filipek et al., 1997; Hynd et al., 1993; Mataro, Garcia-Sanchez, Junque, Estevez-Gonzalez, & Pujol, 1997). In addition, the globus pallidus has been found to be significantly smaller in those with ADHD as well (Aylward et al., 1996; Castellanos et al., 1996; Singer et al., 1993). These structural studies support developmental differences in frontal–striatal structures known to be important in action selection.

The hypothesis that these structural differences were related to deficits in action selection was tested in a study by Casey et al. (1997). They correlated performance on three separate inhibition tasks with measures of PFC and basal ganglia volume. The three inhibition tasks, which tapped response inhibition at different stages of attentional processing, were all impaired in the children with ADHD when compared to controls. Furthermore, PFC, caudate, and globus pallidus volumes correlated significantly with task performance. Of course, this correlation does not prove cause. Such a finding could be a *result* or just a correlate of ADHD.

However, brain structure differences in ADHD are not exclusively in the PFC and basal ganglia. In addition, decreased areas in different regions of the corpus callosum have been observed in several studies (Baumgardner et al., 1996; Castellanos et al., 1996; Giedd et al., 1994; Hynd et al., 1991; Semrud-Clikeman et al., 1994), as well as smaller total cerebral volume and a smaller cerebellum (Castellanos et al., 1996).

Functional neuroimaging, mainly fMRI, has been used in numerous studies to investigate brain activation differences in groups with ADHD in response to the demands of a variety of cognitive control tasks, including several that are well-replicated neuropsychological markers of ADHD, such as go/no-go tasks and the Stroop (see review in Durston & Konrad, 2007). A deficit in frontal–striatal activation is found across studies, consistent with the structural work just reviewed. For instance, the right inferior frontal cortex is a key structure for performance on inhibition tasks, like the stop-signal task (Aron, Robbins, & Poldrack, 2004). These studies have also found cerebellar activation differences consistent with the structural difference in cerebellum found by Castellanos et al. (1996).

Besides frontal–striatal circuits and the cerebellum, white matter structures are also implicated in ADHD and its cognitive deficits. For instance, a key cognitive deficit in ADHD is greater intraindividual variability in RT (SDRT). It is well known that both RT and SDRT decrease with age. Tamnes, Fjell, Westlye, Østby, and Walhovd (2012) found that developmental reductions in SDRT in typical children were correlated with developmental increases in white matter.

There is considerable other evidence for white matter differences in ADHD (e.g., Shaw et al., 2015). These more recent studies are consistent with an earlier meta-analysis of white matter difference in ADHD (van Ewijk, Heslenfeld, Zwiers, Buitelaar, & Oosterlaan, 2012). As discussed in this meta-analysis, previous research has documented a smaller total cerebral volume in ADHD samples ($d = 0.30$–0.64), with decreased white matter accounting for this volume difference. In contrast, cortical grey matter in children with ADHD has a larger volume than that in age-matched controls, consistent with a delay in pruning (Shaw, Lerch, et al., 2006). In their quantitative meta-analysis of nine studies, van Ewijk et al. (2012) found lower fractional anisotropy (FA), a measure of white matter integrity, in five structures: the right and left internal capsule of the basal ganglia, the left cerebellum, the right corona radiata (which overlaps with the superior longitudinal fasciculus), and the forceps minor near the genu of the corpus callosum, all of which have been implicated in previous structural MRI studies of ADHD.

Subsequently, researchers found altered activation of another brain network in ADHD, the default mode network (DMN), in addition to the well-replicated hypoactivation of the frontal–striatal network. The DMN is measured when participants are "at rest," in contrast to other brain networks, which typically have been identified when participants are responding to a task while fMRI data are collected. Going back to the discovery of electroencephalography (EEG) in the 1920s and the use of regional cerebral blood flow in the 1970s, it has long been known that the brain is active while conscious participants are seemingly "at rest." But it has taken the much better spatial resolution of fMRI methods to identify which brain structures produced this resting state activity. Since its description in fMRI data (Raichle et al., 2001), there has been an explosion of research on the DMN.

The DMN includes two key midline brain structures: the medial PFC and the precuneus and the adjacent posterior cingulate cortex, and can include hippocampal structures, as well as some parietal lobe structures. The two key structures in the DMN are consistently activated when one is thinking about oneself: one's thoughts, feelings, and one's relations with other people. Since self-directed thoughts may also include recollections and possible futures, hippocampal structures can be activated as part of the DMN. Activity in the DMN is usually anticorrelated with activity in task-related brain networks, likely reflecting an intuitively plausible trade-off between focusing on oneself and focusing on the task at hand. Obviously, an inability to regulate self-directed thoughts, such as the rumination found in major depression, or the ideas of reference found in schizophrenia, would interfere with adaptive behavior. Hence, there has been a considerable amount of research on the role of the DMN in various psychiatric disorders, including ADHD. Since children with ADHD are by definition exhibiting many off-task behaviors, perhaps they are activating their DMN at inappropriate times.

Castellanos and Proal (2012) reviewed initial evidence for dysregulation of the DMN in ADHD, and argued that models of ADHD needed to go beyond the frontal–striatal model of ADHD that had dominated the field for several decades. Several months later, Cortese at al. (2012) published a meta-analysis of 55 fMRI studies of ADHD in both children and adults. Two key results across both age groups were (1) hypoactivity in frontoparietal executive network and (2) hyperactivity in the DMN. These findings suggest that the *relation* between activity in the central executive network and the DMN may be dysfunctional in ADHD.

In summary, the brain mechanisms of ADHD include changes in dopaminergic and noradrenergic neurotransmission that are remediated by stimulant medications, and well-replicated structural and functional differences in frontal–striatal network known to be important for action selection. But the interaction of this frontal–striatal network with the cerebellum and the DMN are also important, not to mention possible interactions with other resting-state networks. In terms of early brain development, we do not know where or how ADHD starts. Given the genetic heterogeneity we discuss next, as well as the large polygenic contribution, there could be multiple possible starting points that eventually lead to a somewhat similar functional neuroimaging phenotype.

ETIOLOGY

The exact etiology of ADHD is still unknown, and we now know more about the etiology of the majority of learning disorders covered in this book (i.e., ID, ASD, dyslexia, and LI) than we know about the etiology of ADHD. As discussed earlier, some of this relative lack of progress in understanding the etiology of ADHD may derive from its greater heterogeneity at several levels of analysis. In this section, we review genetic and environmental influences on ADHD and evidence for G × E interactions in the etiology of ADHD. We begin with familiality, which is a prerequisite for heritability.

Familiality

The rate of ADHD in families of ADHD male probands has been found to be over *seven* times the rate of the disorder in nonpsychiatric control families (Biederman, Faraone, Keenan, Knee, & Tsuang, 1990); later studies reported a similar increase in risk among relatives of female probands (Faraone et al., 1992; Faraone, Biederman, Keenan, & Tsuang, 1991). Hence, the value for the familiality of ADHD (relative risk of about 7) is on the high end of the range of familialities found in many behaviorally defined disorders, including the other learning disorders covered in this book. Of course, family transmission is not sufficient evidence that genes are involved, but it is a prerequisite for genetic inheritance. Family transmission could be due entirely to the shared family environment (the C term in the ACE model we discussed in Chapter 2). Hence, a different method, such as a twin or adoption study, is needed to determine whether familial transmission is due in whole or in part to inherited genetic variations.

Heritability

A meta-analysis of over 20 twin studies of ADHD found a mean heritability of .76, with the remaining variance accounted for by nonshared environment (Faraone, Spencer, Aleardi, Pagano, & Biederman, 2004). These results indicate that the substantial familiality of ADHD is almost entirely due to genetic influences, but as we discuss below, they do not take into account possible G × E interactions. If present, such interactions will be counted as heritability, in a simple genetic model. A heritability of .76 means that ADHD is one of the more heritable complex behavioral disorders. It is more heritable than RD or major depression, and on par with heritability estimates for ASD.

As reviewed in Thapar, Cooper, Eyre, and Langley (2013), there have been five published adoption studies that report a similarly large heritability of ADHD. Hence, the heritability of ADHD is well established, but as we discuss shortly, finding the actual genes that are involved in the etiology of ADHD has been much more difficult.

Although extreme scores on both the defining dimensions of ADHD, Inatt. and HI, are moderately heritable, this appears *not* to be the case for the HI dimension once the correlation between the two dimensions is accounted for (Willcutt & Pennington, 2000a; Willcutt, Pennington, & DeFries, 2000); that is, extreme scores on the Inatt. dimension are moderately heritable regardless of the level of HI symptoms (i.e., both the Inatt. and C subtypes of ADHD are moderately heritable). However, extreme scores on the HI dimension were *not* significantly heritable (h^2g = .08) when symptoms of Inatt. were covaried. These results suggest that the etiology of the HI presentation is largely nongenetic and differs from the etiology of the other two presentations.

Gene Identification

The earliest molecular evidence for genes that affect ADHD came from genetic syndromes that include ADHD in their phenotype. These include Turner syndrome, which is also associated with math disability (e.g., T. Green et al., 2015), the 22q11 microdeletion that causes velocardiofacial syndrome, which is also associated with schizophrenia (Thapar et al., 2013), as well as virtually all genetic ID syndromes (e.g., Down syndrome, fragile X syndrome, and Williams syndrome; see Chapter 14). However, ADHD symptoms are virtually inevitable in ID, given that executive and attention skills are correlated with IQ.

Identifying actual genes that account for the high heritability of idiopathic ADHD has been frustrating and provides a good illustration of some of the lessons that have been learned in the last 10 years in psychiatric and behavior genetics. Briefly, adaptive behavioral traits such as intelligence, language, self-control, and social skill are continuous, quantitative dimensions, and their etiology is multifactorial and extensively polygenic. In other words, they are quantitative traits such as height and weight, and there are likely hundreds, if not thousands, of gene variants or polymorphisms that influence their development, with each polymorphism only accounting for a very small portion of the phenotypic variance. As we explained in Chapter 2, any common gene variant with a large effect size that adversely affected adaptive traits would quickly be weeded out by natural selection. Hence, only very rare, deleterious mutations would remain in the gene pool. Some of these rare mutations might be sufficient to cause a disorder such as ADHD, but they would necessarily produce a very rare genetic subtype and thus not account for much population variance in the ADHD symptom dimension. Moreover, these rare mutations with a large effect size would be unlikely to be discovered in genomewide association studies (GWAS) using single-nucleotide polymorphisms (SNPs), as explained in Chapter 2, because this genetic method is optimal for detecting *common* variants associated with a trait. Hence, a GWAS of a quantitative trait such as ADHD requires a very large sample size (tens of thousands of affected individuals, or even 100,000) to have enough statistical power to detect a common genetic polymorphism with a very small effect size.

Past GWAS of ADHD, similar to those of dyslexia and LI, have been far too small to detect significant and replicable risk loci. Even when all the existing GWAS of ADHD were combined in a meta-analysis, the total *N* was roughly 3,000 cases, far below the tens of thousands needed (Thapar et al., 2013). Sample collection has been ongoing, however, and during the writing of this book, the first well-powered GWAS of ADHD was disseminated via the preprint website *biorxiv.org* (Demontis et al., 2017). While it is not yet peer-reviewed, it is worth considering a few of the findings from the largest GWAS of ADHD to date. The study included ~20,000 individuals with ADHD and ~35,000 controls. The authors reported 12 genome-wide significant loci, including regions that include the genes *FOXP2* and *DUSP6*. We also discussed *FOXP2* in Chapter 9, because it has been previously associated with speech and language development. This gene was implicated in the early 2000s through a three-generation family with about half of its members affected by severe speech and language disorders (Lai et al., 2001). Through genetic analysis, the cause was localized to an autosomal dominant mutation in the *FOXP2* gene. While *FOXP2* has not been a primary candidate gene previously implicated in the etiology of ADHD (but see Ribasés et al., 2012), there is a high rate of comorbidity between speech and language disorders and ADHD (L. Baker & Cantwell, 1982, 1992; Cantwell & Baker, 1985; Gualtieri, Koriath, Van Bourgondien, & Saleeby, 1983; Love & Thompson, 1988; McGrath et al., 2007). From the current results, it cannot be determined whether *FOXP2* may be pleiotropic for both ADHD and speech–language disorders or whether the genetic association may be due to the comorbidity of speech–language disorders in the sample of individuals with ADHD.

DUSP6 is a particularly interesting gene in relation to ADHD, because it is theorized to play a role in regulating dopamine levels in the synapse. While *FOXP2* and *DUSP6*, and other genes identified in the GWAS, have interesting connections to ADHD and its comorbidities, it is also important to note that none of the well-studied a priori candidate genes, such as *DAT1* and *DRD4* (discussed further below), emerged at the top of the GWAS results (Demontis et al., 2017). More research in large samples will be needed, but at this point it appears that ADHD may be similar to other complex disorders in which a priori candidate genes did not align well with genes that emerged from data-driven GWAS approaches (Duncan et al., 2014). For this reason, the field of psychiatric genetics has increasingly relied on whole-genome, data-driven approaches for initial discovery.

Another genomewide approach to discovery is to include a group of genetically related disorders together in an analysis. ADHD was recently included in a large, adequately powered GWAS of five psychiatric disorders conducted by the Psychiatric Genomics Consortium; the other four disorders were schizophrenia (Schz), bipolar disorder (BPD), major depression (MDD), and ASD. Four risk loci reached genomewide significance (i.e., SNPs on 3p21 and 10q24, and two L-type, voltage-gated calcium channel subunits, *CACNB2*, and *CACNA1C*). The first three of these risk loci affected all five disorders equally, providing a clear example of both pleiotropy and of generalist genes for psychopathology. Using SNP heritability from genomewide complex trait analysis (GCTA), a genetic correlation of .32 was found between ADHD and MDD, consistent with previous results. Also consistent with previous results, there were stronger genetic correlations between Schz and BPD (.68), Schz and MDD (.43) and BPD and MDD (.47) than with ADHD. The least genetic overlap was found between ASD and the other four disorders, namely, only a small genetic correlation between ASD and Schz (.16). These SNP-based bivariate heritability analyses will not detect rare copy number variations (CNVs) that may be shared by two disorders. As discussed later, ADHD *does* share rare CNVs with both ASD and Schz.

Two other molecular methods have been utilized to identify risk genes for ADHD: (1) single-candidate gene association studies, and (2) the use of GWAS data to identify rare CNVs. The first method has generated a great deal of controversy in psychiatric genetics, because single-candidate gene association studies often fail to replicate, as discussed in Chapter 2. As reviewed by Thapar et al. (2013) and by Schachar (2014), the first method has found six candidate genes associated with ADHD. Each gene was a candidate, because it affected neurotransmission, mainly involving specific neurotransmitters already implicated in the pathophysiology of ADHD. But even this requirement for candidacy produced many false-positive results; hence, only well-replicated results are presented here. Moreover, each of these replicated candidate genes has a very small effect sizes (median odds ratio of 1.22), especially relative to the large effect sizes for the familiality and heritability of ADHD discussed earlier. Those six candidates are three dopamine transmission genes: *DRD4, DRD5* and *DAT1*; two serotonin genes: *HTR1B*, and *5-HTT*; and *SNAP-25*, a synaptic vesicle protein also associated with Schz. It remains to be seen whether these genes will also be consistently replicated by large GWAS studies of ADHD. While it is too early to tell at this point, as noted earlier, these genes did not emerge among the very top candidates in the first large-scale GWAS of ADHD (Demontis et al., 2017). Still, further in-depth analysis of variants in these genes will be required to determine if there is a reliable signal in the large GWAS that can be detected for these a priori candidate genes.

Because of their small effect sizes, each candidate gene would only shift an individual's ADHD ratings a tiny amount. With large enough samples, these six candidates could be tested for their additive and interactive effects on risk for ADHD. An interactive effect in the expected negative direction would validate each candidate gene involved in the interaction, as would additive effects. A lack of an additive effect would question the validity of that gene as a risk factor for ADHD.

Regarding CNVs influencing ADHD, several have been identified, and these partially overlap with CNVs influencing ASD and Schz (Thapar et al., 2013). According to Thapar et al. (2013), the phenotype found in ADHD cases with CNVs does not differ from that found in idiopathic ADHD. Interestingly, CNVs do not appear to play a role in the etiology of dyslexia (Gialluisi et al., 2016), so the well-established genetic correlation between ADHD and dyslexia does not appear to be mediated by CNVs. Because each specific CNV is quite rare in the population (because of natural selection, as explained earlier), those associated with ADHD will also only explain a tiny portion of the population variance.

In summary, there is solid evidence (from genetic syndromes, a recent large GWAS, candidate gene association studies, and studies of CNVs) for specific genes that help cause ADHD, but they only account for a very small portion of the known twin study heritability of ADHD (about .76). They also account for a very small portion of the SNP heritabilities of ADHD (.28 in Cross-Disorder Group of the Psychiatric Genomic Consortium et al., 2013; .40 in Pappa et al., 2015). Identifying all the genes that influence ADHD will require much larger GWAS. Incidentally, the large gap between twin and SNP heritability estimates for ADHD is currently unexplained, but it could be due to nonadditive genetic influences, including gene × gene (G × G) and G × E interaction, as well as by the rare genetic syndromes and CNVs discussed earlier (which would not be detected in a GWAS with SNPs).

Environmental Influences

Since the heritability of ADHD is less than 1.0, there must be environmental risk factors, either biological or social, that are part of its etiology. However, proving that a correlated environmental risk factor is actually a *cause* of ADHD is difficult, and some putative environmental risk factors for ADHD have not survived closer scrutiny. Because ADHD is highly familial, some seeming environmental risk factors could be due to gene–environment (G–E) correlation. For instance, since maternal substance use during pregnancy might be elevated because the mother herself has ADHD, we need direct evidence that the substance in question (e.g., nicotine, alcohol, or illegal drugs) actually alters fetal development in a way that produces later ADHD. Postnatal environmental social risk factors face the same interpretive issue. Of the known bioenvironmental correlates of ADHD, including maternal smoking during pregnancy, low birthweight, fetal alcohol exposure, environmental lead, and pediatric head injury, all *but* maternal smoking are currently supported as actually causal (Thapar et al., 2013). Hence, more evidence is needed to determine whether fetal exposure to nicotine is a cause of ADHD.

We do not have evidence that the social environment, in particular, parenting practices, can directly cause ADHD, unless there is severe early social deprivation, such as was present in Romanian orphanages (Thapar et al., 2013). Harsh or inconsistent parenting is associated with ADHD, but the direction of effects could run from the child with ADHD to his or her parents, instead of the reverse, such that children with ADHD evoke harsh or inconsistent practices from their parents. Or parents who themselves have ADHD might be less consistent in their parenting. We do know that child ADHD itself *leads* to increased maternal hostility (Thapar et al., 2013), which is a kind of G–E correlation. At the same time, there is no doubt that the social environment influences the course of ADHD, possibly by interacting with risk alleles for ADHD.

G × E Interactions

Studies of possible G × E interactions in ADHD have focused on replicated risk alleles of dopamine genes interacting with bioenvironmental risk factors (e.g., maternal smoking and drinking alcohol during pregnancy). There have been several such studies, some with positive results, but as far as we know, none of these results has been replicated. If main effects of individual risk alleles are difficult to replicate because the effect size of these risk alleles is so small, replicating a single risk allele by environment interaction will be even more difficult.

We were able to find one adequately powered G × E interaction study of ADHD using a candidate risk allele approach. Martel et al. (2011) tested a G × E interaction between the *DRD4* risk allele and inconsistent parenting (as reported by the child) in a sample of 548 children. They found a significant diathesis–stress G × E interaction for the Inatt. dimension of ADHD, and for ODD; that is, while there were main effects of each risk factor considered separately, children with *both* the G and E risk factors had significantly more symptoms than a pure additive model would predict. This interesting result needs to be replicated.

Twin methods can also test for G × E interaction. They have more power than a single-candidate risk allele approach, because in a twin design, the G term includes *all* the heritable variance in the trait being examined. We tested a G × E interaction for ADHD in a large twin sample, using parent education as the E risk factor, since lower parent education predicts higher levels of ADHD in children (Pennington et al., 2009). Consistent with Martel et al. (2011), we found a significant diathesis–stress G × E interaction; that is, the heritability of ADHD increased as parental education decreased. Parent education, like parent SES, is a broad variable that is correlated with many risk and protective factors; hence, more research is needed to determine whether our finding is specific to parenting or due to some other correlate of parent SES.

DIAGNOSIS AND TREATMENT

Diagnosis

The diagnosis of ADHD is difficult because of the number of confounding conditions that must be excluded, and because objective tests of ADHD are less well developed than those for a learning disorder such as dyslexia. So clinicians should be duly cautious in making this diagnosis. Diagnosis is primarily based on interview and observation to establish history, current symptoms, and the pervasiveness of impairment. Although objective tests for ADHD are not well developed, testing results can often support the diagnosis by identifying underlying cognitive deficits that may be present in ADHD.

Presenting Symptoms

Because the diagnosis is based primarily on symptoms, much of the research on diagnosis has focused on developing lists of critical or primary symptoms and developing behavioral rating scales for parents and teachers that incorporate these critical symptoms. The critical symptoms described in DSM-5 fall into two categories: Inatt. and HI.

Other symptoms that demonstrate an association with ADHD but do not appear to be primary include aggressive behavior, oppositionality, learning disabilities, depression, anxiety, social difficulties, and poor self-esteem.

History

Symptoms of ADHD are usually present from early in life. DSM-5 requires that the symptoms be present by age 12 to make the diagnosis. Nevertheless, if the symptomatic behaviors are not present early in the school years, they may be secondary to academic problems and not reflective of primary ADHD. Therefore, we are more convinced by a history that includes clear examples of inattention, impulsivity, and hyperactivity early in development, as early as preschool. The one exception may be children with the Inatt. subtype of ADHD, whose difficulties with sustained attention may not become problematic until the later school grades, when expectations for focus and attention increase. These children are usually referred later for an evaluation than are children with hyperactive behaviors.

In infancy, symptoms may include a high activity level, less need for sleep, colic, frequent crying, and poor soothability—characteristics that overlap with what is called a "difficult" infant. In toddlerhood, the child with ADHD often has a low sense of danger, an unusual amount of energy, and a tendency to move from one activity to another very quickly. Parents may notice that the child wears out shoes, clothing, and toys faster than other children (Cantwell, 1975).

Children with ADHD often come to clinical attention in the early school years because of the behavior management problems they pose in a classroom setting: frequent talking, getting out of their seats, difficulty keeping their hands to themselves, and problems with finishing schoolwork. While this pattern is prominent in ADHD, we must also recognize that individuals with a more inattentive presentation, especially females, may be more likely to be missed in the early school years. In later school years, organization often becomes particularly problematic for a child with ADHD. He or she may have difficulty turning in homework on time, remembering deadlines, and using good study skills. These weaknesses may impact grades despite the fact that the child appears able to do the work successfully when additional structure is in place. In such cases, poor grades may be mistakenly attributed to "laziness," or "lack of motivation."

In terms of family history, the family studies previously reviewed indicate a greater risk for ADHD in children of parents who themselves had or have ADHD. Therefore, the psychiatric history of the parents is an important piece of diagnostic information.

Behavioral Observations

Because children with ADHD may not manifest their problematic behaviors in a novel or structured situation, the absence of ADHD symptoms in the clinician's office does not necessarily rule out the diagnosis. If such behaviors do occur, they then provide important converging evidence. Fidgetiness, poor attention, daydreaming, impulsive response style, problems persisting with difficult tasks, rushing through work, and making careless mistakes are all behaviors in the clinical setting that are consistent with the diagnosis. Of course, there is a normal developmental course for all of these behaviors, and some fidgeting, impersistence, carelessness, and so forth, would be expected in young children. The question is whether the client exhibits more of these behaviors than would be expected for his or her age, and over time the skilled clinician should develop those "internal norms" that will help to answer this question. Using interviews to collect vicarious behavioral observations from the client's classroom teacher (who has a large sample of behavioral observations from which to draw, as well as a readily available comparison sample of same-age peers) is typically also extremely helpful.

Standardized Behavior Rating Scales

Several different ADHD behavior rating scales are used in clinical practice. Most measures assess the behaviors that are included in DSM diagnostic criteria for ADHD and ask raters to quantify the frequency with which these behaviors occur. The scales vary in the extent to which they ask about other, commonly comorbidity conditions, such as ODD, CD, and learning problems. Rating scales, by themselves, should not be used as the sole source of evidence for a diagnosis of ADHD. However, behavioral ratings can be used in conjunction with evidence from developmental history, interviews about current behavior and impairment, and cognitive testing to support a diagnosis of ADHD. Parents and teachers are frequently asked to give ratings to assess impact across multiple contexts. The child/adolescent, if old enough, can also provide self-reports. Commonly used standardized measures include the Conners Parent or Teacher Rating Scale–Third Edition (Conners, Sitarenios, Parker, & Epstein, 1998), the DuPaul ADHD Rating Scale (DuPaul, Power, Anastopoulos, & Reid, 1998), the Disruptive Behavior Rating Scale (Barkley & Murphy, 2006), the Strengths and Weaknesses of ADHD Symptoms and Normal Behavior (SWAN; J. Swanson, 2011), and the NICHQ Vanderbilt Assessment scales (*www.nichq.org/resource/nichq-vanderbilt-assessment-scales*) (Wolraich, Lambert, Baumgaertel, et al., 2003; Wolraich, Lambert, Doffing, et al., 2003). The SWAN is distinct from the other measures, because it can capture variance at the positive ends of the attention and regulation spectrum, in addition to variance at the symptomatic levels of these dimensions (Arnett, Pennington, et al., 2013).

More global psychosocial assessments also include symptoms associated with ADHD, such as the Attention Problems scale on the CBCL and the Attention Problems and Hyperactivity subscale on the Behavior Assessment System for Children–Third Edition. These scales can be useful screeners, but an ADHD-specific rating scale is recommended for more complete information about the full range of behaviors associated with DSM-5 ADHD.

Case Presentations

Case Presentation 6

Elliot is an 8-year-old third grader. His parents sought an evaluation based on the advice of his teacher, who is concerned that Elliot's inability to focus during class is negatively impacting his progress in school. The teacher has told Elliot's parents that she cannot tell "whether it's a behavior problem or whether it's out of his control." Elliot rushes through classwork, often making careless mistakes or turning in half-completed papers. Although he is a good reader, his writing seems weak compared to that of his peers, in terms of both handwriting and compositional skills. In addition, he has fallen behind his classmates in math "Mad Minutes." Elliot's parents are concerned that his school difficulties are leading to problems with self-esteem and peer relationships. They note that he gets few calls for playdates, and that neighborhood children seem to gravitate to his younger brother rather than to Elliot. In moments of frustration in the last year, Elliot has made comments such as, "I can't do it because I'm an idiot," or "I told you I'm a stupid-head!"

Elliot's prenatal, birth, and early developmental histories are unremarkable. He was an extremely active infant and toddler. His mother described an incident that occurred when Elliot was 12 months old. She heard a loud noise as he was waking from his nap and went upstairs to discover Elliot climbing out of his crib onto a nearby dresser and repeatedly jumping from the dresser back into his crib. Although Elliot's parents had not planned to send him to preschool until he was 4, they enrolled him in a morning program when he turned 3, because his mother "was too exhausted to keep up with him all day." She mentioned that one of her primary criteria for choosing a preschool was how many acres it was on, so that Elliot would have enough room to run and play. Elliot did well in a relatively unstructured preschool environment and seemed well liked by teachers and peers alike. Concerns were first raised in kindergarten, when Elliot got in trouble on several occasions because of difficulty remaining quietly seated on the school bus. His kindergarten report card stated, "Elliot is still learning to listen respectfully, and circle time has been especially challenging for him." Similar concerns continued in first and second grade. Elliot was often placed at a desk away from other children during work times and was described by teachers as "disruptive," "silly," and "loud and fast-moving." Now in third grade, Elliot's difficulties are becoming more apparent in social interactions. He has had two playground altercations this fall that led to visits to the principal. Most recently, he shoved another child during an argument about a soccer game and was sent home for the afternoon. His mother described him as remorseful and apologetic after the incident.

Elliot's mother reports no history of school difficulties. She is a college graduate, currently working part time as a graphic designer. Elliot's father received poor grades in several high school courses but did better in college, "because I finally decided to apply myself." He is now a successful realtor. He is less concerned about Elliot than is his wife, and noted, "He's exactly like I was at that age—he just needs to grow out of it."

A summary of Elliot's diagnostic testing is found in Table 12.1.

DISCUSSION

A diagnosis of ADHD is primarily based on careful interview and observation to establish history and current symptoms, but psychological test results can often help to support the diagnosis. Elliot's case illustrates this pattern well. His early history is consistent with ADHD. He showed signs of hyperactivity even as an infant and toddler. Such symptoms are often observable earlier in development than are symptoms of inattention, because maintaining a high level of focused attention is rarely expected until a child reaches school age. Elliot's school history is suggestive

TABLE 12.1. Test Summary, Case 6

Performance validity
Memory Validity Profile Total   RS = 29
                                 (valid)

General intelligence   **Fluid intelligence**
WISC-V Full Scale IQ   SS = 107   WISC-V Fluid Reasoning Index   SS = 112
                                                    Matrix Reasoning   ss = 11
Crystallized intelligence   Figure Weights   ss = 13
WISC-V Verbal Comprehension Index   SS = 113   WISC-V Visual Spatial Index   SS = 97
  Similarities   ss = 13   Block Design   ss = 10
  Vocabulary   ss = 12   Visual Puzzles   ss = 9

Working memory
WISC-V Working Memory Index   SS = 107
  Digit Span   ss = 11
  Picture Span   ss = 11

Processing speed
WISC-V Processing Speed Index SS = 92
  Coding   ss = 7
  Symbol Search   ss = 10

Academic
Reading   Math
  History   *History*
    CLDQ Reading Scale   43rd %ile   CLDQ Math Scale   74th %ile
  Basic literacy   *Calculation and problem solving*
    WIAT-III Word Reading   SS = 119   WIAT-III Numerical Operations SS = 108
    WIAT-III Pseudoword Decoding SS = 111   Math Problem Solving   SS = 104
    WIAT-III Spelling   SS = 110
                                                    Math fluency
  Reading fluency   WIAT-III Math Fluency   SS = 89
    TOWRE-2 Sight Word Efficiency   SS = 110
    TOWRE-2 Phonemic Decoding Efficiency SS = 113

Attention and executive functions
Attention   *Executive functions*
  Gordon Vigilance Commissions 5th %ile   D-KEFS Trail Making Test
  Gordon Vigilance Total Correct 54th %ile   Visual Scanning   ss = 9
  Vanderbilt Inattention   Number Sequencing   ss = 8
    Parent   RS = 5   Letter Sequencing   ss = 6
    Teacher   RS = 9   Letter–Number Switching   ss = 7
  Vanderbilt Hyperactivity/Impulsivity   D-KEFS Verbal Fluency
    Parent   RS = 4   Letter Fluency   ss = 8
    Teacher   RS = 8   Category Fluency   ss = 11
                                                    D-KEFS Color–Word Interference
                                                      Color Naming   ss = 8
                                                      Word Reading   ss = 12
                                                      Inhibition   ss = 6
                                                      Inhibition/Switching   ss = 7

(continued)

TABLE 12.1. (continued)	
Visual–motor skills	
Beery VMI-6	SS = 85

Note. SS, standard score with mean = 100 and *SD* = 15; ss, scaled score with mean = 10 and *SD* = 3; RS, raw score; %ile, percentile rank; WISC-V, Wechsler Intelligence Scale for Children—Fifth Edition; CLDQ, Colorado Learning Difficulties Questionnaire; WIAT-III, Wechsler Individual Achievement Test—Third Edition; TOWRE-2, Test of Word Reading Efficiency—Second Edition; Gordon, Gordon Diagnostic System; Vanderbilt, NICHQ Vanderbilt Assessment Scales; D-KEFS, Delis–Kaplan Executive Function System; Beery VMI-6, Beery–Buktenica Test of Visual–Motor Integration, 6th Edition.

of difficulties with both ADHD symptom dimensions. Teacher complaints about lack of focus and difficulty completing work relate to inattention. Most of Elliot's behavioral difficulties (shouting out, not remaining seated, shoving another child) can be understood as resulting from impulsivity, and it is clear that his activity level remains very high. His teacher's ratings on the Vanderbilt ADHD rating scale places him in the clinical range (more than six symptoms) on both dimensions, while parent ratings on each dimension fall just under the clinical cutoff point. However, his parents' description of Elliot's behavior is consistent with a diagnosis of attention-deficit/hyperactivity disorder–combined type. Elliot's difficulties may be less impairing in the home than in the school setting. It is also possible that Elliot's father in particular may be underreporting some of Elliot's symptoms, because his own likely ADHD history may increase his tolerance for inattentive and hyperactive behavior.

Although ADHD-related behaviors are not always observable in the structured one-on-one testing environment, Elliot's behavior in testing provided a number of telling observations. Compared to others his age, Elliot had difficulty persisting with difficult tasks and required a great deal of encouragement. When presented with a difficult math problem, for example, he said, "Next!" and tried to turn the page before attempting it. Elliot was fidgety and restless, and played with any objects left out on the testing table, such as pencils or stimulus books. Elliot required three breaks during a 2-hour session. For each break, he typically ran down the hall, got a drink of water, and ran right back. On the morning of the final test session, Elliot was reluctant to start and hid under the table in the waiting room, until his mother convinced him to come out. He commented that he did not want to begin testing: "Those games are too hard and boring."

Several aspects of Elliot's pattern of test results further support a diagnosis of ADHD. First, he made an unusually high number of commission errors on the Gordon Diagnostic System CPT, likely reflecting his impulsive response style. Elliot was aware of many of these errors and often commented aloud on them ("Oops! I did it again"). His weak scores on the inhibition conditions of the Delis–Kaplan Executive Function System (D-KEFS) Color–Word Inhibition are also suggestive of difficulties inhibiting prepotent responses. Second, scores on multiple tests converge to indicate a relative weakness in processing speed (Processing Speed Index of the Wechsler Intelligence Scale for Children–Fifth Edition [WISC-V], D-KEFS Trail Making Test and Color Naming, Wechsler Individual Achievement Test–Third Edition [WIAT-III] Math Fluency), which is a cognitive risk factor for ADHD. These scores cluster around the low-average range. Although many of them are still within normal limits for Elliot's age, they are significantly lower than estimates of either his conceptual reasoning abilities or his untimed math skills. Third, like many children with ADHD, Elliot's handwriting is poor. Fine-motor and organizational difficulties probably relate to his lower score on the Beery–Buktenica Test of Visual–Motor Integration, 6th Edition (VMI-6) test.

Many children with impairing ADHD show mixed results on neuropsychological testing, and this was true of Elliot to a degree; few of his scores fall outside broadly normal limits. In the context of history, current functioning, and observations, however, the diagnosis of ADHD–Combined Type, is warranted.

It is important to screen children with ADHD for dyslexia because of the high degree of comorbidity. In Elliot's case, neither history nor current test results suggest a reading disability; in fact, reading seems to represent a strength for him, one that should be encouraged. Elliot does appear to be experiencing some secondary problems with self-esteem and social relationships as a result of his ADHD. His difficulties with peers appear to relate primarily to impulsivity, and like many children experiencing increasing school failure, his image of himself is suffering. These problems should be carefully monitored as treatment for his ADHD is put in place. If they continue, behavioral intervention (e.g., with a psychologist) may be helpful.

Case Presentation 7

Joan, a 14-year-old girl who is in currently in eighth grade, was referred for an evaluation because of ongoing concerns about her poor performance in school. She has difficulty keeping track of her assignments, turning in her work on time, and staying on task. Her grades have begun to suffer because of these difficulties, and her parents are very concerned about her upcoming transition into high school.

Joan's birth and early development history were uncomplicated. Her mother earned an associate's degree and works as a medical technician, and her father graduated from high school and is a mechanic. Her paternal uncle and his son have been diagnosed with ADHD. Joan's parents first became concerned about her academic progress in early elementary school. Her teachers reported that Joan was a slow worker and often needed to be prompted to finish her work because she was daydreaming or doodling, or staring out the window. The teachers often placed her in the front of the room to facilitate her attention. Her reading skills also lagged behind her peers. In third grade, Joan received extra reading help in the form of a structured, phonics-based reading program. This program reportedly improved her reading accuracy, although Joan continued to be a slow reader. Joan's academic difficulties became even more problematic in middle school because of the increasing homework demands. Her parents observed that Joan was spending much more time on her homework than did her peers. Despite this extra effort, Joan would often forget to turn in assignments she had completed. Currently, Joan's organizational skills continue to be poor, and she has difficulty keeping track of assignments and turning them in on time. Her teachers state that Joan has ongoing difficulties with focus and attention in class, her reading speed continues to be slow, and she has difficulty with writing assignments.

Outside of school, Joan enjoys arts and crafts, listening to music, socializing with friends, and riding her bike. Although her mother is an avid reader who takes weekly trips to the local library, her parents reported that Joan almost never reads for pleasure.

Joan's diagnostic testing is summarized in Table 12.2.

DISCUSSION

Joan's persistent difficulties with sustained attention and organization are consistent with a diagnosis of ADHD—predominantly inattentive subtype. Joan's early difficulties with reading acquisition and persistent fluency weaknesses are suggestive of dyslexia. In terms of history, there is a family history of ADHD. The reading questions from the Learning and Behavior Questionnaire capture Joan's early difficulties with reading.

During the testing sessions, Joan appeared focused and motivated to do well, and her score on an objective performance validity test was above threshold. It is important to note that clinically significant symptoms of inattention may not be evident in a novel one-on-one testing situation, even when they are clinically significant in other settings. Accordingly, an interview with Joan's teacher revealed her significant difficulties with sustained attention and organization at school, consistent with her parents' report. Ratings on the NICHQ Vanderbilt Assessment Scales, a list of the DSM-5 symptoms for ADHD, from Joan's parents and teacher both met symptom criteria for ADHD—predominantly inattentive subtype. Converging evidence for this diagnosis was provided by the test results. On the easier Vigilance subtest of the Gordon Diagnostic System, Joan performed in the average range. However, on the more difficult Distractibility subtest, her scores fell in the below-average to low-average range. This test (like most CPTs) is somewhat insensitive in adolescents, so while normal scores do not rule out ADHD, weaker scores should be carefully considered. Like Elliot, Joan's test results provide convergent evidence for a weakness in processing speed, with scores on most speeded measures clustering around the low-average range (e.g., WISC-V Processing Speed, Comprehensive Test of Phonological Processing Second Edition [CTOPP-2] Rapid Naming, WIAT-III Math Fluency, D-KEFS Trail Making, timed reading measures). Finally, Joan had notable difficulty on D-KEFS Verbal Fluency (Letter Fluency). This test requires a considerable degree of organization in order to generate a large number of responses. In Joan's case, she named words with no phonological or semantic relation. Joan's poor performance on this test in the context of intact verbal conceptual skills likely reflects difficulties with organization. Relatively weak phonological and orthographic skills may also have played a role.

The other important behavioral observation during testing was that although Joan was an accurate reader, she was notably slow. Her history, test results, and observations suggest that she has mild dyslexia for which she has compensated to some degree. Individuals who receive early and effective interventions can often

TABLE 12.2. Test Summary, Case 7

Performance validity
Medical Symptom Validity Test
    Immediate Recognition   RS = 100
    Delayed Recognition   RS = 100
    Consistency   RS = 100
    Paired Associates   RS = 80
    Free Recall   RS = 60
    (valid)

General intelligence
WISC-V Full Scale IQ   SS = 91

Crystallized intelligence
WISC-V Verbal Comprehension Index   SS = 98
    Similarities   ss = 11
    Vocabulary   ss = 8

Working memory
WISC-V Working Memory Index   SS = 94
    Digit Span   ss = 8
    Picture Span   ss = 10

Processing speed
WISC-V Processing Speed Index   SS = 83
    Coding   ss = 5
    Symbol Search   ss = 9

Fluid intelligence
WISC-V Fluid Reasoning Index   SS = 97
    Matrix Reasoning   ss = 11
    Figure Weights   ss = 8
WISC-V Visual Spatial Index   SS = 105
    Block Design   ss = 10
    Visual Puzzles   ss = 12

Academic

Reading
  History
    CLDQ Reading Scale   92nd %ile

  Basic literacy
    WIAT-III Word Reading   SS = 99
    WIAT-III Pseudoword Decoding   SS = 95
    WIAT-III Spelling   SS = 91

  Reading fluency
    TOWRE-2 Sight Word Efficiency   SS = 83
    TOWRE-2 Phonemic Decoding Efficiency   SS = 81
    GORT-5 Fluency   ss = 6

  Reading comprehension
    GORT-5 Comprehension   ss = 9

Math
  History
    CLDQ Math Scale   66th %ile

  Calculation and problem solving
    WIAT-III Numerical Operations   SS = 94
    Math Problem Solving   SS = 102

  Math fluency
    WIAT-III Math Fluency   SS = 80

Oral language

Phonology
  CTOPP-2 Elision   ss = 9
  CTOPP-2 Phoneme Isolation   ss = 7

Verbal processing speed
  CTOPP-2 Rapid Symbolic Naming   SS = 88

Verbal memory
  CTOPP-2 Nonword Repetition   ss = 8
  WRAML-2 Sentence Memory   ss = 9
  WRAML-2 Story Memory   ss = 10
  WRAML-2 Story Memory Delay   ss = 11

(continued)

TABLE 12.2. (continued)

Attention and executive functions

Attention		Executive functions	
Gordon Vigilance Commissions	42nd %ile	D-KEFS Trail Making Test	
Gordon Vigilance Total Correct	65th %ile	Visual Scanning	ss = 7
Gordon Distractibility Commissions	18th %ile	Number Sequencing	ss = 9
Gordon Distractibility Total Correct	9th %ile	Letter Sequencing	ss = 7
Vanderbilt Inattention		Letter–Number Switching	ss = 9
Parent	RS = 9	D-KEFS Verbal Fluency	
Teacher	RS = 8	Letter Fluency	ss = 5
Vanderbilt Hyperactivity/Impulsivity		Category Fluency	ss = 8
Parent	RS = 1		
Teacher	RS = 2		

Note. GORT-5, Gray Oral Reading Tests—Fifth Edition. For other abbreviations, see Table 12.1.

develop solid reading accuracy and comprehension under untimed conditions, although weaknesses in reading fluency, sounding out unknown words, spelling, and proofreading may persist. This profile is evident in Joan's testing results. Most notably, Joan's scores on timed tests of reading (Test of Word Reading Efficiency–Second Edition [TOWRE-2] and Gray Oral Reading Test–Fifth Edition [GORT-5] Fluency) are much lower than her scores on untimed tests. This pattern is also more broadly consistent with her processing speed weaknesses, as described earlier. Processing speed is a shared weakness for dyslexia and ADHD and helps explain their comorbidity. Joan illustrates this pattern well. She continues to show some evidence of a subtle vulnerability in phonological processing skills (e.g., CTOPP-2 Phoneme Elision), but the pattern is not particularly striking or consistent at this point. A more pronounced phonological weakness might have been evident when Joan was younger, especially before she participated in an evidence-based reading intervention.

Taken together, Joan's diagnosis of ADHD–inattentive type explains the referral concerns regarding sustained attention and organization. In the public media, ADHD has come to be associated with primarily hyperactive behaviors, so parents of children with more inattentive symptoms often do not feel that the diagnosis of ADHD applies to their child. In cases such as these, clarification and education about the subtypes of ADHD are often necessary. Joan also shows residual effects of dyslexia, which continue to impact her reading fluency and contribute to her difficulties in efficiently completing academic work.

Treatment

The American Academy of Child and Adolescent Psychiatry (Pliszka, 2007) and the American Academy of Pediatrics (Wolraich et al., 2011) have published practice parameters on ADHD treatment based on available scientific evidence and clinical consensus. Here, we summarize the main points of those recommendations for school-age children and adolescents with ADHD, noting recommendations that differ for preschoolers with ADHD.

The frontline treatment for children and adolescents with ADHD is psychostimulants that have been approved by the U.S. Food and Drug Administration (FDA) to treat ADHD (Pliszka, 2007; Wolraich et al., 2011). The stimulants contain various forms of methylphenidate or amphetamine. The treatments are available in short-acting medications that must be dosed throughout the day (i.e., Adderall, Dexedrine, Focalin, Ritalin) or long-acting forms (i.e., Concerta, Focalin XR [extended release], Adderall XR, Daytrana patch). The use of psychostimulants to treat ADHD is the most thoroughly researched application of psychopharmacology in child psychiatry. The short-term efficacy and safety of these drugs in treating ADHD has now been well established. About 65 to 75% of children with ADHD show a favorable treatment response with psychostimulant medication, which is one of the largest effects for any psychotropic medication in psychiatry (Pliszka, 2007).

The side effects of psychostimulants are generally mild, especially compared to other psychopharmacological treatments, and usually abate with time and changes in dose. The most common side effects include decreased sleep and appetite, weight loss, jitteriness, stomachaches, and headaches. Earlier concerns about clinically significant growth retardation, precipitation of a tic disorder, increased aggression, increased rates of cardiovascular issues, and increased risk of substance abuse, are not supported by research (Pliszka, 2007). There is nonetheless valid concern about the misdiagnosis of ADHD. Not all practitioners prescribing stimulant medication for ADHD have the time or the training to make this demanding differential diagnosis accurately.

The FDA has also approved three nonstimulants for the treatment of ADHD: Strattera (atomoxetine), Intuniv (guanfacine), and Kapvay (clonidine). These medications generally show smaller effect sizes than stimulants, though their effects are still clinically significant. These alternatives may be useful for children who do not tolerate stimulants well, or for those with comorbidities.

In addition to medication options, there are also psychosocial therapies available for ADHD (Pliszka, 2007). Psychosocial treatments for ADHD mainly consist of behavioral intervention techniques for parents and teachers to help them better manage behavior at home and at school. The parent treatments consist of psychoeducation about the nature of ADHD, learning to implement a behavior plan in the home, including using reinforcements and time out, and working with the school to implement similar behavior plans (i.e., the daily report card). Behavior therapy alone can produce improvements in ADHD symptoms, but effects are generally smaller than those with medication for school-age children and adolescents (Pliszka, 2007). Nevertheless, such treatments are particularly important for children who do not respond to medication or whose parents prefer not to use medication.

In preschoolers, behavior therapy is the recommended frontline treatment, because it has been shown to be efficacious in improving behavior (effect sizes ~0.6) (Charach et al., 2013; Mulqueen, Bartley, & Bloch, 2015; Sonuga-Barke, Daley, Thompson, Laver-Bradbury, & Weeks, 2001; Sonuga-Barke, Thompson, Abikoff, Klein, & Brotman, 2006) and because there is more limited information about efficacy and side effects of stimulants in this younger group of children. Thus, at this time, the weight of the evidence supports behavior therapy as the frontline treatment for preschoolers, though medication is not contraindicated (Charach et al., 2013; Greenhill et al., 2006).

The question naturally arises as to whether the combination of psychostimulant and behavioral interventions would be more efficacious than either alone in school-age children and adolescents. A large study funded by the National Institute of Mental Health (NIMH) addressed this question in school-age children ages 7–9 years with ADHD—combined type. This 3-year multimodal treatment of ADHD study (MTA [Multimodal Treatment Study of Children with ADHD] Cooperative Group, 1999) compared four treatment conditions: medication alone, behavioral intervention alone, a combination of the two, and no treatment beyond what is already typically provided in the community. The behavioral intervention was intensive, involving parent training, school intervention, and summer treatment in a camp setting. The medication management was more intensive than what would typically be provided in a community setting. Subjects were randomly assigned to one of the four conditions and treated for 14 months (MTA Cooperative Group, 1999). At the conclusion of the trial, there was a large main effect of medication treatment on ADHD symptoms, for which the addition of the behavioral intervention produced no added benefit for the core symptoms of ADHD. While the addition of behavioral interventions to medication management did not improve core symptoms of ADHD, it did show modest benefits for some other important areas (i.e., oppositionality, internalizing symptoms, teacher-rated social skills, parent–child relations, and reading achievement (MTA Cooperative Group, 1999).

Other studies have converged with the MTA result showing no additive benefit of combination therapy over medication alone for children with relatively uncomplicated ADHD. However adjunctive behavioral therapy is recommended if the child has a less than optimal response to medication, has a comorbid disorder, or experiences additional family stressors (Pliszka, 2007).

The children in the MTA study have now been followed longitudinally to determine the impact of treatment condition on later ADHD and functional outcomes (Jensen et al., 2007; Molina et al., 2009). Approximately half of the treatment advantage of the medication and medication + behavior groups (compared to behavior only and treatment as usual) had dissipated by 10 months following the completion of the trial (MTA Cooperative Group, 2004). The treatment advantage of these groups had entirely dissipated by 3 years after enrollment (Molina et al., 2009) and this lack of a treatment effect remained stable 6 and 8 years following treatment (Molina et al., 2009). It is important to clarify that all four treatment conditions showed an improvement from baseline, but there was no longer a *differential* treatment effect 3 years after enrollment. Thus, the effects of the intensive MTA treatments attenuated over time. It is possible that continued intensive monitoring of medication and its titration may have led to more sustained benefits of medication, but this is speculative (Molina et al., 2009). In the longitudinal part of the trial, the study has become a naturalistic follow-up, with children and families selecting treatments and providers as usual, so selection effects are important to consider.

One important pattern is that adolescents taking medication (as monitored by community providers) were not showing better outcomes compared to those who were unmedicated. This finding raises an ongoing question in the field regarding the long-term efficacy of stimulant medication. Given their results, the MTA authors recommended that decisions about long-term medication use be made on an individual basis, with ongoing monitoring for efficacy, potentially including discontinuations to empirically test the current impact of medications (Molina et al., 2009). They cautioned that discontinuations may be necessary to avoid the default assumption that the medication is continuing to be helpful.

Another active area of investigation is the potential for cognitive training to reduce ADHD symptoms. The premise of this treatment rests on the idea that cognitive risk factors are causal in ADHD, yet, as we discussed earlier, the evidence for this supposition remains mixed. Cognitive training approaches for ADHD have mainly focused on working memory training. Although early studies of working memory training were promising (Klingberg et al., 2005), recent meta-analyses and reviews of this literature have not been as positive (Kofler et al., 2013; Melby-Lervåg & Hulme, 2013; Simons et al., 2016).

With some exceptions, the general pattern has been for computerized working memory training to lead to improvements in working memory tasks (near-transfer), but not improvements in other cognitive, academic, and behavioral domains (far-transfer) (Kofler et al., 2013; Melby-Lervåg & Hulme, 2013; Melby-Lervåg, Redick, & Hulme, 2016; Simons et al., 2016). Because far-transfer effects have been the most difficult to demonstrate and are the most relevant for quality-of-life improvement, there is more skepticism now about the value of cognitive training than when we published the second edition of this book. This skepticism from the developmental disorders literature has been echoed by researchers in the literature on aging, who published an open letter signed by 70 psychologists and neuroscientists asserting the lack of scientific evidence to support claims that cognitive training could prevent or reverse cognitive decline (Stanford Center on Longevity, 2014), though, as a sign of the ongoing controversy in this field, a group of 133 scientists and therapists countered with another open letter (*www.cognitive-trainingdata.org*).

Simons et al. (2016) reported that these differing impressions of the same literature could be resolved by focusing on both the quantity and quality of the studies in the cognitive training literature. They found that many of the studies had methodological issues in design or analysis that precluded strong conclusions. In fact, none of the peer-reviewed studies met all of their criteria for best practices for these intervention studies. Consistent with previous reviews, Simons et al. (2016) concluded that there is evidence for near transfer, but not far transfer of cognitive training interventions. These discussions crossed over into the policy realm when the U.S. Federal Trade Commission charged a major commercial marketer of cognitive training products, Lumos Labs, with "deceptive advertising." The $50 million judgment was settled with a $2 million fine and an agreement to change marketing practices (Associated Press, 2016). Taken together, the weight of the scientific evidence from the most rigorous studies supports the idea that cognitive training can produce near-transfer effects on the trained task, but does not generalize to real-life cognitive demands (far-transfer effects). This conclusion is consistent across the developmental disorders and aging fields.

Another "high tech" but as yet unsupported treatment for ADHD is neurofeedback (also known as EEG biofeedback). Although positive effects have been reported in some individual studies that did not carefully blind raters of ADHD symptoms or that did not include active/sham conditions, more rigorous study designs do not currently support the efficacy of this intervention (Cortese et al., 2016). Biofeedback has shown positive effects for other disorders, and this remains an active area of research, so it is possible that this conclusion could change in the future. For now, however, since these treatments are generally money- and time-intensive and do not appear to offer substantial clinical benefit, we do not recommend them.

Since the previous edition of this book was published, there has been growing support for a number of lifestyle changes that can help mitigate symptoms of ADHD and improve overall functioning. These have recently been reviewed in an excellent book by Nigg (2017) that is intended primarily for parents and the lay public but provides a lot of guidance for practitioners as well. We next briefly summarize the key points related to exercise, sleep, and nutrition. Because all these are generally low-risk lifestyle supports and likely to convey a variety of benefits for physical and psychological health, it seems sensible to recommend them as part of a comprehensive ADHD treatment plan, even if their effects on core ADHD symptoms will be small for most children.

All children (and adults) benefit from regular, moderate to intense aerobic exercise, which conveys not only physical benefits but also positive effects on EFs, learning, and mood. In addition to these main effects, exercise seems to protect against the deleterious effects of stress (quite possibly through epigenetic changes in the brain; Kashimoto et al., 2016). There are good reasons to expect that exercise may be especially important for children with ADHD, and recent studies indicate positive effects of aerobic exercise on ADHD symptoms that were about half as big as those of stimulant medication (Vysniauske, Verburgh, Oosterlaan, & Molendijk, 2016). Further high-quality work is needed to confirm and extend these findings, but this is clearly a very promising line of inquiry.

In many ways, the story about sleep is similar. Everybody needs adequate sleep to support optimal learning, as well as regulation of attention, mood, and behavior. However, most children and adults in our culture do not get the recommended amount of nightly sleep (roughly 11.5 hours for preschoolers, 10 hours for grade school children, 9 hours for adolescents, and 8 hours for adults). Since ADHD is associated with academic and regulatory problems, adequate sleep is probably even more important for children with the disorder than their typically developing peers, yet children with ADHD are at particularly high risk for insufficient sleep. There is a robust correlation between ADHD and sleep problems, most of which is driven by behavioral issues (i.e., the ADHD symptoms making it difficult for children to follow a nightly routine and settle down to sleep). A minority of children who present with apparent ADHD actually have a primary sleep disorder (e.g., obstructive sleep apnea or restless leg syndrome) that has not been adequately treated. Clinicians who diagnose or treat ADHD should regularly screen for sleep difficulties. If there are symptoms of a primary sleep disorder, the child should be referred for further medical workup. In addition, all children, and especially those with ADHD, should practice good *sleep hygiene,* which includes setting a bedtime/waketime schedule that provides sufficient sleep opportunity and practicing a regular bedtime routine that avoids stimulating activities (including viewing the blue light from screens). When behavioral sleep problems are entrenched, children with ADHD and their parents may need short-term support from a mental health provider to address them.

Questions regarding nutrition and ADHD have a long and controversial history. Early claims that ADHD was caused by excessive sugar or food additives and should therefore be treated with restrictive diets (like the Feingold diet) have generally been disproven (Sonuga-Barke et al., 2013). Nigg (2017) argues that in reaction to these strong early claims, the pendulum has now swung too far in the other direction, and many scientists and clinicians do not recognize that there are several ways in which diet can have an impact on ADHD symptoms. First, sufficient intake of omega-3 fatty acids (through diet or high-quality supplements) may reduce ADHD symptoms by a small but significant amount (Hawkey & Nigg, 2014). Second, it does appear that eating a healthy diet that emphasizes fresh produce, protein, and whole grains, and limits sugar, caffeine, processed foods, additives, and pesticides can cause a small improvement in ADHD symptoms at the group level. This small-group effect also includes large effects for some individual children, who may have food sensitivities or allergies (Nigg & Holton, 2014). Third, a minority of children with ADHD may have deficiencies in certain nutrients such as iron, zinc, or vitamin D (all of which have also been linked to sleep difficulties). For these individuals, appropriate supplementation under the care of a physician can have positive impacts on a variety of outcomes, including ADHD symptoms; however, for the majority of children with ADHD, supplementation with these micronutrients is not indicated (Hariri & Azadbakht, 2015).

In summary, psychostimulant treatment of ADHD is the "gold standard" for school-age children and older. The effect size of psychosocial treatments of ADHD is less strong, although these treatments may be helpful when the child does not respond to psychostimulants, when there are complicating comorbidities, or when there are additional environmental stressors. For preschoolers, psychosocial therapy is the frontline treatment, because it has been found to be effective, and because there is more limited information about effectiveness and side effects of stimulants in this younger population, although stimulants are not currently contraindicated. All children benefit from eating a healthy diet and getting adequate exercise and sleep, and these lifestyle factors may be especially important for children with ADHD. Although lifestyle changes have smaller effects than "gold standard" treatments for core ADHD symptoms for most children, there is mounting evidence that they can be clinically meaningful and should be part of a comprehensive ADHD treatment plan.

Table 12.3 provides a summary of current research and evidence-based practice for ADHD.

TABLE 12.3. Summary Table: Attention-Deficit/Hyperactivity Disorder

Definition

- DSM-5 defines ADHD with two distinct but correlated symptom dimensions, inattention and hyperactivity–impulsivity.
- With two dimensions, there are three possible presentations of ADHD: inattentive, hyperactive–impulsive, or combined.
- Hyperactive–impulsive symptoms are more likely to resolve as the child gets older, whereas inattention symptoms are more stable across development.
- There is better empirical support for the construct validity of the inattentive and combined subtypes than for the hyperactive–impulsive subtype.
- There is a potential fourth presentation of ADHD, sluggish cognitive tempo, which is a reliable construct related to but also partly distinct from inattention symptoms.

Prevalence and epidemiology

- ADHD is one of the most common chronic disorders of childhood. Worldwide prevalence estimates are 2.2% in males and 0.7% in females. These estimates are lower than those typically found in the United States.
- Gender ratios in population samples are 3 males:1 female.
- ADHD is a chronic disorder across the lifespan—two out of three children with ADHD continue to have impairing symptoms in adulthood.
- ADHD is found across social classes, racial and ethnic groups, and countries, but with different prevalence.
- Rates of comorbidity in ADHD are as high as 67%, meaning that only 1 in 3 children have "pure" ADHD.

Developmental neuropsychology

- Multiple cognitive deficit models are needed to explain ADHD.
- Even with multiple deficits, the majority of symptom variance in ADHD remains unexplained.
- Neuropsychological theory has been dominated by three competing single-deficit theories—executive disinhibition, state dysregulation, and delay aversion—but advocates of all three theories have moved to multiple-deficit conceptualizations, as no single deficit accounts for the majority of ADHD cases.
- There may be an emotion dysregulation subtype of ADHD that has been underexplored.
- More research is needed to determine whether cognitive deficits in ADHD are causal, as they may be a consequence of the disorder or merely a correlated manifestation of the disorder.

Brain mechanisms

- Neuroimaging studies of ADHD, as for many other developmental disorders, are increasingly focused on distributed brain mechanisms and dynamic models of brain function.
- The brain mechanisms of ADHD include changes in dopaminergic and noradrenergic neurotransmission that are altered by stimulant medications.
- The frontal–striatal dysfunction hypothesis is supported by structural and functional neuroimaging.
- Current imaging studies are examining the relationship between the default mode network and other cognitive networks in ADHD and suggest maladaptive coupling of these dynamic networks.

Etiology

- ADHD is both familial and heritable. A meta-analysis of over 20 twin studies of ADHD found a mean heritability of .76. This large heritability estimate indicates that ADHD is one of the more heritable complex behavioral disorders.
- Molecular genetic research on ADHD has reflected broader trends in psychiatric genetics, with nonreplications of putative candidate genes and an increasing focus on well-powered GWAS that include tens of thousands of participants with ADHD and controls.
- The first large-scale GWAS of ADHD is currently in preprint and has reported 12 significant loci, which include the genes *FOXP2* and *DUSP6*. Both genes have interesting putative connections to ADHD and its comorbidities.
- Large, rare duplications and deletions of genomic regions (also known as copy number variants [CNVs]) have been implicated in ADHD. Several of the CNV regions associated with ADHD are also implicated in ASD, Schz, and ID, suggesting cross-disorder effects.

(continued)

TABLE 12.3. (continued)

- There are several known bioenvironmental correlates of ADHD. Establishing causality is difficult because of potential G–E correlations.
- There is evidence to support a causal role for low birthweight, fetal alcohol exposure, environmental lead, and pediatric head injury in ADHD. More evidence is needed to determine whether fetal exposure to nicotine is a cause of ADHD.
- Although social environments, such as harsh or inconsistent parenting, undoubtedly influence the course of ADHD, we do not have strong evidence that they are causal.
- There is preliminary evidence for diathesis–stress G × E interactions from both molecular and behavioral genetics studies, but more work is needed to replicate these findings before they are considered robust.

Diagnosis

- Diagnosis is primarily based on interview to establish history, current observations and symptom reports from multiple raters, and the pervasiveness of impairment.
- Symptoms typically present early in the school years, though children whose symptoms are primarily in the attentive domain may not experience impairment until later school grades, when attentional demands increase.
- Symptoms may evolve over time and with task demands, such that in the early school years, frequent talking and getting out of one's seat may be a problem, but in later school grades organization and study skills are challenging.
- ADHD behaviors are not always seen in the clinical setting, which is highly structured and novel.
- Commonly used behavior ratings scales include the Conners Rating Scales, the DuPaul ADHD rating scale, the Disruptive Behavior Rating Scale, the Strengths and Weaknesses of ADHD Symptoms and Normal Behavior Rating Scale (SWAN), and the NICHQ Vanderbilt Assessment Scales.

Treatment

- The frontline treatment for school-age children and adolescents is psychostimulants that have been FDA-approved to treat ADHD. The short-term efficacy and safety of these drugs is well-established; 65–75% of children with ADHD show a favorable treatment response.
- The FDA has approved three nonstimulant medications for the treatment of ADHD. These drugs show smaller effect sizes than stimulants, but their effects are still clinically significant.
- Psychosocial treatment can produce reductions in ADHD symptoms, but effects are generally smaller than those with medication for school-age children and adolescents.
- In school-age children and adolescents, the combination of psychosocial treatment and medication does not show added improvement over medication alone for the core symptoms of ADHD, but combination treatment does show benefits for other academic and behavioral skills.
- In preschoolers, psychosocial treatment is the recommended frontline treatment, because it has been shown to be efficacious, and because there is more limited information about efficacy and side effects of stimulants in this younger group of children.
- Cognitive training for ADHD has shown evidence of near transfer, but not far transfer of skills, leading to skepticism about the utility of this approach.
- Lifestyle changes involving exercise, sleep, and nutrition can have a small but meaningful impact on ADHD symptoms.

CHAPTER 13

Autism Spectrum Disorder

CHAPTER SUMMARY

Since the publication of the previous edition of this book, there have been notable advances in our understanding of autism spectrum disorder (ASD), including a major diagnostic reorganization in DSM-5 and progress across multiple levels of analysis—neuropsychological, neural, and genetic. When any field is growing so rapidly, it can be difficult to extract emerging themes, but we will try to highlight areas of consistency across levels of analysis. One consistent theme in this literature is that study designs have become much more sophisticated, with an emphasis on large samples, longitudinal designs, and replication. These investments in rigorous research designs will be able to support stronger conclusions about the underlying deficits and best practices for assessment and treatment.

At the neuropsychological level of analysis, it has been challenging to develop coherent cognitive theories of ASD that can explain both the social–communication impairments, and repetitive and restricted behaviors. The general consensus that existing theories are not comprehensive has resulted in a move toward multiple-deficit theories, consistent with the theoretical evolution of other learning disorders considered in this book. One theory, the "fractionable autism triad hypothesis" holds that the symptom dimensions of ASD have separate etiologies; therefore, a unifying neurobiological theory will be unlikely. If true, this theory necessitates a multiple-deficit framework to explain the features of ASD, though empirical tests of such multiple-deficit models are just beginning in the ASD literature.

The other major developments in the neuropsychology of ASD have been the findings emerging from high-risk, longitudinal designs. One common research design is for studies to recruit the younger infant siblings of children with ASD. These infants at risk for ASD are then followed longitudinally from infancy. For children who go on to develop ASD, these studies can sensitively identify the onset of the first behavioral manifestations of the disorder. Two findings have been somewhat surprising. First, children who go on to develop ASD are difficult to distinguish from controls at 6 months of age, but behavioral differences emerge by 12 months. Second, regressive patterns in ASD seem to be more common than previously thought. These regressive patterns are generally subtle and can only be detected through detailed, longitudinal observations. In contrast, parent-report measures have trouble detecting the subtle regressions in social–communication skills that the research reveals. Together, these findings suggest a renewed focus on regressive effects in autism and will be important for shaping neuropsychological theory going forward.

Replicated findings in the ASD brain imaging literature have long been elusive (with a few exceptions). This pattern continues, but there are some important markers of progress. The field is currently in the process of reevaluating and refining some of the most well-accepted theories in ASD, such as the early brain overgrowth hypothesis and underconnectivity theories. While this might seem like a step backward, we believe it is a marker of progress, because it speaks to technological and methodological advances that are revealing divergent findings from previous work. The reconciliation of these divergent patterns will be important for theoretical refinement in the field. It is too early to say how the literature will coalesce over time, but we are optimistic that consensus findings will be emerging in the next few years. Based on preliminary findings in the current literature, it seems likely that disruptions in the dynamic connectivity of different brain regions, especially cortical–cortical and cortical–subcortical connections, will be revealing.

There are also calls for the brain imaging literature in ASD to expand its range in terms of developmental questions and populations. For example, connectivity studies have largely neglected development, yet it is likely that there are dynamic changes in connectivity over time. Development is also central to this literature because of important questions about whether observed brain correlates are a cause or a consequence of the disorder. In terms of populations, most of the existing ASD literature focuses on male samples with strong cognitive and language skills, while females and individuals with weaker cognitive and language skills are largely excluded from existing studies. Greater inclusion of the full spectrum of individuals with ASD will be important for future neuroimaging work.

Arguably, the genetic level of analysis for ASD has made the most progress in the past decade. While ASD has long been known to have one of the highest heritability estimates among complex neurodevelopmental disorders, some of the first implicated genes and pathways have emerged from the latest genetic methods in the past few years. Not surprisingly, there is evidence for heterogeneity that is both etiological (different genetic causes leading to similar ASD phenotypes) and phenotypic (same genetic risk leading to different phenotypic manifestations) in ASD. The underlying genetic architecture of ASD likely involves hundreds to thousands of genes. Different types of genetic variants have been implicated, including inherited and newly arising (de novo) genetic variants, and variants that are both common and rare in the population. One of the most exciting developments in the past few years has been the coalescing of implicated genetic risk factors into coherent biological pathways that may increase risk for autism, including WNT and MAPK signaling, synaptic signaling, chromatin remodeling, and fragile X pathways.

While genetic factors are clearly important in the etiology of autism, there are environmental risks as well. Pre- and perinatal environmental factors are being actively researched, including paternal and maternal age, *in utero* valproate exposure, maternal infections, obstetric complications, and extreme environmental deprivation. Strong research designs are needed to establish whether these factors are causal or correlational. Of the environmental risks that are being considered, it is important to emphasize that there is rigorous scientific evidence *against* the hypothesis that the measles, mumps, and rubella (MMR) vaccine or thimerosal-containing vaccines cause ASD.

HISTORY

ASD is the most recently recognized learning disorder. The first descriptions of this syndrome (Asperger, 1944/1991; Kanner, 1943) were published about 70 years ago, whereas other childhood disorders, such as dyslexia and attention-deficit/hyperactivity disorder (ADHD), have been in the scientific literature for over a century. This late recognition in the clinical literature presents us with a puzzle. How did earlier generations regard people with ASD, and what treatments did such people receive? Perhaps part of the answer to this puzzle lies in what is a very recent change in social attitudes toward those with severe developmental disabilities, such as autism and intellectual disability (ID). Not very long ago, such individuals were considered essentially untreatable and were institutionalized very early in life. For individuals with ASD with strong intellectual skills, we can speculate that they did not rise to the level of clinical awareness and likely did not receive supportive services.

Public awareness of autism has increased exponentially in the past few decades. Early media portrayals of ASD focused on narrow portrayals (e.g., *Rain Man*), but more recent portrayals have captured the strengths and weaknesses of individuals across the full spectrum (e.g., the biopic *Temple Grandin;* "Max" on the TV series *Parenthood; Autism: The Musical; Life, Animated*). This more balanced portrayal of the full autism spectrum has been important for public education about the heterogeneity in ASD. In addition to these media portrayals, there are also many useful autobiographies that have served to educate the public and have contributed to an active self-advocacy movement among individuals with ASD (e.g., *Thinking in Pictures: My Life with Autism* by Temple Grandin; *Look Me in the Eye: My Life with Asperger's* by John Elder Robison; *The Journal of Best Practices* by David Finch; *The Reason I Jump: The Inner Voice of a Thirteen-Year-Old Boy with Autism* by Naoki Higashida).

ASD, like many of the disorders considered in this book, has been a projective test for theorists; changes in conceptions of the disorder have reflected changes in more general notions about the nature of psychopathology. As we see later in this chapter, autism is still one of the least well understood learning disorders; therefore, it still has a lot to teach us about errors in our conceptual frameworks.

The term *autism* (from the Greek word *autos*, which means "self") was introduced by Bleuler (1911/1950) to describe a symptom of schizophrenia, namely, extreme self-absorption, leading to a loss of contact with external reality. Partly because Bleuler's term *autism* for a symptom of schizophrenia was chosen as the name for this new syndrome, the two disorders were confused. Autism was originally considered to be just another form of childhood schizophrenia. But it is now clear that these are etiologically distinct disorders, with different developmental courses, despite some symptom overlap.

Both Kanner (1943) and Asperger (1944/1991) selected Bleuler's term *autism* to characterize the extreme lack of social awareness in the children they were describing, whether extreme social isolation without speech (the "lives in a shell" quality), or didactic and tangential speech about an obscure subject (e.g., vacuum cleaners or parking garages) of little interest to the listener. The title of Kanner's paper was "Autistic Disturbances of Affective Contact," and he also spoke of "extreme autistic aloneness" (p. 242). The title of Asperger's (1944/1991) paper was "'Autistic Psychopathy' in Childhood." Other features of the syndrome noted by Kanner (1943) included (1) an "obsessive desire for the maintenance of sameness" (p. 245); (2) a fascination with objects; (3) mutism and other language abnormalities, such as echolalia; (4) normal physical appearance; and (5) evidence of preserved intellectual skill, such as a good rote memory or good performance on spatial tasks. Finally, Kanner, good clinician that he was, noted a high frequency of large head circumferences among his 11 patients. As we discuss later, macrocephaly has been consistently reported in children with ASD, so Kanner may have been prescient in this regard, though these macrocephaly findings are receiving renewed scrutiny (see Brain Imaging section below).

Asperger (1944/1991), in his independent description of his different sample of cases strikingly noted many of the same characteristics, the main differences being the better language skills, unusual specialized interests, and somewhat greater social awareness in Asperger's cases (see discussion in Wing, 1991). Indeed, many authors regard the syndromes described by these two men as two points on the same continuum or spectrum. Other experts believe these are two distinct syndromes. This controversy continues to the present day, with DSM-5 favoring the former explanation. We discuss the data bearing on this decision further below.

Although both Kanner (1943) and Asperger (1944/1991) believed their syndromes were of constitutional origin (and Asperger explicitly hypothesized genetic transmission), psychoanalytic theorists (e.g., Bettelheim, 1967; Mahler, 1952) postulated a psychosocial etiology for autism. Even Kanner himself later adopted this view. The psychoanalytic view held that rejecting "refrigerator" mothers caused these children to withdraw from social interaction, and treatment focused on changing parenting. Although it is possible for very extreme environmental deprivation to produce many of the symptoms of autism (Rutter et al., 2007), it is much less plausible that parental coldness could produce such a devastating developmental outcome. Indeed, these psychosocial theories of autism were based only on clinical observations, not on systematic research. Subsequent research has shown that, on average, mothers of children with autism interact with their children at least as much as, if not more, than mothers of typically developing children, most likely because they are trying to engage them (e.g., Kasari, Sigman, Mundy, & Yirmiya, 1988; Watson, 1998). Since parents of a child with atypical development almost inevitably blame themselves for the problem, these erroneous theories undoubtedly increased their guilt and suffering—a fairly striking example of how clinical ignorance can lead to a violation of the Hippocratic maxim: "First, do no harm."

Rimland (1964), a scientist who was also a parent of a child with autism, was among the first to argue that this disorder is neurological rather than psychosocial in origin. A neurological etiology was supported by the association of autism with late-onset seizures (Schain & Yannet, 1960), and certain genetic conditions, such as untreated phenylketonuria. The publication of the first twin studies of autism in the 1970s also helped to turn the tide against these environmental "refrigerator mother" theories. Folstein and Rutter (1977) published the first twin study of autism that reported a higher autism concordance for identical twins compared to fraternal twins. This and other early twin studies of autism were published at a time when environmental theories prevailed, so they made an important contribution by pointing out that a comprehensive theory of the etiology of autism would need to include genetic factors, which were being neglected at that time. These findings have since been replicated across samples and genetic methods (Ronald & Hoekstra, 2011; Tick, Bolton, Happé, Rutter, & Rijsdijk, 2016). Autism turns out to be one of the most heritable learning disorders, with estimates that are consistent with those obtained for schizophrenia and ADHD. Of course, these estimates are not 100%, so there is still room for environmental influences.

The contemporary view of autism emphasizes its biological origin. Current research is focused on identifying the genetic risk factors, the neurological phenotypes, and the resulting changes in neuropsychological development. At the same time, the psychosocial environment remains very important in the development of individuals with autism. Early interventions have shown that the deficits in social behavior found in autism are much more malleable than was previously thought, and that such interventions might lead to "optimal outcomes" (i.e., moving off the autism spectrum), although such optimal outcomes only occur in a minority of cases (Anderson, Liang, & Lord, 2014; Moulton, Barton, Robins, Abrams, & Fein, 2016). We discuss the intervention research further in the last section of this chapter, "Diagnosis and Treatment."

DEFINITION

In DSM-IV (American Psychiatric Association, 1994), autism and Asperger syndrome fell under the broader category of pervasive developmental disorder (PDD), which also included Rett's disorder, childhood disintegrative disorder, and PDD–not otherwise specified (PDD-NOS). This category was significantly revised in DSM-5 (American Psychiatric Association, 2013). In a recent review, Lord and

Bishop (2014) reviewed the evidence behind each of the significant organizational and diagnostic changes for ASD and the following description draws from their analysis. The first major change was that the umbrella term PDD was changed to ASD, and the diagnostic categories under PDD were merged into a single diagnosis of ASD. Although controversial, this change resulted from data that cast doubt on the reliability of subtype diagnoses (Lord et al., 2012). The removal of the category Asperger syndrome was especially controversial, because individuals had come to identify with and form communities associated with this label. Nevertheless, the empirical evidence indicated that most individuals with an Asperger's diagnosis also met criteria for autism in DSM-IV, yet Asperger syndrome was preferred, because it connoted higher cognitive and language skills. In fact, researchers had difficulty distinguishing individuals with high-functioning autism from those with Asperger's (Bennett et al., 2008; Kamp-Becker et al., 2010; South, Ozonoff, & McMahon, 2005; Woodbury-Smith, Klin, & Volkmar, 2005), suggesting that merging these diagnostic categories would be beneficial for advancing research on individuals with ASD who have average to above average cognitive and language abilities.

This decision best serves the research agenda for ASD, but the specific label of *Asperger's* continues to be used in community settings, and the term continues to be important for the prominent "neurodiversity" movement, led by individuals such as John Elder Robison (i.e., Robison, 2007) The neurodiversity movement has been an important voice for inclusion and has advocated against an exclusive focus on "impairment" in favor of an appreciation of strengths that can make important contributions to the community. The neurodiversity movement's focus on appreciating differences has been a powerful message from the disability rights perspective and has been influential in the mental health and educational communities, and beyond.

A second change to the DSM-5 criteria involved moving from three symptom domains (i.e., social, communication, and restricted, repetitive behaviors [RRBs]) to two domains by combining the social and communication symptoms (i.e., social–communication and RRBs). This change was justified by factor analyses showing that social and communication symptoms consistently formed one factor (e.g., Constantino et al., 2004; Frazier, Youngstrom, Kubu, Sinclair, & Rezai, 2008; Mandy, Charman, & Skuse, 2012). DSM-5 also includes a shift from specific symptoms to broader areas of impairment within social–communication: social–emotional reciprocity; nonverbal communication; and developing, maintaining, and understanding relationships and within RRBs: stereotyped or repetitive motor movements; insistence on sameness; restricted, fixated interests; and hyper- or hyporeactivity to sensory input or unusual sensory interests. Each of the broad areas of impairment maps fairly directly to DSM-IV symptoms (Lord & Bishop, 2014) with two exceptions. First, sensory reactivity and sensory interests were added as a domain to RRBs. Second, delayed language acquisition and failure to use verbal language are no longer symptoms of ASD for reasons that we discuss further below. Other than these changes, the organizational change of specifying areas of impairment rather than symptom lists allows for clinical judgment in adapting to contextual variables that influence the manifestation of social behavior, including gender, culture, age, and developmental stage.

A third change is that the age-of-onset criterion was removed entirely. Previously in DSM-IV, an autism diagnosis required an age of onset before age 3 years, with a later age of onset allowed for a diagnosis of PDD-NOS. This change is partly in response to several prospective, longitudinal studies of infant siblings of children with autism that have helped to map the behavioral trajectories of children who will receive a diagnosis of ASD (i.e., Ozonoff et al., 2010). Such careful studies have led to the distinction of the terms *age of onset* and *age of recognition*, since subtle behavioral differences are evident by 12 months between infants who will and will not later receive an ASD diagnosis (Ozonoff et al., 2010). This distinction, coupled with the fact that age of recognition is dependent on contextual and environmental factors, such as race, ethnicity, gender, and socioeconomic status (SES), and the fact that parents' reports of developmental milestones can be inaccurate (Hus, Taylor, & Lord, 2011; Jones, Gliga, Bedford, Charman, & Johnson, 2014; Ozonoff, Iosif, et al., 2011), makes diagnosing subtypes of ASD based on age of onset an untenable task.

A fourth change from DSM-IV is the addition of modifiers that reflect the most common comorbidities of ASD. First, DSM-5 permits diagnosis of ADHD along with ASD. Modifiers for comorbidities with ID and language disorder are also specified. For example, the DSM-IV diagnosis of Asperger's disorder would now be specified as ASD without accompanying intellectual or language impairment. These particular modifiers for intellectual and language impairment are particularly important, because they continue to be the best predictors of later outcome (Howlin, Goode, Hutton, & Rutter, 2004; Sallows & Graupner, 2005). Finally, a fifth change from DSM-IV is that Rett's disorder was dropped, because it can now be defined genetically, so diagnosis no longer needs to rely on behavioral criteria.

Because the ASD diagnosis now requires at least two RRBs, there was concern about children who were previously diagnosed as PDD-NOS because they had social and communication impairments, but not RRBs. Would these children not meet criteria for any diagnosis in DSM-5? The existing data suggest that this problem would not affect many children, as most children with a PDD-NOS diagnosis also had at least a history of RRBs (Lord, Petkova, et al., 2012; Lord et al., 2006). Nevertheless, a new diagnosis of "social (pragmatic) communication disorder" (SCD) was created to address this problem and is grouped with the language disorders. This new diagnosis requires further research, including studies on reliability and validity of assessment measures, well-controlled studies of intervention approaches, and studies of the diagnostic overlap with the full range of neurodevelopmental disorders, including ASD (i.e., Gibson et al., 2013). We also discuss SCD in Chapter 9.

One question about the DSM-5 changes is how they will affect the prevalence of ASD. This question remains controversial, with some studies suggesting that rates are fairly stable (Frazier et al., 2012; Huerta, Bishop, Duncan, Hus, & Lord, 2012) and others suggesting a potential decrease, particularly among individuals with stronger intellectual skills or milder severity (Maenner et al., 2014; McPartland, Reichow, & Volkmar, 2012).

PREVALENCE AND EPIDEMIOLOGY

The increasing prevalence of autism is now regularly discussed in the popular media, as well as the scientific literature. The Centers for Disease Control and Prevention (CDC; 2009, 2012, 2014; Baio et al., 2018; D. Christensen et al., 2016) has released statistics indicating a rate of 1 in 110 children in surveillance year 2006, 1 in 88 in surveillance year 2008, 1 in 68 children in surveillance years 2010 and 2012, and 1 in 59 children in surveillance year 2014 for children age 8 years. These CDC studies rely on education and health records in several states to detect diagnosed cases of ASD, rather than "gold-standard" diagnostic practices using the Autism Diagnostic Interview–Revised (ADI-R) and Autism Diagnostic Observation Schedule–Second Edition (ADOS-2) (see "Diagnosis and Treatment" for more information on these measures). Because these CDC studies did not directly diagnose a random population sample, one can expect that rates would vary according to educational and child health practices in different states, and indeed they did. The highest rates in the most recent CDC report were found in New Jersey (29.3 per 1,000 children) and the lowest rates in Arkansas (13.1 per 1,000 children). Although bioenvironmental risk factors could vary across states, it seems much more likely that the state differences reflect detection differences and not true differences. Moreover, it might also be the case that specific states are known for their autism services, so families move to take advantage of these resources.

A common question both in the lay media and the scientific literature concerns whether rates are *actually* increasing or whether better detection and changes in diagnostic criteria and/or diagnostic substitution are accounting for these increases. In support of the broadening of the diagnostic criteria, previous research indicates that a substantial portion of the increase in prevalence rates is accounted for by children with ASD without ID (D. Christensen et al., 2016; King & Bearman, 2009), suggesting that these children are being identified at higher rates. Additionally, relevant to diagnostic substitution, it is also the case that autism diagnoses are being given to children who, in the past, would have received a diagnosis of ID (King & Bearman, 2009; Polyak, Kubina, & Girirajan, 2015; Shattuck, 2006) or developmental language disorder (Bishop, Whitehouse, Watt, & Line, 2008).

There is also persuasive evidence for better detection. For example, Lundstrom, Reichenberg, Anckarsäter, Lichtenstein, and Gillberg (2015) conducted a study of more than 1 million individuals from the Swedish national patient register. The authors showed that the rates of autism diagnoses increased steadily over a 10-year period from 1993 to 2002. However, using a population-based sample of nearly 20,000 twins, who were tracked over the same period, the authors showed that the twins' autism symptoms, on average, did not increase over that 10-year period. Thus, while autism diagnoses increased over the decade in question, the prevalence of autism symptoms in the population did not change (Lundstrom et al., 2015). This pattern of results argues persuasively for changes in diagnostic practice rather than a true increase in autism symptomatology in the population.

Thus, there is empirical evidence that better detection, broadened diagnostic criteria, and diagnostic substitution are all contributing to these rates. What is not known conclusively is whether these phenomena can account for the entire diagnostic increase, or whether there is still a small rise in prevalence after accounting for these factors.

Even in the midst of these diagnostic increases, it remains the case that diagnostic disparities persist. For example, females with ASD are more likely to be missed (Frazier, Georgiades, Bishop, & Hardan, 2014; Giarelli et al., 2010), and black and Hispanic children, and children from less advantaged backgrounds are also being underidentified (D. Christensen et al., 2016; Mandell & Palmer, 2005; Mandell et al., 2009). These disparities have been attributed to reduced and delayed access to treatment and services (D. Christensen et al., 2016).

The gender ratio in autism is reported to be in the range of 3–4.5:1 (male:female) (Christensen et al., 2016). The reasons for these gender differences are unknown, but a possible "female protective effect" has been reported (Robinson, Lichtenstein, Anckarsäter, Happé, & Ronald, 2013).

Comorbidities

Children with ASD are at risk for multiple comorbidities, most notably ID, language impairment, ADHD, and anxiety disorders. Approximately one-third of individuals with ASD have comorbid ID (Christensen et al., 2016). In the past, this comorbidity was estimated at 50–75%, which speaks to the broadening diagnostic definition of ASD and to the earlier identification and referral to treatment that now occurs. Comorbidity with language impairment is also quite common (Kjelgaard & Tager-Flusberg, 2001). The language phenotypes of children with ASD are also quite diverse and range from children who are minimally verbal (Tager-Flusberg & Kasari, 2013) to children without any structural language difficulties, though pragmatic difficulties are universal. Approximately 30% of individuals with ASD are reported to be minimally verbal (Tager-Flusberg & Kasari, 2013). A consistent finding across a number of studies is that higher IQ and the presence of some communicative speech before age 5 are the best early predictors of a more favorable outcome (Eaves & Ho, 2008; Howlin et al., 2004; Howlin & Moss, 2012).

Before DSM-5, the diagnosis of ASD precluded a diagnosis of ADHD, though there was wide recognition of symptoms of inattention and overactivity that were common in ASD. DSM-5 now permits a comorbid diagnosis of ASD and ADHD, and this comorbidity is an active area of research. This change reflects the high, but not universal, comorbidity between the disorders (estimates from community samples that approximately 1 in 3 children with ASD also have ADHD) (Leitner, 2014; Leyfer, Woodruff-Borden, Klein-Tasman, Fricke, & Mervis, 2006; Simonoff et al., 2008).

Finally, anxiety disorders are quite common in ASD, with estimates reaching as high as 40–50% of individuals with a comorbid anxiety disorder, though these estimates are based on a mix of community-based and clinically referred samples (for reviews, see MacNeil, Lopes, & Minnes, 2009; van Steensel, Bögels, & Perrin,

2011; S. White, Oswald, Ollendick, & Scahill, 2009). Obsessive–compulsive disorder (OCD) is also common in individual with ASD, though the differential diagnosis can be difficult because of the RRBs characteristic of ASD, and because of limited insight to describe whether there are accompanying obsessions.

There are also several medical genetic disorders with well-known etiologies that are associated with a higher risk of autism. The two strongest associations are with tuberous sclerosis and fragile X syndrome (Bailey, Phillips, & Rutter, 1996). Both of these associations can shed light on etiological pathways to ASD. For instance, in the case of fragile X syndrome, recent reports indicate significant overlap between autism-related genetic signals and gene sets consisting of fragile X mental retardation protein (*FMRP*) and the more than 800 genes known to interact with *FMRP* (Iossifov et al., 2012; Samocha et al., 2014). These results point to a specific etiological explanation for the comorbidity of fragile X syndrome and autism.

DEVELOPMENTAL NEUROPSYCHOLOGY

In the previous chapters on specific disorders in Part II of this book, we have reviewed typical development in the impaired domains associated with the disorder. For ASD, we have chosen to forgo this review of typical development, because it is less clear what the specific impaired domain(s) would be in ASD. However, Chapter 9 provides a review of the typical development of both nonverbal and verbal communication that is relevant for understanding the development of autism. Early social development is impaired in ASD, but exactly which aspects are affected remains unclear. Because neuropsychological theory in ASD is arguably less sophisticated than that for many other learning disorders discussed in this book, we focus on challenges for current theories and new ideas and research designs that are leading to further theoretical refinements.

One prominent challenge for neuropsychological theories of ASD is that there are two symptom dimensions, social–communication and RRBs, to explain. To date, there is no consensus cognitive theory of ASD that can explain both symptoms domains (Happé, Ronald, & Plomin, 2006). As a result, neuropsychological theory in ASD has begun to include more multiple-deficit conceptualizations (Happé & Ronald, 2008; Happé et al., 2006; Mandy & Skuse, 2008), consistent with the other learning disorders discussed in this book. Less progress has been made in testing a multiple-deficit model of ASD than in the case of reading disability (RD) and ADHD. Only a handful of studies have empirically tested a multiple-deficit model (e.g., Best, Moffat, Power, Owens, & Johnstone, 2008), though there have been calls for such an approach (e.g., Brunsdon & Happé, 2014). In the neuropsychological review that follows we discuss some of the historically important neuropsychological theories and continue with a new conceptualization of ASD that aligns with the multiple-deficit framework, the fractionable autism triad hypothesis. We end with a discussion of the important contributions of high-risk longitudinal designs to the evolution of neuropsychological theory in ASD.

Neuropsychological Theories of Autism

A successful neuropsychological theory of autism must account for both the social phenotype and RRBs that define the disorder, as well as other features of the disorder, such as comorbidities with language impairment and ID, and the uneven profile of cognitive abilities. The hypothesized primary neuropsychological deficit must also (1) be present before the onset of the disorder, hence very early in development; (2) be pervasive among individuals with the disorder; and (3) be specific to autism. This is a tall order, and there is good agreement among autism researchers that no current neuropsychological theory of autism meets all these criteria (Bailey et al., 1996; Brunsdon & Happé, 2014). Most of the existing theories have approached this problem from a single-deficit perspective, in which a single deficit is hypothesized to account for the full autism phenotype, and each theory has experienced challenges in doing so. While there are breakthroughs happening at the genetic and brain levels of analysis for ASD, it is notable that one of the most striking observations at the neuropsychological level of analysis is that the field is moving away from theories that have been important for past conceptualizations of ASD, because they have failed one or more of the requirements just mentioned.

Historically, the neuropsychological theories of ASD could be grouped into "social" and "nonsocial" theories. The most prominent and longest standing social theory focused on theory of mind (Baron-Cohen, Leslie, & Frith, 1985, 1986; Baron-Cohen et al., 2000). In addition to theory of mind, other social theories focused on social motivation, social orienting, joint attention, imitation, face processing, empathy, and aspects of emotional expression. Some of these deficits, such as those in social orienting and joint attention, are present early in the development of the disorder (Dawson, Webb, Carver, Panagiotides, & McPartland, 2004; Osterling & Dawson, 1994), whereas others (i.e., theory of mind) cannot be measured until later in development. Social theorists took the approach that social deficits are primary, and other manifestations of ASD are downstream effects. Since a great deal of human development depends on social transmission, a child with social impairments would miss much of the input necessary for typical development. Some of the deficits in autism (e.g., in language and IQ) could be seen as secondary to this missing input. While missing this typical input, some individuals with autism may "specialize" in learning other things about the environment, which could explain the savant skills and intense, unusual interests that are sometimes found in this disorder.

The "nonsocial" theories focused on accounting for the restricted and repetitive behaviors and unusual cognitive profiles that are often seen in ASD. The most well-researched and longest standing nonsocial theories were the executive dysfunction theories (Landry & Bryson, 2004; Ozonoff, Pennington, & Rogers, 1991; Russell, 1997; Russell, Jarrold, & Henry, 1996; Wallace et al., 2016). In these theories, limitations in specific cognitive skills, especially attention and executive functions, were hypothesized to interfere with normative social interactions that would then have downstream effects for social development. One example would be a child who has difficulty with cognitive flexibility that interferes with his or her ability to engage in social and play interactions with other children, perhaps because of excessive "rule following" or difficulty with transitions.

In most cases, the social and nonsocial theories were single-deficit conceptualizations of ASD that encountered limitations in explaining both the social and RRB dimensions of the disorder or failed to meet the criteria (discussed earlier) for a neuropsychological theory of ASD. While the theories were often accurate in their descriptions of social and cognitive skills that are impaired in children with ASD, they could not provide a comprehensive neuropsychological explanation of the disorder.

Hence, as discussed earlier in Chapter 4, providing a unifying explanation of all the changes in behavioral development in ASD will likely require us to move beyond neuropsychology to a neurocomputational level of analysis that is tied more closely to the brain mechanisms of this disorder. As we discuss in Chapter 14, we face a similar problem for neuropsychology in trying to explain ID.

Fractionable Autism Triad Hypothesis

In recent years, there has been a reexamination of the assumption that there will be a single unifying explanation for the symptom dimensions of ASD that can be traced across levels of analysis from genetics to brain to cognition and behavior. As an alternative hypothesis, Happé and Ronald (2008) presented the "fractionable autism triad hypothesis," arguing that the three symptom dimensions of ASD from DSM-IV—socialization, communication, RRBs—may have separate etiologies; therefore, a unifying neurobiological theory is unlikely. The first line of evidence to explore in relation to the fractionable autism triad hypothesis is at the behavioral level—whether the symptom dimensions of autism cluster together in population samples. If it is common for individuals in the population to show symptoms associated with one domain and not others, this finding would call into question the existence of a unifying neurobiological cause of autism. One relevant dataset addressing this point comes from the Twins Early Development Study (TEDS) in the United Kingdom (Oliver & Plomin, 2007). This is a longitudinal, population sample of twins where the symptom domains of autism have been measured with the Childhood Asperger Syndrome Test (CAST). Surprisingly, correlations among all three core domains have been quite low (r's = .1–.4) (Ronald, Happé, Bolton, et al., 2006; Ronald, Happé, & Plomin, 2005; Ronald, Happé, Price, Baron-Cohen, & Plomin, 2006). These behavioral correlations have been supported by unexpectedly low genetic correlations among the triad dimensions as well (Happé & Ronald, 2008) reviewed later in "Etiology."

An important insight emerging from the fractionable autism triad hypothesis is that the coherence of the autism symptom dimensions might be weaker than has been presumed over the past few decades of ASD research (Happé & Ronald, 2008). If so, this hypothesis requires that neuropsychological theory will have to explain both why social impairments and RRBs cluster together in ASD, and why these dimensions are relatively independent in population samples.

Longitudinal High-Risk Studies

The challenges inherent in developing a comprehensive neuropsychological theory of ASD have led to a greater appreciation for the developmental unfolding of ASD symptoms. In the past, it was common to use school-age samples of children with ASD in which it was difficult to work out the deficit(s) that are primary and secondary (Elsabbagh & Johnson, 2016). As a result, the field has turned to longitudinal studies of infants at high risk for autism. Although this is a new evolution in the ASD field, there have already been important insights, though a complete explanation of the neuropsychology of autism remains elusive.

The most popular high-risk design has been for studies to recruit later-born infant siblings of children with ASD (for reviews, see Jones et al., 2014; Yirmiya & Charman, 2010; Zwaigenbaum, Bryson, & Garon, 2013). These infant siblings are then followed prospectively beginning as early as 6 months and continuing through the toddler years and beyond (Landa & Garrett-Mayer, 2006; Landa, Gross, Stuart, & Faherty, 2013; Ozonoff et al., 2010; M. Sullivan et al., 2007; Zwaigenbaum et al., 2005). One important insight emerging across several high-risk samples is the finding that group differences are minimal to nonexistent at 6 months of age between infants who will go on to develop ASD and those who will not (Landa et al., 2013; Ozonoff et al., 2010). Of course, these conclusions are limited to behaviors that can be measured at 6 months, such as social orienting and social–communication skills, motor skills, early language skills, temperament, and repetitive behaviors, but it is still remarkable to note that behavioral group differences are difficult to find at 6 months (Jones et al., 2014; Zwaigenbaum et al., 2013). These null results in the first 6 months challenge some social theories of autism, including the imitation and emotion theories, because, as reviewed in Chapter 9, both imitation and emotional exchanges appear very early in typical infant development.

Group differences start to emerge by 12 months for most of the behavioral domains that have been measured. Taking social orienting and social–communication behaviors as an example, Ozonoff et al. (2010) found that gaze to faces, directed vocalizations, and social smiles all showed declining trajectories in the ASD group, whereas the typically developing group showed stable or increasing trajectories for these behaviors from ages 6 to 36 months. These diverging patterns resulted in significant group differences by 12 months for gaze to faces and directed vocalizations, and by 18 months for social smiles, and these group discrepancies continued to widen over time (Ozonoff et al., 2010). These observations call into question the idea first advanced by Kanner (1943) that behavioral signs of ASD are present at birth. In terms of early identification, these results suggest that children with ASD will be more readily distinguished from typically developing and developmentally delayed children in the second year of life (Zwaigenbaum et al., 2013).

Examination of the developmental trajectories in these prospective studies has raised questions about onset subtypes. Traditionally, the early-onset pattern has been thought to be the dominant subtype, with a regressive pattern of onset occurring in about 20% of children (Fombonne, 2001; Lingam et al., 2003). In a third pattern that has also been observed, neither early signs of autism nor regression are present, a pattern known as "developmental plateau" (Hansen et al., 2008; Ozonoff, Heung, Byrd, Hansen, & Hertz-Picciotto, 2008). These previous studies have primarily relied on retrospective parent report, which has several limitations. Prospective studies provide a much stronger design to examine the unfolding of developmental trajectories. In a recent longitudinal, high-risk design, Ozonoff et al. (2010) reported that a surprisingly high 86% of infants who would go on to develop ASD by 36 months experienced a decline in social–communication skills that was unexpected in relation to the typically developing sample. This high rate was contrasted with the fact that only about 20% of parents reported a regression in skills (Ozonoff et al., 2010). This pattern suggests that regression may be more common in ASD than was previously thought, but that this regression is difficult to detect in "real time," so parents' report of regression does not provide a full picture. Given that these parents already have a child with ASD and are likely to be highly informed about ASD-related behaviors, it is striking that parent-report of regression and prospective observations diverged so drastically (Ozonoff et al., 2010). Part of the reason for this discrepancy may be that the losses in social–communication skills were relatively subtle and gradual, making them difficult to detect without the benefit of longitudinal observations from ASD experts (Ozonoff et al., 2010). These results call into question the validity of parent-report measures of regression and suggest that regressive effects in ASD may be far more common than previously thought.

Ozonoff et al. (2010) suggest that the existing categories for onset patterns need revision in light of new data from these prospective studies. They suggest a shift from categorical to continuous definitions of onset. In this model, one anchor of the continuum would be children who experience regression so early that symptoms seem to have been stably present, and the other end of the continuum is anchored by children who experience regression so late that their loss of skills is particularly notable because they had more skills to lose. More work on the regressive patterns in ASD will be needed to understand this important dimension of heterogeneity in the ASD phenotype and will be important for further genetic and neurobiological studies that depend on homogeneous endophenotypes.

Taken together, the high-risk prospective design in ASD has already advanced the literature in terms of understanding the age at which ASD behaviors first manifest and the typical developmental trajectory. The discovery of widespread regression in social–communication in young children with ASD presents an additional challenge for neuropsychological theories of this disorder to explain. Further studies at the neuropsychological level will be necessary to understand the earliest detectable deficits and the developmental unfolding of these deficits that leads to the full ASD phenotype. Such studies could inform early intervention approaches that target the earliest weaknesses and could interrupt the developmental cascade leading to ASD.

BRAIN MECHANISMS

As was seen previously in the section on neuropsychology, there is no consensus, singular cognitive correlate of ASD that can explain the full symptom profile of the disorder, including the social–communication and restricted and repetitive behaviors. We echo this challenge in this section on brain mechanisms, in which there is similarly no consensus brain correlate of ASD that can explain both symptom domains. Still, the literature has advanced considerably in the past 10 years, as marked by larger samples and a greater emphasis on replication. Several well-accepted theories, the early brain overgrowth hypothesis, and underconnectivity theories are undergoing a process of reevaluation and refinement in light of technological and methodological advances, which is a promising marker of progress in the field.

This section includes studies of brain structure and function and connectivity in ASD. Although group differences have been found across neuroimaging modalities, the list of well-replicated findings is very short (Pua, Bowden, & Seal, 2017). It is proposed that etiological heterogeneity has contributed to the mixed findings in the neuroimaging literature. One major area of research is focused on defining more homogeneous phenotypic subgroups of individuals with ASD in order to pinpoint specific neurobiological correlates (i.e., Ecker, 2017). In addition to etiological sources of heterogeneity, sample differences in terms of age and IQ, as well as variation in neuroimaging equipment, methodology, and analysis, also seem to be contributing to difficulties with replication (Pua et al., 2017).

Given these significant sources of variation, increased reliance on meta-analyses and multisite validation and replication studies are critical to progress in the field. This section will draw from several recent meta-analyses and systematic reviews to highlight a few key findings across different neuroimaging modalities: structural, functional, and connectivity studies. A comprehensive review is beyond the scope of this chapter, but the reader is referred to several recent reviews for a fuller discussion (Ecker, 2017; Ecker & Murphy, 2014; Elsabbagh & Johnson, 2016; Hull et al., 2017; Li, Karnath, & Xu, 2017; Mohammad-Rezazadeh, Frohlich, Loo, & Jeste, 2016; Picci, Gotts, & Scherf, 2016; Pua et al., 2017; Rane et al., 2015; Sacco, Gabriele, & Persico, 2015; Yerys & Herrington, 2014). It is also important to note that the existing neuroimaging research tends to focus on male samples with stronger intellectual skills, while female individuals with ASD who have comorbid ID, or who are minimally verbal, are significantly understudied, and there have been recent calls for greater inclusion of individuals from the full spectrum of ASD (Ecker, 2017; Jack & Pelphrey, 2017).

Structural Findings

Historically, one of the best-replicated structural findings has been macrocephaly in about 15–20% of ASD cases (Herbert, 2005; Sacco et al., 2015). As mentioned earlier, Kanner's (1943) original case report noted enlarged head circumferences in 5 of 11 children. This clinical observation has been affirmed by meta-analyses of head circumference and brain size in individuals with ASD (reviewed in Redcay & Courchesne, 2005; Sacco et al., 2015). What change in brain development produces this macrocephaly and how it relates to brain function are currently unknown, though the WNT signaling pathway has recently been implicated through genetic studies (discussed in "Etiology" below). The overgrowth seems to be due to a combination of both grey and white matter, but there are ongoing questions about whether grey or white matter predominate and at which ages (i.e., Hazlett et al., 2005; Redcay & Courchesne, 2005; Sparks et al., 2002).

The emergence of macrocephaly is notable for its unusual developmental trajectory. A meta-analysis of brain size in ASD indicated that, on average, the brains of individuals with ASD are actually slightly smaller at birth, but there is a dramatic period of overgrowth during the first year of life, which then plateaus (Redcay & Courchesne, 2005). As a result, by adulthood, the brain size of most individuals with ASD is within normal limits, because typically developing individuals have "caught up" (Redcay & Courchesne, 2005). This trajectory reveals significant deviations from the normative trajectory for brain growth (Lenroot & Giedd, 2006).

This trajectory in ASD samples has come to be known as the *early brain overgrowth* (EBO) hypothesis. Although this developmental pattern has been replicated by two meta-analyses, a recent paper raises important methodological issues related to the norming of head circumference in typically developing children and calls into question the EBO hypothesis (Raznahan et al., 2013). The authors demonstrate through a systematic review and an analysis of new data that a norming bias may be responsible for the developmental trajectory noted earlier. Two pieces of evidence are most compelling: (1) that a large percentage of typically developing children show the EBO pattern when the questioned norms are used, and (2) that the most rigorous studies using longitudinal, case–control designs studies, which do not depend on norms, find inconsistent support for the EBO hypothesis. Those studies that do find a positive association have a much smaller effect size than in the previous literature and show a later onset of overgrowth during the second year of life (Raznahan et al., 2013). Taken together, the literature regarding the effect size and timing of macrocephaly in ASD has come into question in recent years. Longitudinal case–control studies in epidemiological samples will be necessary to reconcile these conflicting findings (Raznahan et al., 2013). Such work will be important, because defining the timing of brain overgrowth, if it indeed exists, could shed light on disrupted neurodevelopmental mechanisms.

As in the neuropsychological literature, one useful study design that is now being employed to better understand the developmental trajectory of brain growth in ASD is the high-risk family design. A recent study of "high-risk" infant siblings revealed that those who go on to be diagnosed with ASD at 24 months showed "hyperexpansion" of the cortical surface area from ages 6–12 months compared to undiagnosed high-risk siblings and low-risk controls, but no expansion of cortical thickness (Hazlett et al., 2017). The fact that the patterns for cortical surface area and thickness diverge is not too surprising, since cortical surface area and cortical thickness are thought to have distinct cellular and genetic mechanisms (Panizzon et al., 2009; Rakic, 1995). The expansion of cortical surface area in the high-risk ASD siblings was associated with later brain overgrowth in the second year and social deficits (Hazlett et al., 2017). The authors took their findings a step further in developing a machine learning algorithm that used structural brain measurements, especially cortical surface area, at 6 and 12 months to predict ASD diagnosis at 24 months, with 88% sensitivity and 95% specificity (Hazlett et al., 2017). This predictive model based on early brain imaging exceeds the predictive power of existing behavioral algorithms (Chawarska et al., 2014), suggesting that early brain imaging may be clinically useful in early detection efforts (Hazlett et al., 2017). Nevertheless, such clinical translation efforts will require systematic replication and limit testing of the predictive algorithms, particularly in real-world clinical settings in which family history is complicated or unknown, and comorbidity is pervasive.

Structural neuroimaging studies of ASD have also examined whether there are region-specific structural differences in ASD compared to controls. This discussion focuses on the limbic system and frontal–striatal circuity, which have been associated with the social–communication deficits and repetitive behaviors, respectively, that characterize ASD (Ecker, 2017). A host of region-specific volumetric changes in ASD have been reported, though, as in the rest of the neuroimaging literature, findings are generally mixed, and it is difficult to discern patterns (Ecker, 2017; Sacco et al., 2015). Relevant to limbic system, volumetric analyses of the amygdala reveal that it is enlarged relative to controls in some but not all studies (Aylward et al., 1999; Nordahl et al., 2012; Schumann et al., 2004) and that larger increases are associated with more impairment in social–communication skills (Schumann, Barnes, Lord, & Courchesne, 2009). Age seems to be one important factor in the amygdala findings as only young children with ASD show enlargement (Sacco et al., 2015).

In the frontal–striatal system, it has also been shown that individuals with ASD have enlargements in the caudate nucleus, and that this enlargement is related to the severity of repetitive behaviors (Langen et al., 2014; Langen, Durston, Staal, Palmen, & van Engeland, 2007). The connection of these enlargements to symptom dimensions gives important insight into the neural underpinnings of the constellation of ASD symptoms. It is also important to note that disruptions in the limbic and frontal–striatal system are by no means unique to autism (Ecker, 2017). For example, individuals with anxiety disorders have also been reported to have an enlarged amygdala (De Bellis et al., 2000) and the frontal–striatal system has been implicated in ADHD and OCD (Cubillo, Halari, Smith, Taylor, & Rubia, 2012; Marsh, Maia, & Peterson, 2009), among other psychiatric disorders. So an important long-term goal of this literature will be to distinguish neuroimaging correlates that are general to developmental psychopathologies and specific to ASD.

Functional Findings

Task-based functional magnetic resonance imaging (fMRI) studies have typically investigated the two distinct ASD symptom domains separately. The social–communication symptom domain has been explored with tasks targeting social cognition. RRBs have typically not been investigated directly, but because of their association with executive functioning (EF) skills, tasks targeting cognitive control or other executive skills have been hypothesized to be especially relevant to this symptom domain (Pennington & Ozonoff, 1996). In addition, some fMRI studies have used tasks tapping into motor, visual, and language processing. To date, there is no single functional brain correlate of ASD that can explain both of the core symptom domains (Dichter, 2012), so the following discussion focuses separately on the most prominent findings for social processing and cognitive control.

In the social-cognitive domain, face-processing tasks have received the most attention, with a particular focus on the fusiform gyrus, which plays a critical role in face processing. One of the most consistent findings has been underactivation of the fusiform gyrus when viewing faces and facial expressions. Three recent meta-analyses have identified a cluster in the left (and, in some studies, bilateral) fusiform gyrus that shows hypoactivation in functional imaging studies of face processing in ASD compared to controls (Di Martino et al., 2009; Nickl-Jockschat et al., 2015; Nusslock et al., 2012). These meta-analyses illustrate the robustness of the finding, but there have been a few theoretically important failures to replicate this effect, such as when the participant views familiar faces (i.e., Pierce, Haist, Sedaghat, & Courchesne, 2004; Pierce & Redcay, 2008) or when attention is cued to the face (i.e., Hadjikhani et al., 2004).

Although these findings appear contradictory, they might be reconciled by a consideration of the specific experimental paradigm, especially demands on visual attention (Dichter, 2012). Attention to the face might be particularly important in the case of strangers' faces, but less so when the face is familiar or when attention is explicitly cued. In this case, the fusiform gyrus might be deactivated in ASD when an individual views a stranger's faces but not when viewing familiar faces or when his or her attention is explicitly directed to a face. This explanation suggests that the fusiform hypoactivation might be a consequence of how individuals with ASD choose to attend to novel faces rather than a mechanistic cause of their social deficits. Careful longitudinal, functional imaging studies of face processing would be necessary to shed further light on this hypothesis. However, this hypothesis does raise an important point for all brain imaging modalities: the issue of whether the observed brain correlates are a cause or consequence of the disorder. This issue is particularly salient for functional studies of social cognition in ASD, since the experience of living with ASD is associated with reduced social experience that can have consequences for brain development. Only with longitudinal functional imaging studies can the field begin to tease apart the temporal precedence of brain–behavior relationships in ASD.

The functional imaging literature has also focused on EF tasks because of their association with RRBs in ASD (Pennington & Ozonoff, 1996). Typical tasks require working memory, inhibition, interference control, and/or shifting abilities—all skills broadly falling under the umbrella of EF. Comparisons of ASD groups to controls have identified functional differences in frontal regions (most notably the dorsolateral prefrontal cortex and dorsal anterior cingulate cortex) and frontal–striatal regions (Di Martino et al., 2009; Dichter, 2012), which are both important neural substrates for EFs in typically developing individuals. The directionality of the effects has been mixed, however, with some researchers reporting hyperactivation and others reporting hypoactivation of these regions (Di Martino et al., 2009; Dichter, 2012). More work is needed to discern patterns that are unique to specific

EF dimensions and to examine how functional abnormalities in frontal and frontal–striatal regions relate to behavioral manifestations of RRBs.

A last comment about the fMRI findings in ASD concerns sample selection. Compared to the structural studies we discussed earlier and the resting-state connectivity studies we discuss below, fMRI requires task performance in the scanner. Because participants must have minimal motion while in the scanner and the tasks can be complex, such as identifying faces and emotions, and completing EF tasks, samples included in fMRI studies largely represent older individuals with strong intellectual skills (Nusslock et al., 2012). There is also a gender bias, such that many studies recruit all-male or majority-male samples (Nusslock et al., 2012). As such, it is important to remember that fMRI studies of ASD are not representative of the full spectrum of individuals. Moving forward, there is a need for studies to develop task paradigms that can generalize across age and ability levels. Several authors have recently pointed out that developmental issues have been particularly neglected (Di Martino et al., 2009; Dickstein et al., 2013). The first meta-analysis of its kind to compare children and adults with ASD showed developmental differences in regions associated with both social and nonsocial tasks, further highlighting the need for a greater emphasis on developmental trajectories in neuroimaging studies of ASD (Dickstein et al., 2013).

Connectivity

In addition to the structural and functional correlates of ASD that we reviewed earlier, there is also a growing appreciation of the dynamics of neural systems in the brain and a growing awareness that ASD is not likely to be a localized brain disorder, but rather a disorder of multiple brain networks (Gepner & Féron, 2009). One line of evidence supporting this view comes from molecular genetic studies discussed below that have converged on synaptic pathways as one biological process that may be disrupted in ASD (Mohammad-Rezazadeh et al., 2016). Over the past decade, these insights have led to an increased focus on the connectivity of brain networks in ASD (for reviews see Maximo, Cadena, & Kana, 2014; Mohammad-Rezazadeh et al., 2016; Müller et al., 2011; Picci et al., 2016; Rane et al., 2015; Vasa, Mostofsky, & Ewen, 2016; Vissers, Cohen, & Geurts, 2012).

Two hypotheses were advanced in 2004 to explain atypical connectivity in ASD. The "underconnectivity theory" was proposed by Just, Cherkassky, Keller, and Minshew (2004) based on functional activations that were less synchronized in ASD during a language comprehension task. A second conceptual paper by Belmonte et al. (2004) proposed that the long-range underconnectivity observed by Just et al. (2004) might be associated with local overconnectivity. In other words, hyperconnectivity at the local level might impair neural regions' ability to differentiate and connect effectively with more distal regions (Belmonte et al., 2004). Both of these theories posit that long-range connections should show underconnectivity, and a large body of research has been focused on this claim.

Evidence supporting the underconnectivity theory has been accumulating, even leading to the proposal that it is the "first firm finding" in ASD (Hughes,

2007). Studies finding reduced connectivity in the brains of individual with ASD have used both functional (resting-state and task-based) and anatomical (white matter) methods. However, in recent reviews, Müller et al. (2011) and Mohammad-Rezazadeh et al. (2016) have pointed out that the literature does not universally support the underconnectivity theory. Rather, there are a number of studies reporting mixed effects and even overconnectivity in ASD. Müller et al. (2011) set out to examine whether there are inconsistencies in the evidence that may be attributed to important differences in analysis and methodology across the studies. The findings were quite striking in showing specific methodological choices (i.e., whole-brain vs. region of interest analysis, low-pass filtering, task regression) that were highly predictive of whether underconnectivity was found in the study. They argued that the emerging consensus in favor of the underconnectivity theory needs to be reexamined in light of this methodological variation. The authors point out that these methodological choices are not inherently right or wrong, but a greater appreciation of the strengths and limitations of each approach will facilitate a better understanding of the weight of the evidence for the underconnectivity theory (Müller et al., 2011).

Since Müller et al.'s (2011) review, there have been advancements in methodological rigor for functional connectivity studies. Picci et al. (2016) published an updated review of the most recent, well-powered, methodologically advanced studies. In their review of the resting-state functional connectivity literature, the picture of connectivity in ASD is more complicated than either of the original theories proposed by Just et al. (2004) and Belmonte et al. (2004). Picci et al. (2016) described an emerging pattern of underconnectivity in cortical–cortical connections but overconnectivity in subcortical–cortical connections. Picci et al. (2016) also reviewed task-based functional connectivity and found mixed evidence for stronger and weaker connectivity within and across the domains they considered (language, social, EF, visual–spatial).

In summary, the emerging consensus is that the most methodologically advanced studies do not provide unqualified support for Just et al.'s (2004) pervasive underconnectivity theory or Belmonte et al.'s (2004) local overconnectivity/distal underconnectivity theory. Rather, the emerging picture of the dynamic interactions among regions of the brain seems to be quite complex in ASD, and there are likely unexplored modifiers of these dynamics, especially age, sex, and phenotypic characteristics (Picci et al., 2016; Rane et al., 2015; Uddin, Supekar, & Menon, 2013). The question of development is particularly salient in this literature, as many existing ASD studies recruited participants from wide age ranges spanning childhood to adulthood, and there has been very little consideration of changing patterns of connectivity across development (Picci et al., 2016; Uddin et al., 2013). The question of how connectivity differences in ASD relate to behavioral phenotypes is also important. In a recent review, Rane et al. (2015) reported that only 21% of resting-state functional connectivity studies and 28% of diffusion tensor imaging (DTI) studies examined correlations between connectivity findings and behavioral phenotypes.

Although the functional connectivity studies do not provide a simple picture of the dynamics of the ASD brain, there is more consistency among *structural* studies of connectivity (i.e., DTI). Here, there is near universal agreement documenting white matter disruptions and virtually no support for stronger structural connectivity in ASD (Picci et al., 2016). Within these studies, there is evidence that temporal lobe white matter tracts appear to be particularly vulnerable (Picci et al., 2016).

Taken together, the connectivity literature is in a state of reevaluation and refinement. It seems that neither the Just et al. (2004) theory of underconnectivity or the Belmonte et al. (2004) theory of local overconnectivity/distal underconnectivity theory are completely supported. Rather, there is an emerging consensus of reduced connectivity in cortical–cortical connections but overconnectivity in subcortical–cortical connections (Picci et al., 2016; Rane et al., 2015). A similar pattern of reevaluation and refinement of the literature was seen for the early brain overgrowth hypothesis we discussed earlier. That literature also seemed to be converging on an accepted result when a methodological disruption cast doubt on the emerging consensus. It is too early to say how these literatures will coalesce over time, but an increasing focus on replication patterns across the ASD imaging literature, as well as a growing emphasis on methodological consistency, is an important marker of progress in this field. There are also concerted efforts to increase sample sizes through data sharing, a milestone that marked a turning point in the psychiatric genetics field, which also faced large-scale technological challenges and difficulties with replication.

ETIOLOGY

Historically, genetic influences on autism were long doubted, both by psychodynamic theorists and by geneticists, but for different reasons. Psychodynamic theorists postulated that autism was caused by the maternal environment. Geneticists were struck by the apparent lack of both vertical transmission and associated chromosomal anomalies (Rutter, 2000). Ironically, more recent research has documented that autism is one of the most familial and heritable psychiatric diagnoses, with a significant minority of cases associated with chromosomal anomalies or known genetic syndromes. In what follows, we see how research results changed the view that autism was not genetic.

Familiality

Early estimates of the rate of autism in siblings (2–3%) have increased as diagnostic practices have broadened and the methodological rigor of studies has increased. Generally, studies find recurrence rates of ASD given an affected sibling are in the range of 10–15% (Wood et al., 2015). A notable family study conducted by Sandin et al. (2014) is the largest, population-based, longitudinal study of ASD familiality. The authors sampled all births in Sweden between 1982 and 2006 ($N > 2$ million children). They used all siblings (including monozygotic [MZ] and dizygotic [DZ] twins), half-siblings, and cousins to estimate the sibling recurrence risk, and adjusted for potential cohort effects and variation in the length of follow-up for participants in different birth years. Diagnoses were obtained from the national patient register. Children in Sweden undergo routine medical and developmental examinations, including a mandatory developmental assessment at age 4 years. Children with developmental concerns are then referred to a specialized team for diagnostic assessment, and results of the assessment are reported to the national patient register. Results showed that siblings of a child with ASD had a cumulative probability of an ASD diagnosis of 12.9% compared to 1.2% of siblings without an affected family member. This resulted in a sibling recurrence risk of 10.3 (Sandin et al., 2014). The strengths of this sample in terms of size, prospective follow-up, population sampling, and universal screening practices address many of the methodological limitations of existing family studies.

Nevertheless, a complication for population-based approaches like that of Sandin et al. (2014) is the phenomenon of *stoppage,* where families are more likely to stop having more children after having a child with ASD. High-risk longitudinal designs can address this issue, but these studies have fewer participants and so are limited by possible sample selection effects. Thus, converging estimates across different study designs are important. As mentioned previously, a common high-risk design is to study the younger infant siblings of children diagnosed with ASD (Ozonoff et al., 2010). By design, these studies can rule out stoppage. In a recent study of the collaborative Baby Siblings Research Consortium, Ozonoff et al. (2011) reported a higher sibling recurrence rate of 18.7% than did other, previous studies. Infant gender and the presence of multiple affected siblings with ASD were the best predictors of ASD outcome. Taken together, two of the strongest research designs for estimating familiality have obtained estimates in the range of 13–19% for sibling recurrence risk. The fairly close alignment of the rates speaks to the robustness of the finding for at least a 10-fold increased risk for siblings of children with ASD, the highest familiality of all the learning disorders in this book. While this is certainly a notable increase, it is important to communicate these empirical risks to families, as many believe that the risk is actually much larger (Selkirk, Veach, Lian, Schimmenti, & LeRoy, 2009; Whitelaw, Flett, & Amor, 2007).

Studies of family members of individuals with autism have also made it clear that the behavioral phenotype that is transmitted in families is broader than the diagnosis itself (e.g., Piven, 1999). Hence, the familial phenotype may be dimensional rather than categorical. First-degree relatives of probands with autism have increased rates of symptoms of autism, shyness and aloofness, and pragmatic language problems compared to control relatives (Rutter, 2000). Several studies have also found higher rates of anxiety and depressive disorders among relatives of probands with autism. However, these disorders did not cosegregate with the broader autism phenotype (the BAP, which is defined by social and cognitive deficits) and their rate did not increase with the severity of autism in the proband, unlike the BAP (Rutter, 2000). Although individuals with the BAP had higher rates of reading and spelling problems, perhaps because of other cognitive and language problems, a specific reading and spelling problem (i.e., dyslexia) was not more common in such families, nor were intellectual disabilities or seizure disorders, which are increased in probands. Although more work is needed to define the BAP, especially work using neuropsychological markers, these studies are exciting and clearly have implications for what phenotypes are used in molecular studies.

In addition to these more common psychiatric and cognitive problems that are found in relatives, it is also becoming clear that family members of children with autism are also more likely to be diagnosed with severe psychiatric disorders, including schizophrenia and bipolar disorder (P. Sullivan et al., 2012). Recent cross-disorder genetic methods derived from genomewide association studies (GWAS) have also identified cross-disorder genetic sharing. For instance, the genetic correlation between ASD and schizophrenia is significant (r_g = .20), even though the disorders are considered quite distinct (Demontis et al., 2017). This result is consistent with a broader emerging theme of cross-disorder genetic sharing across the psychiatric spectrum (Smoller, 2013b). Such findings suggest that at least a portion of the genetic risk factors for ASD follow a "generalist" pattern (Plomin & Kovas, 2005) and increase risk for myriad psychiatric disorders. It remains to be determined how such "generalist genes" in combination with genes and environments that may be specific to certain disorders combine to shape the phenotype of a child.

Heritability

Studies investigating the heritability of ASD have generally relied on twin studies because adoption studies of autism are less feasible. The first, now classic, twin study of autism was conducted by Folstein and Rutter (1977). The concordance rate in MZ pairs (36%) was significantly greater than that found in DZ pairs (0%). If the phenotype was broadened to include a cognitive or language disorder, these concordance rates became 82 and 10%, respectively. So this study provided evidence that autism was significantly heritable and that the heritable phenotype was broader than the diagnosis of autism itself, consistent with the family studies we just discussed. Such early twin studies were significant in moving the field away from the notion of environmental influences and "refrigerator mothers" (Bettelheim, 1967) as the primary causal factor in ASD. To date, more than 10 published twin studies of ASD have largely reaffirmed strong genetic influences on ASD, with heritability estimates falling in the range of .7–.9 (for reviews, see Ronald & Hoekstra, 2011; Tick et al., 2016). However, in the past few years, two twin studies reported a larger shared environment effect and lower heritability than had been previously reported in ASD, sparking a renewed debate about genetic and environmental contributions to ASD (Frazier, Thompson, et al., 2014; Hallmayer et al., 2011).

Ronald and Hoekstra (2011) and Tick et al. (2016) conducted reviews of the existing twin studies in ASD. The Ronald and Hoekstra (2011) review, which came out before the shared environment debate was emerging, indicated that heritability estimates were strong and consistent across the seven published studies reviewed at that time (heritability ~ .7–.9). They also found that these strong heritability estimates remained when the diagnostic criteria were broadened to include the full spectrum, rather than just autistic disorder (Ronald & Hoekstra, 2011).

Subsequent twin studies emerging after this review showed some notable deviations from the fairly homogeneous heritability estimates in the previous twin studies. Hallmayer et al. (2011) and Frazier, Thompson, et al. (2014) were the first to report a sizable impact of shared environmental effects that questioned previous results showing that genetic influences accounted for the largest proportion of population variance. Hallmayer et al. (2011) reported that shared environmental influences accounted for 58% and genetic influences accounted for 38% of the variance. Frazier, Thompson, et al. (2014) found an even larger effect of shared environment (64–78%, depending on measures). In contrast to these findings, other twin studies continued to find strong genetic influences and no significant effects for shared environment (Colvert et al., 2015; Nordenbæk, Jørgensen, Kyvik, & Bilenberg, 2014). Measurement and sample ascertainment differences, along with differences in the underlying liability threshold model employed, are among the primary hypotheses to explain these mixed results (Colvert et al., 2015).

To better understand this heterogeneity in results, Tick et al. (2016) published a meta-analysis of the current twin literature. Tick and colleagues reanalyzed the individual studies with appropriate corrections for selection and ascertainment, and assuming different liability threshold models. Under different analytic models, heritability estimates ranged from 64 to 91%, and shared environment estimates ranged from 7 to 35%. Despite the variability in these estimates as a function of the threshold model, heritability estimates stayed strong and accounted for the majority of the variance in ASD phenotypes. Even when shared environmental influences were significant, they never exceeded the heritability estimates (Tick et al., 2016). These twin meta-analytic results are also consistent with the largest extended family population study including ~2 million participants, which found moderate heritability (54%) and no significant effect of the shared environment (Sandin et al., 2014). In total, the behavior genetic evidence continues to support genetic influences as the most prominent etiological factor in ASD, with variable evidence for shared environmental effects as a function of the liability threshold model that is chosen. The recent meta-analytic estimates for heritability continue to place ASD among the most heritable psychiatric and developmental disorders.

One limitation of heritability estimates is that they do not provide information on individual risk for ASD. For those estimates, family studies, such as those we discussed in the previous section, are necessary. Hence, in combination, twin and family studies can provide information about risk at both population and individual levels, both useful metrics (Sandin et al., 2014).

In addition to twin studies on the diagnostic category of ASD, there have also been several studies of dimensional autistic trait measures in population samples (reviewed in Ronald & Hoekstra, 2011). The fact that such dimensional traits show a smooth distribution without any discontinuity at the clinical extremes supports the notion that ASD represents an extreme cutoff point on an underlying normal distribution (Constantino & Todd, 2003; Skuse, Mandy, & Scourfield, 2005), consistent with most of the other learning disorders discussed in this book. As a result, researchers have posited that understanding the etiological influences on the full dimensional trait distribution will contribute to our understanding of ASD as well. Ronald et al. (2011) reported in their review that across the 11 twin studies of autistic traits conducted at the time, heritability estimates generally fell in the range of 60–90% for parent and teacher reports on children ages ~7–18 years (Ronald & Hoekstra, 2011). Hence, the estimates of the heritability of autistic traits across the entire distribution are quite similar to estimates of the heritability of the extreme group of individuals with an actual diagnosis of ASD.

Beyond estimating heritability, multivariate twin studies can provide insight about the extent of genetic sharing between the symptom dimensions of ASD (social–communication, RRBs). One consistent and curious finding has been that the symptom dimensions of ASD each have substantial genetic contributions, but these genetic influences are largely specific to the dimension rather than shared. These multivariate twin studies have used general population samples with continuous measures of autistic symptomatology (Hallett, Ronald, Rijsdijk, & Happé, 2010; Robinson et al., 2012; Ronald, Happé, Bolton, et al., 2006; Ronald et al., 2005, 2011; Ronald, Happé, Price, et al., 2006). For example, across ages 7–12 in a large twin sample, the ASD dimensions have shown genetic correlations in the range of ~.20–.50, indicating that the majority of the genetic influences are unique to each dimension rather than shared (Hallett et al., 2010; Robinson et el., 2012; Ronald, Happé, Bolton, et al., 2006; Ronald et al., 2005, 2011; Ronald, Happé, Price, et al., 2006). To further contextualize these findings, it is also important to note that a stronger genetic relationship between social–communication and RRBs has been seen in clinical samples (Frazier, Thompson, et al., 2014), so more work is needed to reconcile these discrepancies.

The fact that genetic influences are showing some specificity to autism dimensions is rather surprising in the context of the larger literature supporting the notion of "generalist genes" across learning and psychiatric disorders. Thus, the fact that the symptom dimensions of a single disorder show relatively low genetic correlations may point to a unique aspect of the genetic architecture of ASD. These genetic findings have led to the hypothesis of a "fractionable autism triad" (Happé & Ronald, 2008; Happé et al., 2006), a model that we discussed earlier in the section on neuropsychology. This model has implications for the design of genetic studies. Under this model, investigators should focus on gene-finding for the specific phenotypic dimensions rather than searching for genes that influence the category of ASD.

The finding of the fractionable autism triad from a genetic perspective is at odds with the more general findings of cross-disorder genetic sharing. For instance, one large multivariate twin study of ASD, Tourette syndrome, ADHD, and developmental coordination disorder found substantial genetic sharing across these disorders (Lichtenstein et al., 2009). In combination with the fractionable autism triad hypothesis, these results suggest that when social–communication and RRBs occur together in the same child (perhaps for distinct genetic reasons), this syndrome is coheritable with other psychiatric disorders (Lichtenstein et al., 2009). This pattern could be observed if the distinct genetic risk factors for either social–communication or RRBs are shared with other psychiatric disorders. Or this pattern might be explained by the relatively small proportion of genetic risk factors shared across social–communication and RRBs also being shared with psychiatric disorders. Clearly, these findings present a puzzle for the field and warrant further multivariate twin studies to reconcile the fractionable autism triad hypothesis with findings of substantial genetic sharing across psychiatric disorders.

Taken together, this growing body of work has expanded well beyond basic questions about the heritability of ASD. Researchers are now using the twin design in innovative ways to address important theoretical questions regarding the shared and specific genetic risk factors for dimensions of ASD.

Gene Findings

Since publication of the previous edition of this book, molecular genetic research in ASD has flourished. Among the learning disorders discussed in this book, ASD clearly leads the field in genetic research and in setting methodological standards for the other developmental disorders to follow. Several excellent reviews and meta-analyses have been published on the genetics of autism, and this section draws on their conclusions (Robinson, Neale, & Hyman, 2015; Betancur, 2011; Bourgeron, 2015; de la Torre-Ubieta, Won, Stein, & Geschwind, 2016; De Rubeis & Buxbaum, 2015; Geschwind & State, 2015; Ronald & Hoekstra, 2011; Vorstman et al., 2017; Willsey & State, 2015).

These studies have now convincingly identified the first associated genes that are leading to hypotheses about implicated biological pathways. The hope is that these biological insights will yield treatment targets in the future. One insight from the genetic research that clearly maps onto behavioral observations is that ASD has a complex, heterogeneous etiology. This complexity involves both etiological heterogeneity (i.e., different genetic risk factors can lead to a similar ASD phenotype) and phenotypic heterogeneity (i.e., the same genetic risk factor may manifest in different developmental phenotypes and in some cases present in unaffected controls).

ASD has been associated with many different types of genetic variation, including both common and rare variants in the population, variants that are inherited or de novo (i.e., arising spontaneously in the offspring), and variants that range in size from a single base-pair change (i.e., single-nucleotide polymorphisms [SNPs]) to large copy number variants (CNVs; i.e., large segments of DNA that are duplicated or deleted) that comprise many thousands to millions of base pairs that are duplicated or deleted (Robinson et al., 2015). Given the complexity of the genetic risk landscape for ASD, it is not surprising that simulations have estimated that there are 600–1,200 ASD risk genes (reviewed in De Rubeis & Buxbaum, 2015). Such simulations stand in stark contrast to previous genetic models of developmental disorders that hypothesized a handful of candidate genes. However, with advances in genetic technology and increasing sample sizes, it is now clear that such estimations were vast underestimates. As of December 2017, there were more than 970 genes included in the Autism Database (AutDB; *http://autism.mindspec.org/autdb/welcome. do*), a resource for tracking the most recent findings in ASD molecular genetics. Although this body of work is impressive, it is important to note that the evidence supporting any individual gene can be quite variable (Vorstman et al., 2017). In what follows, we will divide our discussion into a consideration of recent research on (1) common genetic risk variants and (2) rare genetic risk variants.

Common polygenic risk is estimated to account for 20–50% of genetic liability ASD (Robinson et al., 2015). These values fall short of current twin heritability estimates of ~70–90%, so they suggest that common genetic variation cannot account for all of the genetic risk for ASD. The first GWAS to report significant associations between ASD and common genetic variants (i.e., SNPs) is currently in preprint (Demontis et al., 2017). This study included approximately 18,000 cases and 28,000 controls, and identified five novel genetic loci associated with ASD. Further work is needed to link these genetic variants to implicated genes. Such massive sample sizes are necessary, because the effect sizes of common variants are usually quite small (i.e., orders of magnitude smaller than 1% of the variance).

Work to identify larger effect but rarer genetic variants has also proven to be fruitful. Rare genetic variants are often categorized as inherited or de novo (i.e., a genetic variant that arose spontaneously and is not present in the parents). ASD sample collections fortuitously emphasized trio collections (both parents and child), compared to other psychiatric disorders, which collected more typical case–control samples. The additional effort to collect trios has yielded important insights into the de novo status of genetic variants associated with autism (i.e., without parental DNA, it cannot be determined whether a genetic variant is inherited or newly arising).

The first class of rare variants we discuss is CNVs. In the previous edition of this book, we noted an early study that highlighted an increased rate of de novo CNVs in children with sporadic autism (i.e., the child is affected but parents are not) (Sebat et al., 2007). This work on CNVs was just emerging at the time. Now, it is clear that rare CNVs (both inherited and de novo) do contribute to autism risk (Vorstman et al., 2017). De novo CNVs occur approximately three to four times more frequently in children with autism compared to their unaffected siblings (Ronemus, Iossifov, Levy, & Wigler, 2014). Interestingly, these CNVs are not specific to one disorder but are implicated across developmental and psychiatric phenotypes, including schizophrenia, bipolar disorder, ADHD, ID, and epilepsy (Malhotra & Sebat, 2012; Morrow, 2010). The fact that these CNVs have cross-disorder genetic influences raises important questions about the additional genetic and environmental factors that lead to such diverse outcomes and reinforces the notion of "generalist genes" (Plomin & Kovas, 2005).

An interesting CNV region to highlight is 7q11.23. Deletions of this region have long been known to cause Williams syndrome (WS). Children with WS are notable for their hypersocial phenotype that has sometimes been studied as a contrast to ASD. Children with WS also have generalized intellectual deficits, notable spatial weaknesses, and a relative sparing of language skills in relation to other cognitive skills (Mervis & John, 2010; Pober, 2010). In the past few years, a duplication of this same region of 7q11.23 has also been associated with autism (Sanders et al., 2011), though not exclusively, and other phenotypes such as language impairment have also been detected (Mervis, Morris, Klein-Tasman, Velleman, & Osborne, 2015). Whereas the typical 7q11.23 deletion invariably leads to WS, the

7q11.23 duplication presents with more phenotypic heterogeneity in which ASD is one of many possible manifestations. Despite these complexities, it is very interesting to contrast the 7q11.23 deletion, which has been associated with a hypersocial phenotype to the 7q11.23 duplication that has been implicated in ASD. This pattern might suggest a dosage-sensitive region of the genome that is implicated in sociability, prompting a deeper look at the function of the genes in this region (Malenfant et al., 2012; Schweiger & Meyer-Lindenberg, 2017; Van Hagen et al., 2007). So far, genes in that region, such as *GTF2I* and *GTF2IRD1* have emerged as candidates of interest, but much more work needs to be done to replicate and interpret early findings.

Whole-exome sequencing (i.e., sequencing the bases of every protein-coding segment of DNA) has also been very productive in the autism field (Iossifov et al., 2012; B. Neale et al., 2012; O'Roak et al., 2012; Sanders et al., 2012). De novo mutations, which are predicted to interrupt the function of a gene (loss of function mutations), are approximately twice as likely to occur in children with autism compared to their unaffected siblings (Ronemus et al., 2014). The disrupted genes are now being studied in animal models for new insights into pharmacological and behavioral interventions.

One of the genes emerging from whole-exome sequencing studies of autism is *CHD8* (Chromodomain helicase DNA binding protein 8) (De Rubeis et al., 2014; B. Neale et al., 2012; O'Roak et al., 2012), a gene on chromosome 14q11.2 involved in the WNT signaling pathway, which is important for embryonic central nervous system development, in addition to other biological processes (Vorstman et al., 2017). Further evidence for the importance of this gene pathway in ASD comes from the fact that the binding partners of *CHD8* have also been implicated in ASD. The identification of *CHD8* as a gene of interest for ASD has prompted animal and *in vitro* work to further understand the mechanisms linking this gene to ASD phenotypes. From the animal work, one interesting finding connects *CHD8* to a robust neuroimaging finding in ASD, that of macrocephaly observed in some ASD cases (discussed further in the section "Brain Mechanisms"). This line of animal work finds that disruptions of *chd8* in zebrafish results in macrocephaly, consistent with the phenotypic findings in ASD cases with *CHD8* mutations (Bernier et al., 2014).

From the *in vitro* work, one study (Wang et al., 2015) used CRISPR/Cas9 technology to knock out one copy of *CHD8* in an induced pluripotent stem cell (iPSC), a stem cell that can be induced to differentiate into different types of cells. In this study, Wang et al. (2015) differentiated the iPSCs into neural progenitor cells and neurons. They identified genes that were regulated by *CHD8* by virtue of changes in gene expression in the knockout neurons. These downstream genes clustered into functional pathways important for brain development: cell communication, extracellular matrix formation, and neurogenesis (Wang et al., 2015). These *CHD8* gene targets were also enriched for genes previously implicated in ASD and schizophrenia (Wang et al., 2015), consistent with previous molecular genetics findings indicating genetic overlap between these disorders. Last, the authors reported that genes related to head size and brain volume were also enriched among the targets of *CHD8*, consistent with findings in animal models and ASD cases with *CHD8* mutations (Bernier et al., 2014).

These *in vitro* experiments with *CHD8* illustrate how genetic studies can yield new insights into pathophysiological targets through convergence on specific pathways. Importantly, despite the heterogeneity that is seen at the genetic level of analysis, it appears that there might be more convergence at the level of biological pathways. So, even though a single gene such as *CHD8* will account for a very small minority of cases with ASD, a much larger percentage of cases with ASD might have disruptions to the same pathway, for example, the WNT signaling pathway in which *CHD8* is implicated. So far, similar methods of identifying a gene of interest and its functional connections with other proteins have converged on additional biological processes implicated in ASD, such as disrupted synaptic signaling, chromatin remodeling, MAPK signaling, and interactions with fragile X-associated genes (e.g., *FMR1*) (for a review, see Vorstman et al., 2017). The promise of this work is that greater insight into the disrupted biological processes in ASD will yield new therapeutic targets.

Taken together, researchers estimate that 10–30% of individuals with autism will have a rare inherited or de novo variant that is putatively causal (Vorstman et al., 2017). These findings have led to clinical recommendations from the American Academy of Pediatrics and the American Academy of Child and Adolescent Psychiatry that every child with ASD should have a genetic workup (Committee on Bioethics, Committee on Genetics, & American College of Medical Genetics and Genomics Social, Ethical, and Legal Issues Committee, 2013; D. Miller et al., 2010; Volkmar et al., 2014). Despite this recommendation, there is evidence that clinical implementation is lagging (Cuccaro et al., 2014). Only a minority of families actually receive genetic testing for several reasons, including low referral rates and concerns about costs and relevance. Still, most parents of children with ASD are interested in further genetic information (estimates of 86%) (Cuccaro et al., 2014). However, it should also be appreciated that some parents turn down the opportunity for further genetic testing because of concerns about whether the results will be actionable and/or relevant to health decisions (Cuccaro et al., 2014).

Environmental Influences

Although we emphasized in the previous section the large contributions of genetic influences, both inherited and de novo, we should also emphasize that the heritability of ASD is not 100%, which means that environmental influences do play a role. Based on what we know about the developmental trajectory of ASD, it is not surprising that research is indicating that most environmental risk factors act very early (i.e., pre- or perinatally), as opposed to factors such as parental bonding (i.e., "refrigerator mothers") that played a role in discredited psychoanalytic theories of ASD.

Mandy and Lai (2016) have conducted a comprehensive review of environmental influences on ASD, and this discussion draws from their conclusions. We do not provide a comprehensive review of every putative environmental risk factor; rather, we review a few key environmental factors that illustrate current areas of focus. We first discuss paternal and maternal age as risk factors for ASD as a means of transitioning between the genetic and environmental sections of this chapter, and illustrating complex models of gene–environment interplay. For example, maternal and paternal age might be considered "environmental" factors in the sense that they are external factors to the child, but their action is likely through genetic mechanisms. In a meta-analysis, Hultman, Sandin, Levine, Lichtenstein, and Reichenberg (2011) documented an association between paternal age and ASD. Compared to fathers ages 29 and younger, fathers who were older than 50 years were 2.21 times more likely to have a child with autism. Despite this convincing association, it must also be noted that the impact of these increases is actually quite small when considered from a population perspective. For example, although the statistic we just mentioned seems large (i.e., a doubled risk for autism), because ASD is a fairly rare condition, it does not result in a large increase in risk. If we use a prevalence estimate of 1%, the father who is over 50 now has a 2% risk of having a child with ASD, a trivial level of increase for most families. Hence, the association between paternal age and ASD is reliable, but it is easy for families to be misled by recent headlines on this topic about the magnitude of the effect . For instance, increasing paternal age can only account for a very small proportion of the overall increase in autism prevalence over the past decade.

In their meta-analysis, Hultman et al. (2011) controlled for some important confounds when establishing their association between paternal age and child ASD, most notably, maternal age, parental psychiatric history, perinatal complications, and SES. These covariates rule out a number of alternative hypotheses that could explain the association between paternal age and ASD risk in offspring. A remaining possibility is that increased paternal age is a marker for the broader autism phenotype (Mandy & Lai, 2016), so the association is attributable to genetic risk factors for ASD that are passed on from father to offspring. However, within-family designs have shown that when there are multiple siblings in a family and one child is affected, he or she is more likely to be the youngest, on average (controlling for parity and maternal age) (Hultman et al., 2011). These findings suggest that genetic transmission of the broader autism phenotype from father to offspring is unlikely to be the main genetic mechanism explaining the paternal age effect. Another possibility is related to the finding that older males have a higher rate of de novo mutations in sperm (Kong et al., 2012; Michaelson et al., 2012). As we discussed, de novo mutations are also associated with an increased ASD risk. Hence, this genetic model is the leading hypothesis at this time.

The preceding discussion focused on paternal age, but there is also evidence for an association between ASD and maternal age, even after researchers control for paternal age. In a meta-analysis, Sandin and colleagues (2012) report a relative risk of 1.52 for mothers ages 35 and older compared to those ages 25–29 years. Again, many of the studies controlled for important covariates, such as paternal age, SES, and perinatal factors and obstetric complications. It is currently hypothesized that the mechanisms are distinct for advanced paternal and maternal age. For maternal age, leading hypotheses focus on an increased risk for chromosomal abnormalities (Martin, 2008) and/or epigenetic processes (Sandin et al., 2012).

Emerging evidence also links specific *in utero* drug exposures with increased ASD risk. One of the most convincing findings connects *in utero* valproate exposure, a drug used to treat epilepsy, bipolar disorder, and migraine, with increased ASD risk (Bromley et al., 2013; J. Christensen et al., 2013; G. Williams et al., 2001). When used during pregnancy, exposure to the drug can cause "fetal valproate syndrome" which is associated with generalized developmental delays, including increased risk for ASD (Shallcross et al., 2011; Tomson et al., 2011). As with studies of advanced maternal and paternal age, epidemiological studies of the association between *in utero* valproate exposure and ASD risk need to carefully control for confounders, most notably that epilepsy in the mother is a marker for genetic risk for ASD given the association between ASD and epilepsy. J. Christensen et al. (2013) conducted a whole-population study of Denmark ($N > 600{,}000$ children) with valproate exposure in ~500 children. Results showed a two- to threefold increase in risk, after the authors controlled for important confounders, including the mother's epilepsy, and the association remained when the sample was restricted to mothers with epilepsy. These results suggest a convincing association between valproate and ASD risk, though the risk is not specific to ASD and includes other neurodevelopmental disorders. Intriguingly, further work on valproate exposure in animal models has supported the association and implicated epigenetic modifications to the WNT signaling pathway, a pathway that has also been implicated by genetic risk factors for ASD discussed earlier. This convergence of genetic and environmental risks implicating the same biological pathway is compelling evidence for its etiological importance in ASD (and possibly other neurodevelopmental disorders).

Early reports implicated prenatal infections (i.e., maternal rubella; see Chess, 1971) in the etiology of ASD, but subsequent follow-up indicated an unexpectedly high number of children who recovered from their autism symptoms (Chess, 1977). Nevertheless, there is accumulating evidence that maternal infections can serve as a generalized risk factor for neurodevelopmental disorders, including ASD (see review in Mandy & Lai, 2016). Obstetric complications have also been examined in relation to ASD risk. In a recent meta-analysis, Gardener, Spiegelman, and Buka (2011) found several factors related to perinatal and neonatal health (e.g., fetal distress, birth injury, multiple birth, low birthweight, maternal hemorrhage, summer birth, low 5-minute APGAR, meconium aspiration, and other risk factors) that were significantly associated with ASD risk. However, in many cases, these factors are unlikely to be causal. Rather, the evidence indicates that these obstetric complications are a consequence of an atypically developing fetus (e.g., with congenital malformations or with a greater familial loading for ASD), rather than being etiological themselves (Bailey et al., 1996; Bolton & Griffiths, 1997).

Although the notion of "refrigerator mothers" has been discounted as a cause of autism, there is evidence that *extreme* environmental deprivation, including decreased social stimulation, can produce a phenocopy of ASD (Mandy & Lai, 2016). Such a phenocopy has been found in congenital blindness (R Brown, Hobson, Lee, & Stevenson, 1997; Rogers & Pennington, 1991) and in some orphans (~11–16%) placed in minimally stimulating institutions as infants (Hoksbergen, Ter Laak, Rijk, van Dijkum, & Stoutjesdijk, 2005; A. Levin, Fox, Zeanah, & Nelson,

2015; Rutter et al., 1999, 2007). In the case of the children placed in orphanages, the syndrome has been labeled "quasi-autism" (Rutter et al., 1999), because it differs from idiopathic ASD in a few ways: phenotypic presentation, developmental trajectory, and male:female ratio (1:1). In phenotypic presentation, the children show more flexible communication and more social approach behaviors than is typical in idiopathic ASD. In developmental trajectory, about half of the affected children experience substantial improvements in their symptoms when placed in more enriched environments, while half continue to have persistent ASD symptoms (Mandy & Lai, 2016). Children who are congenitally blind have an even better prognosis, with most no longer qualifying for an ASD diagnosis by adolescence (Mandy & Lai, 2016). The existence of these phenocopies is very important theoretically, because it reminds us that social relatedness is not innate, but rather depends on interactions with a caregiver. Factors that strongly limit those interactions, whether environmental or genetic, can lead to development of the symptoms of ASD. One key question for current research is to identify which early psychological deficits in infants who will develop ASD are the ones that strongly limit their ability to participate in socializing interactions with a caregiver (see discussion in Rogers & Pennington, 1991).

In discussing possible environmental associations with autism, we would be remiss if we did not point out the strong scientific evidence showing *no association* between autism and the MMR vaccine (Madsen et al., 2002) or thimerosal-containing vaccines (Parker, Schwartz, Todd, & Pickering, 2004; Stratton, Gable, McCormick, & Institute of Medicine Immunization Safety Review Committee, 2001), even in children at higher risk of ASD (Jain et al., 2015). A recent meta-analysis, which pooled across five case–control studies and five cohort studies, found no support for a connection between MMR and an increased risk of ASD. Results actually trended towards the MMR vaccine being a protective factor (Taylor, Swerdfeger, & Eslick, 2014). Scientific consensus ruling out the association between MMR and ASD is remarkably strong and consistent, yet myths about the vaccine prevail, with approximately 25% of parents still believing that vaccines cause ASD (Freed, Clark, Butchart, Singer, & Davis, 2010). A recent book by the journalist, Seth Mnookin (2011), entitled *The Panic Virus*, gives an accessible introduction for families to the controversies and evidence.

DIAGNOSIS AND TREATMENT

Diagnosis

Screening and Early Identification

The median age of diagnosis in the United States remains at approximately 4–5 years old (D. Christensen et al., 2016), despite evidence that parents usually report first concerns by age 18–24 months (Zwaigenbaum, 2015). Many families describe a stressful "diagnostic odyssey" involving many different diagnoses before they receive an ASD diagnosis (Zwaigenbaum, 2015). Because the delay from first concerns to

ASD diagnosis may also delay access to specialized, evidence-based intervention for ASD, there is a concerted effort in the field to improve early screening and diagnosis. A multidisciplinary panel of clinical practitioners and researchers recently published a consensus statement on early identification (Zwaigenbaum, 2015). One important consensus point was summarized as follows: "No definitive behavioral or diagnostic markers have yet been identified in infants age <12 months." This consensus aligns with the prospective research we reviewed earlier, in which it has been difficult to find group differences between high-risk and low-risk infants before 12 months of age. Although diagnosis by 12 months is not currently possible, diagnoses are possible and stable in toddlers younger than 2 years (Ozonoff et al., 2015). However, there are children who do not show signs of ASD until 24 or 36 months, so repeated screening is necessary (Ozonoff et al., 2015). Pediatricians are often the first point of contact for parents. Because of this critical role for pediatricians, the American Academy of Pediatrics recommends universal screenings for ASD, using empirically based screening tools, at 18 and 24 months. Children with concerning results of screening should then be referred for a comprehensive developmental evaluation.

The U.S. Preventive Services Task Force published controversial recommendations in 2015 that indicated insufficient evidence to justify screening for ASD in children ages 18–30 months whose parents or health care providers have not raised concerns. There have been forceful rebuttals to this recommendation, which have pointed out the poor diagnostic sensitivity of parent and provider concerns (i.e., Coury, 2015). At this point, the Task Force concluded that there was "insufficient evidence" to justify screening in low-risk children and recommended additional research designs that could provide the evidence. To be clear, the report does not indicate that screenings are not useful, only that there is insufficient evidence. Nevertheless, many in the ASD field strongly disagree with this conclusion and continue to advocate for universal screenings (Coury, 2015), a practice that continues to be supported by the American Academy of Pediatrics as well. We join those advocating for universal screening, because it is low cost and low risk, yet provides important benefits for some children who would be missed if further evaluation was only triggered by parent or provider concerns.

One early screening tool that is widely used is the Modified Checklist for Autism in Toddlers (M-CHAT), which has recently been revised and includes a follow-up component for those who obtain high scores on the initial questions (M-CHAT-R/F; *www.mchatscreen.com*; D. Robins, Casagrande, et al., 2014). The strong sensitivity and specificity (both > .9) of the M-CHAT-R/F was demonstrated in a large sample of low-risk toddlers ages 18–24 months. Physician concern alone had a sensitivity of .24. Results showed that of toddlers identified through the two-stage screener, 47.5% were diagnosed with ASD, and 94.6% with developmental delays. Thus, almost all of the screen-positive cases warranted further evaluation and referral for early intervention. Importantly, universal screening procedures with the M-CHAT-R/F reduced the age of ASD diagnosis by 2 years (D. Robins, Casagrande, et al., 2014).

The Diagnostic Process

Currently, the diagnosis of ASD is based primarily on behavioral observations and history. To date, a definitive neuropsychological test profile does not exist, in part because typical neuropsychological test batteries do not evaluate social cognition in detail. There are cognitive test profiles that would be consistent with ASD, however, and cognitive testing is important to identify strengths and weaknesses in children whose everyday performance may present a confusing picture of their underlying abilities.

Presenting Symptoms

Children are often referred for failure to meet language and motor milestones in the preschool years. A loss of speech or other developmental attainments is particularly telling, though a dramatic regression is quite rare. More subtle regression is actually quite common (86% of high-risk infants), although it may occur so early or so gradually that it does not arouse clinical concern (Ozonoff et al., 2010). In addition, other important symptoms may be mentioned. These include reduced social engagement, reduced or unusual play behavior, nonsocial attachments (e.g., to pieces of string), odd communication (echoing, making up words, mixing up pronouns), motor rituals (rocking, spinning, hand flapping), unusual or repetitive interests (e.g., in timetables, calendars, meteorology, and astronomy), atypical use of objects (spinning, lining up, and close visual inspection), unusual responses to sensory stimuli, and preserved or enhanced areas of function (e.g., precocious reading or excellent rote memory).

History

Symptoms of autism are typically recognized early in development, usually by the toddler years, although children with ASD and strong intellectual skills may not be referred until later at school age. At about 1 year of age, initiation of joint attention and consistent response to name are two social behaviors that reliably discriminate typically developing children from children with ASD. During the toddler years, parents often report having to work hard to engage their child in social games and interactions. Children may show reduced or unusual nonverbal communication, such as reduced eye contact, inappropriate facial expressions, and reduced gesture use. Their language milestones may be delayed, although this is not universally true, and their language may have an odd or repetitive quality. Behavioral outbursts that are triggered by attempts to change a routine or transition to a different activity are common. During preschool, the child's social and play difficulties become more apparent, because the child has consistent opportunities to interact with same-age peers. The child may have limited pretend play skills and prefer parallel or solitary play activities rather than cooperative play. He or she may also fixate on certain toys/activities/interests to the exclusion of others, and these fixations may interfere with peer relationships, because they are not reciprocal. In later school years, social difficulties continue to be an area of weakness, especially in maintaining reciprocal conversations; establishing and maintaining friendships; interpreting humor, sarcasm, and metaphors; and understanding nuanced social interactions characteristic of adolescent peer and romantic relationships.

Behavioral Observations

Evaluating a child with ASD places a heavier than usual burden on the examiner, because the very nature of the disorder can significantly disrupt the relationship with the examiner. It may be difficult to complete some procedures; thus, behavioral observations play a greater role in the diagnostic formulation. These are usually abundant and clinically rich. Observations regarding the child's eye contact, verbal and nonverbal communication (e.g., gesture use and prosody), and social interest and engagement can be diagnostically useful. The examiner will also want to note any restricted interests or repetitive behaviors that present during the session, and how easily the child can adapt to redirection away from these interests or behaviors. The examiner should also note unusual behaviors that may suggest a lack of social awareness or a misreading of the social situation. For instance, a child in our clinic met his examiner for a follow-up session, did not acknowledge the examiner's greeting, and asked if they would be meeting in room 2-5-2 again. He didn't wait for a response and walked down the hall alone while the examiner greeted the parent.

The examiner should also bear in mind that children with ASD are poor at adapting to new situations, so the examining situation itself is likely to be particularly stressful and elicit unusual behaviors. We have seen children with ASD who read everything in sight as a way of coping with this anxiety, or who repetitively sniff pencil shavings or magic markers. The testing environment may also induce rigid and ritualized behaviors in the child, such as insisting on a specific schedule or dictating where examiners and parents will sit and when the examiner can turn the page of a testing booklet. Behavioral observations during neuropsychological testing can also provide converging evidence for a diagnosis by identifying executive deficits and particular cognitive styles that are characteristic of ASD, such as cognitive inflexibility, excessively concrete interpretations, or overfocusing on details in visual–spatial or other tasks.

Autism Assessment Tools

The two main diagnostic tools for ASD are the Autism Diagnostic Observation Schedule–Second Edition (ADOS-2; Lord, Rutter, et al., 2012) and the Autism Diagnostic Interview–Revised (ADI-R; Lord, Rutter, & Le Couteur, 1994). Both are standardized measures that have become the "gold standard" in the ASD field. Both the ADI-R and ADOS-2 have rigorous training procedures to reach reliability standards.

The ADOS-2, a semistructured, play-based assessment, is administered to the individual being assessed for ASD and takes 45 minutes–1 hour. Five modules of the ADOS-2 are designed for different ages and language levels, and include specific social presses and activities. The examiner watches for specific social–communication skills and behaviors during the course of the play session and codes these behaviors on a scale of 0 (*no abnormality*)–3 (*moderate to severe abnormality*). Specific algorithms have been designed to establish cutoffs with optimal sensitivity and specificity (Gotham, Pickles, & Lord, 2009; Gotham, Risi, Pickles, & Lord, 2007). In past iterations of the algorithms, RRBs were not included, but they are now included in the most recent revisions, because they have been shown to improve diagnostic stability. The most recent revision also combines social and communication scores because of previous studies showing that these form a single factor, and are consistent with the current DSM-5 diagnosis that also lumps these domains together. Investigation of the algorithms in a large replication sample showed that sensitivity and specificity for distinguishing children with ASD from those with nonautism diagnoses exceeded .80 for Modules 1–3. The ADOS-2 also makes an additional predictive contribution to ASD diagnosis, above and beyond the ADI-R (Gotham et al., 2009), which is why the two measures are often used in tandem.

The ADI-R is a standardized, semistructured parent interview that takes a few hours to administer. It has an interrater reliability of at least 90%, and both its sensitivity and specificity exceed 90% (Lord et al., 1994). The ADI-R interviews parents about both current behaviors and behaviors when children were 4–5 years old. This latter period can be helpful for assessing older individuals with good intellectual skills who may have shown more typical ASD behaviors in the past. While the diagnostic properties of the ADI-R are quite strong, time and cost concerns are often a barrier to use of this measure in current clinical and research contexts. There is ongoing work to address these concerns. For example, there has been preliminary work on a new measure, the Autism Symptom Interview (ASI), which is based on questions from the ADI-R (Bishop et al., 2017). The ASI is a parent interview that can be administered over the phone in 15–20 minutes. In an initial validation study, the ASI showed promising psychometric properties, particularly when combined with an in-person assessment of the child using the ADOS (Bishop et al., 2017). While the measure is being developed for research applications at this time, it may have clinical utility in the future given further validation.

Clinicians who have not been fully trained in the ADOS-2 and ADI-R may want to use a standardized screening tool to determine whether to refer children with concerning symptoms for a comprehensive ASD diagnostic assessment with a qualified professional. Even clinicians who are trained in "gold standard" measures may often use screening instruments initially to determine whether to move forward with a more time-intensive ASD-specific evaluation. One commonly used parent-report screening measure with acceptable psychometric properties is the Social Communication Questionnaire (SCQ; Berument, Rutter, Lord, Pickles, & Bailey, 1999; Rutter, Bailey, Berument, Lord, & Pickles, 2003). The SCQ comprises questions from the ADI-R. While published papers have supported the psychometric properties of the SCQ, there have also been questions about the validity of this measure because of differences in diagnostic accuracy across studies. A recent meta-analysis revealed that the SCQ's psychometric properties were stronger for the lifetime version and for children > 4 years of age (Chesnut, Wei, Barnard-Brak, & Richman, 2016), highlighting the importance of matching specific measures to the assessment context. For younger children, the M-CHAT has stronger psychometric properties as a screening instrument.

Another measure, the Social Responsiveness Scale—Second Edition (SRS-2; Constantino et al., 2003; Frazier, Ratliff, et al., 2014), is a brief parent- or teacher-report measure designed to assess the severity of autistic traits on a quantitative scale. The psychometric properties of the SRS-2 are strong. The measure relies on a dimensional conceptualization of autistic traits in which ASD is an extreme cutoff point on a continuous distribution (Constantino & Todd, 2003). As a result, it is designed to assess the full range of social–communication and RRBs that occur in the population. The SRS-2 is also appropriate for assessing change in autistic symptoms over time as a result of treatment (Constantino et al., 2003; Frazier, Ratliff, et al., 2014).

Multidisciplinary Assessment

In the previous sections, we have described the tools that are used by psychologists to assess ASD. However, the standard of care is for children to receive a multidisciplinary assessment involving professionals from psychology, speech–language therapy, occupational therapy, physical therapy, and various medical specialties, as appropriate (Volkmar et al., 2014). As part of a multidisciplinary assessment, clinical guidelines from the American Academy of Pediatrics and the American Academy of Child and Adolescent Psychiatry recommend that every child with ASD should also have a genetic workup (Committee on Bioethics, Committee on Genetics, & American College of Medical Genetics and Genomics Social, Ethical, and Legal Issues, 2013; Miller et al., 2010; Volkmar et al., 2014), because it is estimated that 10–30% of individuals with ASD will have an identifiable, putatively causal genetic variant.

Case Presentations

Case Presentation 8

Logan, a 7-year-old boy, is currently in second grade. Logan was referred for an evaluation because of speech–language delays, social difficulties, and behavior problems, including intense outbursts.

There is a family history of speech–language delays and social difficulties. Logan's father reports that he has difficulty making friends and tends to avoid large social gatherings. He works as a computer programmer. Logan's paternal cousin had a speech–language delay but did not experience additional developmental delays. Logan's prenatal and birth history were uncomplicated. His parents first became concerned about his development when Logan was a toddler, because he showed motor and language milestone delays. He did not walk independently until he was 18 months. His first words emerged when he was about 1 year old, but he remained in the single-word stage until he was about 2½ years old. At this time, his parents sought an evaluation through the state's early intervention program. This evaluation described delays in his speech–language, cognitive, motor, social–emotional, and daily living skills. He began receiving in-home speech–language therapy and occupational therapy. When Logan turned age 3 years, he was enrolled in an integrated preschool with special education support. Since that time, Logan has continued to be enrolled in self-contained special education classrooms that provide speech–language and occupational therapy support services. He also continues to receive private speech–language and occupational therapy.

Logan's parents described how, when he was a toddler, it was difficult to know what items he was requesting, and he would often melt down if he did not receive the desired item. To solve this problem, they taught him to point to indicate his request when he was about 1 year old. Although Logan would point to indicate his requests, he very rarely pointed to direct his parents' attention to items. Despite Logan's language delays, his parents do not remember him using any gestures besides pointing to communicate. To get his parents' attention, he would bring interesting items to them, but he tended to be focused on the object more than the social interaction. Logan's parents described his language as unusual at times. As a preschooler, he would get his pronouns mixed up, saying, "Help you," when he meant "Help me." He also repeats phrases and sentences from his favorite movies at unusual times.

Logan's parents' concerns about his social skills did not emerge until he entered preschool, although they report in retrospect that Logan was less socially engaged than their younger daughter. They recall that when Logan was an infant, they had to work hard to get him to smile. When Logan was a toddler, his parents felt that he did not know his name, because he would not always respond to their calls. They worked on Logan's eye contact when he was a toddler and felt that it improved. When Logan was excited about something, he would laugh and flap his hands. His parents thought that this hand-flapping behavior was very unusual.

Logan has had a very difficult time establishing and maintaining friendships. He has particular difficulty playing cooperatively with other children. He prefers to engage in solitary or parallel play. Logan enjoys lining up his toys, and he becomes very upset if someone disturbs them. This rigidity makes it difficult for him to play with other children. Logan does not engage in pretend play with his toys, preferring instead to crash his favorite toy, trains, together.

Behaviorally, Logan began having intense temper tantrums when he was a toddler. His tantrums were usually triggered by transitions or disruption in Logan's routine or agenda. Logan's parents described that he could get "stuck" on an idea or a play activity, and it was very difficult to transition him to another activity even when they provided warnings. Currently, Logan continues to have difficulty with transitions and disruptions in his routine. He likes certain daily routines to be completed in a precise order. If his routine or agenda is disrupted, he often has aggressive behavioral outbursts. Logan's parents also describe him as a child who becomes "obsessed" with items. Currently, he plays with trains to the exclusion of other play materials.

Logan's diagnostic testing is summarized in Table 13.1.

TABLE 13.1. Test Summary, Case 8

Performance validity
Memory Validity Profile Visual   RS = 11
                                         (valid)

General intelligence   **Fluid intelligence**
WISC-V Full Scale IQ   SS = 53   WISC V-Fluid Reasoning Index   SS = 58
                                                            Matrix Reasoning   ss = 2
Crystallized intelligence   Figure Weights   ss = 3
WISC V-Verbal Comprehension Index   SS = 55   WISC V-Visual Spatial Index   SS = 75
    Similarities   ss = 1   Block Design   ss = 5
    Vocabulary   ss = 3   Visual Puzzles   ss = 6

Working memory
WISC-V Working Memory Index   SS = 72
    Digit Span   ss = 6
    Picture Span   ss = 4

Processing speed
WISC-V Processing Speed Index   SS = 45
    Coding   ss = 1
    Symbol Search   ss = 1

Adaptive behavior
Vineland III Adaptive Behavior Composite   SS = 68

Academic
Reading   Math
    Basic literacy   WJ-IV Math Fluency   SS = 56
        WJ-IV Letter Word ID   SS = 70   WJ-IV Calculation   SS = 70
        WJ-IV Word Attack   SS = 72   WJ-IV Applied Problems   SS = 68

    Reading fluency   Spelling
        TOWRE-2 Sight Word Efficiency   SS = 71   WJ-IV Spelling   SS = 60
        TOWRE-2 Phonemic Decoding Efficiency SS = 73

Oral language
Semantics and syntax   *Verbal memory*
    PPVT-4   SS = 59   WRAML-2 Story Memory   ss = 5
    CELF-5 Core Language   SS = 61   WRAML-2 Story Memory Delay   ss = 4
        Sentence Comprehension   ss = 2   CTOPP-2 Nonword Repetition   ss = 5
        Word Structure   ss = 3
        Formulated Sentences   ss = 3
        Recalling Sentences   ss = 5

Attention and executive functions
Executive functions   *Attention*
    TOLDX   Not   Vanderbilt Inattention
                                     completed   Parent   4 of 9
    NEPSY-II Word Generation Semantic   Not   Teacher   5 of 9
                                     completed

(*continued*)

TABLE 13.1. (continued)

		Vanderbilt Hyperactivity/Impulsivity	
		Parent	2 of 9
		Teacher	3 of 9
Visual–spatial skills		**Social communication**	
Beery VMI-6	SS = 46	SCQ	28 of 40 (cutoff = 15)
		ADOS-2—Module 2	
		Social Affect Score	12
		Restricted and Repetitive Behavior	6
		Overall Total	18
		ADOS-2 Classification	Autism (cutoff = 9 for autism; cutoff = 8 for autism spectrum)

Note. SS, standard score with mean = 100 and *SD* = 15; ss, scaled score with mean = 10 and *SD* = 3; RS, raw score; %ile, percentile rank; WISC-V, Wechsler Intelligence Scale for Children—Fifth Edition; WJ-IV, Woodcock–Johnson Tests of Achievement—Fourth Edition; TOWRE-2, Test of Word Reading Efficiency—Second Edition; PPVT-4, Peabody Picture Vocabulary Test—Fourth Edition; CELF-5, Clinical Evaluation of Language Fundamentals—Fifth Edition; CTOPP-2, Comprehensive Test of Phonological Processing—Second Edition; WRAML-2, Wide Range Assessment of Memory and Learning—Second Edition; Vanderbilt, NICHQ Vanderbilt Assessment Scales; ADOS-2, Autism Diagnostic Observation Schedule—Second Edition; SCQ, Social Communication Questionnaire; Beery VMI-6, Beery–Buktenica Test of Visual Motor Integration, Sixth Edition; ToLDX-2, Tower of London DX—2nd Edition; NEPSY-II, NEPSY—Second Edition.

DISCUSSION

Logan's persistent difficulties with social interactions, his verbal and nonverbal communication delays, and his behavioral rigidity are all suggestive of ASD. Several specific behaviors reported in the parent interview are also highly suggestive of this diagnosis. First, Logan did not spontaneously learn to point. Once his parents had taught him to point, he did not use this gesture to initiate joint attention. Logan also showed an inconsistent response to his name, which led his parents to believe that he did not know his own name. Both of these indicators are highly indicative of ASD.

When the examiner first met Logan, he did not respond to her greeting, but he demonstrated interest in the materials. During the testing session, he frequently insisted on continuing with an activity in the manner he initiated. If he was interrupted, Logan became visibly upset. The examiner was able to transition him between tasks by providing ample warnings and structure via visual schedules. Logan's manipulation of the testing materials revealed considerable difficulties with fine-motor control.

Additional behavioral observations were obtained during administration of the ADOS-2, Module 2, a semistructured, play-based interview that provides a series of social situations within which a range of social and communicative behaviors should occur. Module 2 was chosen because it is appropriate for children of any age who are using phrase speech but are not verbally fluent (i.e., using complex sentences to join ideas together.) During the ADOS, Logan had considerable difficulty sustaining social interactions. He did not join in with a play script that the examiner initiated and reverted to functional play by himself. Although he seemed to enjoy the activities of the ADOS-2, he did not share this enjoyment with the examiner. He showed limited gesture use and eye contact. Although Logan generated spontaneous utterances, his language also included immediate echoes of the examiner's language and delayed echoes from his favorite movies. Logan's social–communication difficulties during the ADOS-2 are consistent with his parents' report on the SCQ, which assesses social, communication, and play behaviors and special interests, and helps to determine whether an individual's developmental history is consistent with ASD.

Logan's Full Scale IQ score and his Adaptive Behavior score are consistent with an ID. The fact that Logan's Adaptive Behavior score is considerably stronger than his IQ estimate probably reflects the fact that he has benefited from the interventions and supports he has received through his school and privately. On the Wechsler Intelligence Scale for Children–Fifth Edition (WISC-V), Logan showed some scatter among and within his index scores. His strongest scores were on the Working Memory and Visual Spatial Indices. As previously described, Logan likes to echo language, so he was fairly adept at repeating back information verbatim, such as on the digit span task and on a related subtest, Clinical Evaluation of Language Fundamentals–Fifth Edition (CELF-5) Recalling Sentences. Logan had more difficulty on the backwards and sequencing subtests of the digit span task, on which he repeated all items forward initially and needed to be prompted on every item to reverse the order or sequence the digits. Although this violated standard administration procedures, his performance with prompts was felt to be a more accurate assessment of his abilities, because his tendency to get "stuck" on repeating the items was hindering his performance. This tendency for Logan to get "stuck" was also apparent on the Symbol Search and Matrix Reasoning subtests, in which he fell into a response set of choosing the leftmost items on the page. Logan's tendency to get "stuck" is likely reflective of executive dysfunction. Formal assessment of his EF was limited by his relatively young age, as well as his weak conceptual and language skills.

Another pattern that was evident in the Verbal Comprehension and Fluid Reasoning indices of the WISC-V was that Logan had particular difficulty with abstract reasoning, consistent with his ID. For example, the Similarities subtest requires a higher degree of abstraction than does the Vocabulary subtest. Logan was not able to answer any of the items on the Similarities subtest correctly.

Logan continues to show significant fine-motor delays despite occupational therapy interventions. These fine-motor delays likely affected his performance on timed written tests of this battery (e.g., Processing Speed Index subtests, Woodcock–Johnson IV [WJ-IV] Math Fluency) and on tests requiring precise visual–motor integration (e.g., Beery–Buktenica Test of Visual–Motor Integration). Above and beyond these fine-motor difficulties, Logan showed a tendency to overfocus on the details, to the detriment of the gestalt on both of the visual–spatial tests. This strategy was fairly generalized, as it also characterized his recall on the WRAML-2 Story Memory subtest.

Overall, Logan's academic skills are on par with his cognitive abilities. He shows a relative strength in tasks requiring rote skills, such as word decoding and simple mathematical computations, compared to more integrative and abstract tasks.

Ratings from Logan's parents and teachers on the Vanderbilt NICHQ Rating Scale indicate some difficulties with inattention, although they do not meet the symptom criteria for an ADHD diagnosis. On further interviews, these symptoms were closely related to Logan's behavioral rigidity, which causes him to be distracted and to have difficulty following directions.

In summary, Logan is a child with an ID, but his social difficulties and behavioral rigidity cannot be entirely explained by this diagnosis. He also meets criteria for ASD based on converging evidence from his developmental history, testing results, and clinical observations during the ADOS-2. In Logan's case, the diagnosis of ASD with accompanying intellectual impairment would be appropriate.

Case Presentation 9

Sam, a 9-year-old boy who is currently in fourth grade, was referred for an evaluation because of concerns about his social development and his difficulty adapting to transitions and changes in routine.

Sam's family history is positive for anxiety disorder and depression. His prenatal and birth history were uncomplicated. According to his parents, his early development was typical to advanced, and he met his language and motor milestones within developmental expectations. Sam's parents observed that his language development seemed particularly advanced, because his vocabulary was quite large by the time he was about 1½ years old. During his toddler years, Sam's parents reported that his eye contact was limited, and his facial expression did not always seem appropriate to the situation. For example, Sam's parents described him as very caring and affectionate, but if somebody in his family was hurt or sad, he might not notice and would smile instead of expressing concern. Sam was very interested in the world around him, and he would point out items to his parents, but he did not check back to see whether they were looking at the item with him. Sam would play simple back-and-forth social games, like peekaboo, but he tired of these games quickly and would wander off to play by himself. Sam's response to his name was inconsistent when he was a toddler. If he was engrossed in an activity, his parents would need to work to get his attention, but other times, he would respond immediately.

Sam's parents' first concerns emerged when he was about 2 years old. He began exhibiting severe temper tantrums that occurred almost daily and lasted for about 30 minutes. The triggers for these tantrums were usually when Sam's routine changed or when he did not get what he wanted. Even as a toddler, Sam would latch onto certain routines, then insist that his parents follow them. For example, at bedtime, he requested the same two books to be read to him. If his parents attempted to expand his repertoire, he would get very upset. Currently, Sam continues to have difficulty with transitions and changes in his routine. Although he now throws tantrums only rarely, about once every 6 months, his parents describe that he can have "meltdowns" when something unexpected occurs.

In terms of Sam's academic history, Sam's preschool and kindergarten teachers reported that he excelled academically, but they had concerns about his social development and rigidity. He did not show much interest in other children and typically played alone. He had difficulty playing with other children, because he wanted to be "in charge." For example, he liked to line up cars, then tell the children which cars to play with and what road to take, and so forth. Currently, Sam continues to excel academically, but his social difficulties and rigidity have continued into grade school. His parents describe that he struggles to make and sustain friendships. Sam has a current interest in *Star Wars,* which provides a point of connection with other children, but Sam gets frustrated when the children do not want to play *Star Wars* according to his rules. He likes to use the action figurines to act out the scenes of the movie exactly. He does not like it when children want to pretend or add to the script he has in mind.

In terms of conversations with peers, Sam often does not respond to other children's attempts to initiate conversations, and he does not ask questions of other children. Sam sometimes makes socially inappropriate comments to his peers that isolate him further. For example, when a child gets an answer wrong in class, Sam might say, "Anybody should know that." His parents are puzzled by these statements, because Sam is not mean or rude to children in other contexts. With adults, Sam sometimes does not understand power hierarchies, and he relates to his parents and teachers as if they are his peers. Sam's conversations with adults tend to be less stilted than those with peers, especially if he is permitted to talk about his interest in *Star Wars.* Nevertheless, his parents describe how the conversation is often one-sided, with Sam providing information that he has already told them. They find it difficult to interrupt and redirect him when he is talking about *Star Wars.* They can usually move him off the topic for a couple of minutes, but then he brings the topic back up again. If Sam's parents initiate a conversation that is not about his interest, they find that he is less willing to participate in the conversation.

Although *Star Wars* is Sam's current interest, he has a history of restricted interests in dinosaurs, cars, and trains. His parents indicate that all of these interests have been unusually intense, even though the topics were age-appropriate. For example, regarding *Star Wars,* Sam will only read books about *Star Wars,* even though his parents have tried to interest him in other science-fiction novels. He plays primarily with *Star Wars* action figures, watches the movies repetitively, and prefers to talk about *Star Wars.* His parents find that his interest in *Star Wars* limits his exposure to other age-appropriate topics and toys.

Sam's diagnostic testing is summarized in Table 13.2.

DISCUSSION

Sam's persistent difficulties with reciprocal social and play interactions, his difficulty with transitions, and his restricted special interests are all suggestive of ASD. Sam did not have any delays in his cognitive or language development, so a diagnosis of ASD without intellectual or language impairment is most appropriate in the DSM-5 framework. Previously, the diagnosis of Asperger's disorder (DSM-IV)

TABLE 13.2. Test Summary, Case 9

Performance validity
Medical Symptom Validity Test
    Immediate Recall   RS = 100
    Delayed Recall   RS = 100
    Paired Associates   RS = 100
    Free Recall   RS = 100
    (valid)

General intelligence		**Fluid intelligence**	
WISC-V Full Scale IQ	SS = 129	WISC-V Fluid Reasoning Index	SS = 126
Crystallized intelligence		Matrix Reasoning	ss = 13
WISC-V Verbal Comprehension Index	SS = 124	Figure Weights	ss = 16
Similarities	ss = 13	WISC-V Visual Spatial Index	SS = 122
Vocabulary	ss = 16	Block Design	ss = 17
		Visual Puzzles	ss = 11
Working memory			
WISC-V Working Memory Index	SS = 103		
Digit Span	ss = 12		
Picture Span	ss = 9		
Processing speed			
WISC-V Processing Speed Index	SS = 115		
Coding	ss = 12		
Symbol Search	ss = 13		
Adaptive behavior			
SIB-R	SS = 105		

Academic

Reading		Math	
History		*History*	
CLDQ Reading Scale	43rd %ile	CLDQ Math Scale	44th %ile
Basic literacy		*Basic math/fluency*	
WJ-IV Letter Word ID	SS = 112	WJ-IV Math Fluency	SS = 110
WJ-IV Word Attack	SS = 111	WJ-IV Calculation	SS = 121
WJ-IV Spelling	SS = 122	*Math problem solving*	
Reading fluency		WJ-IV Applied Problems	SS = 116
TOWRE-2 Sight Word Efficiency	SS = 115		
TOWRE-2 Phonemic Decoding Eff	SS = 117		
GORT-5 Fluency	ss = 15		
Reading comprehension			
GORT-5 Comprehension	ss = 13		

Oral language
Verbal memory
  WRAML-2 Sentence Memory   ss = 10
  WRAML-2 Story Memory   ss = 11
  WRAML-2 Story Memory Dely   ss = 12
  CTOPP-2 Nonword Repetition   ss = 10

(continued)

TABLE 13.2. (*continued*)

Attention and executive functions

Attention		Executive functions	
Gordon Vigilance Commissions	63rd %ile	D-KEFS Trail Making Test	
Gordon Vigilance Total Correct	79th %ile	Visual Scanning	ss = 13
Vanderbilt Inattention		Number Sequencing	ss = 14
Parent	RS = 3	Letter Sequencing	ss = 12
Teacher	RS = 2	Letter–Number Switching	ss = 13
Vanderbilt Hyperactivity/Impulsivity		D-KEFS Verbal Fluency	
Parent	RS = 1	Letter Fluency	ss = 13
Teacher	RS = 1	Category Fluency	ss = 11
		WCST	
		Categories Completed	$T = 30$
		Perseverative Errors	$T = 28$

Nonverbal skills and memory		Social communication	
RCFT Copy	2nd–5th %ile	SCQ	18 of 40
Immediate Recall	$T = 35$		(cutoff = 15)
Delayed Recall	$T = 37$	ADOS-2 Module 3	
Beery VMI-6	SS = 85	Social Affect Score	8
		Restricted and Repetitive Behavior	2
		Overall Total	10
		ADOS-2 Classification	Autism (cutoff = 9 for autism; cutoff = 7 for autism spectrum)

Note. T, *T*-score with mean = 50 and *SD* = 15; SIB-R, Scales of Independent Behavior—Revised; TOWL-4, Test of Written Language—Fourth Edition; GORT-5, Gray Oral Reading Test—Fifth Edition; D-KEFS, Delis–Kaplan Executive Function System; WCST, Wisconsin Card Sorting Test; RCFT, Rey Complex Figure Test. For other abbreviations, see Table 13.1.

might have been an appropriate description of Sam's presentation. Although Sam did not have delays in his structural and semantic language development, he does show pragmatic difficulties. Children with strong cognitive and language skills like Sam are often *not* referred for an evaluation, because they perform well in an academic setting. They are often seen as bright children whose social awkwardness is attributable to their high cognitive abilities. Additionally, these children typically interact better with adults than with their peers, because adults are generally more patient with one-sided conversations about the child's special interests and his or her presentation as a "little professor." Moreover, if a child does receive a diagnosis of ASD, often teachers and family members in the child's life are disbelieving of the diagnosis, because they associate ASD exclusively with the lowest-functioning individuals. As such, the family and child may feel unsupported in implementing the interventions that are necessary for the child's optimal development.

On first meeting Sam, his greeting was somewhat unusual. He was standing in the waiting room watching the clock and did not orient when the examiner greeted his mother. He did orient when the examiner explicitly called his name. On another occasion, he asked whether he would be working in the same room, then went ahead to wait in the room by himself while the examiner spoke to his mother. Additional behavioral observations were obtained during administration of the ADOS-2, Module 3, a semistructured, play-based interview that provides a series of social situations within which a range of social and communicative behaviors should occur. Module 3 is appropriate for children and young adolescents who are verbally fluent. During the ADOS-2, Sam showed deficits in his nonverbal and verbal social–communicative behaviors. In the nonverbal realm, his eye contact and repertoire of facial expressions were limited. He occasionally smiled; otherwise, his affect was notably restricted. His gesture use was also limited to contexts in which gestures were prompted (e.g., "Show me" and "Tell me").

In terms of Sam's verbal communication style, his voice quality was loud and high-pitched. His language also had a pedantic quality because of his repeated use of particular words (e.g., *actually*). In fact, speaking with Sam was like talking to a "little professor," because he related to the examiner like a peer (e.g., suggesting ways to increase the efficiency of the testing) and had such a high level of verbal expression and comprehension. Nevertheless, despite these strong verbal skills, Sam had marked difficulty with reciprocal conversations. He was very interested in talking about *Star Wars*, but when the examiner pressed for conversations about other topics, Sam did not respond. A nice strength for Sam, however, was that he was socially motivated to participate in conversations, albeit about his own topics. He also made social bids for the examiner's attention (e.g., saying, "Look"), but these verbalizations were not integrated with eye contact or facial expressions.

Sam's play was notably poor, especially given his strong cognitive scores. He mostly exhibited functional play, such as putting items in the pockets of characters. When the examiner tried to engage him in a reciprocal play interaction, he interrupted and redirected the play toward his own interests.

Sam also showed limited insight into typical social relationships and feelings. When asked what made him feel certain feelings, he referenced his video games (e.g., he feels sad when he cannot complete a level.) His understanding of friendships was also limited. When asked about his friends, he said that he could not remember whether he and another boy were friends. When asked why people get married when they are older, he said it was because they can have cake.

Sam's Full Scale IQ score on the WISC-V fell in the very high range, consistent with teacher reports that Sam is a bright boy who excels at academic work. Among his index scores, Sam did show some scatter. His scores on the Verbal Comprehension, Fluid Reasoning, and Visual Spatial Indices all fell in the very high range, whereas his score on the Processing Speed Index fell in the high average range, and his score on the Working Memory Index fell in the average range. These scores suggest that verbal rote memory may be an area of relative weakness for Sam. Behavioral observations of Sam's performance during the Similarities and Block Design subtests were revealing. On the Similarities subtest, Sam had difficulty deriving the global rule that related the two items together. He had trouble switching from a more detailed strategy (e.g., which letters the words have in common) to a more global strategy, but once he was able to accomplish this switch, he was able to answer the more difficult items correctly. During the Block Design subtest, Sam stated that he was going to make his pattern different, not the same, consistent with observations that he often pursues his own agenda. It was difficult to move him away from this agenda, but once we did so, he was able to complete some of the most difficult patterns. Together these observations reveal a quality of cognitive inflexibility that is often characteristic of ASD. This weakness also emerged on the Wisconsin Card Sorting Test, in which Sam was able to complete the color and figure categories but could not transition to sorting by number. His perseverative errors on this test placed him in the 1st percentile. It is important to note that Sam's fluid reasoning scores were quite discrepant from his score on the Wisconsin Card Sorting Test. Although his abstract problem-solving abilities are above average, he had difficulty using these reasoning abilities in an unstructured task in which social feedback is necessary for solving the problem. This pattern suggests that Sam's rigidity and social difficulties will interfere with his ability to make full use of his abstract problem-solving abilities in some contexts.

A second cognitive style was evident on the WRAML-2 Story Memory, Beery–Buktenica Test of Visual–Motor Integration (Beery VMI), and Rey–Osterrieth Complex Figure Test. On each of these tests, Sam tended to overfocus on details. On the Beery VMI and the Rey, his copies were very detail-oriented, but they often lost the gestalt in the midst of the details. His recall of the Rey was severely fractionated, indicating that he encoded the design in isolated fragments, although there was no evidence for disproportionate loss of information over time. The same pattern was evident on the WRAML-2 Story Memory. On the delayed recall, Sam remembered several details about the story, but he did not recall the global thematic elements. This tendency to overfocus on details is a cognitive style characteristic of some children with ASD.

Sam's scores on the academic tests are consistent with his strong academic performance in school. Historically, he has sometimes struggled with longer written assignments, which is not surprising given his neuropsychological profile. Constructing an essay requires a child to stay focused on a topic and provide relevant details. It is likely difficult for Sam to write about topics that are outside of his special interests, just as it is difficult for him to talk about topics outside of his special interest.

This assessment battery included an assessment for symptoms of inattention and hyperactivity–impulsivity, which are often present in children with ASD. Sam does not seem to be experiencing clinically significant ADHD symptoms at this time. It is also important to include a social–emotional screen for secondary features of internalizing disorders. For example, children with ASD often have anxieties about making friends and being bullied. As these children approach adolescence, they are at increased risk for mood and anxiety problems, especially as they become more sensitive to not "fitting in" socially. Sam does not show secondary mood or anxiety difficulties at this time, but these symptoms should continue to be monitored.

In summary, Sam's persistent social difficulties, restricted interests, and difficulty with change and transitions are consistent with a diagnosis of ASD without language or intellectual impairment. This diagnosis is primarily based on Sam's history and observations of his social–communicative behaviors during testing, although converging evidence was obtained from the neuropsychological testing results. Although Sam excelled on most of the tests, he showed some cognitive inflexibility and a tendency to overfocus on details that is consistent with ASD.

Treatment

ASD alters a child's developmental trajectory. Language, cognitive, and social development all depend on many thousands of hours of learning, which strengthen connections in the relevant neural networks. Since a child with autism has missed much of this natural learning, it would be very surprising if a neurochemical intervention could abruptly reverse the symptoms of autism. However, intensive early interventions targeting these areas of development have been more successful in reversing some of the symptoms of autism.

In terms of pharmacological agents, the U.S. Food and Drug Administration (FDA) has approved two antipsychotics, risperidone and aripiprazole, to treat irritability associated with ASD. Other medications are used to treat associated symptoms, such as stimulants for attention problems and anticonvulsants for seizures. No medications have been approved for treating the core symptoms of ASD.

The most efficacious current treatments are psychosocial, involving intensive early intervention. The short-term goals of these intensive early interventions are to improve social, language, and cognitive skills, and to reduce behaviors that interfere with learning. The long-term goals are to promote adaptive and vocational skills.

In the past 10 years, the treatment literature for ASD has matured, with several randomized controlled trials (RCTs) documenting the efficacy of behavioral interventions for ASD. Advances in early diagnosis have allowed for the development of interventions targeting children <2–3 years (Zwaigenbaum et al., 2015). Zwaigenbaum and a multidisciplinary working group (2015) reviewed this literature and developed consensus recommendations for the field. First, they found strong evidence based on RCTs for the effectiveness of therapies for 2- to 3-year-olds with ASD. The working group advocated that therapy begin as soon as a diagnosis of ASD is "seriously considered" because of evidence of more positive impact with earlier intervention. The working group recommended treatments that blend developmental and behavioral approaches. These include a range of treatment models that fall under the umbrella of naturalistic developmental behavioral interventions (NDBIs; Schreibman et al., 2015). Interventions for ASD can be categorized as comprehensive or targeted. Comprehensive treatment models address a range of skills and abilities, and are delivered as an organized package of components. Comprehensive treatment models that had support from RCTs included the Early Start Denver Model and the UCLA/Lovaas model. Targeted interventions address a more narrow set of weaknesses that are thought to be core to the developmental processes impacted by ASD. Interventions that targeted specific social–communication (i.e., joint engagement), play, and/or imitation skills were also effective in improving outcomes. For example, the joint attention symbolic play engagement and regulation (JASPER) intervention is one example of a targeted intervention that has been tested with an RCT which showed that toddlers improved their joint attention and functional play following a short-term, parent-mediated intervention (Kasari, Gulsrud, Wong, Kwon, & Locke, 2010). The working group also recommended that treatments with children under age 3 years include substantial parent/caregiver involvement in a "cotherapist" model, in which the parent is trained to administer the therapies. Such a model takes advantage of "teachable moments" in daily life by integrating goals with daily routines and facilitating generalization of skills across contexts.

There are several areas for future research on early interventions to address. First, RCTs comparing one treatment approach to another are needed. Additionally, a better understanding of what are the "active ingredients" in multicomponent treatment approaches could improve efficiency of the interventions. Future studies should also continue to test for individual differences in response to intervention, in order to determine which intervention approaches work best for which children and under what conditions.

As children transition to school, treatment models focus on structured educational approaches with explicit teaching. Interdisciplinary teams of providers and family involvement are important to address weaknesses in different domains and to ensure generalization of skills across contexts. The Treatment and Education of Autism and Related Communication Handicapped Children (TEACCH) program is one structured teaching approach with evidence of treatment gains in the small to moderate range depending on the outcome evaluated. Nevertheless, these treatment effects should be considered in the context of a limited pool of available studies (Virues-Ortega, Julio, & Pastor-Barriuso, 2013). While the TEACCH program is a comprehensive structured teaching system, there are also evidence-based recommendations for more focused interventions to address specific behaviors. The National Professional Development Center (NDPC) on ASD has reviewed the research literature and identified 24 practices with a sufficient evidence base (Odom, Collet-Klingenberg, Rogers, & Hatton, 2010). Many of these evidence-based practices can be grouped under the categories of behavioral strategies derived from applied behavior analysis, positive behavioral supports, and structured teaching with visual supports (Odom et al., 2010). In their review, Odom et al. (2010) matched the evidence-based practices with the learning needs of the child—academic, behavior, communication, social, play, transitions—to support the development of individualized education program (IEP) learning goals through evidence-based practices. The NDPC has further supported this work by developing step-by-step guidelines and implementation checklists to guide teachers and practitioners. Importantly, educators in the field have also reviewed these guidelines for realistic implementation given various school settings (Odom et al., 2010) (*http://autismpdc.fpg.unc.edu/evidence-based-practices*). These resources can be very helpful for families and practitioners alike who are working to develop school-based interventions to ensure that children with ASD are making optimal progress toward their learning goals.

Social skills are an important target for school-age children with ASD. Treatments for social skills can be grouped in at least two ways: (1) the age range of the children receiving the therapy and (2) the delivery method of the therapy (parent-mediated, nonparental [teacher, clinician], technological, peers [including siblings], or combined) (Reichow & Volkmar, 2010). Reichow and Volkmar (2010) conducted a best-evidence synthesis of the social skills interventions that were tested with a rigorous research design from 2001–2008. RCTs are still relatively rare in this literature, so their review not only included RCTs, when available, but also examined group comparisons and single-subject designs. The synthesis involved 66 studies including 513 individuals with ASD. Social skills groups for school-age children had enough evidence to be considered an "established evidence-based practice," while video modeling for school-age children could be considered a "promising evidence-based practice" (Reichow & Volkmar, 2010). Other promising practices such as incorporating behavioral techniques in social skills instruction and the use of visual supports, such as social stories, could not be examined independently, because the techniques were used in combination with other intervention methods. The authors noted that this was likely a limitation of the narrowed scope of their review rather than a lack of evidence supporting these techniques. Reichow and Volkmar (2010) also highlighted a lack of research on social skills interventions for adolescents and adults and for individuals of all ages with weaker cognitive and language skills.

Another common treatment target is the EF deficits that are frequently seen in ASD (for a review, see Wallace et al., 2016). We focus here on a recent RCT of the Unstuck and on Target! program (UOT; Cannon, Kenworthy, Alexander, Werner, & Anthony, 2011; Werner & Anthony, 2011; Kenworthy et al., 2014). UOT uses a small-group format to teach self-regulation skills for flexibility, organization, and planning. In conjunction with the child groups, parents are provided instruction in generalizing lessons to the home environment through modeling and supporting flexibility and planning. The program also addresses the importance of flexibility in social interactions. Results from the RCT were quite promising (Kenworthy et al., 2014). Children in third through fifth grade with ASD were randomly assigned to UOT ($N = 47$) or a social skills intervention ($N = 20$) that was matched in intensity. Children in both groups improved in their social skills to an equivalent degree. Both groups also improved in EF skills (following rules, making transitions, being flexible), but the gains of the UOT group were greater. Further research is needed on the UOT program and the children with ASD for whom it is most effective. However, these preliminary results provide a proof of principle that contextually embedded EF training can be an effective intervention approach for children with ASD.

Treatment of children with ASD often involves additional therapies and approaches, including speech–language therapy, occupational therapy, physical therapy, and the management of comorbid disorders, especially medical disorders, ADHD, and anxiety. A full review of these therapies is beyond the scope of this chapter, but we note one promising treatment for anxiety in school-age children with ASD called Facing Your Fears (Reaven, Blakeley-Smith, Culhane-Shelburne, & Hepburn, 2012). This program is a group-based cognitive-behavioral therapy (CBT) intervention. In a randomized trial, Reaven and colleagues showed that 50% of the CBT group but only 9% of the treatment-as-usual group showed clinically meaningful improvement in their anxiety symptoms. Treatment gains were maintained or even enhanced at 3- and 6-month follow-up (Reaven et al., 2012). The Facing Your Fears program shows promise as an evidence-based practice to address clinically impairing anxiety that is frequently comorbid with ASD.

Unfortunately, many treatments offered for ASD are not evidence-based, yet they make broad promises about improvement and even "cures." The FDA has taken action against several companies that have made improper claims, and has recently warned parents about several marketed treatments and provided guidance for how to assess the validity of a treatment (*www.fda.gov/forconsumers/consumerupdates*). The FDA specifically mentioned the following treatments as lacking evidence for their claims—chelation therapies, hyperbaric oxygen therapy, detoxifying clay baths, and various products (i.e., essential oils, raw camel milk)—and reminded parents that there are many others. Similarly the ASD practice parameter from the American Academy of Child and Adolescent Psychiatry (AACAP; Volkmar et al., 2014) mentioned chelation therapies as ineffective and potentially dangerous. The practice parameter also described a number of treatments that have been shown to be ineffective: intravenous infusion of secretin, oral vitamin B_6 and magnesium; gluten-free, casein-free diet, omega-3 fatty acids and oral human immunoglobulin (Volkmar et al., 2014). The FDA has encouraged parents to seek out the advice of a health care professional before buying or using little-known or unproven treatments. While this is always good advice, it is particularly salient for the ASD field in which unproven treatments continue to proliferate and detract from a family's resources and time that could be dedicated to treatments that are known to be effective.

Optimal Outcome

ASD is usually considered a lifelong condition, but there is recent research documenting that a small number of children with ASD might move off the ASD spectrum and display social–communication skills that are within normal limits for their age (Anderson et al., 2014; Fein et al., 2013). These children have been labeled "optimal outcome," and there are still many unanswered questions about this group. One of the leaders of this line of research, Deborah Fein, PhD, noted in a relatively recent paper some of the key questions and controversies: "The existence of this phenomenon, as well as its frequency and interpretation, is still controversial: were they misdiagnosed initially, is this a rare event, did they lose the full diagnosis, but still suffer significant social and communication impairments or did they lose all symptoms of ASD and function socially within the normal range?" (Fein et al., 2013, p. 197). In the past, mainstream opinion has been that the feasibility of a child truly losing an ASD diagnosis over time was unrealistic, so the fact that such children are now being reported and characterized by independent research groups (Anderson et al., 2014; Fein et al., 2013) deserves full scrutiny and consideration. Such children with optimal outcomes, although still relatively rare, might provide insight into effective therapeutics and key predictors of response to treatment.

Fein et al. (2013) define children with *optimal outcome* as those who initially meet full diagnostic criteria for ASD but later no longer display significant autism symptoms and function within the normal intellectual range. They note, however, that optimal outcome does not preclude other weaknesses, such as difficulties with EF, attention, and/or symptoms of anxiety/depression. Research so far suggests: (1) A small percentage of individuals (estimates of 3–10%) initially diagnosed with ASD may later lose the diagnosis (Anderson et al., 2014; Helt et al., 2008; Moulton et al., 2016), and at least a subset of these individuals cannot be accounted for by an initial misdiagnosis; (2) children with higher cognitive functioning and more mild initial symptoms are more likely to fall in the optimal outcome group (Fein et al., 2013); and (3) children in the optimal outcome group compared to a matched ASD group have earlier parent concern, earlier referrals to specialists, and earlier and more intensive intervention, especially applied behavior analysis (ABA) therapy (Orinstein et al., 2014). The implication is that for a subset of children with particular protective factors (some of which we likely have not yet identified), early identification and intensive intervention could lead to optimal outcomes. More prospective, epidemiological research is needed to better define the percent of children who could potentially fall into this optimal outcome category. The available evidence certainly supports current practice recommendations for ASD that strongly recommend early intervention as soon as a diagnosis of ASD is "seriously considered" (Zwaigenbaum et al., 2015). However, some caveats are important. First, the intervention findings have only been documented with a retrospective design, so they cannot prove causality. Based on these exciting initial results, future studies should use more rigorous prospective designs. Second, *most* children with ASD do not display optimal outcomes, even if they are identified early and participate in intensive intervention. Thus, at this point, practitioners should never promise that any intervention will offer a "cure" for any particular individual child. On the other hand, this work in conjunction with the maturing intervention literature we reviewed earlier does provide a more optimistic outlook on ASD treatment than was the case in the past, even as recently as the previous edition of this book.

Table 13.3 provides a summary of current research and evidence-based practice for ASD.

TABLE 13.3. Summary Table: Autism Spectrum Disorder

Definition

- DSM-5 includes a major diagnostic reorganization of ASD.
- The term ASD now encompasses the disorders formerly known in DSM-IV as autism, Asperger's disorder, and PDD-NOS.
- ASD is defined by impairments in two domains: social–communication and RRBs.
- DSM-5 made changes to accommodate the most common comorbidities of ASD. Modifiers specify whether the child has an intellectual disability and/or language disorder. ADHD can now be diagnosed along with ASD.

Prevalence and epidemiology

- Current CDC prevalence estimate is 1 in 59 children.
- Increasing prevalence estimates over the past few decades have been widely reported.
- Better detection, broadened diagnostic criteria, and diagnostic substitution are contributing to prevalence increases. It is still unclear whether these factors account for all of the increase in ASD diagnoses or if there is a much smaller, true increase.
- Gender ratio is 3–4.5 males:1 female.

Developmental neuropsychology

- There is a growing consensus among researchers that a multiple-deficit account will be necessary to explain the full ASD phenotype.
- The "fractionable autism triad hypothesis" proposes that the symptom dimensions of ASD have separate etiologies; therefore, a unifying neurobiological theory of ASD is unlikely.
- Neuropsychological theories of ASD can be grouped into social (i.e., theory of mind) and nonsocial theories (i.e., executive dysfunction, weak central coherence). None of the existing theories of ASD provides a satisfactory account of both the social and nonsocial features of ASD.
- High-risk longitudinal designs have shown that infants with ASD are difficult to distinguish from controls at 6 months, but behavioral patterns start to diverge by 12 months.
- A regressive pattern of development is much more common than previously suspected but is not detected with parent-report measures.

Brain mechanisms

- The neuroimaging literature in ASD continues to have mixed findings that make it difficult to extract replicated results.
- There is no single structural or functional brain correlate of ASD that can explain both of the core symptom domains.
- Macrocephaly has historically been one of the best replicated structural findings in ASD and has led to the "early brain overgrowth hypothesis," which is receiving renewed scrutiny in terms of the timing and effect size of brain overgrowth.
- Region-specific structural differences have been identified in ASD, particularly in the limbic system and the frontal–striatal circuity, which are associated with social–communication and RRBs, respectively.
- Functional studies have primarily focused on social processing and cognitive control. The fusiform gyrus is frequently hypoactivated while viewing faces. Abnormalities are often seen in frontal and frontal–striatal regions during executive tasks, though directionality of effects has been mixed across studies.
- There is an increasing emphasis on the dynamics of the brain in ASD, especially connectivity. Theories of long-range underconnectivity are being reevaluated in light of methodological advances. A more complex picture is emerging that indicates underconnectivity in cortical–cortical connections but overconnectivity in subcortical–cortical connections.
- Studies of structural connectivity consistently find evidence for less robust white matter integrity, with the temporal lobe being particularly vulnerable.

(continued)

TABLE 13.2. (continued)

Etiology

- ASD is one of the most heritable psychiatric diagnoses ($h^2 \sim .70-.90$).
- Sibling recurrence risk is 10–20%.
- The broader autism phenotype, characterized by social and cognitive deficits, runs in families.
- Twin studies find genetic effects to be the most prominent etiological factor in ASD, with variable evidence for shared environmental effects that depend on the sampling and liability model.
- Genetic influences on the social–communication and RRB domains of ASD are surprisingly distinct, leading to the "fractionable autism triad hypothesis."
- Molecular genetic research has flourished in ASD. Advancements in genetic technology have permitted the identification of common and rare, inherited and de novo, and small (one base pair change—SNP or SNV) and large (deletions and duplications—CNV) genetic risk factors associated with ASD.
- Simulations estimate that there will be 800–1,200 ASD risk genes—a much more complex genetic picture than was anticipated.
- Genes implicated in ASD are showing early signs of coalescing into specific biological pathways, including the WNT and MAPK signaling, synaptic signaling, chromatin remodeling, and fragile X pathways.
- Genetic evaluation is recommended for all children with an ASD diagnosis.
- Pre- and perinatal environmental factors are also associated with ASD, including paternal and maternal age, *in utero* valproate exposure, maternal infections, obstetric complications, and extreme environmental deprivation. Strong research designs are needed to establish whether these factors are causal or correlational.
- There is no evidence that the MMR vaccine or thimerosal-containing vaccines cause ASD.

Diagnosis

- The American Academy of Pediatrics recommends universal screenings for ASD, using empirically based screening tools, at 18 and 24 months.
- The M-CHAT has adequate sensitivity and specificity to be used as a screening tool in toddlers ages 18–24 months.
- The ADI-R and ADOS-2 remain the "gold standard" diagnostic tools for ASD. Both have rigorous training procedures to reach reliability standards.

Treatment

- No pharmacological agents have FDA approval for the treatment of core symptoms associated with ASD, though two antipsychotics have been approved for the treatment of associated symptoms (i.e., irritability).
- There are several randomized controlled trials documenting the efficacy of behavioral interventions for young children with ASD, with evidence that earlier intervention is more effective.
- For young children with ASD, consensus recommendations support treatments that blend developmental and behavioral approaches.
- As children transition to school, treatment models should focus on structured educational approaches with explicit teaching.
- Social skills groups for school-age children have amassed enough evidence to be considered an "established evidence-based practice."
- Preliminary evidence suggests that contextually embedded EF training may improve both social and EF skills.
- Unproven treatments continue to proliferate but organizations such as the FDA and the American Academy of Child and Adolescent Psychiatry are more proactive about warning parents.
- Research on "optimal outcome" children who move off the spectrum is ongoing. Many questions about this intriguing minority of children remain.

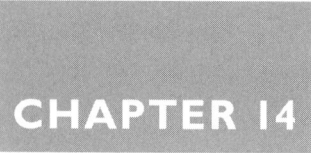

Intellectual Disability

CHAPTER SUMMARY

Unlike the chapters for the other five learning disorders covered in this book, this chapter on intellectual disability (ID) focuses on three genetic syndromes that cause moderate ID: Down syndrome (DS), fragile X syndrome (FXS), and Williams syndrome (WS). This is because much more progress has been made in identifying genetic syndromes that cause moderate ID, compared to mild ID. Each of these three moderate ID syndromes—DS, FXS, and WS—has a somewhat distinct neuropsychological and brain phenotype. Hence, reaching the eventual goal of tracing the developmental pathways that run from a genetic etiology through early brain development and resulting neuropsychology and behavior is much closer in the case of moderate ID than is the case for other learning disorders, partly because each of these syndromes is defined etiologically by its distinct genetic cause, which is necessary and sufficient to cause the syndrome. This homogeneity in genetic etiology is unique when compared to most other learning disorders covered in this book, where it is expected that hundreds to thousands of genes contribute in a massively polygenic fashion, such that no single genetic variation is necessary or sufficient. With a clear genetic etiology as a starting point, mapping developmental pathways across levels of analysis has been more tractable for these syndromes than for the other learning disorders.

After discussing the history and definition of ID, and the etiology of mild ID, we then review what is known about each of these three moderate ID syndromes: DS, FXS, and WS. These three syndromes exemplify the progress that has been made toward a neuroscientific understanding of ID. As we will see, each has a distinctive cognitive *and* social phenotype. The contrasting social phenotypes in these three disorders involve personality dimensions, such as gregariousness, empathy, and social anxiety, which are highly relevant for understanding other behavioral disorders. By tracing the complex developmental pathways that run from genetic alterations through brain development to these distinctive cognitive and social phenotypes, we are learning about the brain mechanisms underlying typical cognitive and social development. As such, ID syndromes can provide a very important universality test for developmental theory. Our review of each syndrome begins with the genetic etiology, then we consider brain mechanisms and neuropsychology. The final clinical portion of the chapter covers the diagnosis and treatment of all of ID, both syndromal and nonsyndromal.

HISTORY

ID, previously called mental retardation, has been recognized since antiquity, as witnessed by the ancient distinction (expressed in pejorative terms) between those who had lost their reasoning ("lunatics") and those who had never developed it ("idiots"). However, in earlier times, those with ID were either neglected or placed in asylums. Efforts to teach individuals with ID, to treat them humanely, and to understand their needs scientifically are much more recent and began with the Enlightenment, although much remains to be done to attain all three goals.

In France in 1799, Jean Itard found an abandoned boy with ID and possibly autism in the forest (Victor, the Wild Boy of Averyon) and attempted to train him using instructional methods already in use with the deaf (Achenbach, 1982). Itard's work with Victor is dramatized in Truffaut's movie, *L'Enfant Sauvage* ("The Wild Child"). Itard succeeded to some extent, showing that training could help those with ID, but Itard eventually abandoned Victor, who lived out his days in lonely custodial care.

Edward Seguin (1812–1880) pursued systematic efforts to train individuals with ID, both in France and the United States (Achenbach, 1982). By the middle of the 19th century, several training schools for individuals with ID were established, and in 1876, the directors of these schools in the United States formed a society that later became the American Association on Mental Retardation (AAMR; Hodapp & Dykens, 1996).

Part of the motivation for Binet and Simon's (1916) development of the first IQ test was to improve the reliability of diagnosing ID, including the three levels of ID distinguished at that time (i.e., moron, imbecile, and idiot, which correspond roughly to mild, moderate, and severe/profound ID). In their 1916 book, they discuss at length the psychometric problems with previous clinical diagnostic methods, mainly used by physicians working in state-funded institutions for people with ID. These earlier diagnostic methods were informal and therefore relied on clinical judgment. As a result, there was often poor agreement across physicians as to whether a patient had ID or not, and if so, what level of ID he or she had, even though these diagnostic decisions had huge consequences for the individuals involved.

Despite the good intentions of Binet and Simon and the founders of the AAMR, training schools for individuals with ID often devolved into deplorable institutions. Widespread acceptance of the "science" of eugenics at the end of the 19th century led to much more hostile attitudes toward those with ID. Eugenics portrayed familial ID as a threat to the gene pool. Such a threat was dramatized by supposedly scientific accounts of extended families with limited intellectual functioning, such as *The Jukes* (Dugdale, 1877) and *The Kallikak Family* (Goddard, 1912). These concerns lead to the reprehensible practice of enforced sterilization of those with ID.

For instance, the Virginia Sterilization Act of 1924 was upheld by the U.S. Supreme Court in 1927 in the famous case of *Buck v. Bell,* which involved a 17-year old female, supposedly with ID. Leading up to the Court's decision, the foster parents of Carrie Buck committed her to the Virginia Colony for Epileptics and Feeble-Minded after she became pregnant from being raped by the couple's nephew! There she became subject to the new sterilization law, whose legality the state of Virginia wanted to test. Chief Justice Oliver Wendell Holmes wrote the majority opinion upholding this sterilization law, concluding with the sentence "three generations of imbeciles are enough." The three generations were Carrie's mother, Carrie, and her newborn daughter, but it is not clear that any of the three actually had ID. Moreover, since very little was actually known about the etiology of ID at the time, such a practice of enforced sterilization was not only ethically but also scientifically questionable.

The contemporary view of the treatment of those with ID is partly a humane reaction against this history of past abuses, and it emphasizes the rights of those with disabilities. An important emphasis is on inclusion and integration into typical life activities—in families, schools, and communities. The AAMR, which has changed its name to the American Association on Intellectual and Developmental Disabilities (AAIDD), promotes these efforts. The AAIDD is the main professional organization in the field of ID; it publishes two journals and supports research, intervention, and social policy efforts in this field. We return to the topic of treatment later in this chapter.

Scientific understanding of some of the causes of ID is actually quite recent. Such causes include genetic syndromes, early neurological insults, polygenic inheritance, and environmental deprivation. Although Down's (1866) description of the syndrome that bears his name is over 140 years old, the genetic basis of Down syndrome was only discovered about 60 years ago (Lejeune, Gauthier, & Turpin, 1959). Our understanding of the molecular basis of FXS, another common genetic cause of ID, is much more recent still. The number of known genetic causes of ID exceeded 100 twenty years ago (Plomin, DeFries, McClearn, & Rutter, 1997), and many more have been more recently discovered by using state-of-the-art genetic methods such as whole-genome sequencing. Other known genetic causes of ID include the bases for phenylketonuria (PKU), Lesch–Nyhan syndrome, tuberous sclerosis, and Prader–Willi, and Angelman syndromes, to name a few.

DEFINITION

The definition of ID provides a good example of the issues involved in dimensional versus categorical conceptions of disorders, as well as the issues involved in etiological versus behavioral definitions. Part of what we call ID (especially mild ID) is on a continuum of intelligence and adaptive functioning, the two constructs used in definitions of ID. Thus, the IQ and adaptive behavior cutoffs for ID, as well as those for the subtypes of ID (i.e., mild, moderate, severe, and profound), are inevitably somewhat arbitrary and have changed over the years.

On the other hand, unlike most of the symptom dimensions considered in this book, there is clear *bimodality* in the lower tail of the IQ distribution, and many cases of moderate or more severe ID are part of a distinct distribution, with distinct etiologies, which we discuss later. Hence, there are many more known ID syndromes than is true for any other learning disorder described in this book. What makes them a syndrome is that they have a distinct etiology that produces a distinctive physical and behavioral phenotype. Nonetheless, the majority of cases of ID are nonsyndromal, although genetic progress continues to reduce this number.

At first glance, it might appear that we should prefer etiological definitions of ID whenever they are available. But since those who share an etiology (e.g., trisomy 21, the cause of Down syndrome) nonetheless vary in their level of cognitive and adaptive functioning, it is not at all clear that etiological definitions should replace behavioral ones, especially for most treatment purposes. Obviously, an individual with Down syndrome, but *not* with ID, needs different services than another individual with Down syndrome and moderate, severe, or profound ID. For any disorder, there is no doubt that etiological definitions help focus research and medical interventions, but short of a medical cure, we continue to need behavioral definitions to guide treatments.

Most current definitions of ID (e.g., such as the one found in DSM-5) require three things: an intellectual deficit, an adaptive behavior deficit, and onset within the developmental period. More specifically, IQ must be approximately 2 *SD*s or more below the mean on an individually administered IQ test (e.g., an IQ of 70 ± 5, on the Wechsler IQ scales, with the confidence interval reflecting measurement error). Hence, an individual with an IQ of 75 (on an IQ test with a mean of 100, an *SD* of 15, and a standard error of the mean [*SEM*] of ± 5) who meets the other two criteria, can be diagnosed as ID according to DSM-5. In contrast, an individual less than 18 years old with an IQ of 65 or less, but with an adaptive behavior score of roughly 80, would not meet diagnostic criteria for ID. Obviously, the progress of such ambiguous cases needs to be monitored after appropriate interventions are implemented to see if the diagnoses change.

Unlike DSM-IV, which used IQ ranges to define the four levels of ID (i.e., mild, moderate, severe, and profound), DSM-5 defines these four levels of severity on the basis of levels of adaptive functioning. The reason for this change is that level of adaptive functioning determines the environmental supports needed by the individual with ID better than IQ does.

Some earlier DSM definitions had a higher IQ cutoff (1 *SD* below the mean), and did not require an adaptive behavior deficit. As a result, about 16% of the population met criteria for ID! Since many such individuals did not have significant social and occupational problems as adults, the validity of this diagnostic definition was questionable. The lower IQ cutoff of 2 *SD*s below the mean plus an adaptive behavior deficit identifies only roughly 1–3% of the general population, compared to the 16% identified earlier. Individuals with IQs that low are much more likely to have problems meeting the demands of everyday life, but even with a lower IQ cutoff, there will inevitably be some false-positive diagnoses. This possibility is especially troublesome in some ethnic minority and low socioeconomic status (SES) groups whose average IQ is below the population mean of 100, likely because of reduced educational opportunities, poorer health care, and other pervasive societal inequities (discussed in Chapter 8).

To illustrate this problem, let us consider a hypothetical group with a mean IQ of 85, a normal distribution of IQ, and an *SD* similar in magnitude to that found in the general population (i.e., 15). In this particular case, about 16% of the subpopulation would fall below an IQ cutoff of 70, again raising questions about the validity of the definition. To eliminate the false-positive problem in some ethnic and SES groups, the adaptive behavior deficit criterion was added to the definition of ID in the 1970s. The combination of the two criteria, an IQ 2 *SD*s below the mean and an equally extreme adaptive behavior deficit, is much more likely to identify individuals who are having significant problems in everyday life because of low intelligence.

In summary, the shifting IQ cutoffs in definitions of ID illustrate that imposing a cutoff on a continuum is somewhat arbitrary. Any cutoff will have a mix of costs and benefits in terms of external validity, clinical benefits to individuals, and social consequences. Moreover, these different uses of the diagnosis will be unlikely to agree on the best cutoff. One can imagine that, as the global economy increasingly demands technological sophistication from workers, arguments for raising the IQ cutoff for ID could become more common again.

Of the three diagnostic criteria for ID, the one that is least well defined is the adaptive behavior deficit. DSM-5 requires that there must be a significant deficit in at least one of three broad areas of adaptive functioning, namely, the conceptual, social, or practical domains. These domains can be assessed with standardized measures such as the Adaptive Behavior Assessment System III (ABAS-3, Harrison & Oakland, 2015), and the Vineland Adaptive Behavior Scales—Third Edition (Vineland-3; Sparrow et al., 2016). These measures have good psychometric characteristics. For example, the ABAS-3 has good test–retest reliability of .82–.89. It is also important to show that the adaptive assessments are clearly measuring something besides IQ. In the case of the ABAS-2, which has high item similarity with the ABAS-3, the correlations with IQ are in the moderate range (.41–.58) (data not available for ABAS-3). In terms of convergent validity, the correlation of the ABAS-3 with the Vineland-2 is .80. This is strong evidence for convergent validity but, of course, this agreement is not perfect, so diagnostic decisions about ID will vary to some extent as a function of which measure of adaptive behavior is used. This diagnostic uncertainty will be greater for individuals with milder deficits in IQ and adaptive behavior (i.e., those with IQs close to 70). Despite this uncertainty, the reliability of the diagnosis of ID is higher than that of many disorders, because it requires the convergence of two separate behavioral criteria, IQ and adaptive behavior, each of which can be highly reliable.

PREVALENCE AND EPIDEMIOLOGY

As the previous discussion makes clear, obviously, the prevalence of ID depends on which cutoffs are used. Using the earlier definition (an IQ that is 2 *SD*s below the mean, an adaptive behavior deficit, and onset before age 18), the prevalence is between 1 and 3% (Hodapp & Dykens, 1996), with the majority having mild ID. The prevalence of the other three subtypes (moderate, severe, and profound) *combined* is 0.4%, or 4 per 1,000 (Hodapp & Dykens, 1996). Thus, depending on which overall prevalence estimate (i.e., 1 or 3%) is used, between 60 and 87% of the total population with ID will have mild ID.

ID is more common in males than in females; the gender ratio is about 1.6 males per female for mild ID and about 1.2/1.0 for severe ID (American Psychiatric Association, 2013). This male predominance is partly due to the large number of X-linked ID syndromes, the most common of which is FXS, which is discussed in more detail below. Because males have only one X chromosome, whereas females have two, they will manifest the phenotype caused by an abnormal gene on their X chromosome, whereas the phenotype in females with the same abnormal gene will be milder (or absent), because they have a normal copy of that gene on their second X chromosome.

Comorbidities

Comorbidity with other psychiatric diagnoses is a common aspect of ID; hence, many individuals with ID have "dual diagnoses," and it is important that they receive appropriate treatment of both their ID and their comorbid disorder. Symptoms of attention-deficit/hyperactivity disorder (ADHD) are very common across most forms of ID.

ETIOLOGY

Nonsyndromal ID

Both genes and environment contribute to the etiology of nonsyndromal ID. For instance, one of the most frequent environmental causes is fetal alcohol syndrome. Both direct and indirect evidence support the conclusion that the etiology of moderate or more severe ID is substantially distinct from the etiology of mild ID. We have already seen that some of these etiologies of moderate or more severe ID are nonfamilial (e.g., DS). Other nonfamilial organic etiologies, such as teratogens, perinatal complications, and postnatal neurological insults (e.g., meningitis and brain injuries) are also much more common in moderate and more severe ID (Hodapp & Dykens, 1996).

Moreover, as mentioned earlier, the lower tail of the IQ distribution is bimodal (Dingman & Tarjan, 1960), which also suggests distinct, nonfamilial etiologies of ID for individuals in the second, smaller distribution. Therefore, one can predict that siblings drawn from probands in this second smaller distribution should *not* be at risk for ID. Consistent with this prediction, the siblings of probands with moderate and more severe ID have a mean IQ of 103 (Nichols, 1984); that is, they have regressed *all* the way back to the population mean, indicating that the etiology of the probands' extreme low IQ scores is nonfamilial; it cannot be due to either genes or environments shared by family members.

In contrast, mild ID is part of the lower tail of the IQ distribution and is clearly familial. In a classic family study of ID (Reed & Reed, 1965), 289 probands with mild ID and their relatives were examined. If mild ID is familial, the mean IQ of siblings of probands with mild ID should *not* regress all the way back to the population mean, unlike the case in moderate or more severe ID. In Reed and Reed (1965), the mean sibling IQ was about 1 *SD* below the population mean (i.e., about 85), thus supporting familiality. A second test of familiality involves transmission from parents to offspring. Reed and Reed (1965) found that if one parent had mild ID, the risk for ID in their children was 20%, whereas if both parents had mild ID, the offspring risk rose to 50%, again supporting familiality.

The distributional and etiological differences between mild and more severe ID have led to a distinction between "organic" and "cultural–familial" ID, which is called the *two group* approach (Hodapp & Dykens, 1996). Pennington (2002) discusses the implicit dualism involved in labeling some disorders "organic" and others not. In the current context, another problem with this distinction is that it might lead one to assume that the familial influences on mild ID are all environmental. Although we do not have a twin or adoption study of probands with mild ID per se, we do know that the overall heritability of IQ is about 50%, and that twin studies of individuals with below average IQs find a similar value (Plomin et al., 1997). In a study of over 3,000 infant twin pairs, Eley et al. (1999) found that the heritability of IQ in the lowest 5% was similar to that in the rest of the sample. So it appears that IQ is similarly heritable across the entire distribution of IQ scores, which would mean that mild ID is about 50% heritable. (As we discussed earlier, moderate, severe, and profound ID are less heritable but can be strongly genetic.)

However, it is also possible that environmental influences could be stronger at the low end of the IQ distribution, because children of parents with low IQs would be exposed to a greater range of environmental adversities, including poorer health care, nutrition, and schools. These possibilities become even more salient when we consider minority groups that are at greater risk for such adversities. Indeed, in two early twin studies, researchers found lower heritability of IQ in children of parents with lower education (i.e., an SES × heritability interaction) (Rowe, Jacobson, & Van den Oord, 1999; Turkheimer, Haley, Waldron, D'Onofrio, & Gottesman, 2003). More recently, there has been mixed support for this finding, with some studies reporting no moderation effect or even a trend in the opposite direction (for a review, see Hanscombe et al., 2012). In a large twin study in the United Kingdom ($N \sim 8,000$ twin pairs), Hanscombe et al. (2012), reported no evidence of a SES × heritability interaction, but they did find consistent support for a SES × shared environment interaction. This result suggests that shared experiences between siblings explain more of the variance in IQ for children raised in lower SES families than for those raised in higher SES families. Hence, the influence of environment on

IQ may differ across environmental circumstances (i.e., an environment × environment interaction).

We next consider the specific genetic mechanisms that operate in DS, FXS, and WS, and also review the neuropsychology and neurology of each syndrome.

Syndromal ID

Before beginning each syndrome section, we present a brief review of the behavioral features of each ID syndrome that are distinctive. While these descriptions of the behavioral phenotype may be useful for understanding the disorder, we must also recognize that there is individual variation within each disorder, so not all features apply to all children.

Down Syndrome

DISTINCTIVE BEHAVIORAL FEATURES

The behavioral phenotype of DS is primarily characterized by the cognitive characteristics that we describe in the neuropsychology section below, most notably, relative weaknesses in speech and language skills and relative strengths in some aspects of visual–spatial processing (an opposite pattern from that seen in WS) (Chapman & Hesketh, 2000; Fidler, 2005). Social skills and social engagement are also areas of relative strength. There is evidence that individuals with DS have relative strengths in adaptive skills compared to individuals with other cognitive disabilities (Chapman & Hesketh, 2000). A unique feature of DS is the early-onset dementia that emerges for many individuals with DS (see discussion below).

GENETIC MECHANISMS AND EPIDEMIOLOGY

DS is the most prevalent (about 1–1.5 per 1,000 live births) form of ID with a known genetic etiology (*nondisjunction* of chromosome 21). Because nondisjunction is sporadic (not familial), the large majority (94%) of cases of DS are nonfamilial, and the most well-documented risk factor for DS is greater maternal age. The genetic etiology of DS involves a whole extra chromosome (thus, possibly an extra dose of the gene products of all its genes), so tracing the developmental pathways from genotype to phenotype is much more difficult in DS than in FXS or WS, in which a more constrained set of genes is involved. Moreover, it has recently become clear that the genetic influences on DS extend beyond the exons (i.e., protein coding regions) on chromosome 21, and include dysregulation of many genes on other chromosomes, as well as changes in epigenetic influences (Dierssen, 2012).

Nonetheless, some progress has been made in refining the DS region on chromosome 21 and relating specific genes in that region to specific DS phenotypes. This progress has come from mouse models of DS (Dierssen, 2012) and from examining patients with different partial trisomies of chromosome 21 (Korbel et al., 2009). Two findings are of particular relevance here, namely, that there is more than one ID region on chromosome 21, unlike what is true for some physical phenotypes in DS, and that the amyloid precursor protein (APP) gene is *not* in an ID region.

The extra dose of APP is strongly implicated as a cause of the high rate of early onset Alzheimer's disease (AD) in adults with DS. Amyloid plaques are part of the characteristic neuropathology of AD and are found in the brains of adult individuals with DS. Hence, most people with DS have two developmentally distinct forms of mental impairment, an early-onset one caused by multiple genes, most not yet identified, and a later-onset dementia caused by APP. Hence, DS is the clearest current example of how research on dementia and a neurodevelopmental ID can complement each other. Recent discoveries in FXS have pointed to a similar connection, as we discuss below.

NEUROPSYCHOLOGY AND NEUROLOGY

Besides low IQ, the neuropsychological phenotype in DS includes below mental-age-level performance on verbal short-term memory (STM) and language skills (e.g., syntax and articulation), verbal and visual–spatial episodic long-term memory (LTM), and certain executive function (EF) tasks (e.g., Zelazo's Dimensional Change Card Sort, which is a "junior" version of the Wisconsin Card Sorting Task (Zelazo, 2006), which elicits perseverative responding in patients with prefrontal cortex [PFC] lesions). Moreover, the *rate* of cognitive development is depressed in children with DS, resulting in slower growth of raw scores than expected based on initial IQ level and hence declining IQ standard scores with age.

The neurological phenotype in children and adults with DS includes (1) microcephaly and (2) differentially smaller volumes of the cerebellum, hippocampus, and PFC, although the PFC finding does not always survive correction for overall brain size. These features all predate the later development of AD in DS, consistent with the fact that the early and late neurological phenotypes have different genetic causes. Very little is known about actual brain development in DS, because there are no longitudinal studies.

Although we can propose plausible brain–behavior relations between the neuroanatomical and neuropsychological phenotypes, such as relating microcephaly to low IQ, decreased hippocampal volumes to episodic LTM deficits, and decreased PFC volume to EF deficits, these associations have not been systematically tested. Dierssen (2012) reviews evidence that (1) the size of the parahippocampal gyrus in individuals with DS predicts IQ and language; (2) that DS and WS have an opposite profile of basal ganglia versus cerebellar morphology (i.e., the basal ganglia are abnormal in WS, whereas the cerebellum is normal; the opposite is found in DS); and (3) that there are dendritic abnormalities in both human patients with DS and mouse models of DS that decrease long-term potentiation (LTP) and increase long-term depression (LTD).

This last finding of LTP decreases and LTD increases is particularly important, because a similar imbalance in synaptic plasticity and homeostasis is also found in WS (Todorovski et al., 2015) and FXS, as we review later. In addition, all three of these syndromes exhibit impairments in LTM (Raitano-Lee, Pennington, & Keenan, 2010). Hence, a unifying neurophysiological explanation of ID is emerging in which the imbalance between LTP and LTD impairs explicit LTM and slows learning (Fernandez & Garner, 2007). As we discussed in Chapter 4, this explicit LTM deficit distinguishes ID from the other learning disorders in this book, which have intact explicit LTM but deficits in implicit LTM (specifically, in procedural and statistical learning).

Fragile X Syndrome

DISTINCTIVE BEHAVIORAL FEATURES

The behavioral phenotype of FXS is strikingly different from that of DS and WS, particularly with regard to social skills. Most males with FXS present with autistic symptoms, including prominent deficits in eye contact, reduced social engagement, and repetitive behaviors. Approximately 30% of boys with FXS qualify for a full diagnosis of autism spectrum disorder (ASD; Hagerman et al., 2009). For those who do not meet full criteria for ASD, shyness and social anxiety are very common. Language delays and ADHD symptoms are also common features in FXS.

GENETIC MECHANISM AND EPIDEMIOLOGY

FXS is the most prevalent *inherited* form of ID, so unlike DS, it is both genetic *and* familial. It has the simplest genetic etiology of these three ID syndromes, because it is a single-gene disorder, in which the *FMR1* gene on the distal end of the long arm of the X chromosome becomes inactivated through methylation.

Because *FMR1* is on the X chromosome, FXS exhibits X-linked inheritance, in which males are more frequently and severely affected than females (because females have two X chromosomes, while males have only one). Despite being a single-gene disorder, the etiology of FXS is not as simple as a classic, Mendelian autosomal single-gene disorder such as PKU. FXS has two important non-Mendelian features that have contributed to changes in our understanding of how genes work. It is an epigenetic disorder, because it results from abnormal gene expression rather than a mutation in the coding portion (exons) of the *FMR1* gene. This change in gene expression results from an accumulation across generations of repetitive, trinucleotide repeats (CGG, in this case) in noncoding portions of the *FMR1* gene. Once the number of CGG repeats reaches a critical threshold of around 200, the whole *FMR1* gene is methylated (by attaching CH_3 molecules to the DNA), resulting in gene inactivation. Hence, the protein produced by that gene, called FMRP (FXS mental retardation protein), which is critical for normal brain and physical development, is unavailable. FMRP is an RNA-binding protein that has a broad role in protein synthesis in the brain and affects dendritic spine maturation, synaptogenesis, and pruning of dendrites and synapses. These three processes are critical for early postnatal brain development, namely, the process of experience-expectant synaptogenesis, and the balance between LTP and LTD.

The second non-Mendelian feature in the genetics of FXS is a parent-of-origin effect mediated by what is called *imprinting*, which also affects gene expression. In the case of FXS, the expansion of the number of CGG repeats is greater when the already-expanded but subthreshold *FMR1* gene is inherited from the mother rather than the father. Because of these non-Mendelian features, full FXS can appear abruptly in a family and appear to be a sporadic mutation.

FMRP binds to specific messenger RNAs (mRNAs) in dendritic spines to down-regulate protein synthesis, so absence of FMRP leads to an excess of these proteins, thus affecting maturation of dendritic spines, and hence synaptogenesis and pruning, and the balance between LTP and LTD. In particular, signaling by the metabotropic glutamate receptor (mGluR) is overactivated by the lack of FMRP, leading to an excess of the AMPA receptor (Garber, Visootsak, & Warren, 2008). Use of an mGluR antagonist has reversed some of the effects of FXS in tissue culture and animal models, so there are pharmacological agents that may be effective in humans and are actively being researched. However, to date, none of the clinical trials in human patients has been successful (Erickson et al., 2017) In summary, there has been considerable progress in understanding how the genetic mutation changes brain development in FXS and how some of these changes may be prevented.

NEUROPSYCHOLOGY AND NEUROLOGY

In contrast to DS and WS, the neuroanatomical phenotype of FXS includes both smaller (cerebellar vermis) and larger brain structures (striatal–frontal), the latter being consistent with reduced synaptic pruning.

Recently, Hoeft et al. (2010) conducted a longitudinal neuroimaging study of boys with FXS from age 1 to age 3 to examine early brain development. Consistent with previous findings, they found a persistent reduction in the volume of the cerebellar vermis in contrast to a wider pattern of increased volumes in both grey and white matter. Specifically, they found a pattern of both early (caudate and fusiform gyri) and later (orbitofrontal cortex [OFC] and basal forebrain) grey matter increases, as well as greater white matter volumes that increased over the two time points in striatal–frontal areas. At a microscopic level, dendritic spines in FXS have been found to be immature and dense (Garber et al., 2008), consistent with the molecular mechanism described earlier.

The neuropsychological phenotype in FXS ID includes (1) decline in IQ with age similar to that described earlier for DS; (2) prominent EF deficits, which are positively correlated in females with FXS with the degree of inactivation of the normal X chromosome; and (3) deficits in LTM (Raitano-Lee et al., 2010). EF deficits are consistent with aspects of the neuroanatomical phenotype, such as the striatal-frontal differences, but this neuropsychological theory has not been systematically tested. A new dementia syndrome resembling Parkinson's disease (PD) has been discovered in seemingly unaffected male FXS carriers once they get older (past age 50 years). This dementia is called FX-associated tremor/ataxia syndrome (Hagerman & Hagerman, 2013). This discovery, similar to the link between DS and AD, demonstrates etiological connections between global disorders in childhood and aging.

In summary, discovery of the *FMR1* gene about 20 years ago has led to dramatic progress in explaining FXS at several levels of analysis that spans gene expression, brain development, neuropsychology, and behavior. Moreover, the alterations in synaptic plasticity found in FXS have helped lead to similar discoveries in DS and WS, and thus an emerging theory of LTP–LTD imbalance across ID syndromes (Fernandez & Garner, 2007). FXS is thus the best understood ID syndrome and arguably even the best understood neurodevelopmental disorder, except for perhaps early treated PKU.

Williams Syndrome

DISTINCTIVE BEHAVIORAL FEATURES

The behavioral phenotype of WS is quite distinctive among the ID syndromes. Individuals with WS are described as having a "hypersocial" personality characterized by high levels of social approach behaviors to familiar individuals *and* strangers alike. Though the social phenotype has been described in the past as the "opposite" of autism, individuals with WS do have pragmatic difficulties that interfere with their ability to make and sustain friendships. While individuals with WS show heightened social approach, they also show heightened rates of generalized and other nonsocial anxiety disorders (Leyfer, Woodruff-Borden, & Mervis, 2009; Leyfer et al., 2006). Children with WS also show marked difficulties in visual–spatial processing in contrast to language skills that are consistent with (or even exceed) expectations based on mental age (an opposite pattern from that seen in DS) (Mervis & John, 2010; Pober, 2010).

GENETIC MECHANISM AND ETIOLOGY

In this section, we draw on a recent review of WS by Mervis and John (2010). WS has a lower prevalence (1 per 7,500 live births) than DS or FXS, and like DS (and unlike FXS), is mostly nonfamilial. It is caused by a usually sporadic, contiguous microdeletion of the chromosomal region 7q11.23 on one of the two copies of chromosome 7 in the child's genotype (a deletion on both copies of the chromosome would be lethal for the fetus). So, WS, like DS, is due to an abnormal dose of normal gene products (deletion in WS and addition in DS), and not to an abnormal gene. This abnormal dose affects at least 25 genes, fewer than in DS (the critical DS region on chromosome 21 contains over 100 genes), but considerably more than FXS, in which only one gene product is absent (in affected males) or reduced (in affected females).

One could reasonably ask why a segment consisting of these 25 or so genes is consistently deleted across different individuals. The reason is that the deleted region is flanked by repetitive sequences, making it more susceptible to crossing-over errors in meiosis. Such errors result in either extra, missing (i.e., deleted), or inverted copies of this region on one chromosome. Individuals with this inversion comprise about 7% of the population and are unaffected carriers who are five times more likely to transmit a deletion, and hence WS, to their children. Thus, in this minority of cases, WS is familial.

There are also occasional partial deletions of the region that have aided in the task of relating specific genes in the deletion region to specific aspects of the WS phenotype. Nearly all genes in the deletion region have been identified and genotype–phenotype relations have been established for some of them. For instance, the *ELN* gene produces *elastin*, a protein important in connective tissue, and a reduced dose of this protein is involved in the cardiac and other connective tissue anomalies in WS. We discuss later the other genes, such as *LIMK1, CYLN2, GTF2I,* and *GTF2IRD1,* implicated in the cognitive phenotype of WS. Across different partial deletions, these two phenotypes, cardiac and cognitive, can dissociate from each other.

In addition, a microaddition syndrome involving an *extra* dose of the same segment of chromosome 7q has recently been described. It is called 7q duplication syndrome (7q11.23dup). This syndrome is the genetic opposite of WS (a 50% dose of the products of the roughly 25 genes on 7q11.23 in WS vs. a 150% dose in 7q11.23dup). Interestingly, the behavioral phenotype of individuals with 7q11.23 dup syndrome, which includes increased rates of autism and severe speech dyspraxia, is roughly the opposite of that found in WS, which is characterized by hypersociability and fluent speech (Sanders et al., 2011; Velleman & Mervis, 2011).

NEUROPSYCHOLOGY AND NEUROLOGY

At the level of brain, WS is characterized by overall microcephaly, as is DS, but the profile of affected structures differs from that found in DS. In WS, reductions are found in the parietal lobule, intraparietal sulcus, and occipital lobe, but not in the cerebellum (which has reduced volume in DS). Although hippocampal volume is not differentially reduced in WS (as it is in DS), the hippocampus exhibits a marked reduction in blood flow on functional neuroimaging scans. The other key functional neuroimaging findings include (1) reduced dorsal stream activity in the parietal lobe and (2) reduced amygdala activation in response to angry or fearful faces, but not to threatening or fearful scenes. These structural and functional neuroimaging findings can be related to two aspects of the neuropsychological phenotype in WS, marked (1) impairment in visual–spatial processing (but not in face and object processing mediated by the ventral visual stream) and (2) social disinhibition, including an increased tendency to approach strangers.

Fan et al. (2016) recently identified and replicated a neuroanatomical phenotype in WS that has high sensitivity and specificity relative to both typical controls and patients with LI, ASD, and focal lesions. This phenotype included well-replicated structural magnetic resonance imaging (MRI) features of WS found in previous studies, including abnormal gyral patterns of the superior parietal and orbital cortices and reduced volumes of subcortical structures, such as the basal ganglia. It would be useful to test the discriminant validity of this neuroanatomical phenotype in WS by examining samples with DS and FXS.

We next describe other features of the neuropsychological phenotype in WS. In addition to a dramatic deficit in visual–spatial processing (which is a relative strength in DS) and social disinhibition, other aspects of the neuropsychological phenotype in WS include (1) a mean and stable IQ of about 60, in contrast to a declining and lower mean IQ in DS and FXS; (2) overall language at mental-age level with concrete vocabulary (e.g., as measured by the Peabody Picture Vocabulary Test [PPVT]) and verbal STM above mental-age level, in contrast to DS; (3) deficits in verbal and spatial LTM (Edgin, Pennington, & Mervis, 2010); and (4) deficits in verbal and spatial working memory (WM) (Edgin et al., 2010). The LTM deficits are consistent with the hypoactivity of the hippocampus we discussed earlier. The social and emotional phenotype is characterized by a paradoxical contrast between exaggerated sociability and empathy, and exaggerated nonsocial anxiety, with the nonsocial anxiety being consistent with the amygdala findings we discussed earlier. This phenotype is paradoxical, because an anxious temperament usually results in reduced social approach.

General versus Specific Deficits Revisited

In closing this section on three ID syndromes, it is important to return to the issue of general versus specific deficits in atypical development. By definition (an IQ score < 70), all three of these ID syndromes have a general deficit in Spearman's general intelligence (g), so we should expect all cognitive skills to be depressed to a certain extent, because all cognitive skills are correlated with g to some degree. As we have demonstrated, each ID syndrome considered here exhibits this global depression in cognitive skills, with some few specific skills being below or above mental age level but none at chronological age level. Hence, these contrasting cognitive profiles across ID syndromes provide evidence for *some* specificity to each syndrome that relates to its etiology, but not evidence for independent cognitive modules.

For instance, it has been claimed that the double dissociation between WS and DS with regard to language versus spatial functions provides support for an independent language module in the brain (Bellugi, Marks, Bihrle, & Sabo, 1988). But neither "spared" skill in either syndrome is anywhere near an age-typical level of performance. So, as we have illustrated many times before, dissociations provide evidence for a degree of specialization in the cortex but not independent processes. The verbal and spatial LTM and WM deficits found in WS in Edgin et al. (2010) were also found in the DS group. These results are important, because they demonstrate that as the cognitive load (or, one might say, loading on g) for a cognitive task increases, the verbal versus spatial dissociation between DS and WS goes down. This result is contrary to the modular view of WS proposed by Bellugi et al. (1988). Also contrary to that view is the fact that overall language is at mental-age, not chronological-age, level in WS, and the contrasting language and spatial skills in WS are nonetheless correlated at about .50.

Given that all ID syndromes exhibit global delays in all cognitive skills, as well as other aspects of development, such as motor and social skills, how useful is the neuropsychological level of analysis in providing an explanation of ID? As we saw in Chapter 13, the same question arises for ASD. For ID, there is emerging evidence that deficits in both explicit and implicit LTM related to an imbalance between LTP and LTD might provide a unifying neuropsychological explanation for ID, but that hypothesis requires further testing. We lack such a unifying neuropsychological explanation for ASD. As we discussed in Chapter 4, eventually we need to move beyond neuropsychology to a neurocomputational level of analysis to fully understand how changes in brain development lead to the changes in behavioral development that define neurodevelopmental disorders, especially ones with more pervasive effects on development, such as ASD and ID.

Summary

In summary, these three genetic IDs illustrate how we can provide a multilevel explanation of a behavioral disorder that links changes in the expression of particular genes to alterations in brain development, which in turn change the development of neuropsychology, and behavior. These three syndromes are part of the nearly 1,000 distinct genetic syndromes that cause ID. The multiplicity of possible genetic causes of ID is consistent with (1) the highly polygenic etiology of normal variations in IQ, and (2) the multiple brain regions that contribute to IQ, as reviewed in Chapter 3.

DIAGNOSIS AND TREATMENT

Diagnosis

As described in this chapter, many genetically based ID syndromes have unique features in their behavioral presentation within the context of general similarities resulting from an ID. We focus in this section on the similarities in presenting symptoms, history, and behavioral observations that can be expected for a child with ID, regardless of the etiology.

Presenting Symptoms

The early presenting symptoms in children with ID are often related to speech–language delays, because language skill is one of the most easily observable aspects of early cognitive development, whereas nonverbal reasoning is more difficult to assess. These children are often identified and treated for speech–language delays before they receive the broader diagnosis of an ID. Global delays achieving developmental milestones such as walking, toileting, and learning to dress oneself are also common. Children who have not yet been identified by school entry will likely raise concern because of learning delays. Parents and teachers may notice that the child is struggling with grade-level work, seems to be learning more slowly than his or her peers, and/or has difficulty mastering new concepts. Parents often ask whether their child has a learning disability or has a particular learning style. At feedback, psychoeducation about the similarities and differences between a specific learning disability and an ID is sometimes helpful for parents to optimally support their child's learning.

The primary presentation of a child with ID may also appear emotional or behavioral in nature. The child may be susceptible to intense outbursts and tantrums, perhaps even exhibiting aggressive behavior. Attentional difficulties are also common. Social–emotional immaturity and social difficulties that impact peer relationships may also be a concern for parents.

History

Children with ID often present with general developmental delays starting in infancy. One of the first developmental tasks of infancy is feeding, which requires coordinated motor movements, so children with ID often have trouble nursing. Motor and language milestones are often delayed. These delayed milestones are often the first trigger for parents to seek out an evaluation and/or therapeutic services. During the toddler years and beyond, the child may exhibit delayed emotion regulation skills and be prone to intense outbursts and temper tantrums. Play behavior during the toddler years will be simpler and more concrete than that of a typically developing child. Additionally, adaptive behavior may begin to show delays during this period, such as difficulty moving toward independence with tasks such as toileting, eating, dressing, and bathing.

When the child enters kindergarten and the grade school years, school difficulties may become more evident. Concerns may be raised about the child's maturity and progress with academic skills. The child will likely have particular difficulty with academic tasks requiring abstract reasoning (e.g., those that emphasize higher-level problem solving as opposed to rote learning). Parents and teachers may observe that the child needs lots of repetition in order to learn new information. And once the information is learned in one context, the child may have difficulty generalizing to other contexts. Parents and teachers often express frustration that the child is able to do certain problems one day but cannot do the same problem the following day. These difficulties with retention and generalization are characteristic of a child with ID. Thus, although a child with ID will be able to learn new material, it will take many repetitions, which may frustrate the child. In this context, it is not surprising that attention difficulties are common in ID, although this issue is not likely to account for the whole of the attention problems in ID. Consistent failure in the school setting may also be an important trigger for the development of comorbid psychopathology, such as anxiety and depression.

It is also important to note that children with ID often develop compensation strategies in the classroom that can mask their difficulties with comprehension. For example, a teacher may check in with a child to see if he or she understands, and the child may respond enthusiastically, "Yes, that is interesting!" Unfortunately, these compensation strategies may result in the child receiving work that is far above his or her academic skills.

Social difficulties often become evident once the child enters the school context. These social difficulties are often secondary to the child's cognitive limitations, because the child is often interested in other children and interactive. However, because the children are at different developmental levels, the maintenance of true friendships can be challenging. The child's language-based difficulties may also impact social relationships. For example, difficulties with language comprehension and expression can make conversations difficult. The child may have trouble following a conversation and say things that seem irrelevant or tangential. Additionally, group-based activities may be particularly problematic, because the child will have difficulty following the quick verbal banter of the children and understanding the evolving structure/rules of games, making the group setting particularly overwhelming.

Behavioral Observations

When working with a child with suspected ID, it is important to look for evidence of dysmorphology that is consistent with known genetic ID syndromes.

During testing, the child may show inordinate difficulty on tasks requiring abstract reasoning and problem solving (matrices), but perform better on more concrete tasks (single-word reading, spelling, simple math computations). This concrete style may also be evident in the child's interpretations of figurative language (e.g., "Hold your horses"), which may be very literal. On the similarities task, the child may have difficulty abstracting similarities and revert to the more concrete strategy of telling what is different about the items.

During conversations, the child's language may be characterized by short, simple utterances. The child may also show a delay in internalization of self-talk, such that he or she talks out loud during tasks to regulate his or her behavior. On the clinician's part, he or she may observe him- or herself slowing down his or her own language, simplifying instructions, and repeating instructions in response to behavioral cues from the child that the information is confusing, overwhelming, or too fast-paced. The child may also show delays in metacognition, such that he or she does not ask for clarification when he or she does not understand instructions.

Case Presentations

Case Presentation 10

Tori, an 8-year-old girl who will be entering second grade in a few weeks, is old for her grade, because she repeated kindergarten due to parent and teacher concerns that she was "immature" and not making expected progress. She has been staffed for special education services under "speech–language disability," and in first grade, she received extra help for literacy and math. Her parents requested this evaluation to get more information about "what is in the way of Tori's learning and how we can help her."

Tori was the result of an uncomplicated pregnancy and birth. APGAR scores were good. Tori had some trouble nursing in the perinatal period, and though her mother had planned on breastfeeding exclusively, Tori's diet had to be supplemented with formula so that she would grow adequately. Parents described her as a happy, easygoing baby but noted that she reached all developmental milestones more slowly than her brother. Tori sat unassisted at 9 months, never crawled, and walked unassisted at 17 months. Language development was quite delayed. Parents report that she had only about 10 words just before she turned 3, used two- to three-word phases at 3, and did not speak in sentences until she was 4 years old. Because of these delays, she was evaluated by the state early intervention program at age 2½ and diagnosed with a language disorder, for which she received regular speech–language therapy.

Tori's parents identified a number of concerns in addition to language development and academic progress. Her father described her as "uncoordinated," and noted that she could not ride a two-wheeled bike and that she struggled to learn routines in her ballet class. Her mother volunteered in Tori's first-grade class once a week and was concerned about social development. By her mother's description, "Tori thinks everybody is her friend and doesn't know when the other kids are being mean to her." Outside of school, Tori enjoys watching Disney movies, then reenacting scenes from them. She also likes listening to music and playing with her stuffed animals.

Tori's parents report no history of learning or academic problems themselves. Her mother completed an Associate's degree and works as a dental assistant. Her father completed a 4-year college degree and works as a banker. Tori has an 11-year-old brother without difficulties.

Tori's diagnostic testing is summarized in Table 14.1.

DISCUSSION

Although Tori's striking language delays could be consistent with a language disorder, her history makes clear that her cognitive limitations extend into the nonverbal realm, and that ID is likely the appropriate diagnosis. Tori's language remains poor for her age, and she certainly will continue to benefit from interventions and support in this area, but her language impairment is not *specific* in the sense that language skill is not discrepant from other intellectual abilities.

From her earliest days, Tori did not quite meet developmental expectations. As a newborn she had difficulty with nursing. A general developmental delay was further evident in the ages at which she met motor and language milestones. In contrast, early social development represented an area of relative strength. By parent report, Tori was interested in others and interactive from an early age. Her current social difficulties are probably secondary to her cognitive limitations. Because her typically developing same-age peers are at a different place in terms of cognitive development, it will be difficult for Tori to develop true friendships with them. If she remains in a regular education classroom, parents and teachers should consider alternative ways for Tori to be exposed to other children functioning at her developmental level (e.g., Special Olympics or other special activities).

The most striking aspect of Tori's test scores is the pervasiveness of her

TABLE 14.1. Test Summary, Case 10

Performance validity
Memory Validity Profile
    Visual Subtest   RS = 12
    (valid)

General intelligence
WISC-V Full Scale IQ   SS = 61

Crystallized intelligence
WISC-V Verbal Comprehension Index   SS = 68
    Similarities   ss = 3
    Vocabulary   ss = 5

Working memory
WISC-V Working Memory Index   SS = 67
    Digit Span   ss = 5
    Picture Span   ss = 3

Processing speed
WISC-V Processing Speed Index   SS = 69
    Coding   ss = 3
    Symbol Search   ss = 6

Fluid intelligence
WISC-V Fluid Reasoning Index   SS = 64
    Matrix Reasoning   ss = 3
    Figure Weights   ss = 4
WISC-V Visual Spatial Index   SS = 72
    Block Design   ss = 6
    Visual Puzzles   ss = 4

Adaptive behavior
ABAS-2
    Global Adaptive Composite (parent)   SS = 62
    Global Adaptive Composite (teacher)   SS = 69

Academic
Reading
    Basic literacy
        WIAT-III Word Reading   SS = 82
        WIAT-III Pseudoword Decoding   SS = 73
        WIAT-III Spelling   SS = 81

    Reading fluency
        TOWRE-2 Sight Word Efficiency   SS = 72
        TOWRE-2 Phonemic Decoding Efficiency   SS = 71
        GORT-5 Fluency   ss = 4

    Reading comprehension
        GORT-5 Comprehension   ss = 4

Math
    Calculation and problem solving
        WIAT-III Numerical Operations   SS = 74
        Math Problem Solving   SS = 66

    Math fluency
        WIAT-III Math Fluency   SS = 79

Oral language
Phonological processing/naming speed
    CTOPP-2 Elision   ss = 4
    CTOPP-2 Phoneme Isolation   ss = 3
    CTOPP-2 Nonword Repetition   ss = 5
    CTOPP-2 Rapid Symbolic Naming   SS = 75

Verbal memory
    WRAML-2 Verbal Learning   ss = 4
    WRAML-2 Verbal Learning Delay   ss = 4
    WRAML-2 Verbal Learning Recognition   ss = 6
    WRAML-2 Story Memory   ss = 5
    WRAML-2 Story Memory Delay   ss = 4
    WRAML-2 Story Memory Recognition   ss = 5

TABLE 14.1. (continued)

Semantics and syntax
    CELF-5 Core Language   SS = 75
        Sentence Comprehension   ss = 5
        Word Structure   ss = 7
        Formulated Sentences   ss = 6
        Recalling Sentences   ss = 4
    PPVT-4   SS = 85

Visual–motor skills
Beery VMI-6   SS = 61

Attention and executive functions

Attention		Executive functions	
Vanderbilt Inattention		ToLDX-2	
Parent	RS = 4	Total Moves	SS = 64
Teacher	RS = 5	Rule Violations	SS ≤ 60
Vanderbilt Hyperactivity/Impulsivity		Total Problem-Solving Time	SS = 74
Parent	RS = 3		
Teacher	RS = 4		

Note. SS, standard score with mean = 100 and *SD* = 15; ss, scaled score with mean =10 and *SD* = 3; RS, raw score; %ile, percentile rank; WISC-V, Wechsler Intelligence Scale for Children—Fifth Edition; ABAS-2, Adaptive Behavior Assessment System—Second Edition; WIAT-III, Wechsler Individual Achievement Test—Third Edition; TOWRE-2: Test of Word Reading Efficiency—Second Edition; GORT-5, Gray Oral Reading Tests—Fifth Edition; CTOPP-2, Comprehensive Test of Phonological Processing—Second Edition; CELF-5, Clinical Evaluation of Language Fundamentals—Fifth Edition; WRAML-2, Wide Range Assessment of Memory and Learning, Second Edition; PPVT-4, Peabody Picture Vocabulary Test—Fourth Edition; Beery VMI-6, Beery–Buktenica Test of Visual Motor Integration, Sixth Edition; Vanderbilt, NICHQ Vanderbilt Assessment Scales; ToLDX-2, Tower of London—DX—Second Edition.

difficulties; she performed in the impaired range on nearly every test given her. Her Full Scale IQ, together with a measure of her adaptive functioning, qualifies her for a diagnosis of mild ID. Like most children with ID, Tori struggles greatly with tasks requiring abstract reasoning or problem solving. This difficulty is evident in her very poor scores on tests such as the Similarities and Matrix Reasoning subtests of the Wechsler Intelligence Scale for Children (WISC), as well as the Tower of London–Drexel University (ToLDX). On the Similarities subtest, Tori's responses were very concrete, even for an 8-year-old. For example, when asked how a shirt and a shoe are alike, she looked at her outfit and said, "They both have yellow on them." In contrast, Tori performed somewhat better on rote tasks, such as basic academic tasks on the Wechsler Individual Achievement Test–Third Edition (WIAT-III), as well as generating morphologically correct utterances on the Word Structure subtest of the Clinical Evaluation of Language Fundamentals–Fifth Edition (CELF-5). Her highest score was on the PPVT, which fell in the low average range. This test often represents a relative strength in children who have received a good deal of environmental language support (e.g., speech–language therapy, enriched home environment).

    Many children with ID have very poor attention. In the supportive, one-on-one testing environment, Tori's attention was adequate. However, parent and teacher ratings indicate that she does have at least some difficulty in this area, although their scores fell below the clinical level. It may be that she has difficulty attending primarily because much of the information she encounters is confusing or otherwise overwhelming to her. However, children with ID can sometimes benefit from both medical and behavioral interventions used for children with ADHD, so parents and teacher should monitor this issue carefully.

The etiology of Tori's difficulties is unclear. Her physical appearance is normal (i.e., not dysmorphic). There is no obvious environmental cause for her delay, such as anoxia or another brain injury, and there is no relevant family history. Based on her parents' occupations and educational levels, Tori's IQ is likely well below theirs. We recommend referring all children with ID of unknown etiology for a genetics evaluation. Sometimes, such an evaluation will identify an underlying genetic syndrome, and this information can be useful to the family from a genetic counseling point of view. In addition, some genetic syndromes associated with ID also correlate with specific medical problems for which the child can then be followed. Rarely, a genetics evaluation will identify an underlying disorder for which there is a known medical treatment (as in the case of some metabolic disorders).

Case Presentation 11

Will, a 7-year-old boy who is currently in second grade, was referred for an evaluation because of learning delays, hyperactivity, anxiety, and poor social skills.

Will's family history is unremarkable. His mother described her pregnancy and delivery as uncomplicated. Will's developmental milestones were delayed, especially his speech–language milestones. He began to walk at 15 months and was very clumsy. It was not until Will was 3 years old that he began to say several words. His medical history includes recurrent otitis media with effusion, which was treated with pressure equalization (PE) tubes when he was 2 years old. During Will's toddler years, his parents became increasingly concerned about his anxiety. He became very anxious in new surroundings and with new people. He would scream and tantrum in these novel settings, and he was difficult to soothe. Will entered preschool when he was 3 years old. At this time, his teachers noted some unusual repetitive behaviors such as hand flapping and sniffing. The teachers also described Will as overactive and distractible. He was susceptible to tantrums and angry outbursts when he was overstimulated. Will's parents described how he struggled to connect with other children. Although he was interested in other children and would approach them, it seemed that he did not know how to act when he approached. He had particular difficulty with making eye contact.

These behavioral and social concerns have continued as Will has progressed into grade school. He continues to struggle with peer relationships and remains very anxious and shy, particularly in social situations. His teachers describe him as hyperactive, with a very short attention span. This year, Will began taking methylphenidate to improve his distractibility and hyperactivity. Will's parents and teachers report that they have seen improvement in these symptoms with the medication.

Despite these improvements, his parents are very concerned that Will is struggling with grade-level work and seems to be learning more slowly than his peers. He currently receives special education pull-out services to support his learning in all academic subjects.

Will's diagnostic testing is summarized in Table 14.2.

DISCUSSION

One of the recommendations from this evaluation was for Will to have genetic testing, because his behavioral phenotype and physical characteristics were characteristic of FXS. The characteristic behavioral phenotype involves language delays, hyperactivity, inattentiveness, autistic-like features (e.g., poor eye contact, hand stereotypies, repetitive behaviors), shyness and social anxiety, and hyperarousal by stimuli. As described, Will's history included many of these features. Will also showed physical features consistent with FXS, including a long face, prominent ears, prominent chin, and hyperextensible finger joints. Genetic testing confirmed a diagnosis of FXS. Will shows a mosaic pattern, with some of his cells having a premutation and the rest of his cells having a full mutation. Hence, a proportion of his cells are able to produce FMRP. As a result, Will is not as severely affected as a typical male with a full mutation that is fully inactivated by methylation. The mean IQ in this most affected group is typically in the moderate range of ID, whereas the mean IQ in mosaic males typically falls in the mild range of ID.

An important rule-out for this case presentation was ASD, since Will shows difficulties with social–communication skills. Although Will shows some features of ASD, his score on the Social Communication Questionnaire fell below the autism screening threshold. This result was consistent with his parents' report that he does show some difficulties relating to other children and making eye contact, but he is interested in other children and seems motivated to interact with them.

Will's Full Scale IQ score and his Adaptive Behavior score are consistent with a mild ID. Although there is some variability within and across tests in the battery, in general, the results highlighted fairly broad-based neuropsychological dysfunction impacting language, visual–spatial skills, fluid reasoning, processing speed, attention, and EF.

Will's academic skills are generally consistent with his cognitive abilities, although the pattern of scores shows some strengths and weaknesses. Children with FXS frequently have trouble with math, and this pattern is evident in Will's scores. In contrast, Will shows relative strengths in single-word reading and spelling.

Will has a history of speech–language delay, and he continues to show weaknesses in understanding the structure and content of language on the CELF-5. Behavioral observations also indicate that Will shows weaknesses in the pragmatics of language. He perseverates on words, phrases, and topics, and shows poor topic maintenance. Consistent with the typical FXS neuropsychological profile, Will shows weaknesses in short-term auditory memory (e.g., WISC-V Digit Span, Comprehensive Test of Phonological Processing, Second Edition [CTOPP-2] Nonword

TABLE 14.2. Test Summary, Case 11

Performance validity
Test of Memory Malingering
    Trial 1   RS = 42
    Trial 2   RS = 47
              (valid)

General intelligence
WISC-V Full Scale IQ   SS = 63

Crystallized intelligence
WISC-V Verbal Comprehension Index   SS = 76
    Similarities   ss = 5
    Vocabulary   ss = 6

Working memory
WISC-V Working Memory Index   SS = 67
    Digit Span   ss = 3
    Picture Span   ss = 5

Processing speed
WISC-V Processing Speed Index   SS = 60
    Coding   ss = 2
    Symbol Search   ss = 4

Fluid intelligence
WISC-V Fluid Reasoning Index   SS = 69
    Matrix Reasoning   ss = 6
    Figure Weights   ss = 3
WISC-V Visual Spatial Index   SS = 64
    Block Design   ss = 6
    Visual Puzzles   ss = 3

Adaptive behavior
ABAS-2
    Global Adaptive Composite (parent)   SS = 68
    Global Adaptive Composite (teacher)   SS = 59

Academic
Reading
    Basic literacy
        WIAT-III Word Reading   SS = 85
        WIAT-III Pseudoword Decoding   SS = 80
        WIAT-III Spelling   SS = 75

    Reading fluency
        TOWRE-2 Sight Word Efficiency   SS = 74
        TOWRE-2 Phonemic Decoding Efficiency   SS = 72
        GORT-5 Fluency   ss = 3

    Reading comprehension
        GORT-5 Comprehension   ss = 4

Math
    Calculation and problem solving
        WIAT-III Numerical Operations   SS = 65
        Math Problem Solving   SS = 68

    Math fluency   SS = 58
        WIAT-III Math Fluency

Oral language
Phonological processing/naming speed
    CTOPP-2 Elision   ss = 5
    CTOPP-2 Nonword Repetition   ss = 3
    CTOPP-2 Rapid Symbolic Naming   SS = 65

Verbal memory
    WRAML-2 Verbal Learning   ss = 5
    WRAML-2 Verbal Learning Delay   ss = 6
    WRAML-2 Story Memory   ss = 7
    WRAML-2 Story Memory Delay   ss = 7

TABLE 14.2. (continued)

Semantics and syntax
    CELF-5 Core Language   SS = 68
    Sentence Comprehension   ss = 4
    Word Structure   ss = 5
    Formulated Sentences   ss = 6
    Recalling Sentences   ss = 2
    PPVT-4   SS = 80

Visual–motor skills
Beery VMI-6   SS = 58

Attention and executive functions

Executive functions		*Attention*	
Vanderbilt Inattention		Gordon Diagnostic System	
Parent	RS = 7	Vigilance Total Correct	z = –0.8
Teacher	RS = 6	Vigilance Total Commissions	z = –3.6
Vanderbilt Hyperactivity/Impulsivity		ToLDX-2	
Parent	RS = 8	Total Moves	SS = 62
Teacher	RS = 8	Rule Violations	SS = 62
BRIEF-2 (parent)	T = 80	Total Problem-Solving Time	SS ≤ 60
Global Executive Composite			

Social communication
SCQ   RS = 10

Note. SCQ, Social Communication Questionnaire. For other abbreviations, see Table 14.1.

Repetition, CELF-5 Recalling Sentences) relative to his memory for more meaningful information such as stories (e.g., Wide Range Assessment of Memory and Learning [WRAML] Story Memory). Will also showed a relative strength on a test of single-word receptive vocabulary, the PPVT-4.

    Children with FXS often show EF deficits that are consistent with some of the behavioral problems characteristic of the syndrome, such as inattention, hyperactivity, impulsivity, and difficulty with transitions. These behavioral characteristics overlap considerably with the symptoms of ADHD, so it is not surprising that Will's parents' and teachers' ratings on ADHD questionnaires met symptom thresholds for an ADHD diagnosis. In fact, Will has begun taking ADHD medication, with beneficial effect. Will's performance on EF tests indicated deficits in planning, inhibition, and mental flexibility (ToLDX and Gordon Diagnostic System). Furthermore, on a parent questionnaire of executive functioning skills in everyday settings (Behavior Rating Inventory of Executive Function–Second Edition [BRIEF-2]), parents reported clinical elevations on all subscales.

    In conclusion, Will is a child with FXS who has a mild ID. He is not as severely affected as some males with FXS, because he shows a mosaic genetic pattern. He shows several behavioral, physical, and neuropsychological features that are characteristic of FXS.

Prevention

Depending on etiology, some forms of ID are preventable. Of course, all cases of ID due to fetal alcohol exposure (as well as other teratogens) are theoretically preventable, although the practicalities remain challenging for a variety of reasons. One of the most impressive prevention studies is the Abecedarian Project, a randomized controlled trial (RCT) of intensive early intervention services that began in 1972. Newborns were enrolled in the study based on a number of environmental risk factors, including poverty and low parental education, but none of the children had known genetic ID syndromes or known neurological disorders. The treatment group received high-quality, coordinated services, including early education, pediatric care, and family social support. The comparison group received nutritional supplements, social services, and low-cost pediatric care. Children in the treatment group showed significantly higher IQ scores beginning at age 18 months and continuing at least until 21 years. The size of the IQ difference was nearly 1 *SD,* which means that substantially fewer children in the treatment group fell below the ID cutoff. Thus, high-quality early intervention can prevent some cases of ID of predominantly environmental etiology (see Ramey, Ramey, & Lanzi, 2007).

A few genetically based forms of ID, most notably metabolic disorders, can be prevented with appropriate medical treatment. Perhaps the best example is PKU. Children with the PKU gene lack the enzyme to metabolize phenylalanine. If they follow a normal diet, the resulting brain damage inevitably leads to ID. However, when babies are identified early and fed a restricted diet, IQ can be normal. Currently, all newborns born in this country are screened for PKU, and it is estimated that thousands of cases of ID have been prevented (National Institutes of Health, 2000).

Treatment

Treatments for ID generally do not remediate the core underlying intellectual deficits, but aim to improve quality of life by reducing associated problems and improving adaptive functioning (Hartley, Horrell, & Maclean, 2007). A key early finding concerned the failure of institutionalization as a treatment for ID. Compared to intellectually disabled individuals raised in their own homes, institutionalized individuals showed a wide range of poor outcomes, including shorter life expectancy (Centerwall & Centerwall, 1960; Dupont, Vaeth, & Videbech, 1986; Shotwell & Shipe, 1964). These findings led to a gradual change in practice, such that people with ID are now likely to live in private homes or in community-based group homes. Although most of these community-based group homes provide dramatically better environments than large institutions, there is little evidence that group living is preferable to semi-independent living. For example, one study found few outcome differences for adults with ID living semi-independently versus those living in group homes; any differences favored semi-independent living, even after researchers controlled for preexisting differences in ability (Stancliffe & Keane, 2000). Such findings have substantial public policy implications because of the higher cost of group homes.

By federal mandate, early intervention services are available to children with global developmental delays during the first 5 years of life. Once children are identified, they can receive services in their home (at no cost to the family) until age 3, then through their public school district until age 5. Early intervention is generally associated with positive outcomes, though results have seldom been as dramatic or long-lasting as providers and parents would hope. Evidence for early intervention as an effective treatment is strongest for children at risk for ID due to environmental factors, such as poverty or prematurity (Ramey et al., 2007). Even among children with genetic ID syndromes, early intervention can have positive effects, but these are more likely to relate to academic outcomes or broader family function than to long-lasting changes in intelligence (Hines & Bennett, 1996).

There has been hope that a better understanding of genetic pathways in ID syndromes such as FXS and DS might lead to rational drug therapies, such as drugs that target glutamate signaling in FXS or cholinegic signaling in DS. Despite initially promising results in animal models, clinical trials in human patients have so far not been successful (for reviews, see Erickson et al., 2017; Fernandez & Edgin, 2016).

Children with ID typically receive a range of supportive behavioral interventions, including occupational and physical therapy, speech–language services, special education, and behavioral interventions. In the past decade, the evidence base for these behavioral interventions has expanded in ID, but it is worth noting that there are fewer RCTs of treatments than in other learning disorders such as dyslexia and ADHD. For example, in a systematic review of interventions for mental health problems in adults with ID, Koslowski et al. (2016) found just 12 controlled studies in the entire literature covering biological, systems, and psychotherapeutic treatments for mental health, behavioral problems, and quality of life. This discrepancy between the treatment literature in ID and other learning disorders is a notable gap and should spur further research on treatments for ID. In what follows we review a sampling of the RCTs that have been conducted across multiple domains of functioning: mental health, cognition, speech–language, and physical activity.

Mental Health

Individuals with ID are at increased risk for psychopathology, including internalizing disorders such as anxiety or depression, and externalizing disorders such as ADHD. Although prevalence estimates vary widely, children with ID are probably four to five times more likely to have a psychiatric disorder than are children with normal-range intellectual abilities (Matson & Laud, 2007). It is important that individuals with ID be assessed and treated for these dual diagnoses.

In the past, there was skepticism about the effectiveness of talk therapies in individuals with ID, and this concern was magnified for cognitive-behavioral (CBT)-based therapies that require a level of abstraction in connecting thoughts to feelings. More recently, there is emerging evidence that CBT can be adapted for the developmental level of individuals with ID. For example, a manualized CBT protocol for mood disorders in adults with ID showed encouraging trends in a recent feasibility RCT (Hassiotis et al., 2011, 2013). While there were no overall group differences between the treatment and control group in the full sample, the treatment did show positive trends for those participants who screened positive for depression (Hassiotis et al., 2013). These results suggest that CBT can be adapted for individuals with ID and should be further studied in large-scale RCTs, particularly those targeting depression.

ADHD is also frequently comorbid with ID. Previous research has suggested that individuals with ID may have a poorer medication response to stimulants than do children with ADHD alone (Aman, Buican, & Arnold, 2003). This finding was recently called into question by a recent randomized, placebo-controlled, double-blind trial of methylphenidate in children with ID (Simonoff et al., 2013). In this trial, the authors addressed many of the design limitations of previous work by following the children for a longer term (16 weeks), including a larger sample (N = 122 children), and establishing optimal dosing regimens (Simonoff et al., 2013). Results showed beneficial effects of the methylphenidate compared to placebo, with effect sizes in the moderate range of 0.39–0.52. IQ did not moderate the treatment effect in their sample of IQ ranging from 30 to 69. Hence, in this study, there was no evidence that lower IQ predicted poorer treatment response, though this null finding might be due to the restriction of range of IQ in the sample. In comparing the effect sizes of stimulants in this ID population (0.39–0.52) with those from the Multimodal Treatment Study of Children with ADHD (MTA) involving typically developing children with ADHD (0.8–0.9), there is some support for the idea that stimulants might be somewhat less effective in the ID population, with the caveat that these studies differed in several meaningful ways that could influence this comparison. Overall, the study by Simonoff et al. (2013) shows that stimulants have clinically significant effects in the ID population when they are appropriately titrated, and so should continue to be recommended for the treatment of co-occurring ADHD.

ID is often accompanied by challenging problem behaviors, such as aggression or self-injurious behavior. The American Psychological Association has identified applied behavior analysis (ABA), a highly structured behavioral treatment, as an empirically supported intervention for problem behaviors in ID. This recommendation is supported by a RCT comparing standard community treatment for ID in the United Kingdom with standard treatment + a specialist behavioral team (Hassiotis et al., 2009). The behavioral team provided treatments using ABA and positive behavioral supports. Results showed that the addition of the specialist behavioral team significantly reduced challenging behaviors (Hassiotis et al., 2009). These results continue to support behavior management strategies as critical to the treatment planning for individuals with ID with challenging behaviors.

Attention–EF

Various behavioral techniques (e.g., computerized training; explicit modeling and practice of WM strategies) have been investigated as potential treatments for the attention and EF challenges associated with ID. Results have been quite similar to those we have previously discussed for computerized training in earlier chapters in Part II of this book. There is some evidence that these techniques lead to modest improvement on the trained task or a limited number of related tasks (i.e., near-transfer), but little to no evidence that the benefits transfer to "real-world" functional outcomes (far-transfer) (F. Conners, Rosenquist, Arnett, Moore, & Hume, 2008; Kirk, Gray, Ellis, Taffe, & Cornish, 2016, 2017; Söderqvist, Nutley, Ottersen, Grill, & Klingberg, 2012).

Speech–Language

An active area of investigation for speech–language development has been the testing of milieu communication treatments (MCTs) for young children with general developmental delay and limited expressive vocabulary (Fey, Yoder, Warren, & Bredin-Oja, 2013; Yoder & Warren, 2002; Yoder, Woynaroski, Fey, & Warren, 2014). One treatment approach that has been rigorously evaluated consists of three components: responsivity education for parents, prelinguistic milieu teaching, and milieu teaching. Responsivity education with parents encourages them to (1) take advantage of opportunities to respond to the child's play or communication bids, (2) verbalize the child's nonverbal communication, (3) expand semantically on topics by following the child's lead, and (4) copy and add structure to the child's vocalizations (i.e., the child says, "Dog," and parent responds, "Yes, it is a dog") (Fey et al., 2013). Prelinguistic milieu teaching is delivered by a clinician through interactions with the child. It is designed to encourage the child's nonverbal communication by arranging the environment and developing routines that press for communication bids from the child, such as coordinated eye gaze, vocalizations, or gestures. Once the child has developed sufficient nonverbal communication skills, the treatment proceeds to milieu teaching that shifts the focus from prelinguistic communication to verbal communication. The treatment builds from the initial stages in which five to 10 words are selected as lexical targets to multiword semantic relations (Fey et al., 2013).

A recent RCT tested the effect of a high-intensity versus lower-intensity dosing of MCT with toddlers with ID with and without DS (Fey et al., 2013; Yoder et al., 2014). The effect of dose was significant in the DS group only. The effect was moderate with the high-dose group, producing 17 words on average compared to 5 words in the low-dose group (Yoder et al., 2014). Given that children with DS have severe and persistent language delays, the fact that increasing intervention intensity yielded greater vocabulary development is an important finding for this group of young children. Interestingly, in the non-DS group, there was not a significant effect of intervention intensity (Yoder et al., 2014). The authors speculated that this result might be due to the mixed etiology of toddlers in this ID group. The authors also pointed to complexities in the language-based intervention literature more broadly, in which increasing intensity has not always yielded better outcomes (Denton et al., 2011; Ukrainetz, Ross, & Harm, 2009). Thus, this study contributes to this literature in questioning the assumption that "more is better" in all cases and reiterates the need for empirical tests of intervention effects at different doses in different groups. One consistent and interesting finding across both groups is that toddlers who had better functional and symbolic play were more likely to benefit from increasing intensity of the intervention, perhaps because they were more engaged with the treatment, or because they were more "ready" to learn particular linguistic skills.

While we have highlighted the recent RCT of the MCT approach, the literature on early speech–language interventions for children with ID is evolving quickly. For example, there are promising variants of MCT for children with ID (Kaiser & Roberts, 2013) and innovative combinations of therapeutic approaches, such as the combination of MCT and the social–communication intervention, JASPER (joint attention, symbolic play, engagement, and regulation) described in Chapter 13 (Wright, Kaiser, Reikowsky, & Roberts, 2013). There is also increasing emphasis on speech–language interventions that address the specific needs of etiological subgroups of children with ID (i.e., DS vs. FXS. vs. WS), because it is clear that the language profiles of these children are quite distinct.

Physical Activity

There is also emerging research on supporting the physical development of children with ID. For example, a home-based treadmill training program appears to be a helpful adjunct to physical therapy in promoting gross motor development in infants with DS (Ulrich, Lloyd, Tiernan, Looper, & Angulo-Barroso, 2008; Wu, Looper, Ulrich, Ulrich, & Angulo-Barroso, 2007). Parents were instructed in how to support prewalking infants in stepping on the treadmill. Compared to a low-intensity group, infants who got more intense treadmill training not only performed better on the trained task but also achieved gross motor milestones (e.g., independent walking) significantly earlier.

Summary

The evidence base for treatment approaches in ID has clearly grown in the past decade and has included more rigorous research designs that can guide clinical practice. Still, the treatment literature in ID is lagging behind the other learning disorders and could benefit from further funding to support large-scale rigorous research designs to answer fundamental questions about the best treatment approaches to meet the diverse needs of individuals with ID.

Table 14.3 provides a summary of current research and evidence-based practice for ID.

TABLE 14.3. Summary Table: Intellectual Disability

Definition

- DSM-5 has three diagnostic criteria: intellectual deficit (70 ± 5), an adaptive behavior deficit, and onset within the developmental period.
- DSM-5 defines severity in terms of adaptive functioning.
- Adaptive functioning deficits are least well defined in the DSM-5 definition.

Prevalence and epidemiology

- The combination of IQ (2 SDs), adaptive, and developmental criteria identifies approximately 1–3% of the general population, with the majority having mild ID.
- ID is more common in males: ~1.6/1 for mild ID and ~1.2/1 for severe ID.
- The male preponderance of ID is partly due to X-linked ID syndromes that differentially impact males. FXS is the most common X-linked ID syndrome.
- Dual diagnoses are common, which means that psychiatric comorbidities frequently accompany ID, especially ADHD.

Etiology of nonsyndromal ID

- The lower tail of the IQ distribution is bimodal, with mild ID reflecting largely familial genetic and environmental influences, and moderate and more severe ID reflecting largely nonfamilial influences.
- Heritability of IQ is approximately .50. The heritability of IQ appears stable across the full distribution of scores, with the exception of moderate and more severe ID.
- Previous studies found that IQ was less heritable in lower SES families (a SES × heritability interaction), but larger-scale studies have not replicated this finding, and instead found that shared environmental influences matter more in lower SES families (a SES × shared environment interaction).

Etiology of DS

- DS is the most prevalent form of ID with a known genetic etiology.
- There has been progress in narrowing the regions of chromosome 21 that are implicated in the DS phenotype. There is more than one ID region on chromosome 21, and the *APP* gene is implicated in the early-onset dementia phenotype.
- The cognitive profile of DS involves weaknesses relative to mental age on verbal short-term memory and language, episodic long-term memory, and EF.
- The rate of cognitive development is slowed, resulting in declining IQ standard scores over time.
- The neurological phenotype in DS includes 1) microcephaly and 2) differentially smaller volumes of the cerebellum, hippocampus, and prefrontal cortex (PFC), although the PFC finding does not always survive correction for overall brain size.
- There is evidence in DS, FXS, and WS of disruptions in synaptic plasticity, specifically, an imbalance between long-term potentiation (LTP) and long-term depression (LTD). This may provide a unifying neurophysiological explanation of the long-term memory and learning deficits in ID.

Etiology of FXS

- Individuals with FXS often present with symptoms of autism and social anxiety.
- FXS is the most prevalent inherited form of ID.
- FXS is a single-gene disorder resulting from disruptions of the *FMR1* gene on the X chromosome.
- Because FXS is X-linked, males are more frequently and severely affected than females.
- The gene product of *FMR1* is called FMRP and is involved in dendritic spine maturation, synaptogenesis, and pruning of dendrites and synapses.
- Although only a single gene is affected, the genetic mechanisms of the disorder are complex involving epigenetic and parent of origin effects.
- The neuroanatomical phenotype of FXS includes both smaller (cerebellar vermis) and larger brain structures (striatal–frontal).
- The neuropsychological phenotype in FXS includes a decline in IQ with age, prominent deficits in EF, and deficits in long-term memory.

(continued)

TABLE 14.3. *(continued)*

Etiology of WS

- Individuals with WS are described as "hypersocial."
  They tend to show relative strengths in language processing and relative weaknesses in visual–spatial processing.
- WS has a lower prevalence than DS and FXS (1 per 7,500 births) and is primarily nonfamilial.
- WS is caused by a sporadic, contiguous microdeletion on chromosome 7 (7q11.23), which involves approximately 25 genes.
- There has been progress in mapping the affected genes to phenotypes: *ELN* is implicated in the cardiac phenotypes and *LIMK1, CYLN2, GTF2I,* and *GTF2IRD1* are most often implicated in the cognitive phenotype.
- Structural brain alterations are observed in WS, including overall microcephaly with specific reductions in the parietal lobule, intraparietal sulcus, and occipital lobe.
- Functional brain alterations are also observed, including reductions in hippocampal activity, in dorsal stream activity in the parietal lobe, and in amygdala activation to angry or fearful faces. The latter two findings map to the visual–spatial processing deficits and social disinhibition that are common features of WS.
- The neuropsychological phenotype is characterized by a mean and stable IQ of ~60, deficits in visual–spatial processing, overall language consistent with mental age with relative strengths in concrete vocabulary and verbal short-term memory, and deficits in verbal and spatial long-term memory and working memory.

Diagnosis

- Speech–language and learning delays are often the primary referral question.
- Early developmental history is likely to include delayed milestones, emotional dysregulation in toddlerhood, delays in abstract play, and adaptive delays.
- In addition to careful history, diagnosis requires individually administered measures of IQ and adaptive functioning.

Prevention

- High-quality early intervention can prevent some cases of ID of predominantly environmental etiology.
- A few genetically based forms of ID, most notably, metabolic disorders, can be prevented with appropriate medical treatment.

Treatment

- The evidence base for treatment approaches in ID has grown in the past decade.
- Institutionalization is not an effective treatment for ID and generally leads to poorer outcomes.
- Increased knowledge of the genetic pathways involved in ID syndromes has led to the development of potential drug therapies. So far, clinical trials in human patients have not been successful.
- CBT can be adapted for developmental level and has shown promising results for depression.
- Stimulants show beneficial effects for treating ADHD in the context of ID. The effect sizes might be slightly reduced relative to children with ADHD alone but still show meaningful clinical impact.
- Applied behavior analysis (ABA), a highly structured behavioral treatment, is an empirically supported intervention for problem behaviors in ID.
- Milieu communication treatments are design to improve language skills in young children with ID. A recent RCT showed beneficial effect for toddlers with DS.

Conclusions

Our goal in this book has been to review our current scientific understanding of learning disorders and to explain how that science translates into best clinical practices, which in turn lead to new scientific questions: the virtuous cycle described in the Preface. Having accomplished these goals, what general conclusions can we draw about the state of the science, and the most important future directions for research and practice? To answer these questions, we discuss the following topics: (1) validity of the multilevel framework used in this book; (2) future research directions at each of the four levels of analysis; and (3) future priorities for translating research into practice.

VALIDITY OF THE MULTILEVEL FRAMEWORK

As we explained in Chapter 1, our approach to explaining the development of learning disorders utilizes a framework that includes four levels of analysis: (1) etiology, (2) brain mechanisms, (3) neuropsychology, and (4) defining symptoms of the disorder. This framework is not specific to learning disorders. Instead, it is relevant for any disorder of behavior, including other psychiatric disorders and neurological disorders (Pennington, 2014). Indeed, with minor modifications, this framework is relevant for any medical disorder. Specifically, for a nonbehavioral disorder such as cancer, we would need to change level (2) to anatomy and level (3) to pathophysiology. Hence, we are definitely embracing an interdisciplinary and, some would say, "medical model" approach to understanding the development of learning disorders. Without addressing all four levels of analysis, we cannot attain a complete scientific understanding of any disorder, or of normal physical and psychological development.

Taking an interdisciplinary approach has necessarily forced the reader *and* the authors out of their comfort zones! It is well beyond the reach of any single scientist or practitioner to be an expert at all four levels of analysis. For instance, it is beyond the ken of virtually all behavioral scientists to see how the development of cilia on neurons might impact language and reading development. Because the key constructs across the two levels of analysis are wildly incommensurate with each other, we need intermediate theoretical constructs to map connections between these two levels of analysis.

Each of the four levels of analysis in our framework has its own set of key constructs, but we are only now beginning to create and test transdisciplinary constructs that map one level of analysis onto another. As we discussed in Chapter 4, neural network models are beginning to provide a way to map connections between brain mechanisms and neuropsychology. We also need to develop ways to map connections between etiological influences (genes, environment, and their interplay) and brain development, which will require advances in developmental biology. The burgeoning field of imaging genetics is also relevant. As research on learning and other behavioral disorders becomes increasingly transdisciplinary, researchers at each level of analysis should be prepared to refine or even discard their favorite constructs. To understand the development of a given behavioral disorder, we will need to abstract away from some of the many details found at each level of analysis. We could map every neuron and every synapse in the developing brain, yet still have no idea how their interaction produces behavior. Even if we could experimentally manipulate a given gene, neurotransmitter, class of synapses, or type of neuron and demonstrate that that manipulation caused a given abnormal behavior, we would still lack a complete explanation of that abnormal behavior. Krakauer, Ghazanfar, Gomez-Marin, MacIver, and Poeppel (2017) discuss this issue and demonstrate why a detailed psychological analysis of the behavior in question will still be needed to go from biological causes to complete explanations.

Hence, while the four-level framework utilized in this book is valid in a broad sense, it will not provide a full explanation of any behavioral disorder without methods for mapping connections between levels of analysis. Such methods will facilitate an iterative process whereby advances at one level provide a new research focus at another.

FUTURE DIRECTIONS AT EACH LEVEL OF ANALYSIS

Etiology

A good example of this transdisciplinary synergy can be found in the important phenomenon of comorbidity, which, as we have demonstrated, is pervasive across learning disorders (and indeed, across all behavioral disorders). Research at the symptom and neuropsychological levels has advanced our understanding of these comorbidities, and behavioral and some molecular genetic studies have demonstrated that shared genes ("generalist genes") play a predominant role in causing comorbidity. Hence, future research aimed at identifying these generalist genes is a high priority.

Having read this book, a skeptic could reasonably ask, "Why keep investigating the molecular genetics of behavioral disorders, since these disorders are so highly polygenic that extremely large samples are required to identify a single risk variant that will only explain a tiny proportion of the variance in the disorder in question?" While this is a valid concern, it is also clear that a single gene identification, even if it accounts for a small percent of the variance in the population or only has a major effect in a small percentage of cases, can nonetheless provide critical insights into biological pathways that are affected in a disorder and lead to new gene discoveries. One example is emerging from the autism field, where gene identifications are coalescing on specific pathways, including synaptic plasticity. Therefore, while any single gene identification contributes modestly to the genetic profile of a disorder, each gene provides a clue into the disrupted biological pathways that are associated with the disorder.

Brain Mechanisms

We felt we encountered the most conflicting findings at this level of analysis, and there are at least three reasons for this confusion. One reason is shared with earlier genetic association studies that produced many conflicting results because they were underpowered. Likewise, many earlier neuroimaging studies of clinical populations, including learning disorders, have been underpowered. In our reviews, we focused on meta-analyses and more recent studies with large sample sizes. A second reason, also shared with genetic association studies, is a failure to distinguish between confirmatory and exploratory analyses. This reason is part of a bigger problem, namely, the lack of a strong theory of the development of brain–behavior relations. We need such a theory to motivate specific hypotheses. A third reason is that neuroimaging methods are developing very rapidly. It is clear that the neuroimaging field, like the genetics field, is moving toward large, collaborative studies, and this will be a positive development for the field in terms of replicating results.

Besides addressing these three problems, another important direction for future neuroimaging studies is to test for neuroimaging phenotypes that are shared by comorbid disorders, just as genetic studies can be strengthened by testing for generalist genes.

Neuropsychology

The methods used at this level of analysis have changed less since the second edition of this book was published, and the maturity of the field has led to much more convergence on key results for each disorder covered in this book. Nonetheless, major puzzles remain. While it is increasingly clear that single cognitive-deficit models of learning disorders are not sufficient, we only have adequate multiple-deficit models for a few of the learning disorders considered here. Probably the most progress has been made for dyslexia, for which we have a good multiple-deficit model of the disorder, as well as its comorbidities. In contrast, multiple-deficit models have hardly been tested for autism, and its neuropsychology remains puzzling. As we discussed in Chapter 13 on autism spectrum disorder (ASD), Brunsdon and Happé (2013) proposed a multiple-deficit model of ASD, because the social and repetitive symptoms that define this disorder appear to have separate etiologies. Attention-deficit/hyperactivity disorder (ADHD) lies somewhere between dyslexia and autism in terms of our neuropsychological understanding. There is strong convergence on a few key neuropsychological results for ADHD, such as a deficit in inhibition, but much of the variance in ADHD symptoms remains unexplained. There is emerging support for a second, key deficit in emotion regulation, but there have been few attempts to test both inhibition and emotion regulation in a multiple-deficit model of ADHD.

One possible reason for less progress in providing neuropsychological models of autism and ADHD could be what is a generic problem in psychiatry; that is, disorders defined by behavioral symptoms instead of cognitive tests (e.g., dyslexia) may exhibit more heterogeneity in terms of underlying neuropsychological and biological causes. In response to this challenge, Insel et al. (2010) proposed the Research Diagnostic Criteria (RDoC) framework, which advocated for research focused on biomarkers instead of the symptom level of analysis used in DSM-5 and earlier DSMs.

However, as we discussed in Chapters 13 and 14, the biggest puzzle for the neuropsychological level of analysis is the one posed by more pervasive disorders such as ASD and intellectual disability (ID), in which there are deficits not only across cognitive domains, but also in social, motor, and adaptive behavior. Even with multiple deficits, it seems unlikely that we will be able to develop a parsimonious neuropsychological model of these disorders. As we discussed in Chapter 4, these disorders will require us to move beyond neuropsychology to a neurocomputational level of analysis that translates brain mechanisms into behavior. Perhaps there is a unifying brain explanation for ID, such as the imbalance between long-term potentiation (LTP) and long-term depression (LTD), discussed in Chapter 14. For ASD, such a unifying brain explanation is not yet in view.

Symptoms

Although diagnostic definitions of learning disorders will continue to evolve, we have fairly strong evidence for the reliability and validity of each of the learning disorders in this book and for the comorbidities of each. Nonetheless, future lumping and splitting is likely as we discover more about underlying mechanisms. In terms of lumping, we already know that a disorder in spelling can be lumped with dyslexia and that a disorder of written language currently lacks discriminant validity, as discussed in Chapter 6. In terms of splitting, we can ask which of these learning disorders have reliable and valid subtypes. The simple answer so far is "None." This issue has probably been researched the most for dyslexia, and so far, we do not have strong support for dyslexia subtypes, such as developmental surface and phonological dyslexia (Peterson, Pennington, & Olson, 2013). Likewise, the validity of the three symptom subtypes of ADHD (inattentive, hyperactive–impulsive, and combined) has been seriously questioned (Willcutt et al., 2012).

Turning to language impairment (LI), it is now clear that the old subtype distinction between receptive and expressive developmental language impairment (which derives from the now questionable distinction between Broca's and Wernicke's acquired aphasias) is *not* valid. Likewise, the subtype distinction between ASD and Asperger syndrome has proven not to be valid, and questions remain as to whether there is a valid subtype distinction between social–communication disorder and ASD. Hence, even as we postulate that heterogeneity may help resolve the puzzles at the neuropsychological level of analysis, the failure to find valid subtypes of these disorders argues against that explanation.

If splitting has not succeeded, has lumping been more fruitful? The simple answer is "yes," as demonstrated by the high level of comorbidity among disorders. While the mechanisms underlying comorbidity are rarely studied directly (see Chapter 5 for a fuller explanation), there are hints across levels of analysis that lumping may improve power for identifying shared risk factors that are common to multiple learning disorders.

FUTURE DIRECTIONS FOR TRANSLATION INTO BEST CLINICAL PRACTICE

As discussed in each of the six chapters on individual learning disorders, big gaps still remain between science and practice. Although the American Academy of Pediatrics (AAP) website provides explicit guidelines for developmental screening by primary care pediatricians, the majority of pediatricians rely on clinical impressions rather than validated screening instruments (Pinto-Martin, Dunkle, Earls, Fliedner, & Landes, 2005). Moreover, disorders that were missed by children's pediatricians are often missed once the children enter school. If pediatricians and schools just implemented what we already know, many more of these children with currently undetected learning disorders would be identified early and receive appropriate preventive treatment. Hence, much work remains to be done to educate primary care pediatricians and teachers of young children about learning disorders.

In addition, as discussed in the second edition of this book (Pennington, 2009), controversial therapies for learning disorders remain quite prevalent, so many identified children are receiving the wrong treatment. The U.S. Food and Drug Administration (FDA) has begun to take a role in warning the public about unvalidated and potentially dangerous medical treatments for autism (e.g., chelation), but it does not regulate behavioral interventions. The Federal Trade Commission (FTC) has taken on some unproven behavioral interventions (e.g., Lumosity and CogMed). The AAP website does periodically review controversial behavioral therapies for learning disorders. More could be done by the FDA, the Centers for Disease Control and Prevention (CDC), the FTC, and various professional organizations, such as the AAP and the American Psychological Association and American Psychiatric Association, to protect the public from wasting time and money on controversial therapies. In addition, both health care providers for children and educators need better training in this area.

In summary, although much has been accomplished in the roughly 10 years since the previous edition of this book appeared (Pennington, 2009), considerable work remains to be done to understand, treat, and eventually prevent learning disorders.

References

Achenbach, T. M. (1982). *Developmental psychopathology*. New York: Wiley.

Achenbach, T. M. (1991). *Manual of the Child Behavior Checklist/4–18 and 1991 Profile*. Burlington: University of Vermont Department of Psychiatry.

Adolphs, R. (2003). Cognitive neuroscience of human social behaviour. *Nature Reviews Neuroscience, 4*(3), 165–178.

Alexander, A. W., & Slinger-Constant, A.-M. (2004). Current status of treatments for dyslexia: Critical review. *Journal of Child Neurology, 19*(10), 744–758.

Ali, N., Pitson, D., & Stradling, J. (1996). Sleep disordered breathing: Effects of adenotonsillectomy on behaviour and psychological functioning. *European Journal of Pediatrics, 155*(1), 56–62.

Aman, M. G., Buican, B., & Arnold, L. E. (2003). Methylphenidate treatment in children with borderline IQ and mental retardation: Analysis of three aggregated studies. *Journal of Child and Adolescent Psychopharmacology, 13*(1), 29–40.

American Psychiatric Association. (1994). *Diagnostic and statistical manual of mental disorders* (4th ed.). Washington, DC: Author.

American Psychiatric Association. (2000). *Diagnostic and statistical manual of mental disorders* (4th ed., text rev.). Washington, DC: Author.

American Psychiatric Association. (2013). *Diagnostic and statistical manual of mental disorders* (5th ed.). Arlington, VA: Author.

Amir, R. E., Van den Veyver, I. B., Wan, M., Tran, C. Q., Francke, U., & Zoghbi, H. Y. (1999). Rett syndrome is caused by mutations in X-linked MECP2, encoding methyl-CpG-binding protein 2. *Nature Genetics, 23*(2), 185–188.

Anderson, D. K., Liang, J. W., & Lord, C. (2014). Predicting young adult outcome among more and less cognitively able individuals with autism spectrum disorders. *Journal of Child Psychology and Psychiatry and Allied Disciplines, 55*, 485–494.

Angold, A., Costello, E. J., & Erkanli, A. (1999). Comorbidity. *Journal of Child Psychology and Psychiatry, 40*(1), 57–87.

Ansari, D. (2010). Neurocognitive approaches to developmental disorders of numerical and mathematical cognition: The perils of neglecting the role of development. *Learning and Individual Differences, 20*(2), 123–129.

Aram, D. M., & Nation, J. E. (1980). Preschool language disorders and subsequent language and academic difficulties. *Journal of Communication Disorders, 13*(2), 159–170.

Aravena, S., Snellings, P., Tijms, J., & van der Molen, M. W. (2013). A lab-controlled simulation of a letter–speech sound binding deficit in dyslexia. *Journal of Experimental Child Psychology, 115*(4), 691–707.

Arnett, A. B., MacDonald, B., & Pennington, B. F. (2013). Cognitive and behavioral indicators of ADHD symptoms prior to school age. *Journal of Learning Disabilities, 46*(6), 500–516.

Arnett, A. B., Pennington, B. F., Friend, A., Willcutt, E. G., Byrne, B., Samuelsson, S., & Olson, R. K. (2013). The SWAN captures variance at the negative and positive ends of the ADHD symptom dimension. *Journal of Attention Disorders, 17*(2), 152–162.

Arnett, A. B., Pennington, B. F., Peterson, R. L., Willcutt, E. G., DeFries, J. C., & Olson, R. K. (2017). Explaining the sex difference in dyslexia. *Journal of Child Psychology and Psychiatry, 58*(6), 719–727.

Arnett, A. B., Pennington, B. F., Willcutt, E. G., DeFries, J. C., & Olson, R. K. (2015). Sex differences in ADHD symptom severity. *Journal of Child Psychology and Psychiatry, 56*(6), 632–639.

Arnett, A. B., Pennington, B. F., Willcutt, E., Dmitrieva, J., Byrne, B., Samuelsson, S., & Olson, R. K. (2012). A cross-lagged model of the development of ADHD Inattention symptoms and rapid naming speed. *Journal of Abnormal Child Psychology, 40*(8), 1313–1326.

Aro, T., Ahonen, T., Tolvanen, A., Lyytinen, H., & de Barra, H. T. (1999). Contribution of ADHD characteristics to the academic treatment outcome of children with learning difficulties. *Developmental Neuropsychology, 15*(2), 291-305.

Aron, A. R., Robbins, T. W., & Poldrack, R. A. (2004). Inhibition and the right inferior frontal cortex. *Trends in Cognitive Sciences, 8*(4), 170-177.

Arsalidou, M., & Taylor, M. J. (2011). Is 2 + 2 = 4?: Meta-analyses of brain areas needed for numbers and calculations. *NeuroImage, 54*(3), 2382-2393.

Asperger, H. (1991). "Autistic psychopathy" in childhood (U. Frith, Trans.). In U. Frith (Ed.), *Autism and Asperger syndrome* (pp. 37-92). Cambridge, UK: Cambridge University Press. (Original work published 1944)

Associated Press. (2016, January 6). Lumosity game developer agrees to $2 million settlement. *The New York Times*, p. B2. Retrieved from *www.nytimes.com/2016/01/06/business/lumosity-game-developer-agrees-to-2-million-settlement.html?mcubz=1*.

Aylward, E. H., Minshew, N. J., Goldstein, G., Honeycutt, N. A., Augustine, A. M., Yates, K. O., . . . Pearlson, G. D. (1999). MRI volumes of amygdala and hippocampus in non-mentally retarded autistic adolescents and adults. *Neurology, 53*(9), 2145-2150.

Aylward, E. H., Reiss, A. L., Reader, M. J., Singer, H. S., Brown, J. E., & Denckla, M. B. (1996). Basal ganglia volumes in children with attention-deficit hyperactivity disorder. *Journal of Child Neurology, 11*(2), 112-115.

Bachevalier, J. (2008). Nonhuman primate models of memory development. In C. A. Nelson & M. Luciana (Eds.), *Handbook of developmental cognitive neuroscience* (2nd ed., pp. 499-508). Cambridge, MA: MIT Press.

Baddeley, A., Gathercole, S., & Papagno, C. (1998). The phonological loop as a language learning device. *Psychological Review, 105*(1), 158-173.

Badian, N. A. (1983). Arithmetic and nonverbal learning. In H. R. Myklebust (Ed.), *Progress in learning disabilities* (Vol. 5, pp. 235-264). New York: Grune & Stratton.

Badian, N. A. (1999). Persistent arithmetic, reading, or arithmetic and reading disability. *Annals of Dyslexia, 49*(1), 43-70.

Bailey, A., Phillips, W., & Rutter, M. (1996). Autism: Towards an integration of clinical, genetic, neuropsychological, and neurobiological perspectives. *Journal of Child Psychology and Psychiatry, 37*(1), 89-126.

Baio, J., Wiggins, L., Christensen, D. L., Maenner, M. J., Daniels, J., Warren, Z., Kurzius-Spencer, M., . . . Dowling, N. F. (2018). Prevalence of autism spectrum disorder among children aged 8 years—Autism and developmental disabilities monitoring network, 11 sites, United States, 2014. *Surveillance Summaries, 67*(6), 1-23.

Baker, E., & McLeod, S. (2011). Evidence-based practice for children with speech sound disorders: Part 1. Narrative review. *Language, Speech, and Hearing Services in Schools, 42*(2), 102-139.

Baker, L., & Cantwell, D. (1982). Developmental, social and behavioral characteristics of speech and language disordered children. *Child Psychiatry and Human Development, 12*(4), 195-206.

Baker, L., & Cantwell, D. (1992). Attention deficit disorder and speech/language disorders. *Comprehensive Mental Health Care, 2*(1), 3-16.

Barkley, R. A. (1996). Attention-deficit/hyperactivity disorder. In E. J. Mash & R. A. Barkley (Eds.), *Child psychopathology* (pp. 63-112). New York: Guilford Press.

Barkley, R. A., & Murphy, K. (2006). *Attention-deficit/hyperactivity disorder: A clinical workbook* (3rd ed.). New York: Guilford Press.

Baron-Cohen, S., Leslie, A. M., & Frith, U. (1985). Does the autistic child have a "theory of mind"? *Cognition, 21*(1), 37-46.

Baron-Cohen, S., Leslie, A. M., & Frith, U. (1986). Mechanical, behavioral and intentional understanding of picture stories in autistic children. *British Journal of Developmental Psychology, 4*, 113-125.

Baron-Cohen, S., Ring, H. A., Bullmore, E. T., Wheelwright, S., Ashwin, C., & Williams, S. C. R. (2000). The amygdala theory of autism. *Neuroscience and Biobehavioral Reviews, 24*, 355-364.

Barquero, L. A., Davis, N., & Cutting, L. E. (2014). Neuroimaging of reading intervention: A systematic review and activation likelihood estimate meta-analysis. *PLOS ONE, 9*(1), e83668.

Bartholomew, D. J., Deary, I. J., & Lawn, M. (2009). A new lease of life for Thomson's bonds model of intelligence. *Psychological Review, 116*(3), 567-579.

Bartlett, C. W., Flax, J. F., Logue, M. W., Vieland, V. J., Bassett, A. S., Tallal, P., & Brzustowicz, L. M. (2002). A major susceptibility locus for specific language impairment is located on 13q21. *American Journal of Human Genetics, 71*(1), 45-55.

Bates, E. A. (1998). Construction grammar and its implications for child language research. *Journal of Child Language, 25*, 462-466.

Bates, E., & Goodman, J. C. (1997). On the inseparability of grammar and the lexicon: Evidence from acquisition, aphasia and real-time processing. *Language and Cognitive Processes, 12*(5-6), 507-584.

Bates, E. A., & MacWhinney, B. (1988). "What is functionalism?" *Papers and Reports on Child Language Development, 27*, 137-152.

Bates, E. A., & Roe, K. (2001). Language development in children with unilateral brain injury. In C. A. Nelson & M. Luciana (Eds.), *Handbook of developmental cognitive neuroscience* (pp. 281-307). Cambridge, MA: MIT Press.

Baumgardner, T. L., Singer, H. S., Denckla, M. B., Rubin, M. A., Abrams, M. T., Colli, M. J., & Reiss, A. L. (1996). Corpus callosum morphology in children with Tourette syndrome and attention deficit hyperactivity disorder. *Neurology, 47*(2), 477-482.

Bavelier, D., & Neville, H. J. (2002). Cross-modal plasticity: Where and how? *National Review of Neuroscience, 3*(6), 443-452.

Beauchamp, M. H., Brooks, B. L., Barrowman, N., Aglipay, M., Keightley, M., Anderson, P., . . . Zemek, R. (2015). Empirical derivation and validation of a clinical case definition for neuropsychological impairment in children and adolescents. *Journal of the International Neuropsychological Society, 21*(8), 596-609.

Becker, S. P., Leopold, D. R., Burns, G. L., Jarrett, M.

A., Langberg, J. M., Marshall, S. A., . . . Willcutt, E. G. (2016). The internal, external, and diagnostic validity of sluggish cognitive tempo: A meta-analysis and critical review. *Journal of the American Academy of Child and Adolescent Psychiatry, 55*(3), 163–178.

Bedard, A. C., Stein, M. A., Halperin, J. M., Krone, B., Rajwan, E., & Newcorn, J. H. (2015). Differential impact of methylphenidate and atomoxetine on sustained attention in youth with attention-deficit/hyperactivity disorder. *Journal of Child Psychology and Psychiatry, 56*(1), 40–48.

Bedny, M., & Saxe, R. (2012). Insights into the origins of knowledge from the cognitive neuroscience of blindness. *Cognitive Neuropsychology, 29*(1-2), 56–84.

Beilock, S. L., Gunderson, E. A., Ramirez, G., & Levine, S. C. (2010). Female teachers' math anxiety affects girls' math achievement. *Proceedings of the National Academy of Sciences of the USA, 107*(5), 1860–1863.

Beitchman, J. H., Hood, J., & Inglis, A. (1990). Psychiatric risk in children with speech and language disorders. *Journal of Abnormal Child Psychology, 18*(3), 283–296.

Bellugi, U., Marks, S., Bihrle, A., & Sabo, H. (1988). Dissociations between language and cognitive functions in Williams syndrome. In D. V. M. Bishop & K. Mogford (Eds.), *Language development in exceptional circumstances* (pp. 177–189). Edinburgh, Scotland: Churchill Livingstone.

Belmonte, M. K., Allen, G., Beckel-Mitchener, A., Boulanger, L. M., Carper, R. A., & Webb, S. J. (2004). Autism and abnormal development of brain connectivity. *Journal of Neuroscience, 24*(42), 9228–9231.

Belsky, J., & Pluess, M. (2009). Beyond diathesis stress: Differential susceptibility to environmental influences. *Psychological Bulletin, 135*(6), 885–908.

Bennett, T., Szatmari, P., Bryson, S., Volden, J., Zwaigenbaum, L., Vaccarella, L., . . . Boyle, M. (2008). Differentiating autism and Asperger syndrome on the basis of language delay or impairment. *Journal of Autism and Developmental Disorders, 38*(4), 616–625.

Berger, H. (1926). Ueber Rechenstörungen bei Herderkrankungen des Brosshirns. *Archiv für Psychiatrie und Nervenkrankheiten, 78,* 238–263.

Bernier, R., Golzio, C., Xiong, B., Stessman, H. A., Coe, B. P., Penn, O., . . . Vulto-van Silfhout, A. T. (2014). Disruptive CHD8 mutations define a subtype of autism early in development. *Cell, 158*(2), 263–276.

Berninger, V. W., Vaughan, K., Abbott, R. D., Begay, K., Coleman, K. B., Curtin, G., . . . Graham, S. (2002). Teaching spelling and composition alone and together: Implications for simple view of writing. *Journal of Educational Psychology, 94*(2), 291–304.

Bernstein, J. H., & Waber, D. P. (1990). Developmental neuropsychological assessment: The systemic approach. In *Neuropsychology: Vol. 17. Neuromethods* (pp. 311–371). Totowa, NJ: Humana Press.

Bernstein, J. H., & Weiler, M. (2000). "Pediatric neuropsychological assessment" examined. In G. Goldstein & M. Hersen (Eds.), *Handbook of psychological assessment* (3rd ed., pp. 263–300). New York: Pergamon.

Berridge, C. W., & Devilbiss, D. M. (2011). Psychostimulants as cognitive enhancers: The prefrontal cortex, catecholamines, and attention-deficit/hyperactivity disorder. *Biological Psychiatry, 69*(12), e101–e111.

Berument, S. K., Rutter, M., Lord, C., Pickles, A., & Bailey, A. (1999). Autism screening questionnaire: Diagnostic validity. *British Journal of Psychiatry, 175,* 444–451.

Best, C. S., Moffat, V. J., Power, M. J., Owens, D. G., & Johnstone, E. C. (2008). The boundaries of the cognitive phenotype of autism: Theory of mind, central coherence and ambiguous figure perception in young people with autistic traits. *Journal of Autism and Developmental Disorders, 38*(5), 840–847.

Best, C. T., McRoberts, G. W., & Goodell, E. (2001). Discrimination of non-native consonant contrasts varying in perceptual assimilation to the listener's native phonological system. *Journal of the Acoustic Society of America, 109,* 775–794.

Betancur, C. (2011). Etiological heterogeneity in autism spectrum disorders: More than 100 genetic and genomic disorders and still counting. *Brain Research, 1380,* 42–77.

Bettelheim, B. (1967). *The empty fortress.* New York: Free Press.

Biederman, J., Faraone, S., Keenan, K., Benjamin, J., Krifcher, B., Moore, C., . . . Steingard, R. (1992). Further evidence for family-genetic risk factors in attention deficit hyperactivity disorder. Patterns of comorbidity in probands and relatives psychiatrically and pediatrically referred samples. *Archives of General Psychiatry, 49*(9), 728–738.

Biederman, J., Faraone, S., Keenan, K., Knee, D., & Tsuang, M. T. (1990). Family-genetic and psychosocial risk factors in DSM-III attention deficit disorder. *Journal of the American Academy of Child and Adolescent Psychiatry, 29*(4), 526–533.

Biederman, J., & Spencer, T. (1999). Attention-deficit/hyperactivity disorder (ADHD) as a noradrenergic disorder. *Biological Psychiatry, 46*(9), 1234–1242.

Binet, A., & Simon, T. (1916). New methods for the diagnosis of the intellectual level of subnormals. In A. Binet & T. Simon (Eds.), *The development of intelligence in children* (pp. 37–90). Baltimore: Williams & Wilkins.

Bishop, D. V. M. (1997). *Uncommon understanding: Development and disorders of language comprehension in children.* Hove, UK: Psychology Press.

Bishop, D. V. M. (2002). Cerebellar abnormalities in developmental dyslexia: Cause, correlate or consequence? *Cortex, 38*(4), 491–498.

Bishop, D. V. M., & Adams, C. (1990). A prospective study of the relationship between specific language impairment, phonological disorders and reading retardation. *Journal of Child Psychology and Psychiatry, 31*(7), 1027–1050.

Bishop, D. V. M., Bishop, S. J., Bright, P., James, C., Delaney, T., & Tallal, P. (1999). Different origin of auditory and phonological processing problems in children with language impairment: Evidence from a twin study. *Journal of Speech, Language and Hearing Research, 42*(1), 155–168.

Bishop, D. V. M., & Edmundson, A. (1987). Language-impaired 4-year-olds: Distinguishing transient from persistent impairment. *Journal of Speech and Hearing Disorders, 52*(2), 156–173.

Bishop, D. V. M., & Hayiou-Thomas, M. E. (2008). Heritability of specific language impairment depends on diagnostic criteria. *Genes, Brain and Behavior, 7,* 365–372.

Bishop, D. V. M., McDonald, D., Bird, S., & Hayiou-Thomas, M. E. (2009). Children who read words accurately despite language impairment: Who are they and how do they do it? *Child Development, 80,* 593–605.

Bishop, D. V. M., Whitehouse, A. J. O., Watt, H. J., & Line, E. A. (2008). Autism and diagnostic substitution: Evidence from a study of adults with a history of developmental language disorder. *Developmental Medicine and Child Neurology, 50,* 341–345.

Bishop, S. L., Huerta, M., Gotham, K., Alexandra Havdahl, K., Pickles, A., Duncan, A., . . . Lord, C. (2017). The Autism Symptom Interview, School-Age: A brief telephone interview to identify autism spectrum disorders in 5- to 12-year-old children. *Autism Research, 10*(1), 78–88.

Bleuler, E. (1950). *Dementia praecox or a group within the schizophrenias* (J. Zinkin, Trans.). New York: International Universities Press. (Original work published 1911)

Blumstein, S. E., & Amso, D. (2013). Dynamic functional organization of language: Insights from functional neuroimaging. *Perspectives on Psychological Science, 8*(1), 44–48.

Bolton, P. F., & Griffiths, P. D. (1997). Association of tuberous sclerosis of temporal lobes with autism and atypical autism. *Lancet, 349*(9049), 392–395.

Boucher, J., Mayes, A., & Bigham, S. (2012). Memory in autistic spectrum disorder. *Psychological Bulletin, 138*(3), 458–496.

Bourgeron, T. (2015). From the genetic architecture to synaptic plasticity in autism spectrum disorder. *Nature Reviews Neuroscience, 16*(9), 551–563.

Bradley, L., & Bryant, P. E. (1983). Categorizing sounds and learning to read: A causal connection. *Nature, 301*(5899), 419–421.

Breaux, K. C. (2009). *Wechsler Individual Achievement Test–Third Edition (WIAT-III): Technical manual.* San Antonio, TX: Pearson.

Breslin, J., Spano, G., Bootzin, R., Anand, P., Nadel, L., & Edgin, J. (2014). Obstructive sleep apnea syndrome and cognition in Down syndrome. *Developmental Medicine and Child Neurology, 56*(7), 657–664.

Bromley, R. L., Mawer, G. E., Briggs, M., Cheyne, C., Clayton-Smith, J., García-Fiñana, M., . . . Baker, G. A. (2013). The prevalence of neurodevelopmental disorders in children prenatally exposed to antiepileptic drugs. *Journal of Neurology, Neurosurgery, and Psychiatry, 84*(6), 637–643.

Bronfenbrenner, U., & Ceci, S. J. (1994). Nature–nurture reconceptualized in developmental perspective: A bioecological model. *Psychological Review, 101*(4), 568–586.

Brooks, B. L. (2010). Seeing the forest for the trees: Prevalence of low scores on the Wechsler Intelligence Scale for Children (WISC-IV). *Psychological Assessment, 22*(3), 650–656.

Brooks, B. L., & Iverson, G. L. (2012). Improving accuracy when identifying cognitive impairment in pediatric neuropsychological assessments. In E. M. S. Sherman & B. L. Brooks (Eds.), *Pediatric forensic neuropsychology* (pp. 66–88). New York: Oxford University Press.

Brown, I. S., & Felton, R. H. (1990). Effects of instruction on beginning reading skills in children at risk for reading disability. *Reading and Writing, 2,* 223–241.

Brown, J. I., Fishco, V. V., & Hanna, G. (1993). *Nelson–Denny reading test: Manual for scoring and interpretation.* Itasca, IL: Riverside.

Brown, R. (1973). *The first language.* Cambridge, MA: Harvard University Press.

Brown, R., Hobson, R. P., Lee, A., & Stevenson, J. (1997). Are there "autistic-like" features in congenitally blind children? *Journal of Child Psychology and Psychiatry, 38*(6), 693–703.

Brown, T. T., Kuperman, J. M., Chung, Y., Erhart, M., McCabe, C., Hagler, D. J., Jr., . . . Dale, A. M. (2012). Neuroanatomical assessment of biological maturity. *Current Biology, 22*(18), 1693–1698.

Bruck, M. (1992). Persistence of dyslexics' phonological deficits. *Developmental Psychology, 28,* 874–886.

Bruner, J. (1981). *Human growth and development.* London: Oxford University Press.

Brunsdon, V. E., & Happé, F. (2014). Exploring the "fractionation" of autism at the cognitive level. *Autism, 18*(1), 17–30.

Buck v. Bell, 274 U.S. 200 (1927).

Butterworth, B. (2005). Developmental dyscalculia. In J. I. D. Campbell (Ed.), *Handbook of mathematical cognition* (pp. 455–469). New York: Psychology Press.

Byrne, B., Coventry, W. L., Olson, R. K., Samuelsson, S., Corley, R., Willcutt, E. G., . . . Defries, J. C. (2009). Genetic and environmental influences on aspects of literacy and language in early childhood: Continuity and change from preschool to grade 2. *Journal of Neurolinguistics, 22,* 219–236.

Byrne, B., Fielding-Barnsley, R., & Ashley, L. (2000). Effects of preschool phoneme identity training after six years: Outcome level distinguished from rate of response. *Journal of Educational Psychology, 92*(4), 659–667.

Cain, K., Oakhill, J., & Lemmon, K. (2004). Individual differences in the inference of word meanings from context. *Journal of Educational Psychology, 96,* 671–681.

Canivez, G. L., Watkins, M. W., & Dombrowski, S. C. (2016). Factor structure of the Wechsler Intelligence Scale for Children–Fifth Edition: Exploratory factor analyses with the 16 primary and secondary subtests. *Psychological Assessment, 28*(8), 975–986.

Canivez, G. L., Watkins, M. W., & Dombrowski, S. C. (2017). Structural validity of the Wechsler Intelligence Scale for Children–Fifth Edition: Confirmatory factor analyses with the 16 primary and secondary subtests. *Psychological Assessment, 29*(4), 458–472.

Cannizzaro, L. A., Chen, Y. Q., Rafi, M. A., & Wenger, D. A. (1994). Regional mapping of the human galactocerebrosidase gene (GALC) to 14q31 by in situ hybridization. *Cytogenetic Cell Genetics, 66*(4), 244–245.

Cannon, L., Kenworthy, L., Alexander, K. C., Werner, M. A., & Anthony, L. (2011). *Unstuck and on Target!: An executive function curriculum to improve* flexibility for children with autism spectrum disorders (research ed.). Baltimore: Brookes.

Cantwell, D. P. (1975). Genetics of hyperactivity. Journal of Child Psychology and Psychiatry, 16(3), 261–264.

Cantwell, D., & Baker, L. (1985). Psychiatric and learning disorders in children with speech and language disorders: A descriptive analysis. Advances in Learning and Behavioral Disabilities, 4, 29–47.

Capano, L., Minden, D., Chen, S. X., Schachar, R. J., & Ickowicz, A. (2008). Mathematical learning disorder in school-age children with attention-deficit hyperactivity disorder. Canadian Journal of Psychiatry, 53(6), 392–399.

Capron, C., & Duyme, M. (1989). Assessment of effects of socio-economic status on IQ in a full cross-fostering study. Nature, 340, 552–554.

Caravolas, M., Volín, J., & Hulme, C. (2005). Phoneme awareness is a key component of alphabetic literacy skills in consistent and inconsistent orthographies: Evidence from Czech and English children. Journal of Experimental Child Psychology, 92, 107–139.

Caron, C., & Rutter, M. (1991). Comorbidity in child psychopathology: Concepts, issues and research strategies. Journal of Child Psychology and Psychiatry, 32(7), 1063–1080.

Carone, D. A., Iverson, G. L., & Bush, S. S. (2010). A model to approaching and providing feedback to patients regarding invalid test performance in clinical neuropsychological evaluations. Clinical Neuropsychologist, 24(5), 759–778.

Carrion-Castillo, A., Franke, B., & Fisher, S. E. (2013). Molecular genetics of dyslexia: An overview. Dyslexia, 19(4), 214–240.

Carrion-Castillo, A., van Bergen, E., Vino, A., van Zuijen, T., de Jong, P. F., Francks, C., & Fisher, S. E. (2016). Evaluation of results from genome-wide studies of language and reading in a novel independent dataset. Genes, Brain and Behavior, 15(6), 531–541.

Carroll, J. B. (1993). Human cognitive abilities: A survey of factor analytic studies. Cambridge, UK: Press Syndicate of the University of Cambridge.

Casey, B. J., Castellanos, F. X., Giedd, J. N., Marsh, W. L., Hamburger, S. D., Schubert, A. B., . . . Rapoport, J. L. (1997). Implication of right frontostriatal circuitry in response inhibition and attention-deficit/hyperactivity disorder. Journal of the American Academy of Child and Adolescent Psychiatry, 36(3), 374–383.

Caspi, A., Sugden, K., Moffitt, T. E., Taylor, A., Craig, I. W., Harrington, H., . . . Poulton, R. (2003). Influence of life stress on depression: Moderation by a polymorphism in the 5-HTT gene. Science, 301(5631), 386–389.

Castellanos, F. X., Giedd, J. N., Marsh, W. L., Hamburger, S. D., Vaituzis, A. C., Dickstein, D. P., . . . Rapoport, J. L. (1996). Quantitative brain magnetic resonance imaging in attention-deficit hyperactivity disorder. Archives of General Psychiatry, 53(7), 607–616.

Castellanos, F. X., & Proal, E. (2012). Large-scale brain systems in ADHD: Beyond the prefrontal–striatal model. Trends in Cognitive Science, 16(1), 17–26.

Castles, A., Wilson, K., & Coltheart, M. (2011). Early orthographic influences on phonemic awareness tasks: Evidence from a preschool training study. Journal of Experimental Child Psychology, 108, 203–210.

Castro-Caldas, A., Petersson, K. M., Reis, A., Stone-Elander, S., & Ingvar, M. (1998). The illiterate brain: Learning to read and write during childhood influences the functional organization of the adult brain. Brain, 121, 1053–1063.

Cattell, R. B. (1943). The measurement of adult intelligence. Psychological Bulletin, 40, 153–193.

Cattell, R. B. (1963). Theory of fluid and crystallized intelligence: A critical experiment. Journal of Educational Psychology, 54, 1–22.

Cattell, R. B., & Horn, J. L. (1978). A check on the theory of fluid and crystallized intelligence with description of new subtest designs. Journal of Educational Measurement, 15(3), 139–164.

Catts, H. W., Compton, D., Tomblin, J. B., & Bridges, M. S. (2012). Prevalence and nature of late-emerging poor readers. Journal of Educational Psychology, 104(1), 166–181.

Catts, H. W., Gillispie, M., Leonard, L. B., Kail, R. V., & Miller, C. A. (2002). The role of speed of processing, rapid naming, and phonological awareness in reading achievement. Journal of Learning Disabilities, 35(6), 509–524.

Centanni, T. M., Booker, A. B., Chen, F., Sloan, A. M., Carraway, R. S., Rennaker, R. L., . . . Kilgard, M. P. (2016). Knockdown of dyslexia-gene Dcdc2 interferes with speech sound discrimination in continuous streams. Journal of Neuroscience, 36(17), 4895–4906.

Centanni, T. M., Booker, A. B., Sloan, A. M., Chen, F., Maher, B., Carraway, R., . . . Kilgard, M. (2013). Knockdown of the dyslexia-associated gene Kiaa0319 impairs temporal responses to speech stimuli in rat primary auditory cortex. Cerebral Cortex, 24(7), 1753–1766.

Centanni, T. M., Chen, F., Booker, A. M., Engineer, C. T., Sloan, A. M., Rennaker, R. L., . . . Kilgard, M. P. (2014). Speech sound processing deficits and training-induced neural plasticity in rats with dyslexia gene knockdown. PLOS ONE, 9(5), e98439.

Centers for Disease Control and Prevention. (2009). Prevalence of autism spectrum disorders—Autism and Developmental Disabilities Monitoring Network, United States, 2006. Morbidity and Mortality Weekly Report, Surveillance Summaries, 58(10), 1–20.

Centers for Disease Control and Prevention. (2012). Prevalence of autism spectrum disorders—Autism and Developmental Disabilities Monitoring Network, 14 Sites, United States, 2008. Morbidity and Mortality Weekly Report Surveillance Summaries, 61(3), 1–19.

Centers for Disease Control and Prevention. (2014). Prevalence of autism spectrum disorder among children aged 8 years—Autism and Developmental Disabilities Monitoring Network, 11 Sites, United States, 2010. Morbidity and Mortality Weekly Report Surveillance Summaries, 63(2), 1–21.

Centerwall, S. A., & Centerwall, W. R. (1960). A study of children with mongolism reared in the home compared to those reared away from home. Pediatrics, 25, 678–685.

Chabris, C. F., Hebert, B. M., Benjamin, D. J.,

Beauchamp, J., Cesarini, D., van der Loos, M., . . . Laibson, D. (2012). Most reported genetic associations with general intelligence are probably false positives. *Psychological Science, 23,* 1314–1323.

Chafetz, M. D. (2008). Malingering on the social security disability consultative exam: Predictors and base rates. *Clinical Neuropsychologist, 22*(3), 529–546.

Chailangkarn, T., Trujillo, C. A., Freitas, B. C., Hrvoj-Mihic, B., Herai, R. H., Yu, D. X., . . . Muotri, A. R. (2016). A human neurodevelopmental model for Williams syndrome. *Nature, 536*(7616), 338–343.

Chandrasekaran, B., Yi, H. G., Blanco, N. J., McGeary, J. E., & Maddox, W. T. (2015). Enhanced procedural learning of speech sound categories in a genetic variant of FOXP2. *Journal of Neuroscience, 35*(20), 7808–7812.

Chang, B. S., Ly, J., Appignani, B., Bodell, A., Apse, K. A., Ravenscroft, R. S., . . . Walsh, C. A. (2005). Reading impairment in the neuronal migration disorder of periventricular nodular heterotopia. *Neurology, 64*(5), 799–803.

Chapman, R. S., & Hesketh, L. J. (2000). Behavioral phenotype of individuals with Down syndrome. *Developmental Disabilities Research Reviews, 6*(2), 84–95.

Charach, A., Carson, P., Fox, S., Ali, M. U., Beckett, J., & Lim, C. G. (2013). Interventions for preschool children at high risk for ADHD: A comparative effectiveness review. *Pediatrics, 131,* e1584–e1604.

Chawarska, K., Shic, F., Macari, S., Campbell, D. J., Brian, J., Landa, R. J., . . . Bryson, S. (2014). 18-month predictors of later outcomes in younger siblings of children with autism spectrum disorder: A baby siblings research consortium study. *Journal of the American Academy of Child and Adolescent Psychiatry, 53,* 1317–1327.

Chazan-Cohen, R., Raikes, H., Brooks-Gunn, J., Ayoub, C., Pan, B. A., Kisker, E. E., . . . Fuligni, A. S. (2009). Low-income children's school readiness: Parent contributions over the first five years. *Early Education and Development, 20*(6), 958–977.

Chesnut, S. R., Wei, T., Barnard-Brak, L., & Richman, D. M. (2017). A meta-analysis of the social communication questionnaire: Screening for autism spectrum disorder. *Autism, 21*(8), 920–928.

Chess, S. (1971). Autism in children with congenital rubella. *Journal of Autism and Developmental Disorders, 1*(1), 33–47.

Chess, S. (1977). Follow-up report on autism in congenital rubella. *Journal of Autism and Childhood Schizophrenia, 7,* 69–81.

Cheung, C. H. M., Fazier-Wood, A. C., Asherson, P., Rijsdijk, F., Kuntsi, J., Ho, C., . . . Interest, C. (2014). Shared cognitive impairments and aetiology in ADHD symptoms and reading difficulties. *PLOS ONE, 9,* e98590.

Chomsky, N. (1959). Review of Skinner's verbal behavior. *Language, 35,* 26–58.

Christensen, D. L., Baio, J., Braun, K. V. N., Bilder, D., Charles, J., Constantino, J. N., . . . Yeargin-Allsopp, M. (2016). Prevalence and characteristics of autism spectrum disorder among children aged 8 years—Autism and Developmental Disabilities Monitoring Network, 11 Sites, United States, 2012. *Morbidity and Mortality Weekly Report, Surveillance Summaries, 65,* 1–23.

Christensen, J., Grønborg, T. K., Sørensen, M. J., Schendel, D., Parner, E. T., Pedersen, L. H., & Vestergaard, M. (2013). Prenatal valproate exposure and risk of autism spectrum disorders and childhood autism. *Journal of the American Medical Association, 309*(16), 1696–1703.

Christopher, M. E., Hulslander, J., Byrne, B., Samuelsson, S., Keenan, J. M., Pennington, B. F., . . . Olson, R. K. (2013). Modeling the etiology of individual differences in early reading development: Evidence for strong genetic influences. *Scientific Studies of Reading, 17*(5), 350–368.

Clark, C., Klonoff, H., & Hayden, M. (1990). Regional cerebral glucose metabolism in Turner syndrome. *Canadian Journal of Neurological Science, 17,* 140–144.

Coghill, D. R., Seth, S., Pedroso, S., Usala, T., Currie, J., & Gagliano, A. (2014). Effects of methylphenidate on cognitive functions in children and adolescents with attention-deficit/hyperactivity disorder: Evidence from a systematic review and a meta-analysis. *Biological Psychiatry, 76,* 603–615.

Cohen Kadosh, R., Soskic, S., Iuculano, T., Kanai, R., & Walsh, V. (2010). Modulating neuronal activity produces specific and long-lasting changes in numerical competence. *Current Biology, 20*(22), 2016–2020.

Colvert, E., Tick, B., McEwen, F., Stewart, C., Curran, S. R., Woodhouse, E., . . . Garnett, T. (2015). Heritability of autism spectrum disorder in a UK population-based twin sample. *JAMA Psychiatry, 72*(5), 415–423.

Committee on Bioethics, Committee on Genetics, & the American College of Medical Genetics and Genomics Social, Ethical, and Legal Issues Committee. (2013). Ethical and policy issues in genetic testing and screening of children. *Pediatrics, 131*(3), 620–622.

Conners, C. K. (2008). *Conners 3rd edition: Manual.* North Tonawanda, NY: Multi-Health Systems.

Conners, C. K. (2014a). *Conners Continuous Performance Test Third Edition (Conners CPT 3).* North Tonawanda, NY: Multi-Health Systems.

Conners, C. K. (2014b). *Conners Kiddie Continuous Performance Test 2nd Edition (K-CPT 2).* North Tonawanda, NY: Multi-Health Systems.

Conners, C. K., Sitarenios, G., Parker, J. D., & Epstein, J. N. (1998). The revised Conners' Parent Rating Scale (CPRS-R): Factor structure, reliability, and criterion validity. *Journal of Abnormal Child Psychology, 26*(4), 257–268.

Conners, F., Rosenquist, C., Arnett, L., Moore, M., & Hume, L. (2008). Improving memory span in children with Down syndrome. *Journal of Intellectual Disability Research, 52*(3), 244–255.

Connery, A. K., Peterson, R. L., Baker, D. A., & Kirkwood, M. W. (2016). The impact of pediatric neuropsychological consultation in mild traumatic brain injury: A model for providing feedback after invalid performance. *Clinical Neuropsychologist, 30*(4), 579–598.

Connery, A. K., & Suchy, Y. (2015). Managing noncredible performance in pediatric clinical assessment. In M. W. Kirkwood (Ed.), *Validity testing in child and adolescent assessment: Evaluating exaggeration, feigning, and noncredible effort* (pp. 145–163). New York: Guilford Press.

Connor, D. F., Steeber, J., & McBurnett, K. (2010). A review of attention-deficit/hyperactivity disorder complicated by symptoms of oppositional defiant disorder or conduct disorder. *Journal of Developmental and Behavioral Pediatrics, 31*(5), 427–440.

Constantino, J. N., Davis, S. A., Todd, R. D., Schindler, M. K., Gross, M. M., Brophy, S. L., . . . Reich, W. (2003). Validation of a brief quantitative measure of autistic traits: Comparison of the social responsiveness scale with the Autism Diagnostic Interview–Revised. *Journal of Autism and Developmental Disorders, 33,* 427–433.

Constantino, J. N., & Gruber, C. P. (2012). *Social Responsiveness Scale–Second Edition (SRS-2).* Torrance, CA: Western Psychological Services.

Constantino, J. N., Gruber, C. P., Davis, S., Hayes, S., Passanante, N., & Przybeck, T. (2004). The factor structure of autistic traits. *Journal of Child Psychology and Psychiatry, 45*(4), 719–726.

Constantino, J. N., & Todd, R. D. (2003). Autistic traits in the general population: A twin study. *Archives of General Psychiatry, 60*(5), 524–530.

Conti-Ramsden, G., Ullman, M. T., & Lum, J. A. (2015). The relation between receptive grammar and procedural, declarative, and working memory in specific language impairment. *Frontiers in Psychology, 6,* 1090.

Cope, N. A., Harold, D., Hill, G., Moskvina, V., Stevenson, J., Holmans, P., . . . Williams, J. (2005). Strong evidence that KIAA0319 on chromosome 6p is a susceptibility gene for developmental dyslexia. *American Journal of Human Genetics, 76*(4), 581–591.

Cortese, S., Ferrin, M., Brandeis, D., Holtmann, M., Aggensteiner, P., Daley, D., . . . Stringaris, A. (2016). Neurofeedback for attention-deficit/hyperactivity disorder: Meta-analysis of clinical and neuropsychological outcomes from randomized controlled trials. *Journal of the American Academy of Child and Adolescent Psychiatry, 55*(6), 444–455.

Cortese, S., Kelly, C., Chabernaud, C., Proal, E., Di Martino, A., Milham, M. P., & Castellanos, F. X. (2012). Toward systems neuroscience of ADHD: A meta-analysis of 55 fMRI studies. *American Journal of Psychiatry, 169*(10), 1038–1055.

Costello, E. J., Angold, A., Burns, B. J., Stangl, D. K., Tweed, D. L., Erkanli, A., & Worthman, C. M. (1996). The Great Smoky Mountains Study of Youth: Goals, design, methods, and the prevalence of DSM-III-R disorders. *Archives of General Psychiatry, 53*(12), 1129–1136.

Coury, D. L. (2015). Babies, bathwater, and screening for autism spectrum disorder: Comments on the USPSTF recommendations for autism spectrum disorder screening. *Journal of Developmental and Behavioral Pediatrics, 36*(9), 661–663.

Crichton, A. (1798). *An inquiry into the nature and origin of mental derangement* (Vol. 2). London: T. Cadell & W. Davies.

Cross-Disorder Group of the Psychiatric Genomic Consortium, Lee, S. H., Ripke, S., Neale, B. M., Faraone, S. V., Purcell, F. M., . . . International Inflammatory Bowel Disease Genetics Consortium. (2013). Genetic relationship between five psyciatric disorders estimated from genome-wide SNPs. *Nature Genetics, 45,* 984–994.

Cubillo, A., Halari, R., Smith, A., Taylor, E., & Rubia, K. (2012). A review of fronto-striatal and fronto-cortical brain abnormalities in children and adults with attention deficit hyperactivity disorder (ADHD) and new evidence for dysfunction in adults with ADHD during motivation and attention. *Cortex, 48*(2), 194–215.

Cuccaro, M. L., Czape, K., Alessandri, M., Lee, J., Deppen, A. R., Bendik, E., . . . Hahn, S. (2014). Genetic testing and corresponding services among individuals with autism spectrum disorder (ASD). *American Journal of Medical Genetics A, 164*(10), 2592–2600.

Culbertson, W., & Zillmer, E. (2005). *Tower of London–Drexel University–Second Edition (ToLDX-2).* Chicago: Multi-Health Systems.

Cunningham, A. E. (1990). Explicit versus implicit instruction in phonemic awareness. *Journal of Experimental Child Psychology, 50*(3), 429–444.

Cunningham, A. E., & Stanovich, K. E. (1998). The impact of print exposure on word recognition. In J. L. Metsala & L. C. Ehri (Eds.), *Word recognition in beginning literacy* (pp. 235–262). Mahwah, NJ: Erlbaum.

Dalmau, J., Tuzun, E., Wu, H. Y., Masjuan, J., Rossi, J. E., Voloschin, A., . . . Lynch, D. R. (2007). Paraneoplastic anti-N-methyl-D-aspartate receptor encephalitis associated with ovarian teratoma. *Annals of Neurology, 61*(1), 25–36.

Dalsgaard, S., Østergaard, S. D., Leckman, J. F., Mortensen, P. B., & Pedersen, M. G. (2015). Mortality in children, adolescents, and adults with attention deficit hyperactivity disorder: A nationwide cohort study. *Lancet, 385*(9983), 2190–2196.

Darki, F., Peyrard-Janvid, M., Matsson, H., Kere, J., & Klingberg, T. (2012). Three dyslexia susceptibility genes, DYX1C1, DCDC2, and KIAA0319, affect temporo-parietal white matter structure. *Biological Psychiatry, 72*(8), 671–676.

Davies, G., Tenesa, A., Payton, A., Yang, J., Harris, S. E., Liewald, D., . . . Deary, I. J. (2011). Genome-wide association studies establish that human intelligence is highly heritable and polygenic. *Molecular Psychiatry, 16,* 996–1005.

Davies, G., Welham, J., Chant, D., Torrey, E. F., & McGrath, J. (2003). A systematic review and meta-analysis of Northern Hemisphere season of birth studies in schizophrenia. *Schizophrenia Bulletin, 29*(3), 587–593.

Dawson, G., Webb, S. J., Carver, L., Panagiotides, H., & McPartland, J. (2004). Young children with autism show atypical brain responses to fearful versus neutral facial expressions of emotion. *Developmental Science, 7,* 340–359.

De Bellis, M. D., Casey, B., Dahl, R. E., Birmaher, B., Williamson, D. E., Thomas, K. M., . . . Hall, J. (2000). A pilot study of amygdala volumes in pediatric generalized anxiety disorder. *Biological Psychiatry, 48*(1), 51–57.

de Jong, C. G., Van De Voorde, S., Roeyers, H., Raymaekers, R., Oosterlaan, J., & Sergeant, J. A. (2009). How distinctive are ADHD and RD?: Results of a double dissociation study. *Journal of Abnormal Child Psychology, 37*(7), 1007–1017.

de la Torre-Ubieta, L., Won, H., Stein, J. L., & Geschwind, D. H. (2016). Advancing the understanding of autism disease mechanisms through genetics. *Nature Medicine, 22*(4), 345–361.

De Rubeis, S., & Buxbaum, J. D. (2015). Recent advances in the genetics of autism spectrum disorder. *Current Neurology and Neuroscience Reports, 15*(6), 36.

De Rubeis, S., He, X., Goldberg, A. P., Poultney, C. S., Samocha, K., Cicek, A. E., . . . Walker, S. (2014). Synaptic, transcriptional and chromatin genes disrupted in autism. *Nature, 515*(7526), 209–215.

De Smedt, B., Noël, M. P., Gilmore, C., & Ansari, D. (2013). How do symbolic and non-symbolic numerical magnitude processing skills relate to individual differences in children's mathematical skills?: A review of evidence from brain and behavior. *Trends in Neuroscience and Education, 2*(2), 48–55.

De Smedt, B., Taylor, J., Archibald, L., & Ansari, D. (2010). How is phonological processing related to individual differences in children's arithmetic skills? *Developmental Science, 13*(3), 508–520.

Deary, I. J., Strand, S., Smith, P., & Fernandes, C. (2007). Intelligence and educational achievement. *Intelligence, 35*(1), 13–21.

DeFries, J. C., Corley, R. P., Johnson, R. C., Vandenberg, S. G., & Wilson, J. R. (1982). Sex-by-generation and ethnic group-by-generation interactions in the Hawaii family study of cognition. *Behavior Genetics, 12*(2), 223–230.

DeFries, J. C., Olson, R. K., Pennington, R. F., & Smith, S. D. (1991). Colorado Reading Project: An update. In D. D. Duane & D. B. Gray (Eds.), *The reading brain: The biological basis of dyslexia* (pp. 53–87). Parkton, MD: York Press.

Dehaene, S. (2003). Acalculia and number processing disorders. In T. E. Feinberg & M. J. Farah (Eds.), *Behavioral neurology and neuropsychology* (2nd ed., pp. 207–215). New York: McGraw-Hill.

Delis, D. C., Kaplan, E., & Kramer, J. H. (2001). *Delis–Kaplan Executive Function System*. San Antonio, TX: Psychological Corporation.

Demonet, J. F., Taylor, M. J., & Chaix, Y. (2004). Developmental dyslexia. *Lancet, 363,* 1451–1460.

Demontis, D., Walters, R. K., Martin, J., Mattheisen, M., Als, T. D., Agerbo, E., . . . Neale, B. M. (2017). Discovery of the first genome-wide significant risk loci for ADHD. Retrieved from *www.biorxiv.org/content/early/ 2017/06/03/ 145581.*

Dennis, M. (2010). Margaret Kennard (1899–1975): Not a "principle" of brain plasticity but a founding mother of developmental neuropsychology. *Cortex, 46,* 1043–1059.

Denton, C. A., Cirino, P. T., Barth, A. E., Romain, M., Vaughn, S., Wexler, J., . . . Fletcher, J. M. (2011). An experimental study of scheduling and duration of "Tier 2" first-grade reading intervention. *Journal of Research on Educational Effectiveness, 4*(3), 208–230.

Deutsch, G. K., Dougherty, R. F., Bammer, R., Siok, W. T., Gabrieli, J. D., & Wandell, B. (2005). Children's reading performance is correlated with white matter structure measured by diffusion tensor imaging. *Cortex, 41,* 354–363.

Di Martino, A., Ross, K., Uddin, L. Q., Sklar, A. B., Castellanos, F. X., & Milham, M. P. (2009). Functional brain correlates of social and nonsocial processes in autism spectrum disorders: An activation likelihood estimation meta-analysis. *Biological Psychiatry, 65*(1), 63–74.

Dichter, G. S. (2012). Functional magnetic resonance imaging of autism spectrum disorders. *Dialogues in Clinical Neuroscience, 14*(3), 319–351.

Dickstein, D. P., Pescosolido, M. F., Reidy, B. L., Galvan, T., Kim, K. L., Seymour, K. E., . . . Barrett, R. P. (2013). Developmental meta-analysis of the functional neural correlates of autism spectrum disorders. *Journal of the American Academy of Child and Adolescent Psychiatry, 52*(3), 279–289.

Dierssen, M. (2012). Down syndrome: The brain in trisomic mode. *National Review of Neuroscience, 13*(12), 844–858.

Dingman, H. F., & Tarjan, G. (1960). Mental retardation and the normal distribution curve. *American Journal of Mental Deficiency, 64,* 991–994.

Docherty, S. J., Davis, O. S. P., Kovas, Y., Meaburn, E. L., Dale, P. S., Petrill, S. A., . . . Plomin, R. (2010). A genome-wide association study identifies mulitiple loci associated with mathematics ability and disability. *Genes, Brain and Behavior, 9,* 234–247.

Dodd, B., Holm, A., Hua, Z., & Crosbie, S. (2003). A normative study of British-speaking children. *Clinical Linguistic Phonology, 17*(8), 617–643.

Donlan, C., Cowan, R., Newton, E. J., & Lloyd, D. (2007). The role of language in mathematical development: Evidence from children with specific language impairments. *Cognition, 103*(1), 23–33.

Dosenbach, N. U., Nardos, B., Cohen, A. L., Fair, D. A., Power, J. D., Church, J. A., . . . Schlaggar, B. L. (2010). Prediction of individual brain maturity using fMRI. *Science, 329*(5997), 1358–1361.

Down, J. L. N. (1866). Observations on ethnic classification of idiots. *Mental Science, 13,* 121–128.

Duchaine, B. C. (2000). Developmental prosopagnosia with normal configural processing. *NeuroReport, 11*(1), 79–83.

Duda, T. A., Casey, J. E., & McNevin, N. (2015). Development of graphomotor fluency in adults with ADHD: Evidence of attenuated procedural learning. *Human Movement Science, 44,* 1–10.

Dugdale, R. L. (1877). *The Jukes.* New York: Putnam.

Duncan, L. E., Pollastri, A. R., & Smoller, J. W. (2014). Mind the gap: Why many geneticists and psychological scientists have discrepant views about gene–environment interaction (GxE) research. *American Psychologist, 69*(3), 249–268.

Dunn, L. M., & Dunn, D. M. (2007). *Peabody Picture Vocabulary Test–Fourth Edition (PPVT 4).* Circle Pines, MN: American Guidance Service.

DuPaul, G. J., Gormley, M. J., & Laracy, S. D. (2013). Comorbidity of LD and ADHD: Implications of DSM-5 for assessment and treatment. *Journal of Learning Disabilities, 46*(1), 43–51.

DuPaul, G. J., Power, T. J., Anastopoulos, A. D., & Reid, R. (1998). *ADHD Rating Scale–IV: Checklists, norms, and clinical interpretation.* New York: Guilford Press.

DuPaul, G. J., Power, T. J., Anastopoulos, A. D., & Reid, R. (2016). *ADHD Rating Scale–5 for Children and Adolescents: Checklists, norms, and clinical interpretation.* New York: Guilford Press.

Dupont, A., Vaeth, M., & Videbech, P. (1986). Mortality and life expectancy of Down's syndrome in Denmark. *Journal of Mental Deficiency Research, 30*(2), 111–120.

Durston, S., & Konrad, K. (2007). Integrating genetic, psychopharmacological and neuroimaging studies: A converging methods approach to understanding the neurobiology of ADHD. *Developmental Review, 27*(3), 374–395.

Eadie, P., Morgan, A., Ukoumunne, O. C., Ttofari Eecen, K., Wake, M., & Reilly, S. (2015). Speech sound disorder at 4 years: Prevalence, comorbidities, and predictors in a community cohort of children. *Developmental Medicine and Child Neurology, 57*(6), 578–584.

Eaves, L. C., & Ho, H. H. (2008). Young adult outcome of autism spectrum disorders. *Journal of Autism and Developmental Disorders, 38*(4), 739–747.

Ebejer, J. L., Coventry, W. L., Byrne, B., Willcutt, E. G., Olson, R. K., Corley, R., & Samuelsson, S. (2010). Genetic and environmental influences on inattention, hyperactivity–impulsivity, and reading: Kindergarten to grade 2. *Scientific Studies of Reading, 14*(4), 293–316.

Ecker, C. (2017). The neuroanatomy of autism spectrum disorder: An overview of structural neuroimaging findings and their translatability to the clinical setting. *Autism, 21*(1), 18–28.

Ecker, C., & Murphy, D. (2014). Neuroimaging in autism—from basic science to translational research. *Nature Reviews Neurology, 10*, 82–91.

Edelman, G. M. (1987). *Neural Darwinism*. New York: Basic Books.

Edgin, J. O., Pennington, B. F., & Mervis, C. B. (2010). Neuropsychological components of intellectual disability: The contributions of immediate, working, and associative memory. *Journal of Intellectual Disability Research, 54*(5), 406–417.

Ehri, L. C. (2015). How children learn to read words. In A. Pollatsek & R. Treiman (Eds.), *The Oxford handbook of reading* (pp. 293–310). New York: Oxford University Press.

Eicher, J. D., Powers, N. R., Miller, L. L., Akshoomoff, N., Amaral, D. G., Bloss, C. S., . . . Casey, B. (2013). Genome-wide association study of shared components of reading disability and language impairment. *Genes, Brain and Behavior, 12*(8), 792–801.

Elder, T. E. (2011). The importance of relative standards in ADHD diagnoses: Evidence based on exact birth dates. *Journal of Health Economics, 29*, 641–656.

Eley, T. C., Bishop, D. V., Dale, P. S., Oliver, B., Petrill, S. A., Price, T. S., . . . Plomin, R. (1999). Genetic and environmental origins of verbal and performance components of cognitive delay in 2-year-olds. *Developmental Psychology, 35*(4), 1122–1131.

Elliott, C. (2007). *Differential Ability Scales* (2nd ed.). San Antonio, TX: Harcourt Assessment.

Elman, J. L., Bates, E. A., Johnson, M. H., Karmiloff-Smith, A., Parisi, D., & Plunkett, K. (1996). *Rethinking innateness: Connectionist perspectives on development*. Cambridge, MA: MIT Press.

Elsabbagh, M., & Johnson, M. H. (2016). Autism and the social brain: The first-year puzzle. *Biological Psychiatry, 80*, 94–99.

Emmert, T. N. (2015). *Examining the effects of mathematics journals on elementary students' mathematics anxiety levels*. Doctoral dissertation, Ohio University, Athens, OH.

Enard, W. (2011). FOXP2 and the role of cortico-basal ganglia circuits in speech and language evolution. *Current Opinion in Neurobiology, 21*, 415–424.

Eppig, C., Fincher, C. L., & Thornhill, R. (2010). Parasite prevalence and the worldwide distribution of cognitive ability. *Proceedings of the Royal Society B: Biological Sciences, 277*(1701), 3801–3808.

Eppig, C., Fincher, C. L., & Thornhill, R. (2011). Parasite prevalence and the distribution of intelligence among the states of the USA. *Intelligence, 39*, 155–160.

Erickson, C. A., Davenport, M. H., Schaefer, T. L., Wink, L. K., Pedapati, E. V., Sweeney, J. A., . . . Hagerman, R. J. (2017). Fragile X targeted pharmacotherapy: Lessons learned and future directions. *Journal of Neurodevelopmental Disorders, 9*(1), 7.

Erskine, H. E., Ferrari, A. J., Nelson, P., Polanczyk, G. V., Flaxman, A. D., Vos, T., . . . Scott, J. G. (2013). Epidemiological modelling of attention-deficit/hyperactivity disorder and conduct disorder for the Global Burden of Disease Study 2010. *Journal of Child Psychology and Psychiatry, 54*(12), 1263–1274.

Evans, T. M., Kochalka, J., Ngoon, T. J., Wu, S. S., Qin, S., Battista, C., & Menon, V. (2015). Brain structural integrity and intrinsic functional connectivity forecast 6 year longitudinal growth in children's numerical abilities. *Journal of Neuroscience, 35*(33), 11743–11750.

Facoetti, A., Corradi, N., Ruffino, M., Gori, S., & Zorzi, M. (2010). Visual spatial attention and speech segmentation are both impaired in preschoolers at familial risk for developmental dyslexia. *Dyslexia, 16*, 226–239.

Fan, C. C., Brown, T. T., Bartsch, H., Kuperman, J. M., Hagler, D. J., Schork, A., . . . Dale, A. (2016). Williams syndrome-specific neuroarchitectural profile and its associations with cognitive features. Retrieved from *www.biorxiv.org/content/early/2016/06/26/060764*. [Epub ahead of print]

Farah, M. J. (2003). Computational modeling in behavioral neurology and neuropsychology. In T. E. Feinberg & J. J. Farah (Eds.), *Behavioral neurology and neuropsychology* (pp. 135–143). New York: McGraw-Hill.

Faraone, S., & Biederman, J. (2016). Can attention-deficit/hyperactivity disorder onset occur in adulthood? *Journal of American Medical Association, 73*(7), 655–656.

Faraone, S., Biederman, J., Chen, W. J., Kricher, B., Moore, C., Sprich, S., & Tsuang, M. T. (1992). Segregation analysis of attention deficit hyperactivity disorder: Evidence for single major gene transmission. *Psychiatric Genetics, 2*, 257–275.

Faraone, S., Biederman, J., Keenan, K., & Tsuang, M. T. (1991). A family-genetic study of girls with DSM-III attention deficit disorder. *American Journal of Psychiatry, 148*(1), 112–117.

Faraone, S., Spencer, T., Aleardi, M., Pagano, C., & Biederman, J. (2004). Meta-analysis of the efficacy of methylphenidate for treating adult attention-deficit/hyperactivity disorder. *Journal of Clinical Psychopharmacology, 24*(1), 24–29.

Farkas, G., & Beron, K. (2004). The detailed age trajectory of oral vocabulary knowledge: Differences by class and race. *Social Science Research, 33*(3), 464–497.

Feigenson, L., Dehaene, S., & Spelke, E. (2004). Core systems of number. *Trends in Cognitive Sciences, 8*(7), 307–314.

Fein, D., Barton, M., Eigsti, I. M., Kelley, E., Naigles, L., Schultz, R. T., . . . Rosenthal, M. (2013). Optimal outcome in individuals with a history of autism. *Journal of Child Psychology and Psychiatry, 54*(2), 195–205.

Fernald, A., Marchman, V. A., & Weisleder, A. (2013). SES differences in language processing skill and vocabulary are evident at 18 months. *Developmental Science, 16*(2), 234–248.

Fernald, A., & Weisleder, A. (2015). Twenty years after "Meaningful Differences," it's time to reframe the "deficit" debate about the importance of children's early language experience. *Human Development, 58*(1), 1–4.

Fernandez, F., & Edgin, J. O. (2016). Pharmacotherapy in Down's syndrome: Which way forward? *Lancet Neurology, 15*(8), 776–777.

Fernandez, F., & Garner, C. C. (2007). Over-inhibition: A model for developmental intellectual disability. *Trends in Neurosciences, 30*(10), 497–503.

Fey, M. E., Yoder, P. J., Warren, S. F., & Bredin-Oja, S. L. (2013). Is more better?: Milieu communication teaching in toddlers with intellectual disabilities. *Journal of Speech, Language, and Hearing Research, 56*(2), 679–693.

Fias, W., Menon, V., & Szucs, D. (2013). Multiple components of developmental dyscalculia. *Trends in Neuroscience and Education, 2*(2), 43–47.

Fidler, D. J. (2005). The emerging Down syndrome behavioral phenotype in early childhood: Implications for practice. *Infants and Young Children, 18*(2), 86–103.

Field, L. L., Shumansky, K., Ryan, J., Truong, D., Swiergala, E., & Kaplan, B. J. (2013). Dense-map genome scan for dyslexia supports loci at 4q13, 16p12, 17q22; suggests novel locus at 7q36. *Genes, Brain and Behavior, 12*(1), 56–69.

Filipek, P. A., Semrud-Clikeman, M., Steingard, R. J., Renshaw, P. F., Kennedy, D. N., & Biederman, J. (1997). Volumetric MRI analysis comparing subjects having attention-deficit hyperactivity disorder with normal controls. *Neurology, 48*(3), 589–601.

Filley, C. M., Heaton, R. K., & Rosenberg, N. L. (1990). White matter dementia in chronic toluene abuse. *Neurology, 40*(1), 532–540.

Fisher, S. E., & DeFries, J. C. (2002). Developmental dyslexia: Genetic dissection of a complex cognitive trait. *Nature Reviews Neuroscience, 3*, 767–780.

Fisher, S. E., Vargha-Khadem, F., Watkins, K. E., Monaco, A. P., & Pembrey, M. E. (1998). Localization of a gene implicated in a severe speech and language disorder. *Nature Genetics, 18*, 168–170.

Fletcher, J. M., Stuebing, K. K., Barth, A. E., Denton, C. A., Cirino, P. T., Francis, D. J., & Vaughn, S. (2011). Cognitive correlates of inadequate response to reading intervention. *School Psychology Review, 40*(1), 3–22.

Fodor, J. A. (1983). *The modularity of mind.* Cambridge, MA: MIT Press.

Folstein, S., & Rutter, M. (1977). Genetic influences and infantile autism. *Nature, 265*(5596), 726–728.

Fombonne, E. (2001). Is there an epidemic of autism? *Pediatrics, 107,* 411–412.

Foti, F., De Crescenzo, F., Vivanti, G., Menghini, D., & Vicari, S. (2015). Implicit learning in individuals with autism spectrum disorders: A meta-analysis. *Psychological Medicine, 45*(5), 897–910.

Fox, J. W., Lamperti, E. D., Eksioglu, Y. Z., Hong, S. E., Feng, Y., Graham, D. A., . . . Walsh, C. A. (1998). Mutations in filamin 1 prevent migration of cerebral cortical neurons in human periventricular heterotopia. *Neuron, 21*(6), 1315–1325.

Franceschini, S., Gori, S., Ruffino, M., Pedroll, K., & Facoetti, A. (2012). A causal link between spatial attention and reading acquisition. *Current Biology, 22*(9), 814–819.

Francis, D. J., Shaywitz, S. E., Stuebing, K. K., Shaywitz, B. A., & Fletcher, J. M. (1996). Developmental lag versus deficit models of reading disability: A longitudinal, individual growth curves analysis. *Journal of Educational Psychology, 88*(1), 3–17.

Frank, M. J., Seeberger, L. C., & O'Reilly R, C. (2004). By carrot or by stick: Cognitive reinforcement learning in parkinsonism. *Science, 306*(5703), 1940–1943.

Frazier, T. W., Georgiades, S., Bishop, S. L., & Hardan, A. Y. (2014). Behavioral and cognitive characteristics of females and males with autism in the Simons Simplex Collection. *Journal of the American Academy of Child and Adolescent Psychiatry, 53*(3), 329–340.

Frazier, T. W., Ratliff, K. R., Gruber, C., Zhang, Y., Law, P. a., & Constantino, J. N. (2014). Confirmatory factor analytic structure and measurement invariance of quantitative autistic traits measured by the Social Responsiveness Scale-2. *Autism, 18,* 31–44.

Frazier, T. W., Thompson, L., Youngstrom, E. A., Law, P., Hardan, A. Y., Eng, C., & Morris, N. (2014). A twin study of heritable and shared environmental contributions to autism. *Journal of Autism and Developmental Disorders, 44*(8), 2013–2025.

Frazier, T. W., Youngstrom, E. A., Kubu, C. S., Sinclair, L., & Rezai, A. (2008). Exploratory and confirmatory factor analysis of the autism diagnostic interview-revised. *Journal of Autism and Developmental Disorders, 38*(3), 474–480.

Frazier, T. W., Youngstrom, E. A., Speer, L., Embacher, R., Law, P., Constantino, J. N., . . . Eng, C. (2012). Validation of proposed DSM-5 criteria for autism spectrum disorder. *Journal of the American Academy of Child and Adolescent Psychiatry, 51*(1), 28–40.

Freed, G. L., Clark, S. J., Butchart, A. T., Singer, D. C., & Davis, M. M. (2010). Parental vaccine safety concerns in 2009. *Pediatrics, 125*(4), 654–659.

Friedman, A. H., Watamura, S. E., & Robertson, S. S. (2005). Movement–attention coupling in infancy and attention problems in childhood. *Developmental Medicine and Child Neurology, 47*(10), 660–665.

Friend, A., DeFries, J. C., Olson, R. K., Pennington, B. F., Harlaar, N., Byrne, B., . . . Keenan, J. M. (2009). Heritability of high reading ability and its interaction with parental education. *Behavioral Genetics, 39,* 427–436.

Fry, A. F., & Hale, S. (1996). Processing speed, working memory, and fluid intelligence. *Psychological Science, 7*(4), 237–241.

Fryer, R. G., & Levitt, S. D. (2013). Testing for racial differences in the mental ability of young children. *American Economic Review, 103*(2), 981–1005.

Fuchs, L. S., Geary, D. C., Compton, D. L., Fuchs, D., Hamlett, C. L., Seethaler, P. M., . . . Schatschneider, C. (2010). Do different types of school mathematics development depend on different constellations of numerical versus general cognitive abilities? *Developmental Psychology, 46*(6), 1731–1746.

Fuchs, L. S., Powell, S. R., Cirino, P. T., Schumacher, R. F., Marrin, S., Hamlett, C. L., . . . Changas, P. C. (2014). Does calculation or word-problem instruction provide a stronger route to prealgebraic knowledge? *Journal of Educational Psychology, 106*(4), 990–1006.

Fuchs, L. S., Powell, S. R., Hamlett, C. L., Fuchs, D., Cirino, P. T., & Fletcher, J. M. (2008). Remediating computational deficits at third grade: A randomized field trial. *Journal of Research on Educational Effectiveness, 1*(1), 2–32.

Fulton, H., Scheffler, R., Hinshaw, S., Levine, P., Stone, S., Brown, T., & Modrek, S. (2009). National variation of ADHD diagnostic prevalence and medication use: Health care providers and education policies. *Psychiatric Services, 60*(8), 1075–1083.

Furlong, M., McLoughlin, F., McGilloway, S., & Geary, D. (2016). Interventions to improve mathematical performance for children with mathematical learning difficulties (MLD). *Cochrane Database of Systematic Reviews, 4*, CD012130.

Fuster, J. M. (1989). *The prefrontal cortex: Anatomy, physiology and neuropsycholgy of the frontal lobe* (2nd ed.). New York: Raven.

Gabay, Y., Thiessen, E. D., & Holt, L. L. (2015). Impaired statistical learning in developmental dyslexia. *Journal of Speech, Language, and Hearing Research, 58*(3), 934–945.

Gabrieli, J. D. (2009). Dyslexia: A new synergy between education and cognitive neuroscience. *Science, 325*(5938), 280–283.

Galaburda, A., & Pascual-Leone, A. (2003). Mechanisms of plasticity and behavior. In T. E. Feinberg & M. J. Farah (Eds.), *Behavioral neurology and neuropsychology* (pp. 57–70). New York: McGraw-Hill.

Galaburda, A. M., Sherman, G. F., Rosen, G. D., Aboitiz, F., & Geschwind, N. (1985). Developmental dyslexia: Four consecutive patients with cortical anomalies. *Annals of Neurology, 18*(2), 222–233.

Gall, F. J. (1835). *On the origin of the moral qualities and intellectual faculties of man, and the conditions of their manifestation*. Boston: Marsh, Capen, and Lyon.

Garber, K. B., Visootsak, J., & Warren, S. T. (2008). Fragile X syndrome. *European Journal of Human Genetics, 16*(6), 666–672.

García, J. R., & Cain, K. (2014). Decoding and reading comprehension. *Review of Educational Research, 84*(1), 74–111.

Gardener, H., Spiegelman, D., & Buka, S. L. (2011). Perinatal and neonatal risk factors for autism: A comprehensive meta-analysis. *Pediatrics, 128*(2), 344–355.

Gargaro, B. A., Rinehart, N. J., Bradshaw, J. L., Tonge, B. J., & Sheppard, D. M. (2011). Autism and ADHD: How far have we come in the comorbidity debate? *Neuroscience and Biobehavioral Reviews, 35*(5), 1081–1088.

Gathercole, S. E., & Baddeley, A. D. (1990). Phonological memory deficits in language disordered children: Is there a causal connection? *Journal of Memory and Language, 29*(3), 336–360.

Gauthier, I., Tarr, M. J., Anderson, A. W., Skudlarski, P., & Gore, J. C. (1999). Activation of the middle fusiform "face area" increases with expertise in recognizing novel objects. *Nature Neuroscience, 2*(6), 568–573.

Geary, D. C. (1994). *Children's mathematical development: Research and practical applications*. Washington, DC: American Psychological Association.

Geary, D. C., Bailey, D. H., & Hoard, M. K. (2009). Predicting mathematical achievement and mathematical learning disability with a simple screening tool: The Number Sets Test. *Journal of Psychoeducational Assessment, 27*(3), 265–279.

Geary, D. C., Hamson, C. O., & Hoard, M. K. (2000). Numerical and arithmetical cognition: A longitudinal study of process and concept deficits in children with learning disability. *Journal of Experimental Child Psychology, 77*, 236–263.

Geary, D. C., Hoard, M. K., Byrd-Craven, J., & DeSoto, M. C. (2004). Strategy choices in simple and complex addition: Contributions of working memory and counting knowledge for children with mathematical disability. *Journal of Experimental Child Psychology, 88*(2), 121–151.

Gelman, R., & Gallistel, C. R. (1986). *The child's understanding of number*. Cambridge, MA: Harvard University Press. (Original work published 1978)

Gepner, B., & Féron, F. (2009). Autism: A world changing too fast for a mis-wired brain? *Neuroscience and Biobehavioral Reviews, 33*(8), 1227–1242.

Gerber, S., Brice, A., Capone, N., Fujiki, M., & Timler, G. (2012). Language use in social interactions of school-age children with language impairments: An evidence-based systematic review of treatment. *Language, Speech, and Hearing Services in Schools, 43*(2), 235–249.

Germano, E., Gagliano, A., & Curatolo, P. (2010). Comorbidity of ADHD and dyslexia. *Developmental Neuropsychology, 35*(5), 475–493.

Geschwind, D. H., & State, M. W. (2015). Gene hunting in autism spectrum disorder: On the path to precision medicine. *Lancet Neurology, 14*(11), 1109–1120.

Gialluisi, A., Newbury, D. F., Wilcutt, E. G., Olson, R. K., DeFries, J. C., Brandler, W. M., . . . Simpson, N. H. (2014). Genome-wide screening for DNA variants associated with reading and language traits. *Genes, Brain and Behavior, 13*(7), 686–701.

Gialluisi, A., Visconti, A., Willcutt, E. G., Smith, S. D., Pennington, B. F., Falchi, M., . . . Fisher, S. E. (2016). Investigating the effects of copy number variants on reading and language performance. *Journal of Neurodevelopmental Disorders, 8*, 17.

Giarelli, E., Wiggins, L. D., Rice, C. E., Levy, S. E., Kirby, R. S., Pinto-Martin, J., & Mandell, D. (2010). Sex differences in the evaluation and diagnosis of autism spectrum disorders among children. *Disability and Health Journal, 3*(2), 107–116.

Gibson, J., Adams, C., Lockton, E., & Green, J. (2013). Social communication disorder outside autism?: A diagnostic classification approach to delineating pragmatic language impairment, high functioning autism and specific language impairment. *Journal of Child Psychology and Psychiatry, 54*(11), 1186–1197.

Giedd, J. N., Castellanos, F. X., Casey, B. J., Kozuch, P., King, A. C., Hamburger, S. D., & Rapoport, J. L. (1994). Quantitative morphology of the corpus callosum in attention deficit hyperactivity disorder. *American Journal of Psychiatry, 151*(5), 665–669.

Giedd, J. N., Shaw, P., Wallace, G. L., Gogtay, N., & Lenroot, K. K. (2006). Anatomic brain imaging studies of normal and abnormal brain development in children and adolescents. In D. Cicchetti & D. J. Cohen (Eds.), *Developmental psychopathology* (Vol. 2, pp. 127–196). Hoboken, NJ: Wiley.

Gillberg, C. (2010). The ESSENCE in child psychiatry: Early symptomatic syndromes eliciting neurodevelopmental clinical examinations. *Research in Developmental Disabilities, 31*(6), 1543–1551.

Gilmore, C., Attridge, N., & Inglis, M. (2011). Measuring the approximate number system. *Quarterly Journal of Experimental Psychology, 64*(11), 2099–2109.

Gioia, G., Isquith, P., Guy, S., & Kenworthy, L. (2015). *Behavior Rating Inventory of Executive Function, Second Edition (BRIEF-2).* Lutz, FL: Professional Assessment Resources.

Gittleman, R., Mannuzza, S., Shenker, R., & Gonagura, N. (1985). Hyperactive boys almost grown up. *Archives of General Psychiatry, 42,* 937–947.

Göbel, S. M., Watson, S. E., Lervåg, A., & Hulme, C. (2014). Children's arithmetic development: It is number knowledge, not the approximate number sense, that counts. *Psychological Science, 25*(3), 789–798.

Goddard, H. H. (1912). *The Kallikak family: A study in the heredity of feeble-mindedness.* New York: Macmillan.

Golding, J., Pembrey, M., & Jones, R. (2001). ALSPAC—the Avon Longitudinal Study of Parents and Children: I. Study methodology. *Paediatric and Perinatal Epidemiology, 15*(1), 74–87.

Goldinger, S. D., & Azuma, T. (2003). Puzzle-solving science: The quixotic quest for units in speech perception. *Journal of Phonetics, 31*(3), 305–320.

González, G. F., Zaric, G., Tijms, J., Bonte, M., Blomert, L., & van der Molen, M. W. (2015). A randomized controlled trial on the beneficial effects of training letter–speech sound integration on reading fluency in children with dyslexia. *PLOS ONE, 10*(12), e0143914.

Goodkind, M., Eickhoff, S. B., Oathes, D. J., Jiang, Y., Chang, A., Jones-Hagata, L. B., . . . Korgaonkar, M. S. (2015). Identification of a common neurobiological substrate for mental illness. *JAMA Psychiatry, 72*(4), 305–315.

Gordon, M., McClure, F., & Aylward, G. (1996). *The Gordon Diagnostic System: Instruction manual and interpretive guide.* DeWitt, NY: Gordon Systems.

Gotham, K., Pickles, A., & Lord, C. (2009). Standardizing ADOS scores for a measure of severity in autism spectrum disorders. *Journal of Autism and Developmental Disorders, 39,* 693–705.

Gotham, K., Risi, S., Pickles, A., & Lord, C. (2007). The autism diagnostic observation schedule: Revised algorithms for improved diagnostic validity. *Journal of Autism and Developmental Disorders, 37*(4), 613–627.

Gottlieb, G. (1991). Experimental canalization of behavioral development: Theory. *Developmental Psychology, 27*(1), 4–13.

Gough, P. B., & Tunmer, W. E. (1986). Decoding, reading, and reading disability. *RASE: Remedial and Special Education, 7*(1), 6–10.

Grant, D. A., & Berg, E. (1948). A behavioral analysis of degree of reinforcement and ease of shifting to new responses in a Weigl-type card-sorting problem. *Journal of Experimental Psychology, 38*(4), 404–411.

Grasby, K. L., Coventry, W. L., Byrne, B., & Olson, R. K. (2017). Little evidence that socioeconomic status modifies heritability of literacy and numeracy in Australia. *Child Development.* [Epub ahead of print]

Grattan, L. M., & Eslinger, P. J. (1991). Frontal lobe damage in children and adults: A comparative review. *Developmental Neuropsychology, 7,* 283–326.

Green, P. (2003). *Manual for the Word Memory Test for Windows.* Edmonton, AB, Canada: Green's.

Green, P. (2004). *Medical Symptom Validity Test (MSVT) for Microsoft Windows: User's manual.* Edmonton, AB, Canada: Green's.

Green, T., Bade Shrestha, S., Chromik, L. C., Rutledge, K., Pennington, B. F., Hong, D. S., & Reiss, A. L. (2015). Elucidating X chromosome influences on attention deficit hyperactivity disorder and executive function. *Journal of Psychiatric Research, 68,* 217–225.

Greenberg, S. (2004). *A multi-tier framework for understanding spoken language.* Mahwah, NJ: Erlbaum.

Greenhill, L. L., Muniz, R., Ball, R. R., Levine, A., Pestreich, L., & Jiang, H. (2006). Efficacy and safety of dexmethylphenidate extended-release capsules in children with attention-deficit/hyperactivity disorder. *Journal of the American Academy of Child and Adolescent Psychiatry, 45,* 817–823.

Greenough, W. T., Black, J. E., & Wallace, C. S. (1987). Experience and brain development. *Child Development, 58*(3), 539–559.

Greven, C. U., Rijsdijk, F. V., Asherson, P., & Plomin, R. (2012). A longitudinal twin study on the association between ADHD symptoms and reading. *Journal of Child Psychology and Psychiatry, 53*(3), 234–242.

Gross-Tsur, V., Manor, O., & Shalev, R. S. (1996). Developmental dyscalculia: Prevalence and demographic features. *Devvelopmental Medicine and Child Neurology, 38*(1), 25–33.

Grove, J., Ripke, S., Als, T. D., Mattheisen, M., Walters, R., Won, H., . . . Anney, R. (2017). Common risk variants identified in autism spectrum disorder. Retrieved from www.biorxiv.org/content/early/2017/11/27/224774.

Gualtieri, C. T., & Hicks, R. E. (1985). Neuropharmacology of methylphenidate and a neural substrate for childhood hyperactivity. *Psychiatric Clinics of North America, 8*(4), 875–892.

Gualtieri, C. T., Koriath, U., Van Bourgondien, M., & Saleeby, N. (1983). Language disorders in children referred for psychiatric services. *Journal of the American Academy of Child and Adolescent Psychiatry, 22*(2), 165–171.

Guenther, F. H. (1995). Speech sound acquisition, coarticulation, and rate effects in a neural network model of speech production. *Psychology Review, 102*(3), 594–621.

Hadjikhani, N., Joseph, R. M., Snyder, J., Chabris,

C. F., Clark, J., Steele, S., . . . Tager-Flusberg, H. (2004). Activation of the fusiform gyrus when individuals with autism spectrum disorder view faces. *NeuroImage, 22*(3), 1141–1150.

Hagerman, R. J., Berry-Kravis, E., Kaufmann, W. E., Ono, M. Y., Tartaglia, N., Lachiewicz, A., . . . Visootsak, J. (2009). Advances in the treatment of fragile X syndrome. *Pediatrics, 123*(1), 378–390.

Hagerman, R. J., & Hagerman, P. (2013). Advances in clinical and molecular understanding of the FMR1 premutation and fragile X-associated tremor/ataxia syndrome. *Lancet Neurology, 12*(8), 786–798.

Halberda, J., & Feigenson, L. (2008). Developmental change in the acuity of the "Number Sense": The Approximate Number System in 3-, 4-, 5-, and 6-year-olds and adults. *Developmental Psychology, 44*(5), 1457–1465.

Hallett, V., Ronald, A., Rijsdijk, F., & Happé, F. (2010). Association of autistic-like and internalizing traits during childhood: A longitudinal twin study. *American Journal of Psychiatry, 167*, 809–817.

Hallgren, B. (1950). Specific dyslexia: A clinical and genetic study. *Acta Psychiatrica et Neurologica Scandinavica, 65*(Suppl.), 1–287.

Hallmayer, J., Cleveland, S., Torres, a., Phillips, J., Cohen, B., Torigoe, T., . . . Risch, N. (2011). Genetic heritability and shared environmental factors among twin pairs with autism. *Archives of General Psychiatry, 68*, 1095–1102.

Halpern, D. F. (2012). *Sex differences in cognitive abilities* (4th ed.). New York: Psychology Press.

Hampshire, A., Highfield, R. R., Parkin, B. L., & Owen, A. M. (2012). Fractionating human intelligence. *Neuron, 76*(6), 1225–1237.

Hannestad, J., Gallezot, J. D., Planeta-Wilson, B., Lin, S. F., Williams, W. A., van Dyck, C. H., . . . Ding, Y. S. (2010). Clinically relevant doses of methylphenidate significantly occupy norepinephrine transporters in humans in vivo. *Biological Psychiatry, 68*(9), 854–860.

Hanscombe, K. B., Trzaskowski, M., Haworth, C. M., Davis, O. S., Dale, P. S., & Plomin, R. (2012). Socioeconomic status (SES) and children's intelligence (IQ): In a UK-representative sample SES moderates the environmental, not genetic, effect on IQ. *PLOS ONE, 7*(2), e30320.

Hansen, R. L., Ozonoff, S., Krakowiak, P., Angkustsiri, K., Jones, C., Deprey, L. J., . . . Hertz-Picciotto, I. (2008). Regression in autism: Prevalence and associated factors in the CHARGE Study. *Ambulatory Pediatrics, 8*(1), 25–31.

Happé, F., & Ronald, A. (2008). The "fractionable autism triad": A review of evidence from behavioural, genetic, cognitive and neural research. *Neuropsychology Review, 18*(4), 287–304.

Happé, F., Ronald, A., & Plomin, R. (2006). Time to give up on a single explanation for autism. *Nature Neuroscience, 9*, 1218–1220.

Hariri, M., & Azadbakht, L. (2015). Magnesium, iron, and zinc supplementation for the treatment of attention deficit hyperactivity disorder: A systematic review on the recent literature. *International Journal of Preventive Medicine, 6*, 83.

Harlaar, N., Butcher, L. M., Meaburn, E., Sham, P., Craig, I. W., & Plomin, R. (2005). A behavioural genomic analysis of DNA markers associated with general cognitive ability in 7-year-olds. *Journal of Child Psychology and Psychiatry, 46*, 1097–1107.

Harlaar, N., Kovas, Y., Dale, P. S., Petrill, S. A., & Plomin, R. (2012). Mathematics is differentially related to reading comprehension and word decoding: Evidence from a genetically sensitive design. *Journal of Educational Psychology, 104*(3), 622–635.

Harrison, A. G., Flaro, L., & Armstrong, I. (2015). Rates of effort test failure in children with ADHD: An exploratory study. *Applied Neuropsychology: Child, 4*(3), 197–210.

Harrison, P., & Oakland, T. (2015). *Adaptive Behavior Assessment System, Third Edition (ABAS-3)*. Torrance, CA: Western Psychological Services.

Hart, B., & Risley, T. R. (1995). *Meaningful differences in the everyday experience of young American children*. Baltimore: Brookes.

Hart, S. A., Petrill, S. A., Thompson, L. A., & Plomin, R. (2009). The ABC's of math: A genetic analysis of mathematics and its links with reading ability and general cognitive ability. *Journal of Educational Psychology, 101*(2), 388–402.

Hart, S. A., Petrill, S. A., Willcutt, E., Thompson, L. A., Schatschneider, C., Deater-Deckard, K., & Cutting, L. E. (2010). Exploring how symptoms of attention-deficit/hyperactivity disorder are related to reading and mathematics performance: General genes, general environments. *Psychological Science, 21*(11), 1708–1715.

Hartley, S. L., Horrell, S. V., & Maclean, W. E. (2007). Science to practice in intellectual disability: The role of empirically supported treatments. In J. W. Jacobson, J. A. Mulick, & J. Rojahn (Eds.), *Handbook of intellectual and developmental disabilities* (pp. 425–443). New York: Springer.

Hassiotis, A., Robotham, D., Canagasabey, A., Romeo, R., Langridge, D., Blizard, R., . . . King, M. (2009). Randomized, single-blind, controlled trial of a specialist behavior therapy team for challenging behavior in adults with intellectual disabilities. *American Journal of Psychiatry, 166*(11), 1278–1285.

Hassiotis, A., Serfaty, M., Azam, K., Strydom, A., Blizard, R., Romeo, R., . . . King, M. (2013). Manualised individual cognitive behavioural therapy for mood disorders in people with mild to moderate intellectual disability: A feasibility randomised controlled trial. *Journal of Affective Disorders, 151*(1), 186–195.

Hassiotis, A., Serfaty, M., Azam, K., Strydom, A., Martin, S., Parkes, C., . . . King, M. (2011). Cognitive behaviour therapy (CBT) for anxiety and depression in adults with mild intellectual disabilities (ID): A pilot randomised controlled trial. *Trials, 12*(1), 95.

Hatcher, J., Snowling, M. J., & Griffiths, Y. M. (2002). Cognitive assessment of dyslexic students in higher education. *British Journal of Educational Psychology, 72*(Pt. 1), 119–133.

Hatcher, P. J., Hulme, C., & Snowling, M. J. (2004). Explicit phoneme training combined with phonic reading instruction helps young children at risk of reading failure. *Journal of Child Psychology and Psychiatry, 45*(2), 338–358.

Hawkey, E., & Nigg, J. T. (2014). Omega-3 fatty acid and ADHD: Blood level analysis and meta-analytic extension of supplementation trials. *Clinical Psychology Review, 34,* 496–505.

Haworth, C. M., Kovas, Y., Harlaar, N., Hayiou-Thomas, M. E., Petrill, S. A., Dale, P. S., & Plomin, R. (2009). Generalist genes and learning disabilities: A multivariate genetic analysis of low performance in reading, mathematics, language and general cognitive ability in a sample of 8000 12-year-old twins. *Journal of Child Psychology and Psychiatry, 50*(10), 1318–1325.

Haworth, C. M., Kovas, Y., Petrill, S. A., & Plomin, R. (2007). Developmental origins of low mathematics performance and normal variation in twins from 7 to 9 years. *Twin Research and Human Genetics, 10*(1), 106–117.

Hayiou-Thomas, M. E., Dale, P. S., & Plomin, R. (2012). The etiology of variation in language skills changes with development: A longitudinal twin study of language from 2 to 12 years. *Developmental Science, 15,* 233–249.

Hazlett, H. C., Gu, H., Munsell, B. C., Kim, S. H., Styner, M., Wolff, J. J., . . . Botteron, K. N. (2017). Early brain development in infants at high risk for autism spectrum disorder. *Nature, 542*(7641), 348–351.

Hazlett, H. C., Poe, M., Gerig, G., Smith, R. G., Provenzale, J., Ross, A., . . . Piven, J. (2005). Magnetic resonance imaging and head circumference study of brain size in autism: Birth through age 2 years. *Archives of General Psychiatry, 62*(12), 1366–1376.

Heath, S. B. (1982). What no bedtime story means: Narrative skills at home and school. *Language in Society, 11*(1), 49–76.

Heaton, R. K., Chelune, G. J., Talley, J. L., Kay, G. G., & Curtiss, G. (1981). *Wisconsin Card Sorting Test manual.* Odessa, FL: Psychological Assessment Resources.

Hebb, D. O. (1949). *The organization of behavior.* New York: Wiley.

Hecaen, H., Angelergues, R., & Houillier, S. (1961). Les varietes cliniques des acalculies au cours des lesions retro-rolandiques: Approache statistique du probleme [The clinical varieties of acalculia with retroplandic lesions: A statistical approach to the problem]. *Revue Neurologique, 105,* 85–103.

Hecht, S. A., Burgess, S. R., Torgesen, J. K., Wagner, R. K., & Rashotte, C. A. (2000). Explaining social class differences in growth of reading skills from beginning kindergarten through fourth-grade: The role of phonological awareness, rate of access, and print knowledge. *Reading and Writing, 12*(1), 99–128.

Helt, M., Kelley, E., Kinsbourne, M., Pandey, J., Boorstein, H., Herbert, M., & Fein, D. (2008). Can children with autism recover?: If so, how? *Neuropsychology Review, 18,* 339–366.

Henschen, S. E. (1925). Clinical and anatomical contributions on brain pathology. *Archives of Neurology and Psychiatry, 13,* 226–249. (Original work published 1919)

Hensler, B. S., Schatschneider, C., Taylor, J., & Wagner, R. K. (2010). Behavioral genetic approach to the study of dyslexia. *Journal of Developmental and Behavioral Pediatrics, 31,* 525–532.

Herbert, M. R. (2005). Large brains in autism: The challenge of pervasive abnormality. *The Neuroscientist, 11*(5), 417–440.

Hickok, G., & Poeppel, D. (2007). The cortical organization of speech processing. *Nature Reviews Neuroscience, 8*(5), 393–402.

Hines, S., & Bennett, F. (1996). Effectiveness of early intervention for children with Down syndrome. *Mental Retardation and Developmental Disabilities Research Reviews, 2*(2), 96–101.

Hiniker, A., Rosenberg-Lee, M., & Menon, V. (2016). Distinctive role of symbolic number sense in mediating the mathematical abilities of children with autism. *Journal of Autism and Developmental Disorders, 46*(4), 1268–1281.

Hinshaw, S. P. (2007). Moderators and mediators of treatment outcome for youth with ADHD: Understanding for whom and how interventions work. *Ambulatory Pediatrics, 7*(1), 91–100.

Hodapp, R. M., & Dykens, E. M. (1996). Mental retardation. In R. J. Mash & R. A. Barkley (Eds.), *Child psychopathology* (pp. 362–389). New York: Guilford Press.

Hoeft, F., Carter, J. C., Lightbody, A. A., Cody Hazlett, H., Piven, J., & Reiss, A. L. (2010). Region-specific alterations in brain development in one- to three-year-old boys with fragile X syndrome. *Proceedings of the National Academy of Science USA, 107*(20), 9335–9339.

Hoff, E. (2003). The specificity of environmental influence: Socioeconomic status affects early vocabulary development via maternal speech. *Child Development, 74*(5), 1368–1378.

Hoffmann, H. (1845). *Der Struwwelpeler: Oder lustige Geschichlen unddrollige Bilder* [Shock-headed Peter: Or pretty stories and funny pictures]. Leipzig, Germany: Insel-Verdag.

Hoksbergen, R., Ter Laak, J., Rijk, K., van Dijkum, C., & Stoutjesdijk, F. (2005). Post-institutional autistic syndrome in Romanian adoptees. *Journal of Autism and Developmental Disorders, 35*(5), 615–623.

Hong, S. E., Shugart, Y. Y., Huang, D. T., Shahwan, S. A., Grant, P. E., Hourihane, J. O., . . . Walsh, C. A. (2000). Autosomal recessive lissencephaly with cerebellar hypoplasia is associated with human RELN mutations. *Nature Genetics, 26*(1), 93–96.

Horn, J. L., & McArdle, J. J. (1992). A practical and theoretical guide to measurement invariance in aging research. *Experimental Aging Research, 18*(3), 117–144.

Horn, J. L., & Noll, J. (1997). Human cognitive capabilities: Gf-Gc theory. In D. P. Flanagan, J. L. Genshaft, & P. L. Harrison (Eds.), *Contemporary intellectual assessment: Theories, tests, and issues* (pp. 53–91). New York: Guilford Press.

Hoskyn, M., & Swanson, H. L. (2000). Cognitive processing of low achievers and children with reading disabilities: A selective meta-analytic review of the published literature. *School Psychology Review, 29*(1), 102–119.

Howlin, P., Goode, S., Hutton, J., & Rutter, M. (2004). Adult outcome for children with autism. *Journal of Child Psychology and Psychiatry, 45*(2), 212–229.

Howlin, P., & Moss, P. (2012). Adults with autism spectrum disorders. *Canadian Journal of Psychiatry, 57*(5), 275–283.

Hu, W., Lee, H. L., Zhang, Q., Liu, T., Geng, L. B., Seghier, M. L., . . . Price, C. J. (2010). Developmental dyslexia in Chinese and English populations: Dissociating the effect of dyslexia from language differences. *Brain, 133*(Pt. 6), 1694–1706.

Huerta, M., Bishop, S. L., Duncan, A., Hus, V., & Lord, C. (2012). Application of DSM-5 criteria for autism spectrum disorder to three samples of children with DSM-IV diagnoses of pervasive developmental disorders. *American Journal of Psychiatry, 169*, 1056–1064.

Hughes, J. R. (2007). Autism: The first firm finding = underconnectivity? *Epilepsy and Behavior, 11*(1), 20–24.

Hull, J. V., Jacokes, Z. J., Torgerson, C. M., Irimia, A., Van Horn, J. D., Aylward, E., . . . Webb, S. J. (2017). Resting-state functional connectivity in autism spectrum disorders: A review. *Frontiers in Psychiatry, 7,* 205.

Hulme, C., Bowyer-Crane, C., Carroll, J. M., Duff, F. J., & Snowling, M. J. (2012). The causal role of phoneme awareness and letter-sound knowledge in learning to read: Combining intervention studies with mediation analyses. *Psychological Science, 23*(6), 572–577.

Hultman, C., Sandin, S., Levine, S., Lichtenstein, P., & Reichenberg, A. (2011). Advancing paternal age and risk of autism: New evidence from a population-based study and a meta-analysis of epidemiological studies. *Molecular Psychiatry, 16*(12), 1203–1212.

Hunt, E. (2011). *Human intelligence.* New York: Cambridge University Press.

Hus, V., Taylor, A., & Lord, C. (2011). Telescoping of caregiver report on the Autism Diagnostic Interview–Revised. *Journal of Child Psychology and Psychiatry, 52*(7), 753–760.

Huttenlocher, P. R., & Dabholchar, A. S. (1997). Regional differences in synaptogenesis in human cerebral cortex. *Journal of Comparative Neurology, 387*(2), 167–178.

Hynd, G. W., Hern, K. L., Novey, E. S., Eliopulos, D., Marshall, R., Gonzalez, J. J., & Voeller, K. K. (1993). Attention deficit-hyperactivity disorder and asymmetry of the caudate nucleus. *Journal of Child Neurology, 8*(4), 339–347.

Hynd, G. W., Semrud-Clikeman, M., Lorys, A. R., Novey, E. S., & Eliopulos, D. (1990). Brain morphology in developmental dyslexia and attention deficit disorder/hyperactivity. *Archives of Neurology, 47*(8), 919–926.

Hynd, G. W., Semrud-Clikeman, M., Lorys, A. R., Novey, E. S., Eliopulos, D., & Lyytinen, H. (1991). Corpus callosum morphology in attention deficit-hyperactivity disorder: Morphometric analysis of MRI. *Journal of Learning Disabilities, 24*(3), 141–146.

Individuals With Disabilities Education Act, 20 U.S.C. § 1400 (2004).

Inglis, M., & Gilmore, C. (2014). Indexing the approximate number system. *Acta Psychologica, 145,* 147–155.

Insel, T., Cuthbert, B., Garvey, M., Heinssen, R., Pine, D. S., Quinn, K., . . . Wang, P. (2010). Research domain criteria (RDoC): Toward a new classification framework for research on mental disorders. *American Journal of Psychiatry, 167*(7), 748–751.

Iossifov, I., Ronemus, M., Levy, D., Wang, Z., Hakker, I., Rosenbaum, J., . . . Leotta, A. (2012). De novo gene disruptions in children on the autistic spectrum. *Neuron, 74*(2), 285–299.

Iuculano, T., Rosenberg-Lee, M., Richardson, J., Tenison, C., Fuchs, L., Supekar, K., & Menon, V. (2015). Cognitive tutoring induces widespread neuroplasticity and remediates brain function in children with mathematical learning disabilities. *Nature Communications, 6,* 8453.

Jack, A., & Pelphrey, K. (2017). Annual Research Review: Understudied populations within the autism spectrum—current trends and future directions in neuroimaging research. *Journal of Child Psychology and Psychiatry and Allied Disciplines, 58*(4) 411–435.

Jackson, A. P., Eastwood, H., Bell, S. M., Adu, J., Toomes, C., Carr, I. M., . . . Woods, C. G. (2002). Identification of microcephalin, a protein implicated in determining the size of the human brain. *American Journal of Human Genetics, 71*(1), 136–142.

Jacobs, R., Harvey, A. S., & Anderson, V. (2007). Executive function following focal frontal lobe lesions: Impact of timing of lesion on outcome. *Cortex, 43,* 792–805.

Jain, A., Marshall, J., Buikema, A., Bancroft, T., Kelly, J. P., & Newschaffer, C. J. (2015). Autism occurrence by MMR vaccine status among US children with older siblings with and without autism. *Journal of the American Medical Association, 313*(15), 1534–1540.

Jakobson, R. (1941). *Kindersprache, aphasie, und allgermeine* [Child language, aphasia, and phonological universals]. Uppsala, Sweden: Almqvist & Wiksell.

Jamieson, J. P., Mendes, W. B., Blackstock, E., & Schmader, T. (2010). Turning the knots in your stomach into bows: Reappraising arousal improves performance on the GRE. *Journal of Experimental Social Psychology, 46*(1), 208–212.

Jensen, P. S., Arnold, L. E., Swanson, J. M., Vitiello, B., Abikoff, H. B., Greenhill, L. L., . . . Hur, K. (2007). 3-year follow-up of the NIMH MTA study. *Journal of the American Academy of Child and Adolescent Psychiatry, 46,* 989–1002.

Jiménez, J. E., Siegel, L. S., O'Shanahan, I., & Ford, L. (2009). The relative roles of IQ and cognitive processes in reading disability. *Educational Psychology, 29*(1), 27–43.

Joanisse, M. F. (2000). *Connectionist phonology.* Doctoral dissertation, University of Southern California, Los Angeles, CA.

Joanisse, M. F. (2004). Specific language impairments in children: Phonology, semantics, and the English past tense. *Current Directions in Psychological Science, 13*(4), 156–160.

Joanisse, M. F. (2007). Phonological deficits and developmental language impairments: Evidence from connectionist models. In D. Mareschal, S. Sirois, G. Westermann, & M. H. Johnson (Eds.), *Neuroconstructionism: Perspectives and prospects* (Vol. 2, pp. 205–229). Oxford, UK: Oxford University Press.

Joanisse, M. F., & Seidenberg, M. S. (2003). Phonology and syntax in specific language impairment: Evidence from a connectionist model. *Brain and Language, 86*(1), 40–56.

Johnson, M. H., & de Haan, M. (2011). *Developmental cognitive neuroscience*. Oxford, UK: Blackwell.

Jones, E. J., Gliga, T., Bedford, R., Charman, T., & Johnson, M. H. (2014). Developmental pathways to autism: A review of prospective studies of infants at risk. *Neuroscience and Biobehavioral Reviews, 39*, 1–33.

Just, M. A., Cherkassky, V. L., Keller, T. A., & Minshew, N. J. (2004). Cortical activation and synchronization during sentence comprehension in high-functioning autism: Evidence of underconnectivity. *Brain, 127*(8), 1811–1821.

Kagan, J., & Snidman, N. (2009). *The long shadow of temperament*. Cambridge, MA: Harvard University Press.

Kail, R. (1991). Development of processing speed in childhood and adolescence. *Advances in Child Development and Behavior, 23*, 151–185.

Kail, R. (1994). A method of studying the generalized slowing hypothesis in children with specific language impairment. *Journal of Speech and Hearing Research, 37*, 418–421.

Kail, R., & Hall, L. K. (1994). Processing speed, naming speed, and reading. *Developmental Psychology, 30*(6), 949–954.

Kaiser, A. P., & Roberts, M. Y. (2013). Parents as communication partners: An evidence-based strategy for improving parent support for language and communication in everyday settings. *Perspectives on Language Learning and Education, 20*(3), 96–111.

Kalff, A. C., De Sonneville, L. M. J., Hurks, P. P. M., Hendriksen, J. G. M., Kroes, M., Feron, F. J. M., . . . Jolles, J. (2005). Speed, speed variability, and accuracy of information processing in 5- to 6-year-old children at risk of ADHD. *Journal of the International Neuropsychological Society, 11*(2), 173–183.

Kamp-Becker, I., Smidt, J., Ghahreman, M., Heinzel-Gutenbrunner, M., Becker, K., & Remschmidt, H. (2010). Categorical and dimensional structure of autism spectrum disorders: The nosologic validity of Asperger syndrome. *Journal of Autism and Developmental Disorders, 40*(8), 921–929.

Kanner, L. (1943). Autistic disturbances of affective contact. *Nervous Child, 2*, 217–250.

Kanwisher, N. (2010). Functional specificity in the human brain: A window into the functional architecture of the mind. *Proceeding of the National Academy of Sciences of the USA, 107*(25), 11163–11170.

Karmiloff-Smith, A., & Thomas, M. S. (2003). What can developmental disorders tell us about the neurocomputational constraints that shape development?: The case of Williams syndrome. *Development and Psychopathology, 15*(4), 969–990.

Kasari, C., Gulsrud, A. C., Wong, C., Kwon, S., & Locke, J. (2010). Randomized controlled caregiver mediated joint engagement intervention for toddlers with autism. *Journal of Autism and Developmental Disorders, 40*, 1045–1056.

Kasari, C., Sigman, M., Mundy, P., & Yirmiya, N. (1988). Caregiver interactions with autistic children. *Journal of Abnormal Child Psychology, 16*, 45–56.

Kashimoto, R., Toffoli, L., Manfredo, M., Volpini, V., Martins-Pinge, M., Pelosi, G., & Gomes, M. (2016). Physical exercise affects the epigenetic programming of rat brain and modulates the adaptive response evoked by repeated restraint stress. *Behavioural Brain Research, 296*, 286–289.

Katusic, S. K., Colligan, R. C., Weaver, A. L., & Barbaresi, W. J. (2009). The forgotten learning disability: Epidemiology of written-language disorder in a population-based birth cohort (1976–1982), Rochester, Minnesota. *Pediatrics, 123*(5), 1306–1313.

Kaufman, A. S., & Kaufman, N. L. (2014). *Kaufman Test of Educational Achievement–Third Edition (KTEA-3) technical and interpretive manual*. Bloomington, MN: Pearson.

Kaufman, S. B., Reynolds, M. R., Liu, X., Kaufman, A. S., & McGrew, K. S. (2012). Are cognitive g and academic achievement g one and the same g?: An exploration on the Woodcock–Johnson and Kaufman tests. *Intelligence, 40*(2), 123–138.

Kaufmann, L., Handl, P., & Thony, B. (2003). Evaluation of a numeracy intervention program focusing on basic numerical knowledge and conceptual knowledge: A pilot study. *Journal of Learning Disabilities, 36*(6), 564–573.

Kaufmann, L., Wood, G., Rubinsten, O., & Henik, A. (2011). Meta-analyses of developmental fMRI studies investigating typical and atypical trajectories of number processing and calculation. *Developmental Neuropsychology, 36*(6), 763–787.

Keller, M. C. (2008). The evolutionary persistence of genes that increase mental disorders risk. *Current Directions in Psychological Science, 17*, 395–399.

Kennard, M. A. (1936). Age and other factors in motor recovery from precentral lesions in monkeys. *American Journal of Physiology, 115*, 138–146.

Kenworthy, L., Anthony, L. G., Naiman, D. Q., Cannon, L., Wills, M. C., Luong-Tran, C., . . . Wallace, G. L. (2014). Randomized controlled effectiveness trial of executive function intervention for children on the autism spectrum. *Journal of Child Psychology and Psychiatry and Allied Disciplines, 55*, 374–383.

Kere, J. (2011). Molecular genetics and molecular biology of dyslexia. *Wiley Interdisciplinary Reviews: Cognitive Science, 4*, 441–448.

Kerr, J. (1897). School hygiene, in its mental, moral, and physical aspects (Howard Medical Prize Essay). *Journal of the Royal Statistical Society, 60*, 613–680.

Kessler, R. C., Avenevoli, S., McLaughlin, K. A., Green, J. G., Lakoma, M. D., Petukhova, M., . . . Merikangas, K. R. (2012). Lifetime co-morbidity of DSM-IV disorders in the US National Comorbidity Survey Replication Adolescent Supplement (NCS-A). *Psychological Medicine, 42*, 1997–2010.

Ketelaars, M. P., Cuperus, J., Jansonius, K., & Verhoeven, L. (2010). Pragmatic language impairment and associated behavioural problems. *International Journal of Language and Communcation Disorders, 45*(2), 204–214.

Kibar, Z., Torban, E., McDearmid, J. R., Reynolds, A., Berghout, J., Mathieu, M., . . . Gros, P. (2007). Mutations in VANGL1 associated with neural-tube defects. *New England Journal of Medicine, 356*(14), 1432–1437.

Kibby, M. Y., Kroese, J. M., Krebbs, H., Hill, C. E., & Hynd, G. W. (2009). The pars triangularis in dyslexia and ADHD: A comprehensive approach. *Brain and Language, 111*(1), 46–54.

King, M., & Bearman, P. (2009). Diagnostic change and the increased prevalence of autism. *International Journal of Epidemiology, 38*, 1224–1234.

Kintsch, W. (1994). The psychology of discourse processing. In A. M. Gernsbacher (Ed.), *Handbook of psycholinguistics* (pp. 721–739). San Diego, CA: Academic Press.

Kirk, H. E., Gray, K. M., Ellis, K., Taffe, J., & Cornish, K. M. (2016). Computerised attention training for children with intellectual and developmental disabilities: A randomised controlled trial. *Journal of Child Psychology and Psychiatry, 57*(12), 1380–1389.

Kirk, H. E., Gray, K., Ellis, K., Taffe, J., & Cornish, K. (2017). Impact of attention training on academic achievement, executive functioning, and behavior: A randomized controlled trial. *American Journal on Intellectual and Developmental Disabilities, 122*(2), 97–117.

Kirkwood, M. W. (2015). *Validity testing in child and adolescent assessment: Evaluating exaggeration, feigning, and noncredible effort*. New York: Guilford Press.

Kirkwood, M. W., Yeates, K. O., Randolph, C., & Kirk, J. W. (2012). The implications of symptom validity test failure for ability-based test performance in a pediatric sample. *Psychological Assessment, 24*(1), 36–45.

Kjelgaard, M. M., & Tager-Flusberg, H. (2001). An investigation of language impairment in autism: Implications for genetic subgroups. *Language and Cognitive Processes, 16*(2), 287–308.

Klingberg, T., Fernell, E., Olesen, P. J., Johnson, M., Gustafsson, P., Dahlstrom, K., . . . Westerberg, H. (2005). Computerized training of working memory in children with ADHD—a randomized, controlled trial. *Journal of the American Academy of Child and Adolescent Psychiatry, 44*(2), 177–186.

Klingberg, T., Hedehus, M., Temple, E., Salz, T., Gabrieli, J. D., Moseley, M. E., & Poldrack, R. A. (2000). Microstructure of temporo-parietal white matter as a basis for reading ability: Evidence from diffusion tensor magnetic resonance imaging. *Neuron, 25*, 493–500.

Knopik, V. S., & DeFries, J. C. (1999). Etiology of covariation between reading and mathematics performance: A twin study. *Twin Research and Human Genetics, 2*(3), 226–234.

Knopik, V. S., Neiderhiser, J. M., DeFries, J. C., & Plomin, R. (2017). *Behavioral genetics* (7th ed.). New York: Worth.

Kochanska, G., Murray, K. T., & Harlan, E. T. (2000). Effortful control in early childhood: Continuity and change, antecedents, and implications for social development. *Developmental Psychology, 36*(2), 220–232.

Kofler, M. J., Rapport, M. D., Sarver, D. E., Raiker, J. S., Orban, S. A., Friedman, L. M., & Kolomeyer, E. G. (2013). Reaction time variability in ADHD: A meta-analytic review of 319 studies. *Clinical Psychology Review, 33*, 795–811.

Kolb, B., Gibb, R., & Gorny, G. (2000). Cortical plasticity and the development of behavior after early frontal cortical injury. *Developmental Neuropsychology, 18*(3), 423–444.

Kolb, B., & Whishaw, I. Q. (1990). *Fundamentals of human neuropsychology* (3rd ed.). New York: Freeman.

Kong, A., Frigge, M. L., Masson, G., Besenbacher, S., Sulem, P., Magnusson, G., . . . Stefansson, K. (2012). Rate of de novo mutations and the importance of father's age to disease risk. *Nature, 488*, 471–475.

Konopka, G., & Roberts, T. F. (2016). Insights into the neural and genetic basis of vocal communication. *Cell, 164*(6), 1269–1276.

Koontz, K. L., & Berch, D. B. (1996). Identifying simple numerical stimuli: Processing inefficiencies exhibited by arithmetic learning disabled children. *Mathematical Cognition, 2*(1), 1–23.

Korbel, J. O., Tirosh-Wagner, T., Urban, A. E., Chen, X. N., Kasowski, M., Dai, L., . . . Korenberg, J. R. (2009). The genetic architecture of Down syndrome phenotypes revealed by high-resolution analysis of human segmental trisomies. *Proceedings of the National Academy of Sciences of the USA, 106*(29), 12031–12036.

Korkman, M., Kirk, U., & Kemp, S. (2007). *NEPSY–Second Edition (NEPSY-II)*. San Antonio, TX: Psychological Corporation.

Kosc, L. (1974). Developmental of dyscalculia. *Journal of Learning Disabilities, 7*, 159–162.

Koslowski, N., Klein, K., Arnold, K., Kösters, M., Schützwohl, M., Salize, H. J., & Puschner, B. (2016). Effectiveness of interventions for adults with mild to moderate intellectual disabilities and mental health problems: Systematic review and meta-analysis. *British Journal of Psychiatry, 209*(6), 469–474.

Kovas, Y., & Plomin, R. (2006). Generalist genes: Implications for the cognitive sciences. *Trends in cognitive sciences, 10*(5), 198–203.

Kovas, Y., & Plomin, R. (2007). Learning abilities and disabilities: Generalist genes, specialist environments. *Current Directions in Psychological Science, 16*(5), 284–288.

Krakauer, J. W., Ghazanfar, A. A., Gomez-Marin, A., MacIver, M. A., & Poeppel, D. (2017). Neuroscience needs behavior: Correcting a reductionist bias. *Neuron, 93*(3), 480–490.

Krishnan, S., Watkins, K. E., & Bishop, D. V. M. (2016). Neurobiological basis of language learning difficulties. *Trends in Cognitive Sciences, 20*(9), 701–714.

Kroeger, L. A., Brown, R. D., & O'Brien, B. A. (2012). Connecting neuroscience, cognitive, and educational theories and research to practice: A review of mathematics intervention programs. *Early Education and Development, 23*(1), 37–58.

Kröger, B. J., Kannampuzha, J., & Neuschaefer-Rube, C. (2009). Towards a neurocomputational model of speech production and perception. *Speech Communication, 51*(9), 793–809.

Kuhl, P. K. (1991). Human adults and human infants show a "perceptual magnet effect" for the prototypes of speech categories, monkeys do not. *Perception and Psychophysics, 50*(2), 93–107.

Kuhl, P. K., & Meltzoff, A. N. (1996). Infant vocalization in response to speech: Vocal imitation and developmental change. *Journal of the Acoustical Society of America, 100*, 2425–2438.

Lai, C. L. E., Fisher, S. E., Hurst, J. A., Vargha-Khadem, F., & Monaco, A. P. (2001). A forkhead-domain gene is mutated in a severe speech and language disorder. *Nature, 413*, 519–523.

Lai, C. L. E., Gerrelli, D., Monaco, A. P., Fisher, S. E., & Copp, A. J. (2003). FOXP2 expression during brain development coincides with adult sites of pathology in a severe speech and language disorder. *Brain, 126*, 2455–2462.

Landa, R. J., & Garrett-Mayer, E. (2006). Development in infants with autism spectrum disorders: A prospective study. *Journal of Child Psychology and Psychiatry, 47*(6), 629–638.

Landa, R. J., Gross, A. L., Stuart, E. A., & Faherty, A. (2013). Developmental trajectories in children with and without autism spectrum disorders: The first 3 years. *Child Development, 84*, 429–442.

Landerl, K., Bevan, A., & Butterworth, B. (2004). Developmental dyscalculia and basic numerical capacities: A study of 8–9-year-old students. *Cognition, 93*(2), 99–125.

Landerl, K., & Moll, K. (2010). Comorbidity of learning disorders: Prevalence and familial transmission. *Journal of Child Psychology and Psychiatry, 51*(3), 287–294.

Landerl, K., Wimmer, H., & Frith, U. (1997). The impact of orthographic consistency on dyslexia: A German–English comparison. *Cognition, 63*, 315–334.

Landry, R., & Bryson, S. E. (2004). Impaired disengagement of attention in young children with autism. *Journal of Child Psychology and Psychiatry, 45*(6), 1115–1122.

Langen, M., Bos, D., Noordermeer, S. D., Nederveen, H., van Engeland, H., & Durston, S. (2014). Changes in the development of striatum are involved in repetitive behavior in autism. *Biological Psychiatry, 76*(5), 405–411.

Langen, M., Durston, S., Staal, W. G., Palmen, S. J., & van Engeland, H. (2007). Caudate nucleus is enlarged in high-functioning medication-naive subjects with autism. *Biological Psychiatry, 62*(3), 262–266.

Larson, K., Russ, S. A., Kahn, R. S., & Halfon, N. (2011). Patterns of comorbidity, functioning, and service use for US children with ADHD, 2007. *Pediatrics, 127*(3), 462–470.

Law, J., Garrett, Z., & Nye, C. (2003). Speech and language therapy interventions for children with primary speech and language delay or disorder. *Cochrane Database of Systematic Reviews, 3*, CD004110.

Lawson, K. R., & Ruff, H. A. (2004). Early attention and negative memotionality predict later cognitive and behavioral function. *International Journal of Behavioral Development, 28*(2), 157–165.

Lee, N. R., Maiman, M., & Godfrey, M. (2016). What can neuropsychology teach us about intellectual disability?: Searching for commonalities in the memory and executive function profiles associated with Down, Williams and fragile X syndromes. In R. M. Hodapp & D. J. Fidler (Eds.), *International review of research in developmental disabilities* (Vol. 51, pp. 1–40). New York: Academic Press.

Leitner, Y. (2014). The co-occurrence of autism and attention deficit hyperactivity disorder in children—what do we know? *Frontiers in Human Neuroscience, 8*, 268.

Lejeune, J., Gauthier, M., & Turpin, R. (1959). [Human chromosomes in tissue cultures.] *Comptes Rendus Hebdomadaires des Seances de l'Académie des Sciences, 248*(4), 602–603.

Lenneberg, E. H. (1967). *Biological foundations of language.* New York: Wiley.

Lenroot, R. K., & Giedd, J. N. (2006). Brain development in children and adolescents: Insights from anatomical magnetic resonance imaging. *Neuroscience and Biobehavioral Reviews, 30*, 718–729.

Leonard, L. B. (2000). *Children with specific language impairment.* Cambridge, MA: MIT Press.

Leonard, L. B. (2014). *Children with specific language impairment* (2nd ed.). Cambridge, MA: MIT Press.

Levin, A. R., Fox, N. A., Zeanah, C. H., & Nelson, C. A. (2015). Social communication difficulties and autism in previously institutionalized children. *Journal of the American Academy of Child and Adolescent Psychiatry, 54*(2), 108–115.

Levin, H. S. (1979). The acalculias. In K. M. Heilman & E. Valenstein (Eds.), *Clinical neuropsychology* (pp. 128–140). New York: Oxford University Press.

Levin, H. S., Eisenberg, H. M., & Benton, A. L. (1991). *Frontal lobe function and dysfunction.* New York: Oxford University Press.

Levy, L. M., Levy, R. I., & Grafman, J. (1999). Metabolic abnormalities detected by 1H-MRS in dyscalculia and dysgraphia. *Neurology, 53*, 639–641.

Lewis, B. A., & Freebairn, L. (1992). Residual effects of preschool phonology disorders in grade school, adolescence, and adulthood. *Journal of Speech and Hearing Research, 35*(4), 819–831.

Lewis, B. A., Freebairn, L. A., Hansen, A., Gerry Taylor, H., Iyengar, S., & Shriberg, L. D. (2004). Family pedigrees of children with suspected childhood apraxia of speech. *Journal of Communication Disorders, 37*(2), 157–175.

Lewis, B. A., Freebairn, L. A., Hansen, A. J., Stein, C. M., Shriberg, L. D., Iyengar, S. K., & Taylor, H. G. (2006). Dimensions of early speech sound disorders: A factor analytic study. *Journal of Communication Disorders, 39*(2), 139–157.

Lewis, B. A., & Thompson, L. A. (1992). A study of developmental speech and language disorders in twins. *Journal of Speech and Hearing Research, 35*(5), 1086–1094.

Lewis, C., Hitch, G. J., & Walker, P. (1994). The prevalence of specific arithmetic difficulties and specific reading difficulties in 9- to 10-year-old boys and girls. *Journal of Child Psychology and Psychiatry, 35*(2), 283–292.

Leyfer, O. T., Woodruff-Borden, J., Klein-Tasman, B. P., Fricke, J. S., & Mervis, C. B. (2006). Prevalence of psychiatric disorders in 4–16-year-olds with Williams syndrome. *American Journal of Medical Genetics B: Neuropsychiatric Genetics, 141*(6), 615–622.

Leyfer, O. T., Woodruff-Borden, J., & Mervis, C. B. (2009). Anxiety disorders in children with Williams syndrome, their mothers, and their siblings: Implications for the etiology of anxiety disorders. *Journal of Neurodevelopmental Disorders, 1*(1), 4–14.

Li, D., Karnath, H.-O., & Xu, X. (2017). Candidate biomarkers in children with autism spectrum disorder: A review of MRI studies. *Neuroscience Bulletin, 33*, 219–237.

Liberman, I. Y., Shankweiler, D., Orlando, C., Harris, K. S., & Berti, F. B. (1971). Letter confusions and reversals of sequence in the beginning reader:

Implications for Orton's theory of developmental dyslexia. *Cortex, 7*(2), 127–142.

Libertus, M. E., Feigenson, L., & Halberda, J. (2011). Preschool acuity of the approximate number system correlates with school math ability. *Developmental Science, 14*(6), 1292–1300.

Lichtenstein, P., Carlstrom, E., Rastam, M., Gillberg, C., & Anckarsater, H. (2010). The genetics of autism spectrum disorders and related neuropsychiatric disorders in childhood. *American Journal of Psychiatry, 167*, 1357–1363.

Lichtenstein, P., Yip, B. H., Bjork, C., Pawitan, Y., Cannon, T. D., Sullivan, P. F., & Hultman, C. M. (2009). Common genetic determinants of schizophrenia and bipolar disorder in Swedish families: A population-based study. *Lancet, 373*, 234–239.

Light, J. G., & DeFries, J. C. (1995). Comorbidity of reading and mathematics disabilities: Genetic and environmental etiologies. *Journal of Learning Disabilities, 28*(2), 96–106.

Light, J. G., DeFries, J. C., & Olson, R. K. (1998). Multivariate behavioral genetic analysis of achievement and cognitive measures in reading-disabled and control twin pairs. *Human Biology, 70*(2), 215–237.

Lingam, R., Simmons, A., Andrews, N., Miller, E., Stowe, J., & Taylor, B. (2003). Prevalence of autism and parentally reported triggers in a north east London population. *Archives of Disease in Childhood, 88*(8), 666–670.

Lobier, M., Dubois, M., & Valdois, S. (2013). The role of visual processing speed in reading speed development. *PLOS ONE, 8*(4), e58097.

Loehlin, J. C. (2000). Group differences in intelligence. In R. Sternberg (Ed.), *Handbook of intelligence* (pp. 176–193). New York: Cambridge University Press.

Logan, J. A. R., Cutting, L., Schatschneider, C., Hart, S. A., Deater-Deckard, K., & Peterill, S. (2013). Reading development in young children: Genetic and environmental influence *Child Development, 84*, 2131–2144.

Lonigan, C. J., & Whitehurst, G. J. (1998). Relative efficacy of parent and teacher involvement in a shared-reading intervention for preschool children from low-income backgrounds. *Early Childhood Research Quarterly, 13*, 263–290.

Lord, C., & Bishop, S. L. (2014). Recent advances in autism research as reflected in DSM-5 criteria for autism spectrum disorder. *Annual Review of Clinical Psychology, 11*, 53–70.

Lord, C., Petkova, E., Hus, V., Gan, W., Lu, F., Martin, D. M., . . . Gerdts, J. (2012). A multisite study of the clinical diagnosis of different autism spectrum disorders. *Archives of General Psychiatry, 69*(3), 306–313.

Lord, C., Risi, S., DiLavore, P. S., Shulman, C., Thurm, A., & Pickles, A. (2006). Autism from 2 to 9 years of age. *Archives of General Psychiatry, 63*(6), 694–701.

Lord, C., Rutter, M., DiLavore, P. C., Risi, S., Gotham, K., & Bishop, S. (2012). *Autism Diagnostic Observation Schedule, Second Edition (ADOS-2)*. Los Angeles: Western Psychological Services.

Lord, C., Rutter, M., & Le Couteur, A. (1994). Autism Diagnostic Interview—Revised: A revised version of a diagnostic interview for caregivers of individuals with possible pervasive developmental disorders. *Journal of Autism and Developmental Disorders, 24*(5), 659–685.

Losen, D. J., & Orfield, G. (2002). *Racial inequity in special education*. Cambridge, MA: Harvard Education Press.

Love, A. J., & Thompson, M. G. (1988). Language disorders and attention deficit disorders in young children referred for psychiatric services: Analysis of prevalence and a conceptual synthesis. *American Journal of Orthopsychiatry, 58*(1), 52–64.

Lubin, A., Simon, G., Noude, O., & De Neys, W. (2015). Inhibition, conflict detection, and number conservation. *Mathematics Education, 47*, 793–800.

Luciano, M., Evans, D., Hansell, N., Medland, S., Montgomery, G., Martin, N., . . . Bates, T. (2013). A genome-wide association study for reading and language abilities in two population cohorts. *Genes, Brain and Behavior, 12*(6), 645–652.

Ludwig, K. U., Roeske, D., Schumacher, J., Schulte-Korne, G., Konig, I. R., Warnke, A., . . . Hoffmann, P. (2008). Investigation of interaction between DCDC2 and KIAA0319 in a large German dyslexia sample. *Journal of Neural Transmission, 115*, 1587–1589.

Lukowski, S. L., Rosenberg-Lee, M., Thompson, L. A., Hart, S. A., Willcutt, E. G., Olson, R. K., . . . Pennington, B. F. (2017). Approximate number sense shares etiological overlap with mathematics and general cognitive ability. *Intelligence, 65*, 67–74.

Lum, J. A. G., Conti-Ramsden, G., Morgan, A. T., & Ullman, M. T. (2014). Procedural learning deficits in specific language impairment (SLI): A meta-analysis of serial reaction time task performance. *Cortex, 51*, 1–10.

Lum, J. A. G., Ullman, M. T., & Conti-Ramsden, G. (2013). Procedural learning is impaired in dyslexia: Evidence from a meta-analysis of serial reaction time studies. *Research in Developmental Disabilities, 34*(10), 3460–3476.

Lundstrom, S., Reichenberg, A., Anckarsäter, H., Lichtenstein, P., & Gillberg, C. (2015). Autism phenotype versus registered diagnosis in Swedish children: Prevalence trends over 10 years in general population samples. *British Medical Journal, 350*, h1961.

Luria, A. (1961). *The role of speech in the regulation of normal and abnormal behavior*. New York: Pergamon Press.

Luria, A. (1966). *Higher cortical functions in man*. New York: Basic Books.

Lynn, R., & Hampson, S. (1986). The rise of national intelligence: Evidence from Britain, Japan and the USA. *Personality and Individual Differences, 7*(1), 23–32.

Lynn, R., & Vanhanen, T. (2006). *IQ and global inequality*. Augusta, GA: Washington Summit.

Lyon, G. R., Shaywitz, S. E., & Shaywitz, B. A. (2003). A definition of dyslexia. *Annals of Dyslexia, 53*, 1–14.

Lyytinen, H., Guttorm, T. K., Huttunen, T., Hämäläinen, J., Leppänen, P. H., & Vesterinen, M. (2005). Psychophysiology of developmental dyslexia: A review of findings including studies of children at risk for dyslexia. *Journal of Neurolinguistics, 18*(2), 167–195.

MacDermot, K. D., Bonora, E., Sykes, N., Coupe, A. M., Lai, C. S., Vernes, S. C., . . . Fisher, S. E.

(2005). Identification of FOXP2 truncation as a novel cause of developmental speech and language deficits. *American Journal of Human Genetics, 76*(6), 1074–1080.

MacDonald, B. (2014). *Comparison of reading development across socioeconomic status in the United States.* Unpublished doctoral dissertation, University of Denver, Denver, CO.

MacDonald, B., Pennington, B. F., Dmitrieva, J., Willcutt, E. G., Samuelsson, S., Byrne, B., & Olson, R. K. (2010). *Understanding cross-cultural difference in rates of ADHD.* Unpublished master's thesis, University of Denver, Denver, CO.

MacNeil, B. M., Lopes, V. A., & Minnes, P. M. (2009). Anxiety in children and adolescents with autism spectrum disorders. *Research in Autism Spectrum Disorders, 3*(1), 1–21.

Maddox, W. T., & Chandrasekaran, B. (2014). Tests of a dual-systems model of speech category learning. *Bilingualism (Cambridge, England), 17*(4), 709–728.

Madsen, K. M., Hviid, A., Vestergaard, M., Schendel, D., Wohlfahrt, J., Thorsen, P., . . . Melbye, M. (2002). [MMR vaccination and autism—a population-based follow-up study] [Article in Danish]. *New England Journal of Medicine, 347,* 1477–1482.

Maenner, M. J., Rice, C. E., Arneson, C. L., Cunniff, C., Schieve, L. A., Carpenter, L. A., . . . Durkin, M. S. (2014). Potential impact of DSM-5 criteria on autism spectrum disorder prevalence estimates. *JAMA Psychiatry, 71*(3), 292–300.

Mahler, M. (1952). On child psychosis and schizophrenia: Autistic and symbiotic infantile psychosis. *Psychoanalytic Study of the Child, 7,* 286–305.

Malenfant, P., Liu, X., Hudson, M. L., Qiao, Y., Hrynchak, M., Riendeau, N., . . . Forster-Gibson, C. (2012). Association of GTF2i in the Williams–Beuren syndrome critical region with autism spectrum disorders. *Journal of Autism and Developmental Disorders, 42*(7), 1459–1469.

Malhotra, D., & Sebat, J. (2012). CNVs: Harbingers of a rare variant revolution in psychiatric genetics. *Cell, 148,* 1223–1241.

Maloney, E. A., & Beilock, S. L. (2012). Math anxiety: Who has it, why it develops, and how to guard against it. *Trends in Cognitive Sciences, 16*(8), 404–406.

Maloney, E. A., Ramirez, G., Gunderson, E. A., Levine, S. C., & Beilock, S. L. (2015). Intergenerational effects of parents' math anxiety on children's math achievement and anxiety. *Psychological Science, 26*(9), 1480–1488.

Maloney, E. A., Risko, E. F., Ansari, D., & Fugelsang, J. (2010). Mathematics anxiety affects counting but not subitizing during visual enumeration. *Cognition, 114*(2), 293–297.

Mampe, B., Friederici, A. D., Christophe, A., & Wermke, K. (2009). Newborns' cry melody is shaped by their native language. *Current Biology, 19*(23), 1994–1997.

Mandell, D. S., & Palmer, R. (2005). Differences among states in the identification of autistic spectrum disorders. *Archives of Pediatrics and Adolescent Medicine, 159*(3), 266–269.

Mandell, D. S., Wiggins, L. D., Carpenter, L. A., Daniels, J., DiGuiseppi, C., Durkin, M. S., . . . Pinto-Martin, J. A. (2009). Racial/ethnic disparities in the identification of children with autism spectrum disorders. *American Journal of Public Health, 99*(3), 493–498.

Mandy, W. P. L., Charman, T., & Skuse, D. H. (2012). Testing the construct validity of proposed criteria for DSM-5 autism spectrum disorder. *Journal of the American Academy of Child and Adolescent Psychiatry, 51*(1), 41–50.

Mandy, W. P. L., & Lai, M.-C. (2016). Annual Research Review: The role of the environment in the developmental psychopathology of autism spectrum condition. *Journal of Child Psychology and Psychiatry and Allied Disciplines, 57,* 271–292.

Mandy, W. P. L., & Skuse, D. H. (2008). Research Review: What is the association between the social-communication element of autism and repetitive interests, behaviours and activities? *Journal of Child Psychology and Psychiatry, 49*(8), 795–808.

Manly, T., Anderson, V., Crawford, J., George, M., & Robertson, I. (2016). *Test of Everyday Attention for Children, Second Edition (TEA-Ch2).* San Antonio, TX: Pearson.

Manolio, T. A., Collins, F. S., Cox, N. J., Goldstein, D. B., Hindorff, L. A., Hunter, D. J., . . . Visscher, P. M. (2009). Finding the missing heritability of complex diseases. *Nature, 461,* 747–753.

Manor, O., Shalev, R. S., Joseph, A., & Gross-Tsur, V. (2001). Arithmetic skills in kindergarten children with developmental language disorders. *European Journal of Pediatric Neurology, 5*(2), 71–77.

Marchman, V. A., Plunkett, K., & Goodman, J. (1997). Overregularization in English plural and past tense inflectional morphology: A response to Marcus (1995). *Journal of Child Language, 24*(3), 767–779.

Mareschal, D., Johnson, M. H., Sirois, S., Spratling, M. W., Thomas, M. S. C., & Westermann, G. (2007). *Neuroconstructivism: I. How the brain constructs cognition.* New York: Oxford University Press.

Marino, C., Mascheretti, S., Riva, V., Cattaneo, F., Rigoletto, C., Rusconi, M., . . . Molteni, M. (2011). Pleiotropic effects of DCDC2 and DYX1C1 genes on language and mathematics traits in nuclear families of developmental dyslexia. *Behavior Genetics, 41*(1), 67–76.

Markey, K. L. (1994). *The sensorimotor foundations of phonology: A computational model of early childhood articulatory and phonetic development.* Doctoral dissertation, University of Colorado, Boulder, CO.

Marsh, R., Maia, T. V., & Peterson, B. S. (2009). Functional disturbances within frontostriatal circuits across multiple childhood psychopathologies. *American Journal of Psychiatry, 166*(6), 664–674.

Martel, M. M., Nikolas, M., Jernigan, K., Friderici, K., Waldman, I., & Nigg, J. T. (2011). The dopamine receptor D4 gene (DRD4) moderates family environmental effects on ADHD. *Journal of Abnormal Child Psychology, 39*(1), 1–10.

Martin, R. H. (2008). Meiotic errors in human oogenesis and spermatogenesis. *Reproductive Biomedicine Online, 16*(4), 523–531.

Martinussen, R., Hayden, J., Hogg-Johnson, S., & Tannock, R. (2005). A meta-analysis of working memory impairments in children with attention-deficit/hyperactivity disorder. *Journal of the American Academy of Child and Adolescent Psychiatry, 44*(4), 377–384.

Mascheretti, S., Trezzi, V., Giorda, R., Boivin, M., Plourde, V., Vitaro, F., . . . Marino, C. (2017). Complex effects of dyslexia risk factors account for ADHD traits: Evidence from two independent samples. *Journal of Child Psychology and Psychiatry, 58*(1), 75–82.

Mataro, M., Garcia-Sanchez, C., Junque, C., Estevez-Gonzalez, A., & Pujol, J. (1997). Magnetic resonance imaging measurement of the caudate nucleus in adolescents with attention-deficit hyperactivity disorder and its relationship with neuropsychological and behavioral measures. *Archives of Neurology, 54*(8), 963–968.

Matson, J. L., & Laud, R. B. (2007). Assessment and treatment psychopathology among people with developmental delays. In J. W. Jacobson, J. A. Mulick, & J. Rojahn (Eds.), *Handbook of intellectual and developmental disabilities* (pp. 507–539). New York: Springer.

Mattarella-Micke, A., Mateo, J., Kozak, M. N., Foster, K., & Beilock, S. L. (2011). Choke or thrive?: The relation between salivary cortisol and math performance depends on individual differences in working memory and math-anxiety. *Emotion, 11*(4), 1000–1005.

Mattes, J. A. (1989). The role of frontal lobe dysfunction in childhood hyperkinesis. *Comprehensive Psychiatry, 21*, 358–369.

Maximo, J. O., Cadena, E. J., & Kana, R. K. (2014). The implications of brain connectivity in the neuropsychology of autism. *Neuropsychology Review, 24*, 16–31.

Mayes, A. K., Reilly, S., & Morgan, A. T. (2015). Neural correlates of childhood language disorder: A systematic review. *Devvelopmental Medicine and Child Neurology, 57*(8), 706–717.

McArthur, G., Eve, P. M., Jones, K., Banales, E., Kohnen, S., Anandakumar, T., . . . Castles, A. (2012). Phonics training for English-speaking poor readers. *Cochrane Database of Systematic Reviews, 12*, CD009115.

McBride-Chang, C., Cho, J.-R., Liu, H., Wagner, R. K., Shu, H., Zhou, A., . . . Muse, A. (2005). Changing models across cultures: Associations of phonological awareness and morphological structure awareness with vocabulary and word recognition in second graders from Beijing, Hong Kong, Korea, and the United States. *Journal of Experimental Child Psychology, 92*(2), 140–160.

McGrath, L. M., Braaten, E. B., Doty, N. D., Willoughby, B. L., Wilson, H. K., O'Donnell, E. H., . . . Hill, E. N. (2016). Extending the "cross-disorder" relevance of executive functions to dimensional neuropsychiatric traits in youth. *Journal of Child Psychology and Psychiatry, 57*(4), 462–471.

McGrath, L. M., Hutaff-Lee, C., Scott, A., Boada, R., Shriberg, L. D., & Pennington, B. F. (2007). Children with comorbid speech sound disorder and specific language impairment have increased rates of attention deficit/hyperactivity disorder. *Journal of Abnormal Child Psychology, 36*, 151–163.

McGrath, L. M., Pennington, B. F., Shanahan, M. A., Santerre-Lemmon, L. E., Barnard, H. D., Willcutt, E. G., . . . Olson, R. K. (2011). A multiple deficit model of reading disability and attention-deficit/hyperactivity disorder: Searching for shared cognitive deficits. *Journal of Child Psychology and Psychiatry, 52*(5), 547–557.

McGrath, L. M., Smith, S. D., & Pennington, B. F. (2006). Breakthroughs in the search for dyslexia candidate genes. *Trends in Molecular Medicine, 12*, 333–341.

McGrath, L. M., Yu, D., Marshall, C., Davis, L. K., Thiruvahindrapuram, B., Li, B., . . . Schroeder, F. A. (2014). Copy number variation in obsessive-compulsive disorder and Tourette syndrome: A cross-disorder study. *Journal of the American Academy of Child and Adolescent Psychiatry, 53*(8), 910–919.

McGrew, K. S., Laforte, E. M., & Schrank, F. A. (2014). *WJ IV Technical Manual*. New York: Houghton Mifflin Harcourt.

McGrew, K. S., & Woodcock, R. W. (2001). *Woodcock–Johnson III technical manual*. Itasca, IL: Riverside.

McKinnon, D. H., McLeod, S., & Reilly, S. (2007). The prevalence of stuttering, voice, and speech–sound disorders in primary school students in Australia. *Language, Speech, and Hearing Services in Schools, 38*(1), 5–15.

McPartland, J. C., Reichow, B., & Volkmar, F. R. (2012). Sensitivity and specificity of proposed DSM-5 diagnostic criteria for autism spectrum disorder. *Journal of the American Academy of Child and Adolescent Psychiatry, 51*(4), 368–383.

Meaburn, E. L., Harlaar, N., Craig, I. W., Schalkwyk, L. C., & Plomin, R. (2008). Quantitative trait locus association scan of early reading disability and ability using pooled DNA and 100K SNP microarrays in a sample of 5760 children. *Molecular Psychiatry, 13*, 729–740.

Melby-Lervåg, M., & Hulme, C. (2013). Is working memory training effective?: A meta-analytic review. *Developmental Psychology, 49*(2), 270–291.

Melby-Lervåg, M., Redick, T. S., & Hulme, C. (2016). Working memory training does not improve performance on measures of intelligence or other measures of "far transfer" evidence from a meta-analytic review. *Perspectives on Psychological Science, 11*(4), 512–534.

Meltzoff, A. N., & Moore, M. K. (1977). Imitation of facial and manual gestures by human neonates. *Science, 198*(4312), 75–78.

Menn, L., Markey, K. L., Mozer, M., & Lewis, C. (1993). Connectionist modeling and the microstructure of phonological development: A progress report. In B. DeBoysson-Bardies (Ed.), *Developmental neurocognition: Speech and face processing in the first year of life* (pp. 421–433). Dordrecht, the Netherlands: Kluwer Academic.

Mervis, C. B., & John, A. E. (2010). Cognitive and behavioral characteristics of children with Williams syndrome: Implications for intervention approaches. *American Journal of Medical Genetics C: Seminars in Medical Genetics, 154*, 229–248.

Mervis, C. B., Klein-Tasman, B. P., Huffman, M. J., Velleman, S. L., Pitts, C. H., Henderson, D. R., Woodruff-Borden, J., . . ., & Osborne, L. R. (2015). Children with 7q11.23 duplication syndrome: psychological characteristics. *American Journal of Medical Genetics Part A, 167*(7), 1436–1450.

Mesulam, M. (1997). Anatomic principles in behavioral neurology and neuropsychology. In T. E. Feinberg & M. J. Farah (Eds.), *Behavioral neurology and neuropsychology* (pp. 55–67). New York: McGraw-Hill.

Meyers, J. E., & Meyers, K. R. (1995). *Rey Complex Figure Test and Recognition Trial professional manual.* Odessa, FL: Psychological Assessment Resources.

Michaelson, J. J., Shi, Y., Gujral, M., Zheng, H., Malhotra, D., Jin, X., . . . Bhandari, A. (2012). Whole-genome sequencing in autism identifies hot spots for de novo germline mutation. *Cell, 151*(7), 1431–1442.

Miciak, J., Fletcher, J. M., Stuebing, K. K., Vaughn, S., & Tolar, T. D. (2014). Patterns of cognitive strengths and weaknesses: Identification rates, agreement, and validity for learning disabilities identification. *School Psychology Quarterly, 29*(1), 21–37.

Miller, A. C., Fuchs, D., Fuchs, L. S., Compton, D. L., Kearns, D., Zhang, W., . . . Kirchner, D. (2014). Behavioral attention: A longitudinal study of whether and how it influences the development of word reading and reading comprehension among at-risk readers. *Journal of Research on Educational Effectiveness, 7,* 232–249.

Miller, D. T., Adam, M. P., Aradhya, S., Biesecker, L. G., Brothman, A. R., Carter, N. P., . . . Ledbetter, D. H. (2010). Consensus statement: Chromosomal microarray is a first-tier clinical diagnostic test for individuals with developmental disabilities or congenital anomalies. *American Journal of Human Genetics, 86,* 749–764.

Miller, G. A. (1963). *Language and communication.* New York: McGraw-Hill.

Miller, T. W., Nigg, J. T., & Miller, R. L. (2009). Attention deficit hyperactivity disorder in African American children: What can be concluded from the past ten years? *Clinical Psychology Review, 29*(1), 77–86.

Mnookin, S. (2011). *The panic virus: A true story of medicine, science, and fear.* New York: Simon & Schuster.

Moeller, K., Pixner, S., Zuber, J., Kaufmann, L., & Nuerk, H.-C. (2011). Early place-value understanding as a precursor for later arithmetic performance—a longitudinal study on numerical development. *Research in Developmental Disabilities, 32*(5), 1837–1851.

Moffitt, T. E., Houts, R., Asherson, P., Belsky, D. W., Corcoran, D. L., Hammerle, M., . . . Caspi, A. (2015). Is adult ADHD a childhood-onset neurodevelopmental disorder?: Evidence from a four-decade longitudinal cohort study. *American Journal of Psychiatry, 172*(10), 967–977.

Mohammad-Rezazadeh, I., Frohlich, J., Loo, S. K., & Jeste, S. S. (2016). Brain connectivity in autism spectrum disorder. *Current Opinion in Neurology, 29*(2), 137–147.

Molenaar, P. C., Boomsma, D. I., & Dolan, C. V. (1993). A third source of developmental differences. *Behavior Genetics, 23,* 519–524.

Molina, B. S. G., Hinshaw, S. P., Swanson, J. M., Arnold, L. E., Vitiello, B., Jensen, P. S., . . . Houck, P. R. (2009). The MTA at 8 years: Prospective follow-up of children treated for combined-type ADHD in a multisite study. *Journal of the American Academy of Child and Adolescent Psychiatry, 48,* 484–500.

Moll, K., Göbel, S. M., Gooch, D., Landerl, K., & Snowling, M. J. (2014). Cognitive risk factors for specific learning disorder: Processing speed, temporal processing, and working memory. *Journal of Learning Disabilities, 49*(3), 272–281.

Morais, J., Cary, L., Alegria, J., & Bertelson, P. (1979). Does awareness of speech as a sequence of phones arise spontaneously? *Cognition, 7*(4), 323–331.

Morgan, P. L., Farkas, G., Hillemeier, M. M., Mattison, R., Maczuga, S., Li, H., & Cook, M. (2015). Minorities are disproportionately underrepresented in special education: Longitudinal evidence across five disability conditions. *Educational Researcher, 44*(5), 278–292.

Morris, R. (1984). *Multivariate methods for neuropsychology—Techniques for classification, identification, and prediction research.* Paper presented at the International Neuropsychological Society Meeting, Houston.

Morrow, E. M. (2010). Genomic copy number variation in disorders of cognitive development. *Journal of the American Academy of Child and Adolescent Psychiatry, 49,* 1091–1104.

Morrow, R. L., Garland, E. J., Wright, J. M., Maclure, M., Taylor, S., & Dormuth, C. R. (2012). Influence of relative age on diagnosis and treatment of attention-deficit/hyperactivity disorder in children. *Canadian Medical Association Journal, 184*(7), 755–762.

Morton, J. (2004). *Understanding developmental disorders: A causal modeling approach.* Oxford, UK: Blackwell.

Morton, J., & Frith, U. (1995). Causal modeling: A structural approach to developmental psychopathology. In D. Cicchetti & D. J. Cohen (Eds.), *Developmental psychopathology* (Vol. 1, pp. 357–390). New York: Wiley.

Moulton, E., Barton, M., Robins, D. L., Abrams, D. N., & Fein, D. (2016). Early characteristics of children with ASD who demonstrate optimal progress between age two and four. *Journal of Autism and Developmental Disorders, 46,* 2160–2173.

Moura, O., Pereira, M., Alfaiate, C., Fernandes, E., Fernandes, B., Nogueira, S., . . . Simões, M. R. (2017). Neurocognitive functioning in children with developmental dyslexia and attention-deficit/hyperactivity disorder: Multiple deficits and diagnostic accuracy. *Journal of Clinical and Experimental Neuropsychology, 39*(3), 296–312.

MTA Cooperative Group. (1999). A 14-month randomized clinical trial of treatment strategies for attention-deficit/hyperactivity disorder. *Archives of General Psychiatry, 56,* 1073–1086.

MTA Cooperative Group. (2004). National Institute of Mental Health Multimodal Treatment Study of ADHD follow-up: 24-month outcomes of treatment strategies for attention-deficit/hyperactivity disorder. *Pediatrics, 113*(4), 754–761.

Müller, R. A., Shih, P., Keehn, B., Deyoe, J. R., Leyden, K. M., & Shukla, D. K. (2011). Underconnected, but how?: A survey of functional connectivity MRI studies in autism spectrum disorders. *Cerebral Cortex, 21,* 2233–2243.

Mulqueen, J. M., Bartley, C. A., & Bloch, M. H. (2015). Meta-analysis: Parental interventions for preschool ADHD. *Journal of Attention Disorders, 19,* 118–124.

Murphy, D. G., DeCarli, C., & Daly, E. M. (1993).

X-chromosome effects on female brain: A magnetic resonance imaging study of Turner's syndrome. *Lancet, 342*(8881), 1197–1200.

Nation, K. (2005). Children's reading comprehension difficulties. In M. J. Snowling & C. Hulme (Eds.), *The science of reading* (pp. 248–265). Oxford, UK: Blackwell.

National Center for Education Statistics. (2011). *The Nation's Report Card: Reading 2011.* Washington, DC: Author.

National Institute for Children's Health Quality. (2002). NICHQ Vanderbilt Assessment. Retrieved from *www.nichq.org/ resource/ nichq-vanderbilt -assessment- scales.*

National Institutes of Health. (2000, October). Phenylketonuria: Screening and management. *NIH Consensus Statement, 17,* 1–27.

National Reading Panel. (2000). Teaching children to read: An evidence-based assessment of the scientific research literature on reading and its implications for reading instruction. Retrieved from *www1.nichd.nih.gov/publications/pubs/nrp/pages/ smallbook.aspx.*

Neale, B. M., Kou, Y., Liu, L., Ma'ayan, A., Samocha, K. E., Sabo, A., . . . Daly, M. J. (2012). Patterns and rates of exonic de novo mutations in autism spectrum disorders. *Nature, 485,* 242–245.

Neale, M. C., & Kendler, K. S. (1995). Models of comorbidity for multifactorial disorders. *American Journal of Human Genetics, 57*(4), 935–953.

Nelson, M., & Denny, E. (1929). *The Nelson–Denny Reading Test for Colleges and Senior High Schools.* New York: Houghton Mifflin.

Nelson, R. J., Benner, G. J., & Gonzalez, J. (2003). Learner characteristics that influence the treatment effectiveness of early literacy interventions: A meta-analytic review. *Learning Disabilities Research and Practice, 18,* 255–267.

Neville, H. J., & Bavelier, D. (2002). Specificity and placticity in neurocogntive development in humans. In M. H. Johnson, Y. Munakata, & R. Gilmore (Eds.), *Brain development and cognition: A reader* (2nd ed., pp. 251–270). Oxford, UK: Blackwell.

Newbury, D. F., Bonora, E., Lamb, J. A., Fisher, S. E., Lai, C. S., Baird, G., . . . Monaco, A. P. (2002). International Molecular Genetic Study of Autism Consortium: FOXP2 is not a major susceptibility gene for autism or specific language impairment. *American Journal of Human Genetics, 70,* 1318–1327.

Newcomer, P. L., & Hammill, D. D. (2008). *Test of Language Development: Primary (TOLD-P:4).* Austin, TX: PRO-ED.

Nichols, P. L. (1984). Twin studies of ability, personality, and interests. *Behavior Genetics, 14,* 161–170.

Nickl-Jockschat, T., Rottschy, C., Thommes, J., Schneider, F., Laird, A. R., Fox, P. T., & Eickhoff, S. B. (2015). Neural networks related to dysfunctional face processing in autism spectrum disorder. *Brain Structure and Function, 220,* 2355–2371.

Nigg, J. T. (2006). *What causes ADHD?: Understanding what goes wrong and why.* New York: Guilford Press.

Nigg, J. T. (2017). *Getting ahead of ADHD: What next-generation science says about treatments that work– and how you can make them work for your child.* New York: Guilford Press.

Nigg, J. T., & Holton, K. (2014). Restriction and elimination diets in ADHD treatment. *Child and Adolescent Psychiatric Clinics of North America, 23*(4), 937–953.

Nigg, J. T., Willcutt, E. G., Doyle, A. E., & Sonuga-Barke, E. J. (2005). Causal heterogeneity in attention-deficit/hyperactivity disorder: Do we need neuropsychologically impaired subtypes? *Biological Psychiatry, 57*(11), 1224–1230.

Nisbett, R. E. (2009). *Intelligence and how to get it.* New York: Norton.

Nittrouer, S. (1996). Discriminability and perceptual weighting of some acoustic cues to speech perception by 3-year-olds. *Journal of Speech and Hearing Research, 39*(2), 278–297.

Nittrouer, S., & Pennington, B. F. (2010). New approaches to the study of childhood language disorders. *Current Directions in Psychology Science, 19*(5), 308–313.

Norbury, C. F., Gooch, D., Wray, C., Baird, G., Charman, T., Simonoff, E., . . . Pickles, A. (2016). The impact of nonverbal ability on prevalence and clinical presentation of language disorder: Evidence from a population study. *Journal of Child Psychology and Psychiatry, 57*(11), 1247–1257.

Nordahl, C. W., Scholz, R., Yang, X., Buonocore, M. H., Simon, T., Rogers, S., & Amaral, D. G. (2012). Increased rate of amygdala growth in children aged 2 to 4 years with autism spectrum disorders: A longitudinal study. *Archives of General Psychiatry, 69*(1), 53–61.

Nordenbæk, C., Jørgensen, M., Kyvik, K. O., & Bilenberg, N. (2014). A Danish population-based twin study on autism spectrum disorders. *European Child and Adolescent Psychiatry, 23*(1), 35–43.

Nordin, V., & Gillberg, C. (1998). The long-term course of autistic disorders: Update on follow-up studies. *Acta Psychiatrica Scandinavica, 97*(2), 99–108.

Norton, E. S., & Wolf, M. (2012). Rapid automatized naming (RAN) and reading fluency: Implications for understanding and treatment of reading disabilities. *Annual Review of Psychology, 63,* 427–452.

Nusslock, R., Almeida, J. R., Forbes, E. E., Versace, A., Frank, E., Labarbara, E. J., . . . Phillips, M. L. (2012). Waiting to win: Elevated striatal and orbitofrontal cortical activity during reward anticipation in euthymic bipolar disorder adults. *Bipolar Disorders, 14*(3), 249–260.

Nye, C., Foster, S. H., & Seaman, D. (1987). Effectiveness of language intervention with the language/ learning disabled. *Journal of Speech and Hearing Disorders, 52*(4), 348–357.

Odom, S. L., Collet-Klingenberg, L., Rogers, S. J., & Hatton, D. D. (2010). Evidence-based practices in interventions for children and youth with autism spectrum disorders. *Preventing School Failure: Alternative Education for Children and Youth, 54,* 275–282.

Oliver, B. R., & Plomin, R. (2007). Twins' Early Development Study (TEDS): A multivariate, longitudinal genetic investigation of language, cognition and behavior problems from childhood through adolescence. *Twin Research and Human Genetics, 10*(1), 96–105.

O'Reilly, R. C., & Munakata, Y. (2000). *Computational explorations in cognitive neuroscience.* Cambridge, MA: MIT Press.

Orinstein, A. J., Helt, M., Troyb, E., Tyson, K. E.,

Barton, M. L., Eigsti, I.-M., ... Fein, D. A. (2014). Intervention for optimal outcome in children and adolescents with a history of autism. *Journal of Developmental and Behavioral Pediatrics, 35,* 247–256.

O'Roak, B. J., Vives, L., Girirajan, S., Karakoc, E., Krumm, N., Coe, B. P., ... Eichler, E. E. (2012). Sporadic autism exomes reveal a highly interconnected protein network of de novo mutations. *Nature, 485,* 246–250.

Orton, S. T. (1925). "Word-blindness" in school children. *Archives of Neurology and Psychiatry, 14,* 582–615.

Orton, S. T. (1937). *Reading, writing, and speech problems in children.* New York: Norton.

Osterling, J., & Dawson, G. (1994). Early recognition of children with autism: A study of first birthday home videotapes. *Journal of Autism and Developmental Disorders, 24*(3), 247–257.

Osterrieth, P. A. (1944). Le test d'une figure complexe: Contribution à l'étude de la perception et de la mémoire [Test of copying a complex figure: Contribution to the study of perception and memory]. *Archives de Psychologie, 30,* 206–356.

Overtoom, C. C., Verbaten, M. N., Kemner, C., Kenemans, J. L., van Engeland, H., Buitelaar, J. K., ... Koelega, H. S. (2003). Effects of methylphenidate, desipramine, and L-dopa on attention and inhibition in children with attention deficit hyperactivity disorder. *Behavioral Brain Research, 145*(1–2), 7–15.

Oyama, S. (1985). *The ontogeny of information.* Cambridge, UK: Cambridge University Press.

Ozonoff, S., Heung, K., Byrd, R., Hansen, R., & Hertz-Picciotto, I. (2008). The onset of autism: Patterns of symptom emergence in the first years of life. *Autism Research, 1*(6), 320–328.

Ozonoff, S., Iosif, A.-M., Baguio, F., Cook, I. C., Hill, M. M., Hutman, T., ... Young, G. S. (2010). A prospective study of the emergence of early behavioral signs of autism. *Journal of the American Academy of Child and Adolescent Psychiatry, 49,* 256–266.

Ozonoff, S., Iosif, A. M., Young, G. S., Hepburn, S., Thompson, M., Colombi, C., ... Rogers, S. J. (2011). Onset patterns in autism: Correspondence between home video and parent report. *Journal of the American Academy of Child and Adolescent Psychiatry, 50,* 796–806.

Ozonoff, S., Pennington, B. F., & Rogers, S. J. (1991). Executive function deficits in high-functioning autistic individuals: Relationship to theory of mind. *Journal of Child Psychology and Psychiatry, 32*(7), 1081–1105.

Ozonoff, S., Young, G. S., Carter, A., Messinger, D., Yirmiya, N., Zwaigenbaum, L., ... Stone, W. L. (2011). Recurrence risk for autism spectrum disorders: A Baby Siblings Research Consortium study. *Pediatrics, 128,* e488–e495.

Ozonoff, S., Young, G. S., Landa, R. J., Brian, J., Bryson, S., Charman, T., ... Stone, W. L. (2015). Diagnostic stability in young children at risk for autism spectrum disorder: A Baby Siblings Research Consortium study. *Journal of Child Psychology and Psychiatry, 56*(9), 988–998.

Palfrey, J. S., Levine, M. D., Walker, D. K., & Sullivan, M. (1985). The emergence of attention deficits in early childhood: A prospective study. *Journal of Developmental and Behavioral Pediatrics, 6*(6), 339–348.

Panizzon, M. S., Fennema-Notestine, C., Eyler, L. T., Jernigan, T. L., Prom-Wormley, E., Neale, M., ... Franz, C. E. (2009). Distinct genetic influences on cortical surface area and cortical thickness. *Cerebral Cortex, 19*(11), 2728–2735.

Papageorgiou, K. A., Smith, T. J., Wu, R., Johnson, M. H., Kirkham, N. Z., & Ronald, A. (2014). Individual differences in infant fixation duration relate to attention and behavioral control in childhood. *Psychological Science, 25*(7), 1371–1379.

Pappa, I., Fedko, I. O., Mileva-Seitz, V. R., Hottenga, J. J., Bakermans-Kranenburg, M. J., Bartels, M., ... Boomsma, D. I. (2015). Single nucleotide polymorphism heritability of behavior problems in childhood: Genome-wide complex trait analysis. *Journal of the American Academy of Child and Adolescent Psychiatry, 54*(9), 737–744.

Paracchini, S., Thomas, A., Castro, S., Lai, C., Paramasivam, M., Wang, Y., ... Monaco, A. P. (2006). The chromosome 6p22 haplotype associated with dyslexia reduces the expression of KIAA0319, a novel gene involved in neuronal migration. *Human Molecular Genetics, 15*(10), 1659–1666.

Park, C. Y., Halevy, T., Lee, D. R., Sung, J. J., Lee, J. S., Yanuka, O., ... Kim, D. W. (2015). Reversion of FMR1 methylation and silencing by editing the triplet repeats in fragile X iPSC-derived neurons. *Cell, 13,* 234–241.

Parker, S. K., Schwartz, B., Todd, J., & Pickering, L. K. (2004). Thimerosal-containing vaccines and autistic spectrum disorder: A critical review of published original data. *Pediatrics, 114*(3), 793–804.

Patros, C. H., Alderson, R. M., Kasper, L. J., Tarle, S. J., Lea, S. E., & Hudec, K. L. (2016). Choice-impulsivity in children and adolescents with attention-deficit/hyperactivity disorder (ADHD): A meta-analytic review. *Clinical Psychology Review, 43,* 162–174.

Patten, E., Belardi, K., Baranek, G. T., Watson, L. R., Labban, J. D., & Oller, D. K. (2014). Vocal patterns in infants with autism spectrum disorder: Canonical babbling status and vocalization frequency. *Journal of Autism and Developmental Disorders, 44*(10), 2413–2428.

Pattison, L., Crow, Y. J., Deeble, V. J., Jackson, A. P., Jafri, H., Rashid, Y., ... Woods, C. G. (2000). A fifth locus for primary autosomal recessive microcephaly maps to chromosome 1q31. *American Journal of Human Genetics, 67*(6), 1578–1580.

Paulesu, E., Demonet, J. F., Fazio, F., McCrory, E., Chanoine, V., Brunswick, N., ... Frith, U. (2001). Dyslexia: Cultural diversity and biological unity. *Science, 291,* 2165–2167.

Pennington, B. F. (1991). *Diagnosing learning disorders: A neuropsychological framework.* New York: Guilford Press.

Pennington, B. F. (2002). *The development of psychopathology: Nature and nurture.* New York: Guilford Press.

Pennington, B. F. (2006). From single to multiple deficit models of developmental disorders. *Cognition, 101*(2), 385–413.

Pennington, B. F. (2009). *Diagnosing learning disorders,*

second edition: A neuropsychological framework. New York: Guilford Press.

Pennington, B. F. (2011, Winter). Controversial therapies for dyslexia. *Perspectives on Language and Literacy,* pp. 7–8.

Pennington, B. F. (2014). *Explaining abnormal behavior: A cognitive neuroscience perspective..* New York: Guilford Press.

Pennington, B. F. (2015). Atypical cognitive development. In L. S. Liben & U. M. Muller (Eds.), *Handbook of child psychology and developmental science* (7th ed., Vol. 2, pp. 995–1042). Hoboken, NJ: Wiley.

Pennington, B. F., & Bishop, D. V. M. (2009). Relations among speech, language, and reading disorders. *Annual Review of Psychology, 60,* 283–306.

Pennington, B. F., & Lefly, D. L. (2001). Early reading development in children at family risk for dyslexia. *Child Development, 72,* 816–833.

Pennington, B. F., Lefly, D. L., Van Orden, G. C., Bookman, M. O., & Smith, S. D. (1987). Is phonology bypassed in normal or dyslexic development? *Annals of Dyslexia, 37,* 62–89.

Pennington, B. F., McGrath, L. M., Rosenberg, J., Barnard, H., Smith, S. D., Willcutt, E. G., . . . Olson, R. K. (2009). Gene × environment interactions in reading disability and attention-deficit/hyperactivity disorder. *Developmental Psychology, 45*(1), 77–89.

Pennington, B. F., & Olson, R. K. (2005). Genetics of dyslexia. In M. J. Snowling & C. Hulme (Eds.), *The science of reading: A handbook* (pp. 453–472). Oxford, UK: Blackwell.

Pennington, B. F., & Ozonoff, S. (1996). Executive functions and developmental psychopathology. *Journal of Child Psychology and Psychiatry, 37*(1), 51–87.

Pennington, B. F., & Peterson, R. L. (2015). Development of dyslexia. In A. Pollatsek & R. Treiman (Eds.), *The Oxford handbook of reading* (pp. 361–376). New York: Oxford University Press.

Pennington, B. F., Santerre-Lemmon, L., Rosenberg, J., MacDonald, B., Boada, R., Friend, A., . . . Olson, R. K. (2012). Individual prediction of dyslexia by single versus multiple deficit models. *Journal of Abnormal Psychology, 121,* 212–224.

Pennington, B. F., Wallach, L., & Wallach, M. (1980). Non-conserver use and understanding of number and arithmetic. *Genetic Psychology Monographs, 101,* 231–243.

Pennington, B. F., & Welsh, M. C. (1995). Neuropsychology and developmental psychopathology. In D. Cicchetti & D. Cohen (Eds.), *Developmental psychopathology* (Vol. 1, pp. 254–290). New York: Wiley.

Pennington, B. F., Willcutt, E., & Rhee, S. H. (2005). Analyzing comorbidity. *Advances in Child Development and Behavior, 33,* 263–304.

Perfetti, C. A. (1998). Learning to read. In P. Reitsma & L. Verhoeven (Eds.), *Literacy problems and interventions* (pp. 15–48). Dordrect, the Netherlands: Kluwer.

Perrachione, T. K., Del Tufo, S. N., Winter, R., Murtagh, J., Cyr, A., Chang, P., . . . Gabrieli, J. D. (2016). Dysfunction of rapid neural adaptation in dyslexia. *Neuron, 92*(6), 1383–1397.

Peters, S. K., Dunlop, K., & Downar, J. (2016). Cortico–striatal–thalamic loop circuits of the salience network: A central pathway in psychiatric disease and treatment. *Frontiers in Systems Neuroscience, 10,* 104.

Petersen, I. T., Bates, J. E., & Staples, A. D. (2015). The role of language ability and self-regulation in the development of inattentive–hyperactive behavior problems. *Developmental Psychopathology, 27*(1), 221–237.

Peterson, R. L., Boada, R., McGrath, L. M., Willcutt, E. G., Olson, R. K., & Pennington, B. F. (2017). Cognitive prediction of reading, math, and attention: Shared and unique influences. *Journal of Learning Disabilities, 50*(4), 408–421.

Peterson, R. L., McGrath, L. M., Willcutt, E. G., Keenan, J. M., Olson, R. K., & Pennington, B. F. (2018). *Exploring academic g: What does a bifactor modeling approach tell us about the structure of academic skills?* Unpublished manuscript.

Peterson, R. L., Pennington, B. F., & Olson, R. K. (2013). Subtypes of developmental dyslexia: Testing the predictions of the dual-route and connectionist frameworks. *Cognition, 126*(1), 20–38.

Peterson, R. L., Pennington, B. F., Shriberg, L. D., & Boada, R. (2009). What influences literacy outcome in children with speech sound disorder? *Journal of Speech, Language, and Hearing Research, 52,* 1175–1188.

Petrill, S. A., Deater-Deckard, K., Schatschneider, C., & Davis, C. (2005). Measured environmental influences on early reading: Evidence from an adoption study [Special issue]. *Scientific Studies of Reading, 9*(3), 237–259.

Phillips, B. M., & Lonigan, C. J. (2009). Variations in the home literacy environment of preschool children: A cluster analytic approach. *Scientific Studies of Reading, 13*(2), 146–174.

Piaget, J. (1952). *The child's conception of number.* London: Routledge & Kegan Paul.

Picci, G., Gotts, S. J., & Scherf, K. S. (2016). A theoretical rut: Revisiting and critically evaluating the generalized under/over-connectivity hypothesis of autism. *Developmental Science, 19,* 524–549.

Pierce, K., Haist, F., Sedaghat, F., & Courchesne, E. (2004). The brain response to personally familiar faces in autism: Findings of fusiform activity and beyond. *Brain, 127*(12), 2703–2716.

Pierce, K., & Redcay, E. (2008). Fusiform function in children with an autism spectrum disorder is a matter of "who." *Biological Psychiatry, 64*(7), 552–560.

Pinker, S. (1994). *The language instinct.* New York: Morrow.

Pinto-Martin, J. A., Dunkle, M., Earls, M., Fliedner, D., & Landes, C. (2005). Developmental stages of developmental screening: Steps to implementation of a successful program. *American Journal of Public Health, 95*(11), 1928–1932.

Piven, J. (1999). Genetic liability for autism: The behavioural expression in relatives. *International Review of Psychiatry, 11*(4), 299–308.

Piven, J. (2001). The broad autism phenotype: A complementary strategy for molecular genetic studies of autism. *American Journal of Medical Genetics, 105*(1), 34–35.

Platt, M., Adler, W., Mehlhorn, A., Johnson, G., Wright, K., Choi, R., . . . Waye, M. (2013).

Embryonic disruption of the candidate dyslexia susceptibility gene homolog Kiaa0319-like results in neuronal migration disorders. *Neuroscience, 248*, 585–593.

Plaut, D. C., & Kello, C. T. (1999). The emergence of phonology from the interplay of speech comprehension and production: A distributed connectionist approach. In B. MacWhinney (Ed.), *The emergence of language* (pp. 381–416). Mahwah, NJ: Erlbaum.

Pliszka, S. (2007). Practice parameter for the assessment and treatment of children and adolescents with attention-deficit/hyperactivity disorder. *Journal of the American Academy of Child and Adolescent Psychiatry, 46*, 894–921.

Plomin, R., DeFries, J. C., Knopik, V. S., & Neiderhiser, J. M. (2013). *Behavioral genetics* (6th ed.). New York: Worth.

Plomin, R., DeFries, J. C., McClearn, G. E., & Rutter, M. (1997). *Behavioral genetics* (3rd ed.). New York: Freeman.

Plomin, R., Haworth, C. M., Meaburn, E. L., Price, T. S., & Davis, O. S. (2013). Common DNA markers can account for more than half of the genetic influence on cognitive abilities. *Psychological Science, 24*, 562–568.

Plomin, R., & Kovas, Y. (2005). Generalist genes and learning disabilities. *Psychological Bulletin, 131*(4), 592–617.

Pober, B. R. (2010). Williams–Beuren syndrome. *New England Journal of Medicine, 362*, 239–252.

Poeppel, D., Emmorey, K., Hickok, G., & Pylkkanen, L. (2012). Towards a new neurobiology of language. *Journal of Neuroscience, 32*(41), 14125–14131.

Pollatsek, A. (2015). The role of sound in silent reading. In A. Pollatsek & R. Treiman (Eds.), *The Oxford handbook of reading* (pp. 185–201). New York: Oxford University Press.

Polyak, A., Kubina, R. M., & Girirajan, S. (2015). Comorbidity of intellectual disability confounds ascertainment of autism: Implications for genetic diagnosis. *American Journal of Medical Genetics B: Neuropsychiatric Genetics, 168*(7), 600–608.

Pontius, A. A. (1973). Dysfunction patterns analogous to frontal lobe system and caudate nucleus syndromes in some groups of minimal brain dysfunction. *Journal of the American Medical Women's Association, 28*(6), 285–292.

Port, R. (2007). How are words stored in memory?: Beyond phones and phonemes. *New Ideas In Psychology, 25*, 143–170.

Posner, M. I., & Rothbart, M. K. (2000). Developing mechanisms of self-regulation. *Development and Psychopathology, 12*(3), 427–441.

Preston, J. L., Felsenfeld, S., Frost, S. J., Mencl, W. E., Fulbright, R. K., Grigorenko, E. L., . . . Pugh, K. R. (2012). Functional brain activation differences in school-age children with speech sound errors: Speech and print processing. *Journal of Speech, Language, and Hearing Research, 55*(4), 1068–1082.

Preston, J. L., Molfese, P. J., Mencl, W. E., Frost, S. J., Hoeft, F., Fulbright, R. K., . . . Pugh, K. R. (2014). Structural brain differences in school-age children with residual speech sound errors. *Brain and Language, 128*(1), 25–33.

Price, G. R., Palmer, D., Battista, C., & Ansari, D. (2012). Nonsymbolic numerical magnitude comparison: Reliability and validity of different task variants and outcome measures, and their relationship to arithmetic achievement in adults. *Acta Psychologica, 140*(1), 50–57.

Pringle-Morgan, W. (1896). A case of congenital word blindness. *British Medical Journal, 2*(1871), 1378.

Pritchard, A. E., Nigro, C. A., Jacobson, L. A., & Mahone, E. M. (2012). The role of neuropsychological assessment in the functional outcomes of children with ADHD. *Neuropsychology Review, 22*(1), 54–68.

Psychiatric GWAS Consortium Bipolar Disorder Working Group. (2011). Large-scale genome-wide association analysis of bipolar disorder identifies a new susceptibility locus near ODZ4. *Nature Genetics, 43*(10), 977–983.

Pua, E. P. K., Bowden, S. C., & Seal, M. L. (2017). Autism spectrum disorders: Neuroimaging findings from systematic reviews. *Research in Autism Spectrum Disorders, 34*, 28–33.

Puolakanaho, A., Ahonen, T., Aro, M., Eklund, K., Leppanen, P. H., Poikkeus, A. M., . . . Lyytinen, H. (2008). Developmental links of very early phonological and language skills to second grade reading outcomes: Strong to accuracy but only minor to fluency. *Journal of Learning Disabilities, 41*, 353–370.

Purvis, K. L., & Tannock, R. (2000). Phonological processing, not inhibitory control, differentiates ADHD and reading disability. *Journal of the American Academy of Child and Adolescent Psychiatry, 39*, 485–494.

Rabiner, D. L., Malone, P. S., & Conduct Problems Prevention Research Group. (2004). The impact of tutoring on early reading achievement for children with and without attention problems. *Journal of Abnormal Child Psychology, 32*(3), 273–284.

Raichle, M. E., MacLeod, A. M., Snyder, A. Z., Powers, W. J., Gusnard, D. A., & Shulman, G. L. (2001). A default mode of brain function. *Proceedings of the National Academy of Sciences of the USA, 98*(2), 676–682.

Raitano-Lee, N., Pennington, B. F., & Keenan, J. M. (2010). Verbal short-term memory deficits in Down syndrome: Phonological semantic, or both? *Journal of Neurodevelopmental Disorders, 2*, 9–25.

Rakic, P. (1995). A small step for the cell, a giant leap for mankind: A hypothesis of neocortical expansion during evolution. *Trends in Neurosciences, 18*(9), 383–388.

Ramey, S. L., Ramey, C. T., & Lanzi, R. G. (2007). Early intervention: Background, research findings, and future directions. In J. W. Jacobson, J. A. Mulick, & J. Rojahn (Eds.), *Handbook of intellectual and developmental disabilities* (pp. 445–463). New York: Springer.

Ramirez, G., & Beilock, S. L. (2011). Writing about testing worries boosts exam performance in the classroom. *Science, 331*(6014), 211–213.

Ramirez, G., Gunderson, E. A., Levine, S. C., & Beilock, S. L. (2013). Math anxiety, working memory, and math achievement in early elementary school. *Journal of Cognition and Development, 14*(2), 187–202.

Ramus, F. (2003). Developmental dyslexia: Specific phonological deficit or general sensorimotor dysfunction? *Current Opinion in Neurobiology, 13*(2), 212–218.

Rane, P., Cochran, D., Hodge, S. M., Haselgrove, C., Kennedy, D., & Frazier, J. A. (2015). Connectivity in autism: A review of MRI connectivity studies. *Harvard Review of Psychiatry, 23*(4), 223–244.

Raschle, N. M., Chang, M., & Gaab, N. (2011). Structural brain alterations associated with dyslexia predate reading onset. *NeuroImage, 57,* 742–749.

Raschle, N. M., Zuk, J., & Gaab, N. (2012). Functional characteristics of developmental dyslexia in left-hemispheric posterior brain regions predate reading onset. *Proceedings of the National Academy of Sciences of the USA, 109*(6), 2156–2161.

Raznahan, A., Wallace, G. L., Antezana, L., Greenstein, D., Lenroot, R., Thurm, A., . . . Swedo, S. E. (2013). Compared to what?: Early brain overgrowth in autism and the perils of population norms. *Biological Psychiatry, 74*(8), 563–575.

Reardon, S. F., & Portilla, X. A. (2016). Recent trends in income, racial, and ethnic school readiness gaps at kindergarten entry. *AERA Open, 2*(3), 1–18.

Reaven, J., Blakeley-Smith, A., Culhane-Shelburne, K., & Hepburn, S. (2012). Group cognitive behavior therapy for children with high-functioning autism spectrum disorders and anxiety: A randomized trial. *Journal of Child Psychology and Psychiatry and Allied Disciplines, 53,* 410–419.

Redcay, E., & Courchesne, E. (2005). When is the brain enlarged in autism?: A meta-analysis of all brain size reports. *Biological Psychiatry, 58*(1), 1–9.

Redcay, E., Haist, F., & Courchesne, E. (2008). Functional neuroimaging of speech perception during a pivotal period in language acquisition. *Developmental Science, 11*(2), 237–252.

Reed, E. W., & Reed, S. C. (1965). *Mental retardation: A family study.* Philadelphia: Saunders.

Reichow, B., & Volkmar, F. R. (2010). Social skills interventions for individuals with autism: Evaluation for evidence-based practices within a best evidence synthesis framework. *Journal of Autism and Developmental Disorders, 40*(2), 149–166.

Reise, S. P., Widaman, K. F., & Pugh, R. H. (1993). Confirmatory factor analysis and item response theory: Two approaches for exploring measurement invariance. *Psychological Bulletin, 114*(3), 552–566.

Reiss, A. L., Freund, L., Plotnick, L., Baumgardner, T., Green, K., Sozer, A. C., . . . Denckla, M. B. (1993). The effects of X monosomy on brain development: Monozygotic twins discordant for Turner's syndrome. *Annals of Neurology, 34*(1), 95–107.

Reiss, A. L., Mazzocco, M. M., Greenlaw, R., Freund, L. S., & Ross, J. L. (1995). Neurodevelopmental effects of X monosomy: A volumetric imaging study. *Annals of Neurology, 38*(5), 731–738.

Report of the Surgeon General. (1999). Children and mental health. *Mental Health,* pp. 124–194. Available at *https://profiles. nlm.nih.gov/ ps/retrieve/Resource Metadata/NNBBHS.*

Rey, A. (1941). L'examen psychologique dans les cas d'encéphalopathie traumatique: Les problems [The psychological examination in cases of traumatic encepholopathy: Problems]. *Archives de Psychologie, 28,* 215–285.

Reynolds, C. R., & Kamphaus, R. W. (2015). *Behavior Assessment System for Children, Third Edition (BASC-3).* Toronto, ON, Canada: PscyhCorp.

Rhee, S. H., Hewitt, J. K., Corley, R. P., Willcutt, E. G., & Pennington, B. F. (2005). Testing hypotheses regarding the causes of comorbidity: Examining the underlying deficits of comorbid disorders. *Journal of Abnormal Psychology, 114*(3), 346–362.

Ribasés, M., Sánchez-Mora, C., Ramos-Quiroga, J. A., Bosch, R., Gómez, N., Nogueira, M., . . . Gross-Lesch, S. (2012). An association study of sequence variants in the forkhead box P2 (FOXP2) gene and adulthood attention-deficit/hyperactivity disorder in two European samples. *Psychiatric Genetics, 22*(4), 155–160.

Rice, M. L., Wexler, K., & Cleave, P. L. (1995). Specific language impairment as a period of extended optional infinitive. *Journal of Speech and Hearing Research, 38*(4), 850–863.

Richlan, F., Kronbichler, M., & Wimmer, H. (2009). Functional abnormalities in the dyslexic brain: A quantitative meta-analysis of neuroimaging studies. *Human Brain Mapping, 30*(10), 3299–3308.

Rimland, B. (1964). *Infantile autism.* New York: Meredith.

Rimrodt, S. L., Peterson, D. J., Denckla, M. B., Kaufmann, W. E., & Cutting, L. E. (2010). White matter microstructural differences linked to left perisylvian language network in children with dyslexia. *Cortex, 46,* 739–749.

Rindermann, H. (2007). The big G-factor of national cognitive ability. *European Journal of Personality, 21,* 767–787.

Ripke, S., Neale, B. M., Corvin, A., Walters, J. T., Farh, K.-H., Holmans, P. A., . . . Huang, H. (2014). Biological insights from 108 schizophrenia-associated genetic loci. *Nature, 511*(7510), 421–427.

Rippon, G., Brock, J., Brown, C., & Boucher, J. (2007). Disordered connectivity in the autistic brain: Challenges for the "new psychophysiology." *International Journal of Psychophysiology, 63*(2), 164–172.

Roberts, J. E., Rosenfeld, R. M., & Zeisel, S. A. (2004). Otitis media and speech and language: A meta-analysis of prospective studies. *Pediatrics, 113*(3), e238–e248.

Robins, D. L., Casagrande, K., Barton, M., Chen, C.-M. A., Dumont-Mathieu, T., & Fein, D. (2014). Validation of the Modified Checklist for Autism in Toddlers, Revised With Follow-up (M-CHAT-R/F). *Pediatrics, 133,* 37–45.

Robins, S., Ghosh, D., Rosales, N., & Treiman, R. (2014). Letter knowledge in parent–child conversations: Differences between families differing in socio-economic status. *Frontiers in Psychology, 5,* 632.

Robinson, E. B., Koenen, K. C., McCormick, M. C., Munir, K., Hallett, V., Happé, F., . . . Ronald, A. (2012). A multivariate twin study of autistic traits in 12-year-olds: Testing the fractionable autism triad hypothesis. *Behavior Genetics, 42,* 245–255.

Robinson, E. B., Lichtenstein, P., Anckarsäter, H., Happé, F., & Ronald, A. (2013). Examining and interpreting the female protective effect against autistic behavior. *Proceedings of the National Academy of Sciences of the USA, 110,* 5258–5262.

Robinson, E. B., Neale, B. M., & Hyman, S. E. (2015).

Genetic research in autism spectrum disorders. *Current Opinion in Pediatrics, 27*(6), 685–691.

Robison, J. E. (2007). *Look me in the eye: My life with Asperger's syndrome.* New York: Crown.

Rodgers, B. (1983). The identification and prevalence of specific reading retardation. *British Journal of Educational Psychology, 53,* 369–373.

Rogers, S. J., & Pennington, B. F. (1991). A theoretical approach to the deficits in infantile autism. *Development and Psychopathology, 27,* 137–163.

Rommelse, N. N., Franke, B., Geurts, H. M., Hartman, C. A., & Buitelaar, J. K. (2010). Shared heritability of attention-deficit/hyperactivity disorder and autism spectrum disorder. *European Child and Adolescent Psychiatry, 19*(3), 281–295.

Ronald, A., Happé, F., Bolton, P., Butcher, L. M., Price, T. S., Wheelwright, S., . . . Plomin, R. (2006). Genetic heterogeneity between the three components of the autism spectrum: A twin study. *Journal of the American Academy of Child and Adolescent Psychiatry, 45*(6), 691–699.

Ronald, A., Happé, F., & Plomin, R. (2005). The genetic relationship between individual differences in social and nonsocial behaviours characteristic of autism. *Developmental Science, 8*(5), 444–458.

Ronald, A., Happé, F., Price, T. S., Baron-Cohen, S., & Plomin, R. (2006). Phenotypic and genetic overlap between autistic traits at the extremes of the general population. *Journal of the American Academy of Child and Adolescent Psychiatry, 45*(10), 1206–1214.

Ronald, A., & Hoekstra, R. A. (2011). Autism spectrum disorders and autistic traits: A decade of new twin studies. *American Journal of Medical Genetics B: Neuropsychiatric Genetics, 156,* 255–274.

Ronald, A., Larsson, H., Anckarsäter, H., & Lichtenstein, P. (2011). A twin study of autism symptoms in Sweden. *Molecular Psychiatry, 16,* 1039–1047.

Ronemus, M., Iossifov, I., Levy, D., & Wigler, M. (2014). The role of de novo mutations in the genetics of autism spectrum disorders. *Nature Reviews Genetics, 15*(2), 133–141.

Roodenrys, S., Koloski, N., & Grainger, J. (2001). Working memory function in attention deficit hyperactivity disordered and reading disabled children. *British Journal of Developmental Psychology, 19,* 325–337.

Rosenthal, R. H., & Allen, T. W. (1978). An examination of attention, arousal, and learning dysfunctions of hyperkinetic children. *Psychological Bulletin, 85*(4), 689–715.

Rothbart, M. K., & Bates, J. E. (2006). Temperment. In N. Eisenberg (Ed.), *Handbook of child psychology: Vol. 3. Social, emotional, and personality development* (6th ed., pp. 99–166). New York: Wiley.

Rothbart, M. K., Derryberry, D., & Posner, M. I. (1994). A psychobiological approach to the development of temperment. In J. E. Bates & T. D. Wachs (Eds.), *Temperament: Individual differences at the interface of biology and behavior* (pp. 83–116). Washington, DC: American Psychological Association.

Rowe, D. C., Jacobson, K. C., & Van den Oord, E. J. (1999). Genetic and environmental influences on vocabulary IQ: Parental education level as moderator. *Child Development, 70*(5), 1151–1162.

Rubinsten, O., & Tannock, R. (2010). Mathematics anxiety in children with developmental dyscalculia. *Behavioral and Brain Functions, 6*(1), 46.

Rucklidge, J. J., & Tannock, R. (2002). Neuropsychological profiles of adolescents with ADHD: Effects of reading difficulties and gender. *Journal of Child Psychology and Psychiatry, 43*(8), 988–1003.

Ruffino, M., Gori, S., Boccardi, D., Molteni, M., & Facoetti, A. (2014). Spatial and temporal attention in developmental dyslexia. *Frontiers in Human Neuroscience, 8,* 331.

Russell, J. (1997). *Autism as an executive disorder.* New York: Oxford University Press.

Russell, J., Jarrold, C., & Henry, L. (1996). Working memory in children with autism and with moderate learning difficulties. *Journal of Child Psychology and Psychiatry, 37*(6), 673–686.

Rutter, M. (2000). Genetic studies of autism: From the 1970s into the millennium. *Journal of Abnormal Child Psychiatry, 28*(1), 3–14.

Rutter, M. (2006). *Genes and behavior: Nature–nurture interplay explained.* Oxford, UK: Blackwell.

Rutter, M., Andersen-Wood, L., Beckett, C., Bredenkamp, D., Castle, J., Groothues, C., . . . O'Connor, T. G. (1999). Quasi-autistic patterns following severe early global privation: English and Romanian Adoptees (ERA) Study Team. *Journal of Child Psychology and Psychiatry, 40*(4), 537–549.

Rutter, M., Bailey, A., Berument, S. K., Lord, C., & Pickles, A. (2003). *Social Communication Questionnaire (SCQ).* Los Angeles: Western Psychological Services.

Rutter, M., Bailey, A., & Lord, C. (2003). *The social communication questionnaire: Manual.* Los Angeles: Western Psychological Services.

Rutter, M., Beckett, C., Castle, J., Colvert, E., Kreppner, J., Mehta, M., . . . Sonuga-Barke, E. (2007). Effects of profound early institutional deprivation: An overview of findings from a UK longitudinal study of Romanian adoptees. *European Journal of Developmental Psychology, 4*(3), 332–350.

Rutter, M., Caspi, A., Fergusson, D., Horwood, L. J., Goodman, R., Maughan, B., . . . Carroll, J. (2004). Sex differences in developmental reading disability: New findings from 4 epidemiological studies. *Journal of the American Medical Association, 291*(16), 2007–2012.

Rutter, M., & Le Couteur, A. (2003). *The Autism Diagnostic Interview–Revised (ADI-R).* Los Angeles: Western Psychological Services.

Rutter, M., & Mahwood, L. (1991). The long-term psychosocial sequelae of specific developmental disorders of speech and language. In M. Rutter & P. Casaer (Eds.), *Biological risk factors for psychosocial disorders* (pp. 233–259). Cambridge, UK: Cambridge University Press.

Rutter, M., & Quinton, D. (1977). Psychiatric disorders: Ecological factors and concepts of causation. In H. McGurk (Ed.), *Ecological factors in human development* (pp. 173–187). Amsterdam: North-Holland.

Rutter, M., Thorpe, K., Greenwood, R., Northstone, K., & Golding, J. (2003). Twins as a natural experiment to study the causes of mild language delay: I: Design; twin-singleton differences in language, and obstetric risks. *Journal of Child Psychology and Psychiatry, 44*(3), 326–341.

Sacco, R., Gabriele, S., & Persico, A. M. (2015). Head

circumference and brain size in autism spectrum disorder: A systematic review and meta-analysis. *Psychiatry Research: Neuroimaging, 234*(2), 239–251.

Saffran, J. R., Aslin, R. N., & Newport, E. L. (1996). Statistical learning by 8-month-old infants. *Science, 274*(5294), 1926–1928.

Saffran, J. R., Johnson, E. K., Aslin, R. N., & Newport, E. L. (1999). Statistical learning of tone sequences by human infants and adults. *Cognition, 70*(1), 27–52.

Sallows, G. O., & Graupner, T. D. (2005). Intensive behavioral treatment for children with autism: Four-year outcome and predictors. *American Journal of Mental Retardation, 110*(6), 417–438.

Salthouse, T. A. (1991). Age and experience effects on the interpretation of orthographic drawings of three-dimensional objects. *Psychology of Aging, 6*(3), 426–433.

Samocha, K. E., Robinson, E. B., Sanders, S. J., Stevens, C., Sabo, A., McGrath, L. M., . . . Daly, M. J. (2014). A framework for the interpretation of de novo mutation in human disease. *Nature Genetics, 46*, 944–950.

Samyn, V., Roeyers, H., Bijttebier, P., Rosseel, Y., & Wiersema, J. R. (2015). Assessing effortful control in typical and atypical development: Are questionnaires and neuropsychological measures interchangeable?: A latent-variable analysis. *Research in Developmental Disabilities, 36*, 587–599.

Sanders, S. J., Ercan-Sencicek, A. G., Hus, V., Luo, R., Murtha, M. T., Moreno-De-Luca, D., . . . State, M. W. (2011). Multiple recurrent de novo CNVs, including duplications of the 7q11.23 Williams syndrome region, are strongly associated with autism. *Neuron, 70*(5), 863–885.

Sanders, S. J., Murtha, M. T., Gupta, A. R., Murdoch, J. D., Raubeson, M. J., Willsey, A. J., . . . State, M. W. (2012). De novo mutations revealed by whole-exome sequencing are strongly associated with autism. *Nature, 485*, 237–241.

Sandin, S., Hultman, C. M., Kolevzon, A., Gross, R., MacCabe, J. H., & Reichenberg, A. (2012). Advancing maternal age is associated with increasing risk for autism: A review and meta-analysis. *Journal of the American Academy of Child and Adolescent Psychiatry, 51*(5), 477–486.

Sandin, S., Lichtenstein, P., Kuja-Halkola, R., Larsson, H., Hultman, C. M., & Reichenberg, A. (2014). The familial risk of autism. *Journal of the American Medical Association, 311*, 1770–1777.

Sarkar, A., & Cohen Kadosh, R. (2016). Transcranial electrical stimulation and numerical cognition. *Canadian Journal of Experimental Psychology, 70*(1), 41–58.

Scammacca, N., Roberts, G., Vaughn, S., & Stuebing, K. K. (2015). A meta-analysis of interventions for struggling readers in grades 4–12: 1980–2011. *Journal of Learning Disabilities, 48*(4), 369–390.

Scammacca, N., Vaughn, S., Roberts, G., Wanzek, J., & Torgeson, J. K. (2007). *Extensive reading interventions in grades K–3 from research to practice.* Portsmouth, NH: Research Corporation, Center on Instruction.

Scarborough, H. S. (1990). Very early language deficits in dyslexic children. *Child Development, 61*, 1728–1743.

Scarborough, H. S. (1991a). Antecedents to reading disability: Preschool language development and literacy experiences of children from dyslexic families. *Reading and Writing, 3*(3), 219–233.

Scarborough, H. S. (1991b). Early syntactic development of dyslexic children. *Annals of Dyslexia, 41*, 207–220.

Scarborough, H. S. (1998). Early identification of children at risk for reading disabilities: Phonological awareness and some other promising predictors. In B. K. Shapiro, P. J. Accardo, & A. J. Capute (Eds.), *Specific reading disability: A view of the spectrum* (pp. 75–119). Timonium, MD: York Press.

Scarborough, H. S., & Dobrich, W. (1994). On the efficacy of reading to preschoolers. *Developmental Review, 14*(3), 245–302.

Scarborough, H. S., Dobrich, W., & Hager, M. (1991). Preschool literacy experience and later reading achievement. *Journal of Learning Disabilities, 24*, 508–511.

Scarr, S., & McCartney, K. (1983). How people make their own environments: A theory of genotype greater than environment effects. *Child Development, 54*, 424–435.

Scerri, T. S., Macpherson, E., Martinelli, A., Wa, W. C., Monaco, A. P., Stein, J., . . . Snowling, M. J. (2017). The DCDC2 deletion is not a risk factor for dyslexia. *Translational Psychiatry, 7*(7), e1182.

Schachar, R. (2014). Genetics of attention deficit hyperactivity disorder (ADHD): Recent updates and future prospects. *Current Developmental Disorders Reports, 1*(1), 41–49.

Schain, R. J., & Yannet, H. (1960). Infantile autism: An analysis of 50 cases and a consideration of certain relevant neurophysiologic concepts. *Journal of Pediatrics, 57*, 560–567.

Scharff, C., & Haesler, S. (2005). An evolutionary perspective on FoxP2: Strictly for the birds? *Current Opinion in Neurobiology, 15*, 694–703.

Schizophrenia Working Group of the Psychiatric Genomics Consortium. (2014). Biological insights from 108 schizophrenia-associated genetic loci. *Nature, 511*(7510), 421–427.

Schrank, F. A., McGrew, K. S., & Mather, N. (2014a). *Woodcock–Johnson IV Tests of Achievement.* Rolling Meadows, IL: Riverside.

Schrank, F. A., McGrew, K. S., & Mather, N. (2014b). *Woodcock–Johnson IV Tests of Oral Language.* Rolling Meadows, IL: Riverside.

Schrank, F. A., McGrew, K. S., & Mather, N. (2014c). *Woodcock–Johnson IV Tests of Cognitive Abilities.* Rolling Meadows, IL: Riverside.

Schreibman, L., Dawson, G., Stahmer, A. C., Landa, R. J., Rogers, S. J., McGee, G. G., . . . Halladay, A. (2015). Naturalistic developmental behavioral interventions: Empirically validated treatments for autism spectrum disorder. *Journal of Autism and Developmental Disorders, 45*, 2411–2428.

Schumann, C. M., Barnes, C. C., Lord, C., & Courchesne, E. (2009). Amygdala enlargement in toddlers with autism related to severity of social and communication impairments. *Biological Psychiatry, 66*(10), 942–949.

Schumann, C. M., Hamstra, J., Goodlin-Jones, B. L., Lotspeich, L. J., Kwon, H., Buonocore, M. H., . . . Amaral, D. G. (2004). The amygdala is enlarged in children but not adolescents with autism: The hippocampus is enlarged at all ages. *Journal of Neuroscience, 24*(28), 6392–6401.

Schweiger, J. I., & Meyer-Lindenberg, A. (2017). Common variation in the GTF2I gene: A promising neurogenetic mechanism for affiliative drive and social anxiety. *Biological Psychiatry, 81*(3), 175–176.

Sebat, J., Lakshmi, B., Malhotra, D., Troge, J., Lese-Martin, C., Walsh, T., . . . Wigler, M. (2007). Strong association of de novo copy number mutations with autism. *Science, 316*(5823), 445–449.

Sekar, A., Bialas, A. R., de Rivera, H., Davis, A., Hammond, T. R., Kamitaki, N., . . . McCarroll, S. A. (2016). Schizophrenia risk from complex variation of complement component 4. *Nature, 530*(7589), 177–183.

Selkirk, C. G., Veach, P. M., Lian, F., Schimmenti, L., & LeRoy, B. S. (2009). Parents' perceptions of autism spectrum disorder etiology and recurrence risk and effects of their perceptions on family planning: Recommendations for genetic counselors. *Journal of Genetic Counseling, 18*(5), 507–519.

Semel, E., Wiig, E. H., & Secord, W. A. (2003). *Clinical Evaluation of Language Fundamentals–Fourth Edition*. San Antonio, TX: Psychological Corporation.

Semrud-Clikeman, M., Biederman, J., Sprich-Buckminster, S., Lehman, B. K., Faraone, S. V., & Norman, D. (1992). Comorbidity between attention deficit hyperactivity disorder and learning disability: A review and report in a clinically referred sample. *Journal of the American Academy of Child and Adolescent Psychiatry, 31*(3), 439–448.

Semrud-Clikeman, M., Filipek, P. A., Biederman, J., Steingard, R., Kennedy, D., Renshaw, P., & Bekken, K. (1994). Attention-deficit hyperactivity disorder: Magnetic resonance imaging morphometric analysis of the corpus callosum. *Journal of the American Academy of Child and Adolescent Psychiatry, 33*(6), 875–881.

Sénéchal, M. (2015). Young children's home literacy. In A. Pollatsek & R. Treiman (Eds.), *The Oxford handbook of reading* (pp. 397–414). New York: Oxford University Press.

Sexton, C. C., Gelhorn, H. L., Bell, J. A., & Classi, P. M. (2012). The co-occurrence of reading disorder and ADHD: Epidemiology, treatment, psychosocial impact, and economic burden. *Journal of Learning Disabilities, 45*(6), 538–564.

Shalev, R. S., & Gross-Tsur, V. (2001). Developmental dyscalculia. *Pediatric Neurology, 24*(5), 337–342.

Shallcross, R., Bromley, R. L., Irwin, B., Bonnett, L., Morrow, J., & Baker, G. (2011). Child development following in utero exposure: Levetiracetam vs sodium valproate. *Neurology, 76*(4), 383–389.

Shallice, T. (1988). *From neuropsychology to mental structure*. New York: Cambridge University Press.

Shanahan, M. A., Pennington, B. F., Yerys, B. E., Scott, A., Boada, R., Willcutt, E. G., . . . DeFries, J. C. (2006). Processing speed deficits in attention deficit/hyperactivity disorder and reading disability. *Journal of Abnormal Child Psychology, 34*(5), 585–602.

Shattuck, P. T. (2006). The contribution of diagnostic substitution to the growing administrative prevalence of autism in US special education. *Pediatrics, 117*, 1028–1037.

Shatz, C. J. (1992). The developing brain. *Scientific American, 267*(3), 60–67.

Shaw, P., Eckstrand, K., Sharp, W., Blumenthal, J., Lerch, J. P., Greenstein, D., . . . Rapoport, J. L. (2007). Attention-deficit/hyperactivity disorder is characterized by a delay in cortical maturation. *Proceedings of the National Academy of Sciences of the USA, 104*, 19649–19654.

Shaw, P., Greenstein, D., Lerch, J., Clasen, L., Lenroot, R., Gogtay, N., . . . Giedd, J. (2006). Intellectual ability and cortical development in children and adolescents. *Nature, 440*(7084), 676–679.

Shaw, P., Lerch, J., Greenstein, D., Sharp, W., Clasen, L., Evans, A., . . . Rapoport, J. (2006). Longitudinal mapping of cortical thickness and clinical outcome in children and adolescents with attention-deficit/hyperactivity disorder. *Archives of General Psychiatry, 63*(5), 540–549.

Shaw, P., Sudre, G., Wahton, A., Weingart, D., Sharp, W., & Sarlis, J. (2015). White matter microstructure and the variable adult outcome of childhood attention deficit hyperactivity disorder. *Neuropharmacology, 40*(3), 746–754.

Shaywitz, S. (2003). *Overcoming dyslexia: A new and complete science-based program for reading problems at any level*. New York: Knopf.

Shaywitz, S. E., Escobar, M. D., Shaywitz, B. A., Fletcher, J. M., & Makuch, R. (1992). Evidence that dyslexia may represent the lower tail of a normal distribution of reading ability. *New England Journal of Medicine, 326*, 145–150.

Shaywitz, S. E., Shaywitz, B. A., Fletcher, J. M., & Escobar, M. D. (1990). Prevalence of reading disability in boys and girls: Results of the Connecticut Longitudinal Study. *Journal of the American Medical Association, 264*(8), 998–1002.

Sherman, E., & Brooks, B. (2015). *Memory Validity Profile (MVP)*. Lutz, FL: Psychological Assessment Resources.

Shneidman, L. A., Arroyo, M. E., Levine, S. C., & Goldin-Meadow, S. (2013). What counts as effective input for word learning? *Journal of Child Language, 40*(3), 672–686.

Shneidman, L. A., & Goldin-Meadow, S. (2012). Language input and acquisition in a Mayan village: How important is directed speech? *Developmental Science, 15*(5), 659–673.

Shotwell, A. M., & Shipe, D. (1964). Effect of out-of-home care on the intellectual and social development of mongoloid children. *American Journal of Mental Deficiency, 90*, 693–699.

Shrank, F. A., McGrew, K. S., & Mather, N. (2014). *Woodcock-Johnson IV*. Rolling Meadows, IL: Riverside.

Shriberg, L. D., Aram, D. M., & Kwiatkowski, J. (1997). Developmental apraxia of speech: I. Descriptive and theoretical perspectives. *Journal of Speech, Language, and Hearing Research, 40*(2), 273–285.

Shriberg, L. D., Tomblin, J. B., & McSweeny, J. L. (1999). Prevalence of speech delay in 6-year-old children and comorbidity with language impairment. *Journal of Speech Language and Hearing Research, 42*(6), 1461–1481.

Siegel, L. S. (1992). An evaluation of the discrepancy definition of dyslexia. *Journal of Learning Disabilities, 25*(10), 618–629.

Siegler, R. S., & Booth, J. L. (2004). Development of

numerical estimation in young children. *Child Development, 75,* 428–444.

Silani, G., Frith, U., Demonet, J. F., Fazio, F., Perani, D., Price, C., . . . Paulesu, E. (2005). Brain abnormalities underlying altered activation in dyslexia: A voxel based morphometry study. *Brain, 128,* 2453–2461.

Simms, V., Gilmore, C., Sloan, S., & McKeaveney, C. (2017). Interventions to improve mathematics achievement in primary school-aged children: A systematic review. Retrieved from *https://campbellcollaboration.org/library/improving-mathematics-achievement-primary-school-children.html*.

Simonoff, E., Pickles, A., Charman, T., Chandler, S., Loucas, T., & Baird, G. (2008). Psychiatric disorders in children with autism spectrum disorders: Prevalence, comorbidity, and associated factors in a population-derived sample. *Journal of the American Academy of Child and Adolescent Psychiatry, 47*(8), 921–929.

Simonoff, E., Taylor, E., Baird, G., Bernard, S., Chadwick, O., Liang, H., . . . Sharma, S. P. (2013). Randomized controlled double-blind trial of optimal dose methylphenidate in children and adolescents with severe attention deficit hyperactivity disorder and intellectual disability. *Journal of Child Psychology and Psychiatry, 54*(5), 527–535.

Simons, D. J., Boot, W. R., Charness, N., Gathercole, S. E., Chabris, C. F., Hambrick, D. Z., & Stine-Morrow, E. A. (2016). Do "brain-training" programs work? *Psychological Science in the Public Interest, 17*(3), 103–186.

Sims, D. M., & Lonigan, C. J. (2013). Inattention, hyperactivity, and emergent literacy: Different facets of inattention relate uniquely to preschoolers' reading-related skills. *Journal of Clinical Child and Adolescent Psychology, 53*(42), 208–219.

Sing, C. F., & Reilly, S. L. (1993). Genetics of common diseases that aggregate, but do not segregate in families. In C. F. Sing & C. L. Hanis (Eds.), *Genetics of cellular, individual, family and population variability* (pp. 140–161). New York: Oxford University Press.

Singer, H. S., Reiss, A. L., Brown, J. E., Aylward, E. H., Shih, B., Chee, E., . . . et al. (1993). Volumetric MRI changes in basal ganglia of children with Tourette's syndrome. *Neurology, 43*(5), 950–956.

Sirin, S. R. (2005). Socioeconomic status and academic achievement: A meta-analytic review of research. *Review of Educational Research, 75*(3), 417–453.

Sjowall, D., Roth, L., Lindqvist, S., & Thorell, L. B. (2013). Multiple deficits in ADHD: Executive dysfunction, delay aversion, reaction time variability, and emotional deficits. *Journal of Child Psychology and Psychiatry, 54*(6), 619–627.

Skinner, B. F. (1957). *Verbal behavior.* New York: Appleton-Century-Crofts.

Skuse, D. H., Mandy, W. P. L., & Scourfield, J. (2005). Measuring autistic traits: Heritability, reliability and validity of the Social and Communication Disorders Checklist. *British Journal of Psychiatry, 187*(6), 568–572.

Slot, E. M., van Viersen, S., de Bree, E. H., & Kroesbergen, E. H. (2016). Shared and unique risk factors underlying mathematical disability and reading and spelling disability. *Frontiers in Psychology, 7,* 803.

Smith, L. S., Roberts, J. A., Locke, J. L., & Tozer, R. (2010). An exploratory study of the development of early syllable structure in reading impaired children. *Journal of Learning Disabilities, 43*(4), 294–307.

Smith, S. D., Gilger, J. W., & Pennington, B. F. (2001). Dyslexia and other specific learning disorders. In D. L. Rimoin, J. M. Conner, & R. E. Pyeritz (Eds.), *Emery and Rimoin's principles and practice of medical genetics* (pp. 2827–2865). New York: Churchill Livingstone.

Smith, S. D., Pennington, B. F., Boada, R., & Shriberg, L. D. (2005). Linkage of speech sound disorder to reading disability loci. *Journal of Child Psychology and Psychiatry, 46*(10), 1057–1066.

Smoller, J. W. (2013a). Disorders and borders: Psychiatric genetics and nosology. *American Journal of Medical Genetics B: Neuropsychiatric Genetics, 162*(7), 559–578.

Smoller, J. W. (2013b). Identification of risk loci with shared effects on five major psychiatric disorders: A genome-wide analysis. *Lancet, 381,* 1371–1379.

Snow, C. E., Burns, M. S., & Griffin, P. (1998). *Preventing reading difficulties in young children.* Washington, DC: National Academy Press.

Snowball, A., Tachtsidis, I., Popescu, T., Thompson, J., Delazer, M., Zamarian, L., . . . Kadosh, R. C. (2013). Long-term enhancement of brain function and cognition using cognitive training and brain stimulation. *Current Biology, 23*(11), 987–992.

Snowling, M. J., Bishop, D. V. M., & Stothard, S. E. (2000). Is preschool language impairment a risk factor for dyslexia in adolescence? *Journal of Child Psychology and Psychiatry, 41*(5), 587–600.

Snowling, M. J., Gallagher, A., & Frith, U. (2003). Family risk of dyslexia is continuous: Individual differences in the precursors of reading skill. *Child Development, 74,* 358–373.

Snowling, M. J., & Hulme, C. (2011). Evidence-based interventions for reading and language difficulites: Creating a virtuous circle. *British Journal of Educational Psychology, 81,* 1–23.

Snowling, M. J., & Melby-Lervåg, M. (2016). Oral language deficits in familial dyslexia: A meta-analysis and review. *Psychological Bulletin, 142*(5), 498–545.

Söderqvist, S., Nutley, S. B., Ottersen, J., Grill, K. M., & Klingberg, T. (2012). Computerized training of non-verbal reasoning and working memory in children with intellectual disability. *Frontiers in Human Neuroscience, 6,* 271.

Sonuga-Barke, E. J., Brandeis, D., Cortese, S., Daley, D., Ferrin, M., Holtmann, M., . . . Döpfner, M. (2013). Nonpharmacological interventions for ADHD: Systematic review and meta-analyses of randomized controlled trials of dietary and psychological treatments. *American Journal of Psychiatry, 170*(3), 275–289.

Sonuga-Barke, E. J., Daley, D., Thompson, M., Laver-Bradbury, C., & Weeks, A. (2001). Parent-based therapies for preschool attention-deficit/hyperactivity disorder: A randomized, controlled trial with a community sample. *Journal of the American Academy of Child and Adolescent Psychiatry, 40,* 402–408.

Sonuga-Barke, E. J., Taylor, E., Sembi, S., & Smith, J. (1992). Hyperactivity and delay aversion–I. The effect of delay on choice. *Journal of Child Psychology and Psychiatry, 33*(2), 387–398.

Sonuga-Barke, E. J., Thompson, M., Abikoff, H., Klein, R., & Brotman, L. M. (2006). Nonpharmacological interventions for preschoolers with ADHD: The case for specialized parent training. *Infants and Young Children, 19,* 142–153.

South, M., Ozonoff, S., & McMahon, W. M. (2005). Repetitive behavior profiles in Asperger syndrome and high-functioning autism. *Journal of Autism and Developmental Disorders, 35*(2), 145–158.

Sparks, B., Friedman, S., Shaw, D., Aylward, E., Echelard, D., Artru, A., . . . Dawson, G. (2002). Brain structural abnormalities in young children with autism spectrum disorder. *Neurology, 59*(2), 184–192.

Sparrow, S. S., Cicchetti, D. V., & Saulnier, C. A. (2016). *Vineland Adaptive Behavior Scales–Third Edition (Vineland-3)*. Toronto, ON, Canada: PsychCorp.

Specific Language Impairment Consortium. (2002). A genomewide scan identifies two novel loci involved in specific language impairment. *American Journal of Human Genetics, 70*(2), 384–398.

Specific Language Impairment Consortium. (2004). Highly significant linkage to the SLI1 locus in an expanded sample of individuals affected by specific language impairment. *American Journal of Human Genetics, 74*(6), 1225–1238.

Sporns, O., & Zwi, J. D. (2004). The small world of the cerebral cortex. *Neuroinformatics, 2*(2), 145–162.

Squire, L. R. (1987). *Memory and brain.* New York: Oxford University Press.

Stamm, J. S., & Kreder, S. V. (1979). Minimal brain dysfunction: Psychological and neuropsychological disorders in hyperkinetic children. In M. S. Gazzaniga (Ed.), *Handbook of behavioral neurology: Vol. 2. Neuropsychology* (pp. 119–150). New York: Plenum Press.

Stancliffe, R. J., & Keane, S. (2000). Outcomes and costs of community living: A matched comparison of group homes and semi-independent living. *Journal of Intellectual and Developmental Disability, 25*(4), 281–305.

Stanford Center on Longevity. (2014). A consensus on the brain training industry from the scientific community. Retrieved from http://longevity3.stanford.edu/blog/ 2014/10/15/the- consensus-on-the- brain-training- industry-from- the-scientific- community.

Stanovich, K. E. (1986). Matthew effects in reading: Some consequences of individual differences in the acquisition of literacy. *Reading Research Quarterly, 21,* 360–406.

Stanovich, K. E. (2005). The future of a mistake: Will discrepancy measurement continue to make the learning disabilities field a pseudoscience? *Learning Disability Quarterly, 28*(2), 103–106.

Starkey, G. S., & McCandliss, B. D. (2014). The emergence of "groupitizing" in children's numerical cognition. *Journal of Experimental Child Psychology, 126,* 120–137.

Starkey, P., & Cooper, R. G. (1980). Perception of numbers by human infants. *Science, 210*(4473), 1033–1035.

Starkey, P., & Cooper, R. G. (1995). The development of subitizing in young children. *British Journal of Developmental Psychology, 13*(4), 399–420.

Stein, C. M., Millard, C., Kluge, A., Miscimarra, L. E., Cartier, K. C., Freebairn, L. A., . . . Iyengar, S. K. (2006). Speech sound disorder influenced by a locus in 15q14 region. *Behavior Genetics, 36*(6), 858–868.

Stein, C. M., Schick, J. H., Taylor, H., Shriberg, L. D., Millard, C., Kundtz-Kluge, A., . . . Iyengar, S. K. (2004). Pleiotropic effects of a chromosome 3 locus on speech-sound disorder and reading. *American Journal of Human Genetics, 74*(2), 283–297.

Stern, D. N. (1985). *The interpersonal world of the infant: A view from psychoanalysis and developmental psychology.* New York: Basic Books.

Stiles, J., Brown, T. T., Haist, F., & Jernigan, T. L. (2015). Brain and cognitive development. In L. S. Liben & R. M. Lerner (Eds.), *Handbook of child psychology and developmental science* (pp. 9–62). Hoboken, NJ: Wiley.

Stiles, J., Reilly, J. S., Levine, S. C., & Trauner, D. A. (2012). *Neural plasticity and cognitive development: Insights from children with perinatal brain injury.* New York: Oxford University Press.

Still, G. F. (1902). Some abnormal psychical conditions in children. *Lancet, 1,* 1008–1012, 1077–1082, 1163–1168.

Stoodley, C. J. (2015). The role of the cerebellum in developmental dyslexia. In P. Mariën & M. Manto (Eds.), *The linguistic cerebellum* (pp. 199–222). London: Academic Press.

Stothard, S. E., Snowling, M. J., Bishop, D. V. M., Chipchase, B. B., & Kaplan, C. A. (1998). Language-impaired preschoolers: A follow-up into adolescence. *Journal of Speech, Language, and Hearing Research, 41*(2), 407–418.

Stratton, K., Gable, A., McCormick, M. C., & Institute of Medicine Immunization Safety Review Committee. (2001). *Immunization Safety Review: Thimerosal-containing vaccines and neurodevelopmental disorders.* Washington, DC: National Academies Press.

Strauss, A., & Lehtinen, L. (1947). *Psychopathology and education of the brain-injured child.* New York: Grune & Stratton.

Stuebing, K. K., Barth, A. E., Molfese, P. J., Weiss, B., & Fletcher, J. M. (2009). IQ is not strongly related to response to reading instruction: A meta-analytic interpretation. *Exceptional Child, 76,* 31–51.

Stuebing, K. K., Barth, A. E., Trahan, L. H., Reddy, R. R., Miciak, J., & Fletcher, J. M. (2015). Are child cognitive characteristics strong predictors of responses to intervention?: A meta-analysis. *Review of Educational Research, 85*(3), 395–429.

Stuebing, K. K., Fletcher, J. M., Branum-Martin, L., & Francis, D. J. (2012). Evaluation of the technical adequacy of three methods for identifying specific learning disabilities based on cognitive discrepancies. *School Psychology Review, 41*(1), 3–22.

Stuebing, K. K., Fletcher, J. M., LeDoux, J. M., Lyon, G. R., Shaywitz, S. E., & Shaywitz, B. A. (2002). Validity of IQ-discrepancy classifications of reading disabilities: A meta-analysis. *American Educational Research Journal, 39*(2), 469–518.

Stuss, D. T., & Benson, D. F. (1986). *The frontal lobes.* New York: Raven Press.

Sullivan, E. L., Holton, K. F., Nousen, E. K., Barling, A. N., Sullivan, C. A., Propper, C. B., & Nigg, J.

T. (2015). Early identification of ADHD risk via infant temperament and emotion regulation: A pilot study. *Journal of Child Psychology and Psychiatry, 56*(9), 949–957.

Sullivan, M., Finelli, J., Marvin, A., Garrett-Mayer, E., Bauman, M., & Landa, R. J. (2007). Response to joint attention in toddlers at risk for autism spectrum disorder: A prospective study. *Journal of Autism and Developmental Disorders, 37*(1), 37–48.

Sullivan, P. F., Daly, M. J., & O'Donovan, M. (2012). Genetic architectures of psychiatric disorders: The emerging picture and its implications. *Nature Reviews Genetics, 13*(8), 537–551.

Sullivan, P. F., Magnusson, C., Reichenberg, A., Boman, M., Dalman, C., Davidson, M., . . . Långström, N. (2012). Family history of schizophrenia and bipolar disorder as risk factors for autism. *Archives of General Psychiatry, 69*(11), 1099–1103.

Supekar, K., Iuculano, T., Chen, L., & Menon, V. (2015). Remediation of childhood math anxiety and associated neural circuits through cognitive tutoring. *Journal of Neuroscience, 35*(36), 12574–12583.

Sur, M., & Rubenstein, J. L. (2005). Patterning and plasticity of the cerebral cortex. *Science, 310*(5749), 805–810.

Suskind, D. L., Leffel, K. R., Graf, E., Hernandez, M. W., Gunderson, E. A., Sapolich, S. G., . . . Levine, S. C. (2016). A parent-directed language intervention for children of low socioeconomic status: A randomized controlled pilot study. *Journal of Child Language, 43*(2), 366–406.

Swanson, H., Mink, J., & Bocian, K. (1999). Cognitive processing deficits in poor readers with symptoms of reading disabilities and ADHD: More alike than different? *Journal of Educational Psychology, 91*, 321–333.

Swanson, J. (2011). Strengths and Weaknesses of ADHD-Symptoms and Normal-Behavior Rating Scale (SWAN). Retrieved from www.attentionpoint. com/x_upload/ media/images/swan- description-questions.pdf.

Sylva, K., Scott, S., Totsika, V., Ereky-Stevens, K., & Crook, C. (2008). Training parents to help their children read: A randomized control trial. *British Journal of Educational Psychology, 78*, 435–455.

Szalkowski, C. E., Booker, A. B., Truong, D. T., Threlkeld, S. W., Rosen, G. D., & Fitch, R. H. (2013). Knockdown of the candidate dyslexia susceptibility gene homolog Dyx1c1 in rodents: Effects on auditory processing, visual attention, and cortical and thalamic anatomy. *Developmental Neuroscience, 35*(1), 50–68.

Tager-Flusberg, H., & Kasari, C. (2013). Minimally verbal school-aged children with autism spectrum disorder: The neglected end of the spectrum. *Autism Research, 6*(6), 468–478.

Tallal, P., & Piercy, M. (1973). Developmental aphasia: Impaired rate of nonverbal processing as a function of sensory modality. *Neuropsychologia, 11*, 389–398.

Tamnes, C. K., Fjell, A. M., Westlye, L. T., Østby, Y., & Walhovd, K. B. (2012). Becoming consistent: Developmental reductions in intraindividual variability in reaction time are related to white matter integrity. *Journal of Neuroscience, 32*(3), 972–982.

Tanaka, H., Black, J. M., Hulme, C., Stanley, L. M., Kessler, S. R., Whitfield-Gabrieli, S., et al. (2011). The brain basis of the phonological deficit in dyslexia is independent of IQ. *Psychological Science, 22*(11), 1442–1451.

Tannock, R. (2013). Rethinking ADHD and LD in DSM-5: Proposed changes in diagnostic criteria. *Journal of Learning Disabilities, 46*(1), 5–25.

Tannock, R., Martinussen, R., & Frijters, J. (2000). Naming speed performance and stimulant effects indicate effortful, semantic processing deficits in attention-deficit/hyperactivity disorder. *Journal of Abnormal Child Psychology, 28*(3), 237–252.

Taylor, L. E., Swerdfeger, A. L., & Eslick, G. D. (2014). Vaccines are not associated with autism: An evidence-based meta-analysis of case-control and cohort studies. *Vaccine, 32*(29), 3623–3629.

Terband, H., Maassen, B., Guenther, F. H., & Brumberg, J. (2014). Auditory–motor interactions in pediatric motor speech disorders: Neurocomputational modeling of disordered development. *Journal of Communication Disorders, 47*, 17–33.

Terband, H., van Brenk, F., & van Doornik-van der Zee, A. (2014). Auditory feedback perturbation in children with developmental speech sound disorders. *Journal of Communication Disorders, 51*, 64–77.

Thapar, A., Cooper, M., Eyre, O., & Langley, K. (2013). Practitioner Review: What have we learnt about the causes of ADHD? *Journal of Child Psychology and Psychiatry, 54*(1), 3–16.

Thompson, D. W. (1917). *On growth and form*. Cambridge, UK: Cambridge University Press.

Thompson, L. A., Detterman, D. K., & Plomin, R. (1991). Associations between cognitive abilities and scholastic achievement: Genetic overlap but environmental differences. *Psychological Science, 2*, 158–165.

Thorpe, K., Rutter, M., & Greenwood, R. (2003). Twins as a natural experiment to study the causes of mild language delay: II. Family interaction risk factors. *Journal of Child Psychology and Psychiatry, 44*(3), 342–355.

Tick, B., Bolton, P., Happé, F., Rutter, M., & Rijsdijk, F. (2016). Heritability of autism spectrum disorders: A meta-analysis of twin studies. *Journal of Child Psychology and Psychiatry and Allied Disciplines, 57*, 585–595.

Tiffin-Richards, M., Hasselhorn, M., Woerner, W., Rothenberger, A., & Banaschewski, T. (2008). Phonological short-term memory and central executive processing in attention-deficit/hyperactivity disorder with/without dyslexia—evidence of cognitive overlap. *Journal of Neural Transmission, 115*(2), 227–234.

Todorovski, Z., Asrar, S., Liu, J., Saw, N. M., Joshi, K., Cortez, M. A., . . . Jia, Z. (2015). LIMK1 regulates long-term memory and synaptic plasticity via the transcriptional factor CREB. *Molecular and Cellular Biology, 35*(8), 1316–1328.

Tomasello, M., & Brooks, P. J. (1999). Early syntactic development: A construction grammar approach. In M. Barrett (Ed.), *The development of language* (pp. 161–190). New York: Psychology Press.

Tombaugh, T. N. (1996). *Test of Memory Malingering: TOMM*. North Tonawanda, NY: Multi-Health Systems.

Tomblin, J. B., Records, N. L., Buckwalter, P., Zhang,

X., Smith, E., & O'Brien, M. (1997). Prevalence of specific language impairment in kindergarten children. *Journal of Speech, Language, and Hearing Research, 40*(6), 1245–1260.

Tomblin, J. B., Smith, E., & Zhang, X. (1997). Epidemiology of specific language impairment: Prenatal and perinatal risk factors. *International Journal of Language and Communication Disorders, 30*(4), 325–343; quiz 343–344.

Tomson, T., Battino, D., Bonizzoni, E., Craig, J., Lindhout, D., Sabers, A., . . . EURAP Study Group. (2011). Dose-dependent risk of malformations with antiepileptic drugs: An analysis of data from the EURAP epilepsy and pregnancy registry. *Lancet Neurology, 10*(7), 609–617.

Toplak, M. E., West, R. F., & Stanovich, K. E. (2013). Practitioner Review: Do performance-based measures and ratings of executive function assess the same construct? *Journal of Child Psychology and Psychiatry, 54*(2), 131–143.

Torgesen, J. K. (2005). Recent discoveries on remedial interventions for children with dyslexia. In M. J. Snowling & C. Hulme (Eds.), *The science of reading: A handbook* (pp. 521–537). Malden, MA: Blackwell.

Torgesen, J. K., Wagner, R. K., & Rashotte, C. A. (2012). *Test of Word Reading Efficiency–Second Edition (TOWRE-2)*. Austin, TX: PRO-ED.

Torppa, M., Lyytinen, P., Erskine, J., Eklund, K., & Lyytinen, H. (2010). Language development, literacy skills, and predictive connections to reading in Finnish children with and without familial risk for dyslexia. *Journal of Learning Disabilities, 43*, 308–321.

Tosto, M. G., Petrill, S. A., Halberda, J., Trzaskowski, M., Tikhomirova, T. N., Bogdanova, O. Y., . . . Kovas, Y. (2014). Why do we differ in number sense?: Evidence from a genetically sensitive investigation. *Intelligence, 43*, 35–46.

Trevarthen, C. (1979). Communication and cooperation in early infancy: A description of primary intersubjectivity. In M. Bullowa (Ed.), *Before speech: The beginning of human communication* (pp. 321–347). London: Cambridge University Press.

Trzaskowski, M., Davis, O. S., DeFries, J. C., Yang, J., Visscher, P. M., & Plomin, R. (2013). DNA evidence for strong genome-wide pleiotropy of cognitive and learning abilities. *Behavior Genetics, 43*(4), 267–273.

Turken, U., Whitfield-Gabrieli, S., Bammer, R., Baldo, J. V., Dronkers, N. F., & Gabrieli, J. D. (2008). Cognitive processing speed and the structure of white matter pathways: Convergent evidence from normal variation and lesion studies. *NeuroImage, 42*(2), 1032–1044.

Turkheimer, E., Haley, A., Waldron, M., D'Onofrio, B., & Gottesman, I. I. (2003). Socioeconomic status modifies heritability of IQ in young children. *Psychological Science, 14*(6), 623–628.

Uddin, L. Q., Supekar, K., & Menon, V. (2013). Reconceptualizing functional brain connectivity in autism from a developmental perspective. *Frontiers in Human Neuroscience, 7*, 1–11.

Ukrainetz, T. A., Ross, C. L., & Harm, H. M. (2009). An investigation of treatment scheduling for phonemic awareness with kindergartners who are at risk for reading difficulties. *Language, Speech, and Hearing Services in Schools, 40*(1), 86–100.

Ullman, M. T., & Pierpont, E. I. (2005). Specific language impairment is not specific to language: The procedural deficit hypothesis. *Cortex, 41*(3), 399–433.

Ullman, M. T., & Pullman, M. Y. (2015). A compensatory role for declarative memory in neurodevelopmental disorders. *Neuroscience and Behavioral Reviews, 51*, 205–222.

Ulrich, D. A., Lloyd, M. C., Tiernan, C. W., Looper, J. E., & Angulo-Barroso, R. M. (2008). Effects of intensity of treadmill training on developmental outcomes and stepping in infants with Down syndrome: A randomized trial. *Physical Therapy, 88*(1), 114–122.

van Bergen, E., van Zuijen, T., Bishop, D., & de Jong, P. F. (2017). Why are home literacy environment and children's reading skills associated?: What parental skills reveal. *Reading Research Quarterly, 52*(2), 147–160.

Van Den Heuvel, C., Thornton, E., & Vink, R. (2007). Traumatic brain injury and Alzheimer's disease: A review. *Progress in Brain Research, 161*, 303–316.

van den Heuvel, M. P., Stam, C. J., Kahn, R. S., & Hulshoff Pol, H. E. (2009). Efficiency of functional brain networks and intellectual performance. *Journal of Neuroscience, 29*(23), 7619–7624.

van der Maas, H. L., Dolan, C. V., Grasman, R. P., Wicherts, J. M., Huizenga, H. M., & Raijmakers, M. E. (2006). A dynamical model of general intelligence: The positive manifold of intelligence by mutualism. *Psychological Review, 113*(4), 842–861.

van Ewijk, H., Heslenfeld, D. J., Zwiers, M. P., Buitelaar, J. K., & Oosterlaan, J. (2012). Diffusion tensor imaging in attention deficit/hyperactivity disorder: A systematic review and meta-analysis. *Neuroscience and Biobehavioral Reviews, 36*(4), 1093–1106.

van Lieshout, M., Luman, M., Buitelaar, J., Rommelse, N., & Oosterlaan, J. (2013). Does neurocognitive functioning predict future or persistence of ADHD?: A systematic review. *Clinical Psychology Review, 33*(4), 539–560.

Van Orden, G. C., Pennington, B. F., & Stone, G. O. (2001). What do double dissociations prove? *Cognitive Science, 25*, 111–172.

van Steensel, F. J., Bögels, S. M., & Perrin, S. (2011). Anxiety disorders in children and adolescents with autistic spectrum disorders: A meta-analysis. *Clinical Child and Family Psychology Review, 14*(3), 302–317.

Vande Voort, J. L., He, J. P., Jameson, N. D., & Merikangas, K. R. (2014). Impact of the DSM-5 attention-deficit/hyperactivity disorder age-of-onset criterion in the US adolescent population. *Journal of the American Academy of Child and Adolescent Psychiatry, 53*(7), 736–744.

Vargha-Khadem, F., Gadian, D. G., Watkins, K. E., Connelly, A., Van Paesschen, W., & Mishkin, M. (1997). Differential effects of early hippocampal pathology on episodic and semantic memory. *Science, 277*(5324), 376–380.

Vasa, R. A., Mostofsky, S. H., & Ewen, J. B. (2016). The disrupted connectivity hypothesis of autism spectrum disorders: Time for the next phase in research. *Biological Psychiatry: Cognitive Neuroscience and Neuroimaging, 1*(3), 245–252.

Vaughn, S., Denton, C. A., & Fletcher, J. M. (2010). Why intensive interventions are necessary for students with severe reading difficulties. *Psychology in the Schools, 47*(5), 432–444.

Vaughn, S., Linan-Thompson, S., Kouzeanani, K., Bryant, D. P., Dickson, S., & Blozis, S. A. (2003). Reading instruction grouping for students with reading difficulties. *Remediation Research Quarterly, 24,* 301–315.

Velleman, S. L., & Mervis, C. B. (2011). Children with 7q11.23 duplication syndrome: Speech, language, cognitive, and behavioral characteristics and their implications for intervention. *Perspectives in Language and Learning Education, 18*(3), 108–116.

Vellutino, F. R. (1979a). *Dyslexia: Theory and research.* Cambridge, MA: MIT Press.

Vellutino, F. R. (1979b). The validity of perceptual deficit explanations of reading disability: A reply to Fletcher and Satz. *Journal of Learning Disabilities, 12*(3), 160–167.

Vellutino, F. R., Scanlon, D. M., Small, S. G., & Fanuele, D. P. (2006). Response to intervention as a vehicle for distinguishing between children with and without reading disabilities: Evidence for the role of kindergarten and first-grade interventions. *Journal of Learning Disabilities, 39,* 157–169.

Vicari, S. (2004). Memory development and intellectual disabilities. *Acta Paediatrica Supplement, 93*(445), 60–63; discussion 63–64.

Virues-Ortega, J., Julio, F. M., & Pastor-Barriuso, R. (2013). The TEACCH program for children and adults with autism: A meta-analysis of intervention studies. *Clinical Psychology Review, 33*(8), 940–953.

Vissers, M. E., Cohen, M. X., & Geurts, H. M. (2012). Brain connectivity and high functioning autism: A promising path of research that needs refined models, methodological convergence, and stronger behavioral links. *Neuroscience and Biobehavioral Reviews, 36*(1), 604–625.

Volkmar, F., Siegel, M., Woodbury-Smith, M., King, B., McCracken, J., & State, M. (2014). Practice parameter for the assessment and treatment of children and adolescents with autism spectrum disorder. *Journal of the American Academy of Child and Adolescent Psychiatry, 53,* 237–257.

Volkow, N. D., Fowler, J. S., Wang, G., Ding, Y., & Gatley, S. J. (2002). Mechanism of action of methylphenidate: Insights from PET imaging studies. *Journal of Attention Disorders, 6*(Suppl. 1), S31–S43.

Volkow, N. D., Wang, G. J., Tomasi, D., Kollins, S. H., Wigal, T. L., Newcorn, J. H., . . . Swanson, J. M. (2012). Methylphenidate-elicited dopamine increases in ventral striatum are associated with long-term symptom improvement in adults with attention deficit hyperactivity disorder. *Journal of Neuroscience, 32*(3), 841–849.

Vorstman, J. A., Parr, J. R., Moreno-De-Luca, D., Anney, R. J., Nurnberger, J. I., Jr., & Hallmayer, J. F. (2017). Autism genetics: Opportunities and challenges for clinical translation. *Nature Reviews Genetics, 18,* 362–376.

Vygotsky, L. S. (1979). *Mind in society: The development of high mental processes.* Cambridge, MA: Harvard University Press.

Vysniauske, R., Verburgh, L., Oosterlaan, J., & Molendijk, M. L. (2016). The effects of physical exercise on functional outcomes in the treatment of ADHD: A meta-analysis. *Journal of Attention Disorders.* [Epub ahead of print]

Wadsworth, S. J., Corley, R., Hewitt, J., & DeFries, J. (2001). Stability of genetic and environmental influences on reading performance at 7, 12, and 16 years of age in the Colorado Adoption Project. *Behavior Genetics, 31*(4), 353–359.

Wadsworth, S. J., DeFries, J. C., Fulker, D. W., & Plomin, R. (1995). Cognitive ability and academic achievement in the Colorado Adoption Project: A multivariate genetic analysis of parent–offspring and sibling data. *Behavior Genetics, 25*(1), 1–15.

Wadsworth, S. J., DeFries, J. C., Willcutt, E. G., Pennington, B. F., & Olson, R. K. (2015). The Colorado Longitudinal Twin Study of Reading Difficulties and ADHD: Etiologies of comorbidity and stability. *Twin Research and Human Genetics, 18*(6), 755–761.

Wadsworth, S. J., Olson, R. K., & DeFries, J. C. (2010). Differential genetic etiology of reading difficulties as a function of IQ: An update. *Behavior Genetics, 40,* 751–758.

Wagner, R. K., Puranik, C. S., Foorman, B., Foster, E., Wilson, L. G., Tschinkel, E., & Kantor, P. T. (2011). Modeling the development of written language. *Reading and Writing, 24*(2), 203–220.

Wagner, R. K., & Torgesen, J. K. (1987). The nature of phonological processing and its causal role in the acquisition of reading skills. *Psychological Bulletin, 101,* 192–212.

Wagner, R. K., Torgesen, J. K., Rashotte, C. A., & Pearson, N. A. (2013). *Comprehensive Test of Phonological Processing: CTOPP2.* Austin, TX: PRO-ED.

Wahlsten, D. (2012). The hunt for gene effects pertinent to behavioral traits and psychiatric disorders: From mouse to human. *Developmental Psychobiology, 54,* 475–492.

Wallace, G. L., Yerys, B. E., Peng, C., Dlugi, E., Anthony, L. G., & Kenworthy, L. (2016). Assessment and treatment of executive function impairments in autism spectrum disorder. *International Review of Research in Developmental Disabilities, 51,* 85–122.

Walley, A. C. (1993). The role of vocabulary development in children's spoken word recognition and segmentation ability. *Developmental Review, 13,* 286–350.

Wang, P., Lin, M., Pedrosa, E., Hrabovsky, A., Zhang, Z., Guo, W., . . . Zheng, D. (2015). CRISPR/Cas9-mediated heterozygous knockout of the autism gene CHD8 and characterization of its transcriptional networks in neurodevelopment. *Molecular Autism, 6,* 55.

Waschbusch, D. A. (2002). A meta-analytic examination of comorbid hyperactive–impulsive–attention problems and conduct problems. *Psychological Bulletin, 128*(1), 118–150.

Watson, L. R. (1998). Following the child's lead: Mothers' interactions with children with autism. *Journal of Autism and Developmental Disorders, 28,* 51–59.

Weber, A., Fernald, A., & Diop, Y. (2017). When cultural norms discourage talking to babies: Effectiveness of a parenting program in rural Senegal. *Child Development, 88*(5), 1513–1526.

Wechsler, D. (1997a). *Wechsler Adult Intelligence Scale–Third Edition: Administration and scoring manual*. San Antonio, TX: Psychological Corporation.

Wechsler, D. (1997b). *Wechsler Intelligence Scale for Children–Third Edition*. San Antonio, TX: Psychological Corporation.

Wechsler, D. (2003). *WISC-IV: Technical and interpretive manual*. San Antonio, TX: Psychological Corporation.

Wechsler, D. (2008). *Wechsler Adult Intelligence Scale–Fourth Edition: Technical and interpretive manual*. San Antonio, TX: Psychological Corporation.

Wechsler, D. (2011). *Wechsler Abbreviated Scale of Intelligence–Second Edition (WASI-II)*. San Antonio, TX: Psychological Corporation.

Wechsler, D. (2012). *Wechsler Preschool And Primary Scale of Intelligence–Fourth Edition (WPPSI-IV)*. San Antonio, TX: Psychological Corporation.

Wechsler, D. (2014). *Wechsler Intelligence Scale for Children–Fifth Edition (WISC-V): Technical and interpretive manual*. Bloomington, MN: Pearson Clinical Assessment.

Weiler, M. D., Bernstein, J. H., Bellinger, D. C., & Waber, D. P. (2000). Processing speed in children with attention deficit/hyperactivity disorder, inattentive type. *Child Neuropsychology, 6*(3), 218–234.

Weisleder, A., & Fernald, A. (2013). Talking to children matters: Early language experience strengthens processing and builds vocabulary. *Psychological Science, 24*(11), 2143–2152.

Werker, J. F., & Tees, R. C. (1984). Cross-language speech-perception—evidence for perceptual reorganization during the first year of life. *Infant Behavior and Development, 7*, 49–63.

West, G., Vadillo, M. A., Shanks, D. R., & Hulme, C. (2018). The procedural learning deficit hypothesis of language learning disorders: We see some problems. *Developmental Science, 21*(2), 1–13.

Westby, C. E., & Cutler, S. K. (1994). Language and ADHD: Understanding the bases and treatment of self-regulatory deficits. *Topics in Language Disorders, 14*(4), 58–76.

Westermann, G., & Miranda, E. R. (2004). A new model of sensorimotor coupling in the development of speech. *Brain and Language, 89*, 393–400.

White, K. R. (1982). The relation between socioeconomic status and academic achievement. *Psychological Bulletin, 91*(3), 461–481.

White, S. W., Oswald, D., Ollendick, T., & Scahill, L. (2009). Anxiety in children and adolescents with autism spectrum disorders. *Clinical Psychology Review, 29*, 216–229.

Whitelaw, C., Flett, P., & Amor, D. J. (2007). Recurrence risk in autism spectrum disorder: A study of parental knowledge. *Journal of Paediatrics and Child Health, 43*(11), 752–754.

Wiederholt, J., & Bryant, B. R. (2013). *Gray Oral Reading Test–Fifth Edition*. Austin, TX: Psychological Corporation.

Wiig, E. H., Semel, E., & Secord, W. A. (2013). *Clinical Evaluation of Language Fundamentals–Fifth Edition (CELF-5)*. Bloomington, MN: NCS Pearson.

Wilder, R. L. (1968). *Evolution of mathematical concepts*. New York: Wiley.

Wilkinson, G. S., & Robertson, G. J. (2006). *Wide Range Achievement Test–Revision 4*. Wilmington, DE: Jastak Associates.

Willcutt, E. (2014). Behavioral genetic approaches to understand the etiology of comorbidity. In S. H. Rhee & A. Ronald (Eds.), *Behavior genetics of psychopathology* (pp. 231–252). New York: Springer.

Willcutt, E. G., Betjemann, R. S., McGrath, L. M., Chhabildas, N. A., Olson, R. K., DeFries, J. C., & Pennington, B. F. (2010). Etiology and neuropsychology of comorbidity between RD and ADHD: The case for multiple-deficit models. *Cortex, 46*(10), 1345–1361.

Willcutt, E. G., Boada, R., Riddle, M. W., Chhabildas, N., DeFries, J. C., & Pennington, B. F. (2011). Colorado Learning Difficulties Questionnaire: Validation of a parent-report screening measure. *Psychological Assessment, 23*(3), 778–791.

Willcutt, E. G., Nigg, J. T., Pennington, B. F., Solanto, M. V., Rohde, L. A., Tannock, R., . . . Lahey, B. B. (2012). Validity of DSM-IV attention deficit/hyperactivity disorder symptom dimensions and subtypes. *Journal of Abnormal Psychology, 121*(4), 991–1010.

Willcutt, E. G., & Pennington, B. F. (2000a). Comorbidity of reading disability and attention-deficit/hyperactivity disorder: Differences by gender and subtype. *Journal of Learning Disabilities, 33*(2), 179–191.

Willcutt, E. G., & Pennington, B. F. (2000b). Psychiatric comorbidity in children and adolescents with reading disability. *Journal of Child Psychology and Psychiatry, 41*, 1039–1048.

Willcutt, E. G., Pennington, B. F., Boada, R., Ogline, J. S., Tunick, R. A., Chhabildas, N. A., & Olson, R. K. (2001). A comparison of the cognitive deficits in reading disability and attention-deficit/hyperactivity disorder. *Journal of Abnormal Psychology, 110*(1), 157–172.

Willcutt, E. G., Pennington, B. F., & DeFries, J. C. (2000). Twin study of the etiology of comorbidity between reading disability and attention-deficit/hyperactivity disorder. *American Journal of Medical Genetics, 96*(3), 293–301.

Willcutt, E. G., Pennington, B. F., Olson, R. K., Chhabildas, N. A., & Hulslander, J. L. (2005). Neuropsychological analyses of comorbidity between reading disability and attention deficit hyperactivity disorder: In search of the common deficit. *Developmental Neuropsychology, 27*, 35–78.

Willcutt, E. G., Pennington, B. F., Olson, R. K., & DeFries, J. C. (2007). Understanding comorbidity: A twin study of reading disability and attention deficit/hyperactivity disorder. *American Journal of Medical Genetics B: Neuropsychiatric Genetics, 144*(6), 709–714.

Willcutt, E. G., Pennington, B. F., Smith, S. D., Cardon, L. R., Gayan, J., Knopik, V. S., . . . DeFries, J. C. (2002). Quantitative trait locus for reading disability on chromosome 6p is pleiotropic for attention-deficit/hyperactivity disorder. *American Journal of Medical Genetics, 114*(3), 260–268.

Willcutt, E. G., Petrill, S. A., Wu, S., Boada, R., DeFries, J. C., Olson, R. K., & Pennington, B. F.

(2013). Implications of comorbidity between reading and math disability: Neuropsychological and functional impairment. *Journal of Learning Disabilities, 46*(6), 500–516.

Willcutt, E. G., Sonuga-Barke, E. J., Nigg, J. T., & Sergeant, J. A. (2008). Developments in neuropsychological models of childhood psychiatric disorders. In T. Banaschewski & L. A. Rohde (Eds.), *Advances in biological psychiatry* (Vol. 24, pp. 195–226). Basel, Switzerland: Karger.

Williams, G., King, J., Cunningham, M., Stephan, M., Kerr, B., & Hersh, J. H. (2001). Fetal valproate syndrome and autism: Additional evidence of an association. *Developmental Medicine and Child Neurology, 43*(3), 202–206.

Williams, K. T. (2007). *Expressive Vocabulary Test–Second Edition*. Minneapolis, MN: Pearson Assessments.

Willsey, A. J., & State, M. W. (2015). Autism spectrum disorders: From genes to neurobiology. *Current Opinion in Neurobiology, 30,* 92–99.

Wing, L. (1991). The relationship between Asperger's syndrome and Kanner's autism. In U. Frith (Ed.), *Autism and Asperger syndrome* (pp. 93–121). New York: Cambridge University Press.

Wise, B. W., Ring, J., & Olson, R. K. (2000). Individual differences in gains from computer-assisted remedial reading. *Journal of Experimental Child Psychology, 77*(3), 197–235.

Wolf, M., & Bowers, P. G. (1999). The double-deficit hypothesis for the developmental dyslexias. *Journal of Educational Psychology, 91,* 415–438.

Wolraich, M., Brown, L., Brown, R. T., DuPaul, G. J., Earls, M. F., Feldman, H. M., . . . Visser, S. (2011). ADHD: Clinical practice guideline for the diagnosis, evaluation, and treatment of attention-deficit/hyperactivity disorder in children and adolescents. *Pediatrics, 128,* 1007–1022.

Wolraich, M., Lambert, E. W., Baumgaertel, A., Garcia-Tornel, S., Feurer, I. D., Bickman, L., & Doffing, M. A. (2003). Teachers' screening for attention deficit/hyperactivity disorder: Comparing multinational samples on teacher ratings of ADHD. *Journal of Abnormal Child Psychology, 31*(4), 445–455.

Wolraich, M., Lambert, W., Doffing, M. A., Bickman, L., Simmons, T., & Worley, K. (2003). Psychometric properties of the Vanderbilt ADHD diagnostic Parent Rating Scale in a referred population. *Journal of Pediatric Psychology, 28*(8), 559–568.

Woo, Y. J., Wang, T., Guadalupe, T., Nebel, R. A., Vino, A., Del Bene, V. A., . . . Fisher, S. E. (2016). A common CYFIP1 variant at the 15q11.2 disease locus is associated with structural variation at the language-related left supramarginal gyrus. *PLOS ONE, 11*(6), e0158036.

Wood, C. L., Warnell, F., Johnson, M., Hames, A., Pearce, M. S., McConachie, H., & Parr, J. R. (2015). Evidence for ASD recurrence rates and reproductive stoppage from large UK ASD research family databases. *Autism Research, 8*(1), 73–81.

Woodbury-Smith, M., Klin, A., & Volkmar, F. (2005). Asperger's syndrome: A comparison of clinical diagnoses and those made according to the ICD-10 and DSM-IV. *Journal of Autism and Developmental Disorders, 35*(2), 235–240.

Wright, C. A., Kaiser, A. P., Reikowsky, D. I., & Roberts, M. Y. (2013). Effects of a naturalistic sign intervention on expressive language of toddlers with Down syndrome. *Journal of Speech, Language, and Hearing Research, 56*(3), 994–1008.

Wu, J., Looper, J., Ulrich, B. D., Ulrich, D. A., & Angulo-Barroso, R. M. (2007). Exploring effects of different treadmill interventions on walking onset and gait patterns in infants with Down syndrome. *Developmental Medicine and Child Neurology, 49*(11), 839–945.

Wynn, K. (1992). Addition and subtraction by human infants. *Nature, 358*(6389), 749–750.

Wynn, K. (1998). Psychological foundations of number: Numerical competence in human infants. *Trends in Cognitive Science, 2,* 296–303.

Xiao, Y., Friederici, A. D., Margulies, D. S., & Brauer, J. (2016). Longitudinal changes in resting-state fMRI from age 5 to age 6 years covary with language development. *NeuroImage, 128,* 116–124.

Yang, J., Benyamin, B., McEvoy, B. P., Gordon, S., Henders, A. K., Nyholt, D. R., . . . Visscher, P. M. (2010). Common SNPs explain a large proportion of the heritability for human height. *Nature Genetics, 42,* 565–569.

Yang, J., Lee, S. H., Goddard, M. E., & Visscher, P. M. (2011). GCTA: A tool for genome-wide complex trait analysis. *American Journal of Human Genetics, 88*(1), 76–82.

Yeates, K. O. (2010). Traumatic brain injury. In K. O. Yeates, M. D. Ris, H. G. Taylor, & B. F. Pennington (Eds.), *Pediatric neuropsychology* (pp. 112–146). New York: Guilford Press.

Yerys, B. E., & Herrington, J. D. (2014). Multimodal imaging in autism: An early review of comprehensive neural circuit characterization. *Current Psychiatry Reports, 16*(11), 496.

Yirmiya, N., & Charman, T. (2010). The prodrome of autism: Early behavioral and biological signs, regression, peri- and post-natal development and genetics. *Journal of Child Psychology and Psychiatry and Allied Disciplines, 51,* 432–458.

Yoder, P. J., & Warren, S. F. (2002). Effects of prelinguistic milieu teaching and parent responsivity education on dyads involving children with intellectual disabilities. *Journal of Speech, Language, and Hearing Research, 45*(6), 1158–1174.

Yoder, P. J., Woynaroski, T., Fey, M., & Warren, S. (2014). Effects of dose frequency of early communication intervention in young children with and without Down syndrome. *American Journal on Intellectual and Developmental Disabilities, 119*(1), 17–32.

Yoshimasu, K., Barbaresi, W. J., Colligan, R. C., Killian, J. M., Voigt, R. G., Weaver, A. L., & Katusic, S. K. (2011). Written-language disorder among children with and without ADHD in a population-based birth cohort. *Pediatrics, 128*(3), e605–e612.

Young, C. B., Wu, S. S., & Menon, V. (2012). The neurodevelopmental basis of math anxiety. *Psychological Science, 23*(5), 492–501.

Zametkin, A. J., & Rapoport, J. L. (1986). The pathophysiology of attention deficit disorders. In B. B. Lahey & A. E. Kadzin (Eds.), *Advances in clinical child psychology* (pp. 177–216). New York: Plenum Press.

Zaric, G., González, G. F., Tijms, J., van der Molen, M. W., Blomert, L., & Bonte, M. (2014). Reduced neural integration of letters and speech sounds in dyslexic children scales with individual differences in reading fluency. *PLOS ONE, 9*(10), e110337.

Zelazo, P. D. (2006). The Dimensional Change Card Sort (DCCS): A method of assessing executive function in children. *Nature Protocols, 1*(1), 297.

Zemunik, T., & Boraska, V. (2011). Genetics of type I diabetes. In D. Wagner (Ed.), *Type I diabetes–Pathogenesis, genetics, and immunotherapy* (pp. 529–548). London: InTech Open.

Zheng, X., Flynn, L. J., & Swanson, H. L. (2013). Experimental intervention studies on word problem solving and math disabilities: A selective analysis of the literature. *Learning Disability Quarterly, 36*(2), 97–111.

Ziegler, J. C., Bertrand, D., Toth, D., Csepe, V., Reis, A., Faisca, L., . . . Blomert, L. (2010). Orthographic depth and its impact on universal predictors of reading: A cross-language investigation. *Psychological Science, 21,* 551–559.

Zorzi, M., Barbiero, C., Facoetti, A., Lonciari, I., Carrozzi, M., Montico, M., . . . Ziegler, J. C. (2012). Extra-large letter spacing improves reading in dyslexia. *Proceedings of the National Academy of Sciences of the USA, 109,* 11455–11459.

Zuijen, T. L., Plakas, A., Maassen, B. A., Maurits, N. M., & Leij, A. (2013). Infant ERPs separate children at risk of dyslexia who become good readers from those who become poor readers. *Developmental Science, 16*(4), 554–563.

Zwaigenbaum, L. (2015). Early identification of autism spectrum disorder: Recommendations for practice and research. *Pediatrics, 136*(Suppl. 1), S10–S40.

Zwaigenbaum, L., Bauman, M. L., Choueiri, R., Kasari, C., Carter, A., Granpeesheh, D., . . . Natowicz, M. R. (2015). Early intervention for children with autism spectrum disorder under 3 years of age: Recommendations for practice and research. *Pediatrics, 136,* S60–S81.

Zwaigenbaum, L., Bryson, S., & Garon, N. (2013). Early identification of autism spectrum disorders. *Behavioural Brain Research, 251,* 133–146.

Zwaigenbaum, L., Bryson, S., Rogers, T., Roberts, W., Brian, J., & Szatmari, P. (2005). Behavioral manifestations of autism in the first year of life. *International Journal of Developmental Neuroscience, 23*(2), 143–152.

Index

Note. *f* or *t* following a page number indicates a figure or a table.

Academic achievement, country differences in, 98–99
Academic *g*, cognitive *g* and, 48–49
Academic skills
   automatic, 70
   complex *versus* basic, 70–71
   development of, 69–70
   individual *versus* group differences in, 94–95
   "simple" models of, 70–71, 71*t*
   tests of, 88*t*
Acalculia, subtypes of, 192–193
ACE model of gene–environment interplay, 17–18, 103–104
Achievement gaps, 93–107
   and analysis of group differences, 95–97, 95*f*
   country differences and, 95*f*, 97–99, 97*f*
   evidence for, 101–102
   individual *versus* group differences and, 94–95
   policy implications, 105–106
   racial/ethnic differences and, 100–101
   reasons for, 102–105
   sex differences and, 99–100
   socioeconomic status and, 100–101
   studies of, 101–102
Acquired lesions, brain plasticity and, 33–37
Adaptive functioning, tests of, 88*t*
ADHD: *see* Attention-deficit/hyperactivity disorder (ADHD)
Age discrepancy, specific learning disorder and, 73–74

Alzheimer's disease, genetic variants and, 21, 22*f*
American Association on Intellectual and Developmental Disabilities (AAIDD), 314
Amygdala, acquired lesions in, 36
Anarithmetia, primary, 192, 202
Anxiety disorders, ASD and, 266–267
Aphasia, Wernicke–Lichtheim–Geschwind model and, 133
APOE-4 risk variant, Alzheimer's disease and, 21
Applied behavior analysis (ABA), for intellectual disability, 338
Approximate number sense
   heritability of, 206–208
   in infants, 197
Approximate relative numerosity, 192
ASD + ADHD comorbidity, neuroimaging studies of, 63
Asperger, H., 260–262
Asperger syndrome, 262
   DSM-5 and, 263
Assessment, 77–92
   common quandaries and confusions, 89–92
      etiology, 89–90
      severity, 90–91
      specificity, 91–92
   common tests used in, 87*t*–89*t*
   holistic approach to, 79
   HOT mnemonic and, 79
   observations in, 81–82
   overall approach to, 78–79

Assessment *(cont.)*
  patient history in, 79–81
  test results in, 82–89
    base-rate variability, 86
    battery selection, 85–86
    performance validity, 82–85
Atomoxetine (Straterra), for ADHD, 232
Attention
  early development of, 225–226
  tests of, 87t–88t
Attention-deficit/hyperactivity disorder (ADHD), 217–257
  adult-onset controversy and, 222
  behavior rating scales and, 243
  behavioral observations, 242–243
  brain mechanisms, 217–218, 219, 230–235
    neuroimaging of, 233–235
    transmitters, 231–233
  case presentation 6, 243–244, 245t–246t, 246–247
  case presentation 7, 247–248, 249t–250t, 250
  chapter summary, 217–218
  cognitive predictors, 217
  cognitive risk factors, 51t
  comorbidities, 223–224
    with ASD, 220–221
    with dyslexia, 157, 163
    with ID, 317
    with mathematics disorder, 191, 209–210, 211t–212t, 212–213
  country differences in, 221–222
  definitions, 220–221
  development
    early, 224–227
    later, 227–230
  developmental neuropsychology, 224–230
    early development, 224–227
    later development, 227–230
  diagnosis, 218, 241–243
  in DSM-5, 56, 219, 220–221
  environmental influences, 240
  etiology, 218, 236–241
    familiality in, 236
    G × E interactions in, 240–241
    gene identification in, 237–240
    heritability in, 236–237
  genetic influences, 219
  genetic overlap with dyslexia, 10
  GWAS and, 237–238
  history, 218–219, 241–242
  molecular genetics studies of, 60–61
  neuroimaging phenotype of, 40t
  presenting symptoms, 241
  prevalence and epidemiology, 221–224
  processing speed in, 65
  single-deficit theories of, 227–228
  sluggish cognitive tempo and, 221
  speech and language disorders and, 111, 238
  subtypes, 220–221
  summary table, 256t–257t
  symptoms of, in intellectual disability, 237
  treatment, 218, 219, 250–255
    lifestyle changes in, 254–255
    medications in, 231–232, 251–253
    with neurofeedback, 254
    psychosocial therapies in, 251–252
Autism spectrum disorder (ASD), 258–311
  assessment tools, 292–294
  brain imaging studies of, 259
  brain mechanisms, 271–278
    connectivity, 276–278
    functional findings, 274–276
    structural findings, 272–274
  case presentation 8, 294–295, 296t–297t, 297–299
  case presentation, 9, 299–300, 301t–302t, 302–305
  chapter summary, 258–260
  cognitive risk factors for, 51t
  comorbidities, 220–221, 266–267
  contemporary view, 262
  definition, 262–264
  developmental neuropsychology, 267–271
    fractionable autism triad hypothesis, 269, 282
    longitudinal high-risk studies, 270–271
    neuropsychological theories, 268–269
  diagnosis, 289–294
  etiology, 278–289
    environmental influences, 286–289
    familiality, 278–280
    gene findings, 283–286
    heritability, 280–283
  genetic analysis in, 19, 259–260
  history, 260–262
  lack of evidence for vaccine causation, 289
  language impairments in, 120
  molecular genetics studies of, 60–61
  multiple-deficit theories of, 12, 258
  mutation–selection model and, 20–21
  neuroimaging phenotype of, 40t, 272–278
  neuropsychological studies of, 42, 267–271

versus PLI, 114
    prevalence and epidemiology, 265–267
    psychoanalytic view of, 261–262
    public awareness of, 260
    "refrigerator" mother theory, 261–262
    regressive effects in, 259
    restricted, repetitive behaviors and, 263–264, 267–269, 274–275
    screening/early identification, 289–290
    social cognition in, 41–42, 268, 270–271
    speech and language disorders and, 111
    summary table, 310*t*–311*t*
    treatment, 305–309
Automaticity, in complex nonacademic skills, 70

B

Babbling, infant, 122
    delayed onset of, 112, 128
    speech development and, 123–126
Basal ganglia, acquired lesions in, 36
Behavior
    genetic *versus* environmental factors in, 16
    neurodevelopmental disorders and, 8, 8*f*
    proximal causes of, 15
    species-typical, 15
Behavioral genetics
    in etiology of RD, 171–172
    in etiology of RD + ADHD, 59–60
    in etiology studies, 16–17
Behavioral observations
    in ADHD, 242–243
    in assessment, 81–82
    in autism spectrum disorder, 292
    in dyslexia, 177–178
    in intellectual disability, 328
    in language impairment, 144–145
    in math disability, 209
    in speech and language disorders, 144–145
    in speech sound disorder, 145
Behaviorism, language development and, 120
Brain development
    atypical, 25, 26*t*, 27–28
    cognitive development and, 37–39
    connectionist models of, 37–39
    connectivity analyses of, 28–29
    neurodevelopmental disorders and, 8, 8*f*
    and proximal causes of behavior, 15
    stages of, 25–28, 26*t*
    summary, 26*t*

Brain mechanisms, 24–40; *see also* Brain-behavior development models; Pathophysiology of learning disorders
    connectivity studies of, 276–278
    generalist genes hypothesis and, 62–64
    in ADHD, 217–218, 230–235
        fMRI studies of, 234–235
        neuroimaging studies of, 233–235
        neurotransmitters, 231–233
    in ASD, 271–278
    in Down syndrome, 320
    in dyslexia, 169–170
    in Fragile X syndrome, 322–323
    future directions for analysis, 345
    in mathematics disorder, 191, 201–204
    neuroimaging studies of, 136–137
    in speech and language development, 132–137
    in speech disorders, 112
    in Williams syndrome, 324
    structural versus functional connectivity in, 28–29
Brain plasticity, 24
    acquired lesions and, 33–37
    limits on, 34–37
    and models of brain-behavior development, 30–37
    neurodevelopmental disorders and, 6–7
    sign language acquisition and, 136
    variations in, 40
Brain-behavior development models, 29–37
    brain plasticity in, 30–37
    comparing/contrasting, 30–33
    connectivity analyses and, 28
    interactive specialization model, 29, 31–33 (*see also* Interactive specialization model)
    maturational model, 29–30
    neocortical specialization in, 31–33
    predictive significance of, 33
    skill learning model, 30, 32
Brain-behavior problem, theoretical gaps in, 42
Broca's aphasia, 133
Buck v. Bell, 314

C

Calculation
    automaticity in, 70
    development of, 198–199

Candidate gene association studies, of ADHD, 239
Case presentations
  for ADHD, 243–250
  for ASD, 294–305
  for intellectual disability, 328–335
  for language impairment (LI), 145–149
  for mathematics disorder, 209–213
  for reading disability, 178–186
  for speech and language disorders, 145–152
  for speech sound disorder, 149–152
Categorical disorders, 14
CHD8 gene, in ASD, 285–286
Childhood apraxia of speech (CAS), 15, 112
  babbling in, 128–129
  deficit in, 118
  familiality of, 137–138
  gene mutation in, 112–113
  genetic factors in, 138–139
  presenting symptoms, 143
  versus SSD, 114–115
Chomsky, N., language development theory of, 118, 120–121, 123, 127
CNTNAP2 gene, 16
Cognitive constructs
  neuropsychology and, 50–51
  versus psychometric constructs, 48t
Cognitive deficits, general *versus* specific, 48–49
Cognitive development
  comparisons of models, 29–33
  connectionist models of, 37–39
  functional networks and, 38–39
  integration with brain development, 37–39
  memory systems in, 5
Cognitive g, academic g and, 48–49
Cognitive processing, types of, 37–38
Cognitive risk factors, 51, 51t
Cognitive skills, individual *versus* group differences in, 94–95
Cognitive-behavioral therapy (CBT), for intellectual disability, 337–338
Cognitive-deficit model, single *versus* multiple, 11, 201, 224, 345
Communication
  nonhuman, 117–118
  nonverbal, 122–123
Comorbidity, 54–68; *see also* RD + ADHD comorbidity
  ADHD and, 219, 221, 223–224, 229, 238, 243, 247, 250, 251, 255, 256t
  ASD, 264, 266–267, 268, 274, 310t
  current study limitations, 55
  defined, 54
  homotypic *versus* heterotypic, 55–56
  ID, 317, 341t
  and insights into learning disorders, 10–13, 11f
  learning disorders and, 10–13, 11f
  mathematics disorder and, 191, 194, 196, 197, 210, 216t
  neuroimaging studies of, 63
  prevalence of, 54
  reading disability and, 163, 182,
  research challenges of, 55–56
  speech and language disorders and, 112–113, 116–117, 131, 138, 139, 142, 143, 155t
  theoretical models of, 56
Computerized training
  connectionist model and, 37
  for working memory, 213, 253, 338–339
Congenital aphasia, 113
Connectionist models of cognitive development, 37–39
Connectivity studies of brain, 276–278
Conservation of number concept, 193
Counting, development of, 198–199
Country differences, environmental factors in, 99
Cross-cultural factors, dyslexia and, 162–163
Cytogenesis, development and pathological conditions, 26t

D

Default mode network (DMN), in ADHD, 235
Deterministic epigenesis, 30, 33
Developmental aphasia/dysphasia, 113
Developmental coordination disorder, neuroimaging phenotype of, 40t
Developmental dyscalculia, 192–193
Developmental history, 80, 143–144, 176, 241–242, 291–292, 327–328
Developmental prosopagnosia, 10
Diagnoses
  limitations and benefits of, 77–78
  person-first language and, 78
Diagnostic and Statistical Manual of Mental Disorders (DSM-IV)
  ADHD in, 220, 221
  ASD in, 262–264
  intellectual disability in, 315

mathematics disorder in, 194–195
and "splitting" of specific learning disorders, 72
Diagnostic and Statistical Manual of Mental Disorders (DSM-5)
  ADHD in, 220–221
  ADHD subtypes in, 56
  ASD in, 262–264
  basic *versus* complex academic skills in, 72
  versus DSM-IV, 72
  dyslexia in, 158–160
  intellectual disability in, 315–316
  language disorder (language impairment) in, 114
  learning disorders in, 3, 69–74
  and "lumping" of specific learning disorders, 72–73
  mathematical disorder in, 195
  social communication disorder (pragmatic language impairment) in, 114
Diffusion tensor imaging (DTI), 28
Discourse, 118
  defined, 119*t*
  processing, 119
Disorders
  categorical *versus* noncategorical, 14
  distal causes, 15, 24
  proximal causes, 24
DNA segments, recombination of, 19
DNA variations, molecular methods for measuring, 18–19
Down syndrome, 312
  characteristics and findings, 319–321
  LTM impairment in, 43–44
  microcephaly in, 25
Dual-stream model of speech processing, 133–135
Dyscalculia, 70, 190–216
Dysgraphia, 70

E

Early brain overgrowth (EBO) hypothesis, in ASD, 272–273
Early Symptomatic Syndromes Eliciting Neurodevelopmental Clinical Evaluations (ESSENCE), 67
Educational history, 80
Effortful control, 224–227
Embryogenesis, 25
Emotional functioning, tests of, 88*t*
Entrenchment, 31

Environmental influences; *see also* Gene-environment interplay
  in ADHD, 240
  in ASD, 286–289
  DSM-5 exclusions of, 90
  in dyslexia, 160, 175–176
  group achievement differences and, 94
  and group differences in cognitive skills, 99
  in intellectual disability, 318
  literacy development and, 161–162
  in speech and language disorders, 140–142
Epigenesis
  deterministic, 30, 33
  probabilistic, 33
ESSENCE (Early Symptomatic Syndromes Eliciting Neurodevelopmental Clinical Evaluations), 67
Ethnicity
  ADHD and, 222
  group differences in LD and, 100–105
Etiology, 14–23
  of ADHD, 236–241
  of ASD, 278–289
  behavioral genetics approach to, 16–17
  defined, 14
  distal factors in, 15
  gene-environment interplay and, 17–18
  of ID, 317–326
  of mathematics disorder, 204–209
  missing heritability problem and, 19–22, 22*f*
  molecular genetics approach to, 18–19
  of reading disability, 171–176
  risk factors, 15
  of speech and language disorders, 137–142
  studies of, 96
Eugenics movement, 313–314
Evidence-based practice in assessment: *see* Assessment
Executive function
  acquired lesions and, 35
  ADHD and, 218, 224, 227, 229
  ASD and, 274–277, 298, 307, 309
  intellectual disability and, 320, 322, 333, 335, 338
  tests of, 87*t*–88*t*

F

Face-processing tasks, in ASD, 275
Familiality
  in ADHD, 236
  in ASD, 278–280

Familiality *(cont.)*
  in dyslexia, 177
  in intellectual disability, 313–314, 318
  in mathematics disorder, 204–205
  in speech and language disorders, 137–138
Family history, heritable disorders and, 80–81
Fluid and crystallized intelligence, 45–46, 85, 87*t*
Fluid intelligence, age-related changes in, 47
FOXP2 gene
  breakthrough discoveries and, 15–16
  explicit to implicit learning transition and, 44
  in language impairments, 139–140
  in speech and language disorders, 112–113
Fractionable autism triad hypothesis, 269, 282
Fragile X syndrome, 7, 14, 19, 24, 27, 37, 43, 90, 204, 209, 237, 267, 312
  characteristics and findings, 321–323
  LTM impairment in, 43
Fusiform face area (FFA), 30

G

g factor
  academic *versus* cognitive, 48–49
  neuropsychology of, 49–50
G × E interactions: *see* Gene–environment interplay
G–E correlations, types of, 18
Gene mutations, in microcephaly, 25
Gene variants, identifying, 24
Gene–environment interplay
  ACE model of, 17–18
  in ADHD, 240–241
  in ASD, 287
  examples of, 18
  in RD, 171–172
Generalist genes hypothesis, RD + ADHD comorbidity and, 59–60, 62–64, 344–345
  in mathematics disorder, 205–208
Genetic correlation, RD + ADHD and, 59
Genetic disorders, ASD risk and, 267
Genetic influences
  in ADHD, 219, 237–240
  in ASD, 281–286
  in dyslexia
  in Down syndrome, 319–320
  in dyslexia, 160

in fragile X syndrome, 321–322
in language development, 138–140
in mathematics disorder, 191, 204–206
in Williams syndrome, 323–324
Genetic risk factors, 15
Genetic sharing, cross-disorder, in RD + ADHD, 61–62
Genetics
  behavioral, 16–17
  molecular, 18–19
Genome
  individual differences in, 19
  as recipe *versus* blueprint, 16
Genomewide association studies (GWAS), 19–22, 22*f*
  of ADHD, 237–238
  of ASD, 284
  of mathematics disorder, 208
  of RD, 173–174
Genomewide complex trait analysis (GCTA), missing heritability and, 22
Grey matter, cognitive development and, 38
Group differences
  analyzing, 95–97, 95*f*
  by country, 95*f*, 97–99, 97*f*
  policy implications of, 105–106

H

Handwriting, automaticity in, 70, 74
Health, in analysis of group differences, 99
Hearing mutism, 113
Heritability
  of ADHD, 236–237
  of approximate number sense, 206–208
  of ASD, 280–283
  of mathematics disorder, 205–206
  misunderstandings about, 16–17
  of RD, 171
  of speech and language disorders, 138–140
Heritability estimates, derivation of, 17
Heritable disorders, family history and, 80–81
Hickok and Poeppel model, 133–135
Hippocampus, acquired lesions in, 36
Holmes, O. W., 314
HOT (History, Observations, Test Results) mnemonic, in assessment, 79
Human Connectome Project, 28
Human language, 117–132; *see also* Language
  definitions and components, 117–120, 119*t*
  development models of, 125–128, 126*f*, 127*f*

development of
  atypical, 128–132
  typical, 120–128
hierarchy of, 37–38, 119t, 121
infant learning of, 121–125
structural, 118–119, 119t
written, 119–120

I

Individuals with Disabilities Education Act (IDEA)
  dyslexia and, 158
  specific learning disorder and, 75
Intellectual disability (ID), 312–342; *see also* Down syndrome; Fragile X syndrome; Williams syndrome
  ADHD symptoms in, 237
  candidate genes for, 19
  case presentation 10, 328–329, 330t–331t, 331–332
  case presentation 11, 332–333, 334t–335t, 335
  chapter summary, 312–313
  cognitive risk factors for, 51t
  comorbidities, 317
  current treatment of, 314
  deficits in, 10
  definitions, 314–316
  diagnosis, 326–328
  diagnostic criteria in, 316
  early interventions for, 337
  environmental influences, 318–319
  etiology, 317–326
    for nonsyndromal ID, 317–319
    for syndromal ID, 319–326
  general *versus* specific deficits in, 325–326
  history, 313–314
  IQ cutoff problems and, 315–316
  LTM impairment in, 43–44
  neuropsychological studies of, 42
  prevalence and epidemiology, 317
  prevention, 336
  speech and language disorders and, 111
  summary table, 341t–342t
  syndromal
    Down syndrome, 319–321
    fragile X syndrome, 321–323
    Williams syndrome, 323–325
  treatment, 336–340
  two-group approach to, 318

Intelligence
  fluid *versus* crystallized, 45–46
  hierarchical model of, 44–46, 45f
  instruments for measuring, 45
  tests of, 87t
Interactive specialization model
  acquired lesions and, 34–37
  brain development and, 136
  cognitive development and, 29–33, 38
  Hickok and Poeppel model and, 135
  nature–nurture debate and, 40
IQ
  country differences in, 98–99
  dyslexia and, 160
  grey and white matter development and, 28, 37
  specific learning disorder and, 73–74
IQ gaps
  early language experience and, 104
  SES and ethnicity and, 102
IQ testing, country differences in, 98
Itard, J., 313

K

Kanner, L., 260–262
KE family
  CAS and, 138–139
  speech dyspraxia and, 10, 15–17
Kennard principle, 34

L

Language; *see also* Human language
  tests of, 87t
  written, *versus* oral language development, 163–164
Language acquisition device (LAD), 121
Language development, *FOXP2* gene, 15–16
Language disorders, candidate genes for, 19
Language impairment (LI), 112; *see also* Pragmatic language impairment (PLI)
  versus ASD, 143
  behavioral observations, 144–145
  case presentation, 145–146, 147t–148t, 148–149
  cognitive risk factors for, 51t
  comorbidities
    with dyslexia, 157, 163
    with mathematics disorder, 191
  deficit in, 118

Language impairment *(cont.)*
  definitions of, 115
  developmental hypotheses of, 129–132
  familiality of, 137–138
  heritability of, 138
  implicit LTM impairment in, 43
  versus intellectual disability, 143
  IQ- *versus* age-discrepancy in, 115–116
  LTM impairment in, 43
  neuroimaging studies of, 136–137
  neuropsychological studies of, 42
  patient history, 143–144
  versus pragmatic language impairment, 114
  presenting symptoms, 142–143
  prevalence, 116–117
  specific, history of, 113
  treatment, 153–154
Language input, parent-to-child, 140–142
L-dopa, for ADHD, 232
Learning, developmental process of, 38
Learning disabilities, *versus* learning disorders, 4
Learning disorders
  brain mechanisms of *(see* Brain mechanisms)
  classification based on explicit *versus* implicit LTM, 43–44
  cognitive-deficit model of, 11–12, 11f
  comorbidity among, 69
  defining, 4
  development of, 3
  in DSM-5, 3
  early learning deficit in, 43–44
  and explicit *versus* implicit memory, 4–5
  implementing DSM-5 framework for, 75
  and insights from comorbidity, 10–13, 11f
  localized *versus* distributed features of, 39
  lumping and splitting of, future directions for, 346–347
  multilevel model of, 7–9, 8f
    future directions for, 344–347
    validity of, 343–344
  multiple-deficit model of, 9–10
  neuroimaging phenotypes of, 38–40, 40t
  nosology of, 3
  "pure" *versus* mixed cases of, 9–10
  scientific method for understanding, 3
  simple *versus* complex, 69
  single-deficit model of, 9–10
  timing of onset, 80
  translation into clinical practice, future directions for, 347–348
  types of, 4

Left inferior frontal gyrus, neuroimaging phenotype of, 40t
Left inferior parietal sulcus, neuroimaging phenotype of, 40t
Lesions, acquired
  brain plasticity and, 33–37
  current evidence on, 34
Leukodystrophies, 27
Lexical structuring of phonology, 126
Lexicon, 118
  defined, 119t
  delayed acquisition of, 128
  development of, 126–127
Lifestyle, ADHD and, 254–255
Lissencephaly, 25, 26t
Listening comprehension, 71
Literacy development, milestones in, 164–165
Long-term memory (LTM), explicit *versus* implicit, 4–5
  deficits in, 43–44
  in learning disorder classification, 43–44
Long-term potentiation (LTP), in ID syndromes, 44

M

Macrocephaly, in ASD, 272–273
Major depression, molecular genetics studies of, 60
Math anxiety, 214–215
Mathematical problem solving
  DSM-5 criteria for, 71, 72t
  "simple" model of, 71, 71t
Mathematics, developmental milestones in, 197–200
Mathematics disorder (MD), 4, 19, 48, 190–216
  age- *versus* IQ-discrepancy definitions of, 195
  approximate *versus* symbolic number sense and, 190
  brain mechanisms, 201–204
  case presentation 5, 209–210, 211t–212t, 212–213
  chapter summary, 190–191
  cognitive risk factors for, 51t
  comorbidities, 191, 196
    with ADHD, 209–210, 211t–212t, 212–213
  definitions, 194–195
  developmental neuropsychology, 196–201
  diagnosis and treatment, 209–215

diagnostic validity of, 73
etiology, 204–209
  approximate number sense heritability, 206–208
  generalist genes in, 205–206
  molecular genetics and, 208
fMRI studies of, 203–204
history, 191–194
multiple-deficit model of, 196–197
neuroimaging studies of, 201–203
prevalence and epidemiology, 195–196
specific *versus* general predictors of, 200–201
summary table, 216*t*
treatment, 213–215
validation of, 74
Maturational model of brain–behavior development, 29–33
  acquired lesions and, 34–37
Medical model, concerns about, 77, 90
Medications
  for ADHD, 231–232, 251–253
  nonstimulant, for ADHD, 251
Memory; *see also* Long-term memory (LTM)
  explicit *versus* implicit, 4–5
  phonological, 127, 131
  procedural, 131–132
  working, 46–47 (*see also* Working memory)
Mendelian diseases, genetic variants and, 21, 22*f*
Mental health disorders, neuroimaging studies of, 63–64
Mental retardation: *see* Intellectual disability (ID)
Methylphenidate (MPH/Ritalin), for ADHD, 231–232
Microcephaly, gene mutations in, 25, 26*t*
Milieu communication treatments (MCTs), for intellectual disability, 339–340
Minority disproportionate representation (MDR), 105–106
Missing heritability problem, 19–22, 22*f*
MMR vaccine, lack of evidence for ASD association, 289
Molecular genetics, 18–19
  in ASD, 283–286
  in etiology of RD + ADHD, 60–61
  in mathematics disorder, 208
  in RD, 172–175
  revolution in, 23
  in speech–language disorders, 139–140
Morphemes, 118
  defined, 119*t*

Movement–attention coupling, early development of, 226
MPH (methylphenidate/Ritalin), for ADHD, 231–232
Multiple-deficit models, 12
  of ADHD, 229
  of ASD, 267
  comorbidity and, 54–55, 65–66, 66*f*
  of language impairment, 132
  of mathematics disorder, 196–197
  of RD, 167
Mutation–selection model, 20–21
Mutualism, psychological *g* and, 49
Myelination, development and pathological conditions, 26*t*

N

National Institute of Mental Health (NIMH), Research Domain Criteria initiative of, 64
Nature–nurture debate, 16
  brain–behavior models and, 40
Neocortex
  function localization in, 31–32
  plasticity of, 34–37
Neural adaptation, in dyslexic *versus* skilled readers, 170
Neurodevelopmental disorders
  brain plasticity and, 6–7
  heterotypic continuity in, 5–7
  learning disorders as subset of, 4
  physical bases of, 7
Neuroimaging phenotypes, of learning disorders, 38–40, 40*t*; *see also* Brain mechanisms
Neuronal migration, 25–26
Neuropsychology, 41–53
  ADHD and developmental neuropsychology, 224–230
  advances in, 42–43
  ASD and developmental neuropsychology, 267–271
  cognitive constructs and, 50–51
  defined, 42
  future directions for analysis, 345–346
  of *g* factor, 49–50
  and general *versus* specific cognitive deficits, 48–49
  learning disorder studies in, 8, 8*f*, 42–43
  mathematics disorder and developmental neuropsychology, 196–201

Neuropsychology *(cont.)*
   versus psychological explanations, 51–53
   psychometric cognitive constructs and, 44–47, 45f, 48t
   of RD + ADHD, 57–58
   RD and developmental neuropsychology, 163–169
   role of, 41
   speech and language disorders and developmental neuropsychology, 117–132
Neuroscience, *versus* neuropsychology/psychology, 52–53
Neurotransmitters, in ADHD, 231–233
No Child Left Behind Act of 2001 (NCLB), 100
Nonacademic skills, complex, 71
Number concepts, automaticity in, 70
Numerosity
   approximate relative, 192
   and developmental milestones in mathematics, 197–200
Nutrition, ADHD and, 255

O

Orthographic learning hypothesis, reading problems and, 168–169

P

Parental influences, in ASD, 287–289
Parent–child verbal engagement, cross-cultural and subcultural variations in, 140–142
Pathophysiology of learning disorders, 24
   brain development and, 25–28, 26t
   and brain–behavior development models, 29–37
   and integration of brain and cognitive development, 37–39
   structural/functional connectivity and, 28–29
Patient history, in assessment, 79–81
Patterns of strengths and weaknesses model (PSW), specific learning disorder and, 75
Periventricular nodular heterotopia (PNH), 25–26, 26t
Person-first language, diagnoses and, 78

Phenotypes, brain, 24
Phenylketonuria (PKU), early-treated, 37
Phoneme awareness
   in dyslexia, 187
   learning disorders and, 12
Phonemes, 118
   defined, 119t
Phonological awareness, and solving of arithmetic problems, 199
Phonological memory, 127
Phonological memory hypothesis, 131
Phonological processing deficit, dyslexia and, 159, 165–168
Phonology
   development of, 123–128
   lexical structuring of, 126
Physical activity, Down syndrome and, 340
Piaget, J., conservation of number concept of, 193
Plasticity: *see* Brain plasticity
Poor comprehenders, 70, 72, 72t, 156
Pragmatic language impairment (PLI), 112; *see also* Language impairment (LI)
   versus ASD, 114
   deficit in, 118
   familiality of, 137–138
   versus language impairment, 114
   presenting symptoms, 143
Pragmatics, 118, 120
   ADHD and, 111
Prefrontal cortex (PFC)
   acquired lesions in, 35–36
   neuroimaging phenotype of, 40t
   synaptic pruning in, 27–28
Probabilistic epigenesis, 33
Procedural memory hypothesis, 131–132
Processing speed, 46–47
   age-related changes in, 47
   in RD and ADHD, 65
   tests of, 87t–88t
Prosody, 118
   defined, 119t, 120
   development of, 122
Prosopagnosia, developmental, 10
Psychiatric disorders
   in families of children with autism, 280
   molecular genetics studies and, 23
   neuroimaging studies of, 63–64
   salience network in, 64
Psychology, analysis levels in, 51–52
Psychometric cognitive constructs, 44–47, 45f, 48t

Psychometric constructs, *versus* cognitive constructs, 48*t*
Psychometric *g*, 48–49
Psychostimulants, for ADHD, 251–252

R

Race
   ADHD and, 222
   group differences in LD and, 100–105
RD + ADHD comorbidity, 56–65
   etiology of, 59–65
      behavioral genetics perspective, 59–60
      cross-disorder genetic sharing in, 61–62
      generalist genes hypothesis in, 59–60, 62–64
      molecular genetics perspective, 60–61
      neuroimaging and, 64–65
   multiple-deficit models and, 65–66, 66*f*
   neuroimaging studies of, 63–65
   neuropsychology of, 57–58
Reading, single-word, 70–71, 71*t*, 72*t*
Reading comprehension, "simple" models of, 70–71, 71*t*
Reading development, G–E correlation in, 18
Reading disability (RD) (dyslexia), 70, 156–189
   best neuropsychological model of, 157
   brain mechanisms, 169–170
   candidate genes for, 19
   case presentation 3, 178–179, 180*t*–181*t*, 181–182
   case presentation 4, 182, 183*t*–184*t*, 184–186
   chapter summary, 156–157
   cognitive risk factors for, 51*t*
   comorbidities, 157
      with mathematics disorder, 191
   definitions, 156, 158–160
   developmental, early hypothesis of, 10
   developmental neuropsychology, 163–169
      and milestones in literacy development, 164–165
   diagnosis, 176–178
   diagnostic validity of, 73
   etiology, 157, 171–176
      behavioral genetics and, 171–172
      environmental factors, 175–176
      molecular genetics and, 172–175
   family risk design and, 165–167
   G–E correlation and, 18
   genetic overlap with ADHD, 10
   genetic risk factors in, 139–140
   heterotypic continuity in, 5–7
   history, 157–158
   implicit LTM impairment in, 43
   IQ- *versus* age-discrepancy in, 160
   LTM impairment in, 43–44
   and memorization of math facts, 199
   multiple-deficit models and, 12
   neuroimaging phenotype of, 40*t*, 157
   neuropsychology of, 165–169
   patient history, 176
   prevalence and epidemiology, 160–163
      comorbidities, 163
      cross-cultural findings, 162–163
      socioeconomic status and, 161–162
   processing speed in, 65
   reading errors in, 177–178
   sampling bias in studies of, 95
   summary table, 188*t*–189*t*
   treatment, 186–188
   validation of, 74
Referrals, 78–79
Research Domain Criteria initiative (RDoC), 64
Resource allocation hypothesis, 70–71
Response-to-intervention (RTI), specific learning disorder and, 75–76
Restricted, repetitive behaviors (RRB), 263–264, 267–269, 274–275, 282–283
Rett syndrome, 27, 37
Ritalin (methylphenidate/MPH), for ADHD, 231–232, 251

S

Salience network, in psychiatric disorders, 64
Sampling biases, in dyslexia studies, 95
Sampling theory, psychological *g* and, 49
Schizophrenia
   immune system gene mutations and, 27–28
   molecular genetics studies of, 60
   mutation–selection model and, 20–21
Seguin, E., 313
Self-control, early development of, 224–225
Self-talk, overt *versus* internalized, 226
Semantic acalculia, pure, 202
Semantic dyscalculia, 192–193
Semantics, 118
   defined, 119*t*
Sign language, brain plasticity and, 136

Single-word reading, 70–71, 71*t*, 72*t*; *see also* Reading disability (RD) (dyslexia)
Skill learning model of brain–behavior development, 29–33
  acquired lesions and, 34–37
Skinner, B. F., language development theory of, 120
Sleep disorders, 81
  ADHD and, 254–255
Sluggish cognitive tempo (SCT), ADHD and, 221
SNP heritability estimates, 19–22
  for mathematics disorder, 208
Social cognition, development of, 42
Social communication disorder (SCD): *see* Pragmatic language impairment (PLI)
Social functioning, tests of, 88*t*
Socioeconomic status
  group differences and, 100–105
  literacy development and, 161–162
  parent–child language input and, 140–141
  role of, 80
Special education, poor/minority representation in, 106
Specific language impairment, history of, 113
Specific learning disorder, 69–76
  academic skills included in, 69–70
  and definition of *specific* in DSM-5 *versus* DSM-IV, 73
  DSM-5 "lumping" of, 72–73
  in DSM-5 *versus* DSM-IV, 69, 72–73
  in DSM-5 *versus* IDEA, 75
  full clinical picture of, 74
  IQ and age discrepancies and, 73–74
  research on, 72
  RTI and, 75–76
  and simple models of academic skills, 70–71, 71*t*
Specificity, 91–92
Speech, childhood apraxia of: *see* Childhood apraxia of speech (CAS)
Speech and language disorders, 111–115
  behavioral observations, 144–145
  brain mechanisms, 132–137, 134*f*
  case presentation 1, 145–146, 147*t*–148*t*, 148–149
  case presentation 2, 149–150, 151*t*–152*t*, 152
  chapter summary, 111–113
  cognitive risk factors and, 112
  comorbidities, 112
    with ADHD, 238

definitions, 114–116
developmental neuropsychology of, 117–132
diagnosis, 142–145
etiology, 112–113, 137–142
  environmental influences, 140–142
  familiality, 137–138
  gene locations, 138–140
  heritability, 138
history of, 113
prevalence and epidemiology, 116–117
summary table, 155*t*
treatment, 153–154
Speech disorders, 128–129; *see also* Childhood apraxia of speech (CAS); Speech sound disorder (SSD)
  candidate genes for, 19
Speech language development, milieu communication treatments and, 339–340
Speech perception/production, dual-stream model of, 112
Speech processing, dual-stream model of, 133–135
Speech sound disorder (SSD), 6, 10, 112
  babbling in, 128–129
  behavioral observations, 145
  versus CAS, 114–115
  case presentation, 149–150, 151*t*–152*t*, 152
  cognitive risk factors for, 51*t*
  comorbidities
    with dyslexia, 163
    with RD, 157
  deficit in, 118
  definitions of, 115
  familiality of, 137–138
  genetic overlap with dyslexia, 10
  genetic risk factors in, 139–140
  heritability of, 138, 141–142
  multiple-deficit models and, 12
  neuroimaging studies of, 136–137
  neuropsychological studies of, 42
  patient history, 144
  presenting symptoms, 143
  prevalence, 116–117
  treatment, 153–154
Spelling
  automaticity in, 70
  as isolated learning disorder, 72
Spina bifida, 26*t*
Sterilization, enforced, 314
Strephosymbolia, 158
Subitizing, 197

Synaptogenesis, development and pathological conditions, 26*t*, 27
Syntax, 118
  acquisition of, 127
  defined, 119*t*

T

Tests, 82–92
  of academic skills, 88*t*
  of attention, processing speed, executive functions, 87*t*–88*t*
  base-rate variability and, 86, 89
  battery selection and, 85–86
  of crystallized/fluid intelligence, 87*t*
  of language, 87*t*
  performance validity and, 82–85, 87*t*
  of social, emotional, adaptive functioning, 89*t*
Transactional processes, G–E correlation example, 18
Transcription
  automaticity in, 70
  "simple" model of, 71, 71*t*
Traumatic brain injury (TBI), 4
Turner syndrome, 202, 203, 204, 209, 237
Twin studies, GWAS data and, 21–22

V

Vaccines, lack of evidence for ASD association, 289
Virginia Sterilization Act of 1924, 314

Visual attentional deficits, reading difficulties and, 167

W

Wechsler Intelligence Scale for Children-IV, *versus* WISC-V, 45–46
Wechsler Intelligence Scale for Children-V, 44–46, 45*f*
Wernicke–Lichtheim–Geschwind model, 112, 133, 134*f*
Wernicke's aphasia, 133
White matter
  in ADHD, 234
  cognitive development and, 38
  disorders of, 36
  IQ and, 28, 37
  neuroimaging phenotype of, 40*t*
  processing speed and, 47
Williams syndrome, 7, 10, 237, 312
  characteristics and findings, 323–325
  gene deletions in, 284
    LTM impairment in, 43–44
    microcephaly in, 25
Working memory, 46–47
  age-related changes in, 47
  computerized training for, 213, 253, 338–339
Writing disorders, epidemiological studies of, 74
Writing skills
  assessment of, 74–75
  "simple" model of, 71